BABY 411

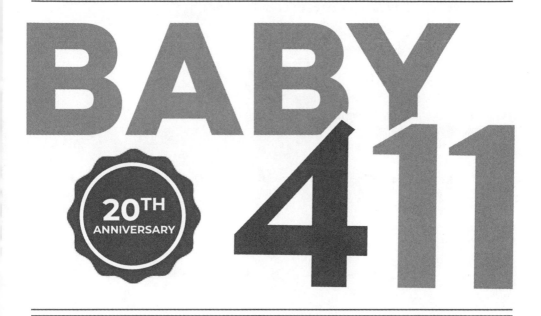

20TH ANNIVERSARY

YOUR BABY, BIRTH TO AGE 1

10th edition

T0037873

DR. ARI BROWN AND DENISE FIELDS

Copyright Page and Low-Impact Pilates Workout

Saxophone, lead guitar by Denise Fields
Drums, rhythm guitar and interior layout by Alan Fields
Cover/interior design and keyboard solo by Sol Marketing
Backing harmony vocals and keyboards by Andy and Julia Brown
Percussion and additional guitar by Ben and Jack Fields
Index by New West Indexing
Band photography by Tracy Trahar

To order this book, order online at Baby411.com or call 1-800-888-0385. Questions or comments? Please call the authors at (303) 442-8792. Or fax them a note at (303) 442-3744. Or write to them at Windsor Peak Press, 436 Pine Street, Boulder, CO 80302. E-mail us at authors@baby411.com. Baby 411 is a registered trademark of Windsor Peak Press.

The latest info on this book is online at www.Baby411.com

Distributed to the book trade by Ingram Publisher Services, (866) 400-5351

Library Cataloging in Publication Data

Brown, Ari, M.D.
Fields, Denise
    Baby 411: Clear Answers & Smart Advice for Your Baby's First Year/ Ari Brown, M.D. and Denise Fields
    632 pages. Includes index.
    ISBN 978-1-889392-72-1

    1. Infants. 2. Child rearing. 3. Infants—Care.

Child Care—Handbooks, manuals, etc. 2. Infants' supplies—Purchasing—United States, Canada, Directories. 3. Children's paraphernalia—Purchasing—Handbooks, manuals. 4. Product Safety—Handbooks, manuals. 5. Consumer education.
    649′.122′0296—dc20. 2024.

Version 10.1

Do you have an old copy of this book? Check our web site at Baby411.com to make sure you have the most current version.

Baby 411 Medical Advisory Board

Steven Adair, DDS, MS
Pediatric Dentist
Professor and Chair, Pediatric Dentistry
Medical College of Georgia

Mark T. Brown, MD, FACS
Ear, Nose, and Throat Specialist

Jose C. Cortez, MD
Pediatric Urologist
Dell Children's Medical Center
Austin, TX

Lewis First, MD, FAAP
Professor and Chair
University of Vermont Department of Pediatrics
Burlington, VT

Corinne Frank, Esq.
Professional Mother

Kiran Hahn, RN, IBCLC
Certified Lactation Consultant
Austin, TX

Linda Hill, RN, IBCLC
Certified Lactation Consultant
Midland, TX

Randy Kunik, DDS
Orthodontist and Cosmetic Dentist
Austin, TX

Paul Offit, MD, FAAP
Director, Vaccine Education Center
Children's Hospital of Philadelphia
Philadelphia, PA

Edward Peters, MD, FAAAI
Allergist, Pulmonologist
Allergy & Asthma Assoc. of Austin
Austin, TX

Sidney Seidman, MD, FAAP
Pediatrician
Baltimore, MD

Gabriella Shaughnessy, RNC, BS, IBCLC
Manager, OB Education
Hoag Memorial Hospital
Newport Beach, CA

Shelley Solka, MS, CCC-SLP
Speech Language Pathologist
Austin, TX

Helina Teshome, RN, IBCLC
Certified Lactation Consultant
Austin, TX

Karen L. Wright, MD
Pediatric Cardiologist
Children's Cardiology Associates
Austin, TX

Bridget E. Young, PhD, CLC
Research Assistant Professor of Pediatrics,
Allergy and Immunology, University of
Rochester School of Medicine and Dentistry;
BabyFormulaExpert.com

Mark Zamutt, RPh.
Pharmacist, Austin, TX

R. Jeff Zwiener, MD
Medical Director, Pediatric
Gastroenterology
Dell Children's Medical Center
Austin, TX

ACKNOWLEDGMENTS

So how'd a pediatrician like me end up writing three books with over a million copies in print and founding a multimedia national parenting brand? I ponder that myself every once in a while!

As we put the finishing touches on the tenth edition of *Baby 411*, it makes me look back on the past 20 years. Boy, time flies. I was perfectly content with life as I knew it prior to 2002. I had a great pediatric practice with the nicest families I could ever dream of. And I found child advocacy for my local and state medical societies to be very rewarding.

Then I had a conversation that changed my life. Alan and Denise Fields were long-time friends and bestselling authors of *Baby Bargains*. Based on our collective experiences, we came to the following conclusion: despite the surplus of parenting books, today's parents needed help.

The Information Age led parents to more questions than answers. The Fields were experts in writing books but did not go to medical school (maybe a wise decision!). I could answer all the questions, but I didn't have the time (or so I thought) or the skill (I learned along the way) to write a book. But I had a passion to educate parents—just like I did in my office every day.

"Write a couple chapters and send them to us," said my friends.

So I did.

"We like it," said my friends/future co-author/editors/publishers. "Give us 15 chapters by Thanksgiving."

"But that's a chapter a week!" I protested.

"Yep. Welcome to the book business."

Jotting down ideas between seeing patients, pulling an all-nighter to write the sleep chapter, and missing a few bedtime stories with my own kids . . . *Baby 411* was born. *Toddler 411* and *Expecting 411* followed to complete the trilogy.

Since the first edition was published, many aspects of pediatric healthcare have changed and so have the ways new parents access that information. Just do a quick Google search on starting solid foods, for example. It's no wonder parents are confused about what to do! And then the pandemic showed up . . . as if keeping a baby healthy wasn't already scary enough as a new parent.

So, in retrospect, writing the first edition of *Baby 411* was the easy part. Revising the book every couple of years, creating a companion educational video series and online community to keep up with the the pace of medicine has been the challenge. But I am committed to this mission of helping new parents in the office (I still see patients every day) and on a larger stage through these platforms. And, I wouldn't change a thing.

Hearing from our readers keeps me energized, so keep those notes and messages coming— I love hearing from you!

I owe many thanks to the Fields for believing in me and in this project.

A big shout out to my mom for always being there for me. I miss you! I also thank my sister and brothers for their grassroots marketing efforts, giving books to everyone they know, and approaching random pregnant women in Costco parking lots across the country. (I swear I had nothing to do with this idea.)

To my patients and their parents. You are my inspiration. Thank you for sharing your experiences to help other families. You teach me everyday!

I thank the citizens of Austin and the Austin medical community for their extraordinary encouragement. I am so proud to call you my friends, neighbors, and colleagues. I vow to Keep Austin Weird.

Thank you, American Academy of Pediatrics and Parents Magazine/Parents.com for your support over all these years.

And finally, I dedicate this book to Andy and Julia. I love you so much and am so very proud to be your mom. 　　　　　　　　　　　　　　　　　　— *Ari Brown, M.D.*

OVERVIEW

SECTION ONE: 3-2-1 BABY! PREPARING FOR THE NEW ONE I

Your baby is here! This section explores your baby's first few days . . . plus how to survive the first two weeks. Next we tackle finding a pediatrician, explaining newborn screening tests and other timely topics. What are the insider tips to scheduling appointments and what to do on weekends and holidays when your baby is sick. Also in this section: parenting 101 and navigating the world of child care.

SECTION TWO: CARE & FEEDING 77

How do you care for your newborn? The first part of this section explores bathing your newborn, diaper rash and other fun hygiene issues. Next, let's talk nutrition and growth—what do growth charts mean? What does your baby need to eat for the first year? We'll break down nutrition into separate chapters that focus on liquids and solids. We'll take a deep dive on breastfeeding, with troubleshooting tips to overcome common challenges and we will de-mystify all the baby formula options for you. Next, we'll discuss how to tell when your baby is ready for solid foods, including advice on baby-led weaning and preventing food allergies. The last chapter in this section is titled "The other end"—everything you wanted to know about baby poop and more!

SECTION THREE: SLEEP, MILESTONES, & SOOTHING YOUR BABY 223

Let's talk sleep—this section will give you the scoop on your baby's sleep (or lack thereof). We'll talk about setting up good habits and explain all those truly annoying catch phrases like wake windows, sleep regressions, and cry it out. Look no further because we have all the answers you need to get a good night's sleep (when the times comes). Next, we'll look at how your baby will develop, including milestones and social/emotional growth. Finally, we'll share the most important advice of all: how to soothe a newborn and calm your little one as they grow up.

SECTION FOUR: SICKNESS & HOW TO AVOID IT! 315

Here, we'll discuss vaccinations—real talk on the routine vaccination schedule, plus flu and COVID-19 shots. Yes, we'll hit all the controversies head on, armed with science and facts. This section also covers the most common infections and diseases, with separate chapters devoted to such topics as the com- mon cold, bacterial infections, COVID-19, and more. And we'll share some key safety tips.

SECTION FIVE: FIRST AID—TOP 12 PROBLEMS & SOLUTIONS 431

What should you do when your baby gets sick? This section will give you advice on taking your baby's vital signs and what to have in a first aid kit. We'll hit the Top 12 problems and solutions for newborns, including fever, rashes, trauma and more.

SECTION SIX: THE REFERENCE LIBRARY 485

This section includes detailed information on medicines, complementary therapies, lab tests, the glossary, references and footnotes.

TABLE OF CONTENTS

Introduction..xv

SECTION ONE: 3-2-1 BABY! PREPARING FOR THE NEW ONE

Chapter 1

BIRTH DAY

Cutting the Cord and Your Baby's To Do List 4
    Should We Wait to Cut the Cord? 4
    Does My Baby Need To Study For His APGARs? 5
Your Baby's First Physical Exam 6
Getting To Know You: Your Baby's 1st Days..13
    What's THAT In My Baby's Diaper? 14
    Why is My Baby Shrinking? 15
More tests and procedures: hearing screen, newborn screening 16
That Wasn't in the Birth Plan!..18
    The 411 on Jaundice..19
Optional: Cord Blood Banking & Circumcision..22
The Baby 411 Two-Week Survival Guide..29
    Partner 411: Tips & Advice 36
    The Baby Blues..37
    The Handy Feeding And Elimination Table..38
Special Situations: Pre-term Babies, Twins, Adoption..............................39

Chapter 2

YOU & YOUR BABY'S DOC: INSIDER TIPS & ADVICE

Selecting a Doctor..47
The Schedule Of Well Baby Checkups 55
9 Screening Tests..56
Insider Tip: The Best Time To Schedule An Appointment...............................59
What To Do: Evening and Weekends..61

Chapter 3

PARENTHOOD

Parenting 101 64
Childcare..66
    Weighing The Options For Childcare..67
    Balancing Work & Baby 73

SECTION TWO: CARE & FEEDING

Chapter 4

HYGIENE: THE SPA TREATMENT

The First Manicure 79
When Can I Use Diaper Wipes?..80
How Often Do I Clean The Belly Button?..80
Diaper Rash: 5 Tips & Tricks..81
Bathing Baby 82
Cradle Cap...84
Eczema: Advice And Tips..85
Insect Repellent and Sunscreen..86
The Boy Parts..87
The Girl Parts..89
Mouth care: Thrush, Teething, and Drool..90

Chapter 5

NUTRITION & GROWTH

What Growth Charts Mean 93
How Infants Grow (Height, Head Size, Weight)...............................93
Flat Heads & Tummy Time...96
Calories & Nutrition For The First Year...98
The Big Picture: Nutrition For The First Year..................................100
Feeding Schedules, Or Lack Thereof...101
Special Concerns: Dropping Down The Growth Chart....................102
Does My Baby Need A Vitamin Supplement? 103
Fluoride: Does Baby Need A Supplement?......................................107
Can Babies Eat Too Much?..108
Calcium, Fiber, Zinc And Iron 110
Happy Birthday! You're One! Food guidelines and hunger strikes 111

Chapter 6

LIQUIDS

Breast Milk..114
    The Advantages Of Breast Milk..114
    The Hardest Hurdles Are Up Front...115
    Day-By-Day Guide...117
    The First Night At Home 120
    Top 10 Tips To Survive The First Two Weeks...............................121
    Is It Ok to Supplement With Formula?...124
    Top 8 Breastfeeding Problems and Solutions 130
    Troubleshooting: When Breastfeeding Goes Wrong 133

Sore Nipples: 6 Tips For Relief 138
Expressing Milk: Breast Pumps, How to Serve Breastmilk................141
Mom Considerations: Diet, Medications...145
Breastfeeding and Cow Milk Protein Allergy.....................................146
Special Situations: Adoptions, Twins, Preemies 151
Weaning: The Guide 154
The Big Picture: Breastfeeding For The First Year.............................155
Formula...157
What formula do you recommend? 157
Handy Table of Formula Options...162
European? Organic? Goat Milk Based? DIY?.....................................167
Powder Vs. Liquid: Which Formula is Best? 170
Bottles: Which Are Best?...172
The Big Picture: Formula Feeding For The First Year 172
Other Liquids: Water, Juice, Milk..173

Chapter 7

SOLIDS

How To Tell When Your Baby Is Ready?..180
How to Start Solid Foods..182
Baby-Led Weaning...182
Fearless Feeding Ideas 184
Six Months & Beyond: More Food And Textures 190
Food Allergy: Introducing Foods And Food Allergy Prevention..............193
Celiac Disease..198
The Big Picture For Liquid And Solid Nutrition 202

Chapter 8

THE OTHER END

What Is Normal Newborn Poop?...204
The Top 5 Worrisome Poops...205
5 Trade Secrets For Constipation Relief 206
Older Babies: Solid Foods = Solid Poop..207
Fun Fiber Foods 207
Spit Up, Regurgitation, And Vomit 210
What Is Gastresophageal Reflux (GER)? 210
Tricks Of The Trade: Treating GER 212
Quiz: Does Your Baby Have GERD?...214
Top 5 Worries About Vomit 216
Urine And Bladder Infections 218
Burping, Hiccups, And Gas..220

SECTION THREE: DEVELOPMENTAL MILESTONES, SOOTHING AND TEMPERAMENT

Chapter 9

SLEEP

All You Need to Know Is Here! (You Don't Need More Experts!)........ ...225
The Science Of Sleep 226
How Long Should Newborns Sleep?...227
Sleep Safety Tips: SIDS And Other Dangers 234
Our Warning on Sleep Devices: Loungers, DockATot, and Merlin......240
The Snoo And How Long Is Too Long to Swaddle?.......................241
Family Bed: Pros & Cons..242
Sleeping Solo: Pros & Cons...243
Two To Four Months: Setting Up Good Habits..............................244
Top 10 Commandments For Establishing A Healthy Sleep Routine.........244
Four To Five Months: The Big Transition.......................................246
Crying-It-Out: Let's Discuss.. 247
Undoing Bad Habits 248
Top 10 Mistakes Parents Make With Infant Sleep..........................249
It's Not A Sleep Regression, It's a Sleep Progression....................250
Dream Feeds?.. 251
Sleep Crutches: Pacifiers And Night Feedings............................ 251
3 Approaches Explained 253
Gradual vs Rapid Training..257
Naps And "Wake Windows"...260
Special Situations: Multiples And Preemies..................................263

Chapter 10

DEVELOPMENTAL MILESTONES

How Do I Know My Baby Is Developing Normally?....................................267
Bookmark this page! Our Milestones Checklist 268
Failing Milestones: What To Do...273
What Is Autism And When Do I Worry?...273
Other Developmental Differences..278
How Your Baby Learns 280
Your Baby's Social And Emotional Growth 282
Promoting Your Baby's Development By Age...............................283
   Birth to Two Months..283
   Two to Four Months...284
   Four to Six Months...285
   Six to Nine Months..287
   Nine to 12 Months..289
Sign Language..289

Screen Time: Do Media Use And Babies Mix?...................................291
Good Toys And Books...295

Chapter 11

TEMPERAMENT & SOOTHING

Getting To Know Your Baby's Temperament..................................297
The 3 Rules Of Cry Management...301
10 Tips For Soothing Newborns...301
Pacifiers: The Great Binky Debate 302
What Is Colic And What Can I Do About It?..................................305
Self-Regulation And Discipline... 308
Planting The Seeds Of Discipline..309
11 Steps For Raising a Self-Regulated Child.................................311
Special Situations: Separation Anxiety, Thumb Sucking..............312

SECTION FOUR: SICKNESS & HOW TO AVOID IT!

Chapter 12

VACCINATIONS

Infectious Diseases And Vaccines: History and Present Day................. 318
The Top 15 Vaccine Questions 321
The Childhood Vaccination Schedule..330
Special Section: COVID-19 Vaccine. 340
Vaccine Controversies...342
Vaccine Additives: What are They?...345
Real Talk: Delayed Or Spaced-Out Childhood Vaccines............................347

Chapter 13

COMMON INFECTIONS

What Are Viruses?...352
The Common Cold...357
What Are Bacteria?...360
Antibiotic Resistance...363
Viral Infections: Flu, Croup, RSV, and more..................................365
Special section: COVID-19..366
Bacterial Infections: Food Poisoning, Pneumonia and more.....................371
Feeling Itchy? Ringworm, Scabies, Pinworms, and Head Lice. 375
Special Feature: Ear Infections..378
7 Risk Factors For Ear Infections 379
The Infection Hit Parade...385
When Your Child Can Return To Childcare....................................388

Chapter 14
COMMON DISEASES

Eyes: Lazy Eye...389
Lungs: Asthma..390
Heart: Murmurs..384
Blood: Anemia, Sickle Cell Disease, Iron Deficiency, Lead Exposure.......395
Skin: Eczema 398
Muscles/Bones: Intoeing, Bow-Legged, Flat Feet, Torticollis....................400
Endocrine: Diabetes...403
Allergies: Seasonal, Environmental..404
Genitals: Penile Adhesions, Labial Adhesions..405
What's That Smell? Unusual Odors 406

Chapter 15
SAFETY

The Top Eco Hazards 408
Food Safety...410
    Formula..410
    Nitrates..414
    Fish And Mercury 416
Home Safety 418
    How to Prevent Drowing...418
    Cleaning Products, Carpeting, Pesticides..419
    Pesticides, Radon...421
    Baby Proofing...422
    Baby Product and Toy Safety 424
    28 Tips for Reducing Hazards..429

SECTION FIVE: FIRST AID—TOP 12 PROBLEMS & SOLUTIONS
Chapter 16
FIRST AID

Tips For Calling The Doctor After-Hours...433
Your First Aid Kit 435
How To Take Your Baby's Vital Signs 435
The Most Frequent Emergencies 437
    Abdominal Pain...437
    Allergic Reaction...439
    Bleeding And Bruising..440
    How To Avoid Food-Poisoning...444

Burns 445
Breathing Problems (Respiratory Distress) 446
Labored Breathing...446
Everything You Wanted To Know About Croup 447
Choking Emergencies: 4 Tips 449
Cough & Congestion...450
Diarrhea 453
How To Tell If Your Baby Is Dehydrated 454
Vomiting 456
Eye Problems: Pink Eye, Blocked Tear Ducts................................459
Fever: A Special Section 461
10 Things To Do When Your Baby Has A Fever.............................465
How To Take Your Baby's Temperature...466
Poisoning 470
Rashes 471
Seizures..476
Does It Need Stitches?...476
Trauma: Injuries To The Head, Neck, Back, Eyes 479

SECTION SIX: THE REFERENCE LIBRARY

Appendix A: Medications..487
Appendix B: Complementary Medicines...513
Appendix C: Lab Work & Tests 519
Appendix D: Glossary...529
Appendix E: References...549
Appendix F: Footnotes 559
Index...569
How To Reach The Authors, Baby411.com 610
Our Other Books: Toddler 411, Expecting 411................................612

ICONS

 Helpful Hint

 Reality Check

 Bottom Line

 Red Flags

 Feedback from the Real World

 Old Wives Tale

 Insider Secrets

 New Parent 411

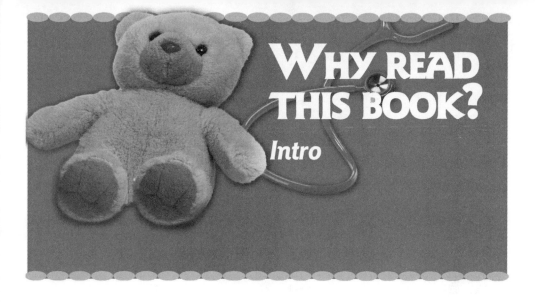

WHY READ THIS BOOK?

Intro

WHAT'S IN THIS CHAPTER

◆ **MEET THE AUTHORS**

◆ **HOW TO USE THIS BOOK**

◆ **NO ADS! NO PLUGS!**

◆ **SHOW US THE SCIENCE**

elcome to the world of parenthood. Yes, having a baby is both exciting . . . and terrifying.

Soon, you'll be responsible for taking care of this little urchin 24/7, with no time off for good behavior. We've been in your shoes—and NOTHING can prepare you for parenthood (even Dr. Brown's training as a pediatrician)! You have been given a precious gift and you don't want to screw it up. And that can lead to some real anxiety!

Once your baby is born, your thoughts will be swimming with dozens of questions, often at 2 AM . . . from the mundane (what's THAT in my baby's diaper?) to the serious (Why won't my baby stop crying? Should I call the doctor?).

That's why we are here. Think of us as your sherpa guide as you climb Mt. Everest Baby. You need detailed, up-to-date info about taking care of your baby—we've got it. You want straight answers on hot topics like vaccines, COVID-19 and how to get your baby to sleep through the night—again, we're there.

Yes, we realize there are many other experts (and non-experts!) who have multimedia platforms all promising to reveal the secrets to taking care of your baby. So, why turn to us for help? Well, let's introduce ourselves and then you'll know you have come to the right place.

Hi, I'm Dr. Ari Brown! I've been a pediatrician for over 25 years--and I see babies and new parents like you every day in my office. I did my pediatric residency training at Harvard Medical School/Boston Children's Hospital and I have served as a spokesperson for the American Academy of

Pediatrics and a medical advisor for *Parents Magazine* for most of my career. I love sharing my knowledge and I'm committed to advocating for kids and their parents.

But, my most important credential is that I'm a parent, too. I have been in your shoes and I KNOW what you're feeling--your hopes, dreams, and fears...and that sheer panic when you are up at 2 AM with a baby who is screaming non-stop. I know what you're worried about and what keeps you up at night--both physically and mentally. I'll hold your hand and we'll get through this together. Over the years, I've helped many new parents like you navigate this amazing (and at times, really challenging) journey.

View me as your best friend, who will always give you real talk and have your back...but I also happened to go to medical school, which turns out to be pretty helpful!

I love my job--because I get to watch your babies grow and YOU grow as parents.

And with this 20th Anniversary Edition of Baby 411 and over a million copies in print, I am truly honored to say I have helped an entire generation of parents with my authentic, clear, and relatable voice.

Hi, I'm Denise Fields! I have over 30 years of experience as a consumer advocate. As the co-author of *Baby Bargains* and *Baby 411*, I've been featured on Oprah and in the Wall Street Journal. I add my experience as both a mom and author—many of the questions we get on our social media hit the same hot button issues you'll see here.

One thing we have both learned: no one is the perfect parent. We are all just doing our best and we all make mistakes.

We'll give you the science-based facts you need to feel confident as a new parent, combined with the empathy that only another parent can have.

Here's the best advice we can give you:

1. Trust Yourself. You won't miss something serious going on with your baby. We promise. We know it will feel that way when you are up with a feverish baby.

2. Rely on Accurate Sources. Some information isn't reliable and some may be outdated--babies haven't changed in the past 20 years, but what we have learned about them has. Dr. Brown's superpower is that she is really good at breaking down all the science jargon and medical research and explaining it to families. She's also seen it all over the years!

You should also trust your pediatrician to guide you with the latest evidence-based advice.

There's so much information and so much to learn, it can be overwhelming. Your friends with babies have already warned you, but you are about to be really busy and really exhausted. If we're being honest, there is NO WAY you can fully understand exactly what that means yet....But trust us, you will soon enough.

In all the excitement of bringing a baby into the world, it's easy to get caught up in the whirlwind of shopping, birth-planning, and reading up on pregnancy. Let's just say you won't have time to read once your baby is born, so take advantage of the time you have now to learn about your baby's health and development.

While you're out there taking a crash course with Dr. Google, we can help you make sense of the endless supply of confusing, sometimes concerning, or even contradictory information coming from everyone. There is no shortage of opinion or judgment swirling around babies and parenting...But let's be clear: Parenting should be guilt-free and you should never feel judged.

We know it is tempting to solve every problem by doing a quick internet search, but it can cause more stress than it alleviates when you convince yourself that your baby has a horrible disease and you end up in a panic spiral. Dr. Brown can do what Dr. Google can't: Curate the latest science-based advice and explain it to you. Parenting is much more than just Googling an answer, it's about putting it in context. That's why our books, videos, and online community are life-savers for new parents.

We encourage you to join our community and keep up with breaking news. Find it all at linktr.ee/AriBrownMD

You've got this....and we are going to ensure you feel that way. So, relax and enjoy the journey. Happy parents lead to happy babies.

How to Use this Book

Instructions: Open cover. Start reading.

Just kidding! We realize you know how to read a book, but let's go over a few details on how to get the most out of *Baby 411*.

First, let's talk about BIG UGLY LATIN WORDS. You can't discuss baby's health without whipping out the Latin. To keep the jargon from overwhelming you, we have a handy glossary at the end of this book. When you see a **LATIN WORD** in bold small caps, turn to the back to get a quick definition.

Second, if you flip through the chapters, you'll note boxes with Dr. B's opinion. As it sounds, these are her *opinions* on several hot button issues. Feel free to disagree with these thoughts, but they are based on years of seeing real-world patients and talking with parents. Unlike some other parenting books, we think readers deserve to know where the line is drawn between fact and opinion. You can then decide what works for you and your family.

Finally, let's talk footnotes—we've footnoted the sources used throughout this book. These references are in Appendix F in the back of the book.

What? No one paid you to recommend a treatment?

Yes, it's true. No pharmaceutical company has paid the authors to plug their products or treatment in this book. The opinions in this book are those of Denise Fields and Dr. Brown—in the latter case, based on her training and experience practicing pediatric medicine. If we recommend a product or treatment, it is because we believe in it!

Show us the Science!

The goal of *Baby 411* is to provide you with the most up-to-date medical info on your baby. We're talking state-of-the-art when it comes to your baby's health and nutrition.

Our mantra is SHOW US THE SCIENCE! Before we recommend a particular treatment, parenting method or medicine, we expect there to be good science behind it.

Exhibit A: COVID-19. The pandemic has proven why following the science is mission critical! And, sadly, social media algorithms complicate what gets pushed into our news feed. It's easy to get an incomplete or worse, inaccurate picture on an important health topic because one can find a junk science article on just about any topic that supports a position we may have.

What is good science? Good scientific research is conducted by reputable researchers and published in a major medical journal, like the *New England Journal of Medicine*. Good science is based on a large enough sample to be statistically significant—and verified by peers before it is published.

Here's the take-home message: as your guides in Baby Health Land, we hope to steer you toward the *good* science when making decisions for your baby.

What's New In This Edition?

As usual, we just can't leave well enough alone! Like every new edition, you can be sure you are reading the most recent research and data on every child health topic. The big old elephant in the room since our last edition is COVID-19. We'll cover the latest on the virus and the vaccine as we go to print, but follow us on our social media channels for updates.

We explain the latest research on food allergies and how to prevent them. And, we discuss the newest baby formulas on the market and black market (stay tuned for some straight talk on buying European formula online).

We've also expanded our content on safety. Just because a baby product is on the market, does not mean it's safe or recommended by pediatricians (hello, infant loungers and recliners). And we'll share lots of practical tips on how to make your baby's world a safe place to explore.

Baby411.com: Advice, Updates & More

Pop by linktr.ee/AriBrownMD for all sorts of goodies—educational videos, advice, updates and more. Our famous Rash-o-Rama lets you see pictures of common rashes. And don't forget to like us on Instagram (@aribrownmd), Facebook (facebook.com/expecting411) and follow us on Twitter (@baby411) for the latest breaking news on infant health, reader questions and answers and more. Find the handy QR code on the back page for access to even more content!

Major Legal Disclaimer

No medical book about babies is complete without that ubiquitous legal disclaimer . . . so here's ours:

The information we provide in this book is intended to help families understand their baby's medical issues. It is NOT intended to replace the advice of your doctor. Before you start any medical treatment, always check in with your baby's doctor who can counsel you on the specific needs of your baby.

We have made a tremendous effort to give you the most up-to-date medical info available. However, medical research is constantly providing new insight into pediatric healthcare. That's why we stay connected on social media to give you the latest breaking updates (and why you should also discuss your baby's medical care with your baby's doc).

Okay, enough of the introductions—let's get rolling. First up: preparing for your new baby. You've got decisions to make . . . we'll discuss this first.

Section 1

3-2-1 Baby!

Preparing for the New One

BIRTH DAY

Chapter 1

"Giving birth is like taking your lower lip and forcing it over your head."
~ Carol Burnett

WHAT'S IN THIS CHAPTER

◆ **CUTTING THE CORD, LITERALLY**

◆ **DETAILS OF YOUR BABY'S FIRST PHYSICAL EXAMINATION**

◆ **VITAMIN K, EYE OINTMENT**

◆ **YOUR BABY'S FIRST MEAL**

◆ **THE FIRST FEW DAYS WITH YOUR NEWBORN**

◆ **MORE TESTS AND PROCEDURES**

◆ **THIS WASN'T IN THE BIRTH PLAN**

◆ **JAUNDICE**

◆ **OPTIONAL TESTS AND PROCEDURES**

◆ **GOING HOME/2 WEEK SURVIVAL GUIDE**

◆ **SPECIAL SITUATIONS: PREEMIES, ADOPTION**

Birth Day is finally here—the most incredible day of your life. You have prepared the nursery and taken the childbirth class, breastfeeding class, and baby care class. Hopefully, you've also met with your pediatrician (see Chapter 2, "You and Your Baby's Doc"). So you're ready, right?

There is no way anyone can prepare you for this, but this chapter will guide you through your baby's first days of life. Let's leave the giving birth part to the pregnancy books (see our other book, *Expecting 411*) . . . Instead, we'll focus on what happens once your baby is born. This chapter will give you an overview of your newborn, head to toe. It also includes a handy two-week survival guide, which you will want to bookmark!

Many people are not aware of this, but your baby's healthcare begins with their first check up right after birth. Why, you may ask? Because entering the world is a big transition. Babies who are still inside the womb may have certain medical problems that do not show themselves until they take their first breath of fresh air. It is very helpful in the world of modern day medicine to have ultrasounds, lab tests, and amniocentesis to get a glimpse of potential problems in your baby—but they don't cover every issue.

Also in this chapter, we'll explain a few decisions you should make before giving birth. You may desire additional tests and procedures for your baby post-delivery, which are only options if you plan ahead. And we will address the unique issues related to having a premature baby or adopting a newborn.

This chapter will also cover things you don't have in your birth plan, such as delivering a premature baby or one who needs some additional medical attention after delivery.

That is a ton of ground to cover, so let's start with your baby's first moment of life.

Cutting the Cord, and Your Baby's To Do List

Q. Can my partner cut the umbilical cord?

Yes. But, your partner is also allowed to say no—especially if the sight of blood induces nausea or fainting.

If your partner wants to cut the baby's cord, this event occurs after the baby has come out and after your practitioner has placed two clamps (about one inch apart) on the cord. (Don't worry, your doc will give the cue).

Your partner cuts the cord with a pair of scissors (provided by your practitioner) between the two clamps. The umbilical cord is a little rubbery so it often takes a few snips to complete the job. It also can spray blood—you've been warned!

Q. I've been told that we should wait to cut the umbilical cord. Why?

The American Congress of Obstetricians and Gynecologists (ACOG) advises that for routine deliveries, there is no rush to cut the cord. Studies show that by waiting at least 30–60 seconds after delivery to place two clamps (aka medical clothespins) and cut the umbilical cord, more blood flows from the placenta to the newborn. That extra blood boosts a baby's iron stores for several months, which prevents anemia.

The downsides? Delayed cord clamping and cutting reduces the odds of having enough umbilical cord blood to store. It also increases the chance of a newborn becoming jaundiced in the first few days of life (see **JAUNDICE** later in this chapter). And if your baby is in distress and there is a concern for his health, the obstetrician (OB) needs to cut the cord right away and hand the baby over to the pediatric team for immediate care.

Bottom line: Wait to cut the cord unless a medical reason requires a quick snip!

Q. When does the OB collect blood for cord blood banking?

Within minutes after delivery. So, if this is something you want to do (it's optional), you need to plan ahead for it. We'll discuss optional tests and procedures later in this chapter.

Here is how it typically goes. The baby comes out and your practitioner (usually) puts them right up on mom's chest. If a couple wants to bank their baby's cord blood, your practitioner places two clamps on the cord right after delivery and the cord is cut (either by your partner or by your practitioner).

Once the cord is cut, your practitioner places a needle into the largest vessel in the umbilical cord to drain as much blood as possible into a bag or syringe. The goal is to get as much blood as possible before the vessels spasm and the placenta begins to separate from the wall of the uterus. Once that happens, no more blood flows through the umbilical cord.

Q. When will I be able to hold the baby for the first time?

If the delivery goes smoothly and the baby is doing well, you can hold your baby pretty soon after the big entrance.

Your baby will be covered in blood and white cheesy stuff (**VERNIX**) and sometimes poop (**MECONIUM**). In other words, they are all wet. And that means they are going to get cold pretty fast. So, the staff needs to vigorously dry your baby off with towels first and either places them skin to skin on your chest or put them on a small exam table that has a heater (warming table). The vigorous rubdown stimulates your baby to breathe and gets their circulation going. The delivery team staff also suctions their mouth and nose to remove thick secretions.

The team will do a quick assessment (see APGAR test below), and then you get to snuggle for the first time together.

Q. Does my baby need to study for the Apgar test?

No. They probably won't score a perfect "10" either—those foreign judges are so critical of the dismount. Just kidding. The Apgar test determines which babies need extra help adjusting to life outside the womb. They are given a score from zero to ten. Your baby's **A**ppearance (color), **P**ulse (heart rate), **G**rimace (reaction to stimulation), **A**ctivity (tone), and **R**espiration rate are assessed at one minute of life and again at five minutes. Babies who endure difficult deliveries often have low (less than five) Apgar scores at one minute then perk up (greater than seven) at five minutes. The babies that don't rise in their scores may need observation and assistance by medical staff. Rest assured, low Apgar scores do NOT correlate with low SAT scores and future intelligence.

Reality Check

If the baby has an immediate problem (such as trouble breathing), they may get whisked over to the warming table in your delivery suite or even off to the neonatal intensive care unit.

If your newborn has an urgent health issue, the hospital may ask a neonatologist (newborn intensive care specialist) or a staff pediatrician in the hospital to care for your baby immediately.

If you deliver at a birthing center or at home and there is a problem, your baby would need to be transported to the nearest medical facility via ambulance.

This is very unsettling if you have a perfect vision planned of those first moments together with your newborn. If this should happen to you, remember that your baby's health is the utmost priority. Even if you don't get to bond in those precious minutes right after delivery, you still have time later—and we promise it won't impact your long-term relationship with your child.

Q. When is my baby examined for the first time?

Your baby will be examined several times, so be prepared. If you deliver at a hospital, the delivery healthcare staff performs the first overall exam on your baby after you have a little bond- ing time. The staff measures the baby's weight, length, and head circumference. They also place an ID band on the ankle as well as a security clip. Eye ointment and a Vitamin K shot are routinely administered at this point. We'll explain the importance of these two therapies in the section to follow. Your baby will eat a first meal, and then while you are getting cleaned up (childbirth is pretty messy), your baby will be observed for the first couple of hours in the nursery. That is when they will have a complete head to toe exam by the nursery staff. Your baby's heart rate, respiratory rate, body temperature, and oxygen level is monitored. That's the time your baby also gets any blood drawn for lab tests should any be necessary (blood sugar, blood count, blood culture). Your baby can get cleaned up after proving they can maintain their body temperature.

After all those hurdles, your baby is ready to join you in your postpartum room.

The nursery staff notifies your baby's doctor about the birth. The doctor will examine the baby and visit with mom and dad (that's you—has a nice ring to it) within 24 hours of the birth and then daily until you are discharged home. If your personal pediatrician does not make hospital rounds, a pediatrician on the hospital staff will take care of these initial exams.

Reality Check

If you deliver at a birthing center or at home, the midwife/practitioner does the initial and follow up examinations of your baby; the pediatrician meets your baby at two weeks of age. (Alternatively, your pediatrician may enter the scene at two months of age if the midwife handles the two-week visit).

Q. Tell me about the baby's first exam. What are you looking for?

Bear with us—this stuff is a little dry, but we think it will help you to understand what your doctor is doing. It will also make you appreciate how fortunate you are to have a baby who makes an A+ on their first exam!

Vital Signs

This includes heart rate (pulse), breathing rate (respiratory rate), body temperature, and weight. Abnormalities can indicate infection, dehydration, and heart/lung abnormalities. These are checked at least every eight hours. Babies are weighed daily. Input (length of breastfeeding/amount of formula) and output (number of pees and poops) are also documented.

The Head

◆ Shape of the head. The head may look cone-shaped initially, but it rounds out after a few weeks. The skull bones often overlap right after delivery (that's what allows the baby's head to leave the birth canal) so there may be a firm ridge present. Those ridges go away in the first week of life.

◆ Bruises from the trauma of delivery caused by forceps, vacuum, or pushing on your pelvic bones for two-plus hours. Big bruises can take six to eight weeks to resolve (see **CEPHALHEMATOMA**)

◆ Soft spot. The soft spot (**ANTERIOR FONTANELLE**) in the middle of the skull is open with room for the brain to grow (see **CRANIOSYNOSTOSIS**). There is also a very small soft spot on the back of the skull called the posterior fontanelle, which is sometimes large enough to feel at birth.

The Eyes

◆ Red reflex. Doctors use a special light to see the baby's red reflex (the "red eye" you see in flash photography pictures). **CATARACTS** and eye tumors (see **RETINOBLASTOMA**) are two problems doctors are trying to catch here.

◆ Broken blood vessel. **SUBCONJUNCTIVAL HEMORRHAGES** are broken blood vessels in one or both eyes that can happen when the baby is pushed through the birth canal.

These are common and go away in a few weeks.

◆ Tear ducts. Many newborns get clogged tear ducts (see **NASOLACRIMAL DUCT OBSTRUCTION**). The ducts are narrow and cause the tears to get goopy and make the eye look infected. This can come and go for your baby's entire first year of life. We'll cover this issue later in Chapter 15, "First Aid" in the eye problems section.

Reality Check

Newborns can only see 8 to 12 inches in front of them. They can see you if you bring their face up close to yours. They frequently look cross-eyed for the first two months. And by the way, we cannot predict true eye color until about six months of life.

The Ears

◆ Eardrums are checked, as well as abnormal formations of the outer part of the ears (see **PREAURICULAR PITS**, **SKIN TAGS**).

◆ A hearing test should be performed on all newborns. No, we don't ask them to raise their hand when they hear the beep. The baby wears headphones and we measure the electrical activity of the brain when a noise is made. (See **BAER**). We'll discuss more about hearing screening in the Tests section of this chapter.

The Nose

◆ Can baby breathe through their nose (see **CHOANAL ATRESIA**)? By the way, all babies have stuffy noses at birth and continue to have nasal congestion for the next four to six weeks (see **NEWBORN NASAL CONGESTION**).

The Mouth

◆ Formation of the mouth. A doctor will check to make sure the roof of the mouth (palate) has formed and the funny thing hanging in the back of the mouth (uvula) is there (see **CLEFT LIP** and **CLEFT PALATE**). Some babies are born with white pimples on the roof of their mouths (see **EPSTEIN'S PEARLS**) that go away on their own.

◆ Tongue. Your baby's tongue is checked for a forked tip or any trouble in moving it. This is called a tongue tie or a tight frenulum (see **ANKYLOGLOSSIA**). This can be a significant issue when it comes to successful and comfortable breastfeeding (see more in Chapter 6, "Liquids"), so it is important to identify this abnormality shortly after birth.

◆ Gums. Many babies have white pimples on the gums that go away on their own. These are not teeth—the first tooth usually comes out between six to 12 months of age. However, every once in a blue moon (I've never had a patient with one in 25 years), a baby is born with a tooth. These are called **NATAL TEETH.** They usually fall out on their own, but occasionally need to be pulled.

The Throat

◆ Breathing. Occasionally, babies make unusual noises when breathing. Some babies are born with floppy breathing tubes (see **LARYNGOMALACIA**) that they will outgrow. This squeaky noise really concerns parents (because it sounds strange), but is usually of no consequence.

The Neck and Shoulders

◆ These areas are checked for any unusual lumps, bumps, or cysts (see **BRANCHIAL CLEFT CYST**).

◆ If birth was difficult (big baby, small mommy), the collarbone can break (see **CLAVICLE FRACTURE, SHOULDER DYSTOCIA**).

◆ Can your baby turn its head to each side? Some babies will have a stiff neck muscle that limits head motion (see **TORTICOLLIS**).

The Chest

◆ Doctors look for any signs of labored breathing (see **RESPIRATORY DISTRESS**). Adults breathe 12 times per minute at an even rate. Newborns breathe 30 to 40 times per minute and have episodes of **PERIODIC BREATHING**. So, your baby will breathe rapidly several times, p-a-u-s-e, then breathe again. That pause will seem like an eternity to you. It is normal. Signs of respiratory distress are:

1. A pause between two breaths that lasts 15-20 seconds (see **APNEA**).
2. Baby is consistently breathing over 60 times per minute. (see **TACHYPNEA OF NEWBORN**)
3. Baby's ribs are sucking in at each breath, nostrils are flaring, grunting noises are heard (see **RETRACTIONS, RESPIRATORY DISTRESS**)

The Heart and Circulation

◆ Murmurs (unusual noises), irregular heartbeats, fast or slow heart rate, unusual discoloration (pale or dusky blue). Many heart problems, especially severe defects (see **CONGENITAL HEART DISEASE**) are now detected on fetal ultrasounds. However, doctors listen carefully with their good old stethoscopes to pick up abnormalities.

◆ Baby's pulses are carefully checked, particularly those in the groin area (femoral pulses). The main blood vessel (aorta) supplying oxygen rich blood to the body can have kinks and narrowings (see **COARCTATION OF AORTA**) causing a weakened pulse in the groin. Most hospitals routinely assess for potential heart defects by checking a newborn's oxygen supply with a non-invasive monitoring device.

◆ A normal, benign murmur is often heard in the first 24 hours of life, as the newborn's circulation transitions from that of the fetus. This murmur, often called a **TRANSITIONAL MURMUR** resolves within the first few days and does *not* represent a problem.

◆ Purple hands and feet (see **ACROCYANOSIS**) are due to newborn circulation. Your baby is merely attempting to adapt to life outside the womb. This is normal and can last from weeks to sometimes months, especially after exposure to cold, or following a bath.

The Abdomen

◆ Your baby's doctor will feel the belly to check the size of the liver and spleen. The belly should be soft and not hurt to touch. Abnormally large body organ size can be caused by problems metabolizing foods (see **METABOLIC STORAGE DISEASE**) or poor heart function (see **CONGESTIVE HEART FAILURE**). Abnormal fullness or distention alerts doctors to look for **ABDOMINAL TUMORS**.

◆ Firm or full bellies may be a sign of abnormal intestine formation (see **MALROTATION**, **DUODENAL ATRESIA**). An abnormal exam and problems feeding—that is, vomiting, especially bile, will be a tip off to investigate things further.

◆ A baby is expected to pass one stool called **MECONIUM** in the first 24 hours of life. If a baby doesn't poop on Day 1, we evaluate for abnormal anus formation (see **HIRSCHSPRUNG'S DISEASE, ANAL ATRESIA**) or poor stool formation that can be seen in cystic fibrosis (see **MECONIUM PLUG, CYSTIC FIBROSIS**).

◆ Sometimes the belly button (umbilicus) pops out. This is the extreme form of an "outty" (see **UMBILICAL HERNIA**) and often resolves on its own.

Factoid: Your doc will check the umbilical cord stump to make sure the cord had two umbilical arteries and one vein. In rare cases, cords have only one umbilical artery—this can be a sign of kidney malformation. Your doctor may order an ultrasound of your baby's kidneys to rule that out.

 Old Wives Tale

Placing a coin or a Band-Aid on the belly button will help the "outty" belly button go in. FALSE. Time is the best therapy.

The Genitals
Boys

◆ For boys, the baby's doctor makes sure both testes are in the scrotum. Occasionally, one or both testes will not make the pilgrimage south (see **UNDESCENDED TESTES**).

◆ For boys, the fullness of the scrotum is also checked. Many boys are born with extra fluid in the scrotum that goes away over the first six months of life. (see **HYDROCELE**) The other thing that causes fullness is a hernia—part of the intestine that has pushed into the scrotum (see **INGUINAL HERNIA**). Cool doctor trick: we can tell the difference by shining a light on the scrotum. Fluid (hydrocele) is light and intestine (hernia) is dark.

Normal penis

◆ For boys, the baby's doctor will make sure the opening (urethra) is at the tip of the penis. The opening can abnormally develop on the undersurface of the penis shaft (see **HYPOSPADIAS,** see picture at right) or on topside (see **EPISPADIAS**). Boys with this problem are not routinely circumcised because the foreskin is needed to surgically correct it around six months of age.

Hypospadias

GIRLS

◆ For girls, the vagina and urethra (the holes tucked inside the lips) are checked. The lips (labia minora) can be stuck together (see **LABIAL ADHESION**). Usually, you see some white mucousy fluid (see **VAGINAL DISCHARGE**). This is normal. Occasionally, newborn girls also have some vaginal bleeding (see What's That in My Baby's Diaper? question in the "Getting to Know You" section later in this chapter). New parent alert—you need to learn how to clean this area well. (See Chapter 4, "Hygiene" in the "Girl Parts" section for details.)

BOTH SEXES

◆ When the clitoris looks too large, or the penis looks too small, your doctor will evaluate for problems with the baby's hormones or chromosomes. (see **AMBIGU-OUS GENITALIA**)

◆ Breast or nipple enlargement: For both sexes, the breasts can be swollen due to Mom's hormones passing through to baby. It is temporary and they shrink back down on their own. We repeat: both baby girls and boys can have transient breast tissue. The man boobs will not last for very long and your newborn daughter will not need to wear a sports bra for several years. No worries! And just to really freak you out, a baby's breast will also occasionally secrete milk (called Witch's Milk) in the first weeks of life.

◆ Accessory (or **SUPRANUMERARY**) nipples: About one in 40 babies will have extra nipples. They are usually brown and flat and just look like a birthmark. They're not functional and don't cause any problems.

The Kidneys and Bladder

◆ Expect the baby to pee (urinate) once in the first 24 hours of life. We start investigating if this does not occur.

◆ Abnormal formation of the passageway from the kidneys to the bladder (see **VESI-COURETERAL REFLUX, POSTERIOR URETHRAL VALVES**) can occur in rare occasions. An evaluation for this is done if a baby develops a bladder or kidney infection. (see **URINARY TRACT INFECTION, PYELONEPHRITIS**)

The Spine and Nervous System

◆ Your baby's doctor will look for dimples or tufts of hair near the buttocks. Abnormalities on the skin can be a clue to a spine abnormality underneath the skin (see **SACRAL DIMPLE, NEURAL TUBE DEFECT, SPINA BIFIDA**).

◆ Also checked: the newborn's unique reflexes that fade over the first six months of life. It tells us their brain and nerves are coordinated. (see **CEREBRAL PALSY**) These reflexes include: *Rooting* (turning the head when the cheek is rubbed), *Sucking* (automatically sucking on objects placed in the mouth), *Palmar Grasp* (closing fingers on object placed on the palm), and *Moro* (body startles when head is dropped back).

The Arms and Legs (Extremities)

◆ Do both arms move? A weakness of the nerves causes a limp arm. (see **ERB'S PALSY**)

◆ Many people are familiar with purebred dogs with hip problems. Humans can have similar problems. We check the hips by rotating them in and out. If there is a concern, we'll order an ultrasound to look at the hips. Breech babies have a slightly increased risk of this disorder. (see **HIP DYSPLASIA**)

◆ Rarely, babies will have extra fingers and toes, and some that are fused together (see **POLYDACTYLY, SYNDACTYLY**).

? ?

BIRTH DAY

◆ A severe deformity (see **CLUB FOOT**) makes the bottoms of the feet face each other and requires casting. This occurs in about 1 in 1000 births.

The Skin

◆ Brown birthmarks: Moles (see **CONGENITAL NEVUS**) and light brown oval shaped areas (see **CAFÉ AU LAIT SPOTS**) are permanent markings and rarely are related to other medical problems.

◆ Purple birthmarks: These marks (see **PORT WINE STAINS**) are permanent and can be quite large. If they are located on the face, your baby's doctor will look for other medical problems (see **STURGE-WEBER SYNDROME**).

◆ Red birthmarks: These marks (see **STRAWBERRY HEMANGIOMA**) may be seen at birth, or by the first month of life. They start out flat, grow much larger and become raised. These particular marks shrink and go away by the age of ten.

◆ More red birthmarks: Red marks known as stork bites and angel kisses (see **NEVUS FLAMMEUS, FLAT ANGIOMATA**) are on the back of the neck or eyelids and fade over the first few months of life. When your baby gets mad at you, they turn even redder.

◆ Blue, bruise-like marks: These spots (see **MONGOLIAN SPOTS**) are found on the buttocks or back of babies of Asian or African ancestry or those with darker skin. They fade over several years.

◆ Yellow skin: This is a whole topic in itself—see **JAUNDICE** in the "Getting to Know You" section later in this chapter.

Go to our web site Baby411.com for pictures of all of these common birthmarks. Click on "Bonus Material".

Reality Check

Newborns are really rashy. Most rashes will come and go. You'll have a window of "photo opportunity" from two to three weeks of age when their skin is clearer. Then more rashes crop up at four to eight weeks of age. These are all due to fluctuating hormone levels. No matter what you do, they will go away. A good thing to remember is your baby could care less. The names are listed below. For details, refer to the glossary. (see **ERYTHEMA TOXICUM, MILIA, MILIARIA, NEONATAL ACNE, PUSTULAR MELANOSIS**). For pictures of these rashes, check out our web site Baby411.com (click on "Bonus Material.")

Q. Why do all babies get a shot of Vitamin K?

Vitamin K is essential for blood clotting. Most newborns have a deficiency in Vitamin K because it does not efficiently cross the placenta while fetuses are in the womb. Babies who are born with a severe Vitamin K deficiency can have significant bleeding into vital organs (such as the brain, see **VKDB OR VITAMIN K DEFICIENCY BLEEDING**). Since time is of the essence, it makes more sense to give all babies Vitamin K than to test them all and find out too late who really needed it.

Some parents have decided to decline the Vitamin K shot for their baby. Why? Natural parenting proponents cast suspicion on the Vitamin K shot, saying the shot itself is too invasive. Others question the additives and preservatives in the shot.

BIRTH DAY

We highly recommend the Vitamin K shot—there can be serious consequences if you skip it. Vanderbilt University Medical Center reported five babies in Nashville needlessly experienced brain hemorrhages when their parents opted out of this extremely safe and simple vitamin injection. No, the shot does not cause leukemia, autism, or any other malady. What about giving the Vitamin K dose orally? Giving an oral Vitamin K supplement is not an effective alternative to prevent this potentially tragic problem. *(Schulte)*

Q. Why do all babies get eye ointment?

Having a baby is messy. Some mothers carry bacteria that can lead to serious eye infections in the baby. Again, it makes more sense to treat every baby immediately than to test every mother at delivery and figure out which baby needs it. Antibiotic ointment has low risk with great benefit. While some countries have stopped routinely using eye ointment moved towards screening moms for infection, it is still the norm and standard of care in the U.S. to simply treat all newborns.

Q. When do I get to feed the baby for the first time?

Assuming all is well after vaginal delivery and baby doesn't need to go to the nursery for any reason, you can start feeding your baby right away. If you have a C-section, you may be able to nurse in the recovery room. If not, you can nurse when you reach your postpartum room a few hours later.

Some babies want to eat immediately. It is easy to tell because they start moving their lips and sticking out their tongues. They are usually very alert for the first hour of life (and then they just want to get some shut-eye for a few hours). So, it is best to try to get in a feeding while you have the opportunity.

But some babies are coughing and sneezing to try to get all the fluid out of their lungs. They have little desire to feed. Don't worry if your baby doesn't want to eat right away. Breathing is a higher priority than eating, so they will need to get the hang of it first (remember, they just learned how to do this at delivery).

Whether you are nursing or formula feeding, those first feeding moments can be awkward since you probably have no idea what you are doing. Don't be embarrassed to ask for help. Your baby is very forgiving.

Q. Do I "room-in" with my baby at the hospital?

Yes. Once you and your baby get cleaned up after delivery, and all the initial assessments

NEW PARENT 411: WHY DO ALL THESE TESTS?

Some parents feel uncomfortable with all the poking and prodding their newborn endures. Trust us—there is a method to the madness. Your doctor wants to make sure you are taking home a healthy baby! Remember the key rule to all these tests: if it weren't important, we wouldn't be doing it!

? ?

BIRTH DAY

are complete, your family will move to a postpartum suite if you deliver at a hospital. Hospitals encourage mother and baby stay in the same room ("rooming in") to help with bonding and to make breastfeeding successful. This will allow you to learn your baby's hunger cues and nurse before your baby is screaming and demanding to be fed.

However, we should warn you that babies are very noisy sleepers. Try not to obsess over every squeak your baby makes. You need sleep to recover from the delivery and produce milk. However, the hospital staff can baby-sit your newborn in the nursery for a few hours while you get some shut-eye.

If you have a vaginal delivery, expect to spend 48 hours at the hospital before heading home. If you have a C-section, plan to be recovering for three to four days before discharge home.

Getting to Know You: Your Baby's First Few Days

After your baby passes the first exam, the fun is just beginning—it's time for you the parent to get to know your new family addition. Let's talk about what you'll experience for the first few hours . . . and days. This section will cover changing those first diapers and more.

Q. How often will my baby need to eat?

Eight is the magic number.

If you do that math, you might think that means that your baby will need to eat every three hours over a 24-hour day. Sorry, newborns do not follow any type of schedule. There is a time and place to begin routines and schedules, but that happens around two to three months of age. Be patient.

Newborns like to cluster feed. They may want to eat every 90 minutes for two or three feedings, then take a snooze for two or three hours. Unfortunately, those cluster feedings often occur during the hours you would like to be asleep. But somehow, they usually get to the minimum requirement of eight feedings a day. Why do we let them be in charge? A newborn that eats "on-demand," eats better than one who is awakened and told that it is time to eat.

NEW PARENT 411: BIRTH TRAUMA

This is what happens when your baby is larger than your pelvis can handle or just simply doesn't want to leave the womb. Your newborn's head may be pressed against your pelvic bones for 2 hours or may have had forceps or a vacuum applied to their head. The result: a huge bruise on his head caused by bleeding just under the skin that clots and looks rather dramatic. (see baby411.com for a great picture).

Because the skin is also injured, a scab will form and peel off (like a sunburn). The blood clot will get hard and leave a lump for up to eight weeks. Not to worry, none of this is permanent.

Your baby will be very sleepy in the first couple of days of life, so feedings will be relatively short (5-10 minutes per breast on Day 1, 10-15 mins per breast on Day 2) or low volume (0.5-1 ounce or 15-30 ml if formula feeding). But as long as they get to the magic number of feedings, they are probably getting enough to eat and your milk supply is getting revved up if you are breastfeeding.

Check out Chapter 6, "Liquids" for more details on nursing.

Insider Secrets

Nursing feels like having a mini-vacuum attached to your nipple. So, it's no surprise that new moms feel a little discomfort with nursing until they get used to that sensation. But if it hurts more than 10-20 seconds beyond the initial latch, break the suction seal, reposition the baby, and try again. If you have a bad latch, you will pay for it. See Chapter 6, "Liquids", for more tips.

Q. Why am I being asked to track my baby's feedings and diapers?

Keeping track of feedings—both duration of feeds and the number of feeds—is very important in the first week of life to be sure breastfeeding is going well and your baby is getting their nutritional needs met. See Chapter 6, "Liquids" for more details.

Additionally, monitoring diapers (both pee and poop) tells us that your baby is meeting their nutritional needs because what goes in is what comes out. For the first four days, we expect to see the same number of wet and poopy diapers as your child's age (that is, one pee and one poop on Day 1, four pees and four poops by Day 4). The poop also changes in color and in texture over the first few days, signaling that your baby is actually eating and eliminating their body garbage properly. We'll want you to describe what you see in that diaper as well—entertaining, no?

For feeding and diaper tracking as well as lots of other great information, we highly recommend the Glow Baby app (free on iOS and Android). After you get the green light from your baby's doctor, you can stop tracking these things.

Q. What's THAT in my baby's diaper?

We've got an entire chapter (Chapter 8 "The Other End") with accompanying pictures on our website dedicated to poop (yippee!) but let's give you a brief primer on what you'll be seeing in those first few diapers.

◆ *Black tar poop.* The official name is **MECONIUM.** Doctors expect one of these poops in the first day of life. If you see more, congratulations—you're on your way to being a diaper changing pro. See Chapter 8, "The Other End," Newborn Poop section for details.

◆ *Brick dust.* Babies should urinate (pee) at least once in the first day as well. If your baby is hovering around that 10% weight loss (see box in this section, Why is My Baby Shrinking?), you may see a red-orange brick dust spot in the diaper (see **URIC ACID CRYSTALS**). You'll think it is blood, but take a closer look. Blood gets absorbed into the diaper since it's a liquid. The crystal powder sits on the surface. It just means your baby needs to drink. For a great picture of this, go to Baby411.com/bonus and click on the Visual Library.

◆ **Blood**. Baby girls will have a "period" thanks to Mom's hormones. Don't worry, they don't get the PMS to go with it! This should only happen in the first month of life and not again until puberty.

◆ **Gel balls.** This did not come out of your baby. It is your super absorbent diaper. When the volume of urine (pee) exceeds the diaper absorbency, the gels rise to the surface. Your baby is not an alien and it is not a health hazard.

Q. My baby sleeps all the time. Were my prayers answered?

Wait until the baby gets home . . . you will find out then! All babies sleep through their first two days of life. They have been through the same experience as their Mom. They realize they have left the womb about the exact moment you take them home (if you deliver vaginally). It is not the magic of the nursery nurse's touch (although you will feel inadequate when faced with a screaming baby). Newborns don't have the skills to pull it together and settle down. You will need to figure out what soothes your baby. We will give you all the secrets to soothing your baby in Chapter 11, "Temperament & Soothing" and answer all of your sleep questions in Chapter 9, "Sleep."

Q. I am getting a lot of different advice from nurses and lactation specialists—who is right?

Everyone, sort of. You will meet many health care professionals in your baby's first few days. They will all have different approaches to the same child health issues. To avoid frustration and confusion, realize that there are many ways, for example, to position a baby to nurse. Just take it all in, then figure out what works for you and your child.

More Tests & Procedures

Q. What other procedures and tests are done on my baby?

Before your baby is discharged home, they will have a hearing screening test, a newborn metabolic screen (blood test), and a bilirubin blood test to assess for jaundice. Read on for more information about each test. It is also standard of care for all babies to receive a Hepatitis B vaccination.

NEW PARENT 411: WHY IS MY BABY SHRINKING?

The shrinking baby phenomenon! No, it's not a headline ripped from the tabloids. Babies travel out of the womb with extra baggage. They have about 10% more fluid than their bodies need. Over the first few days of life, they will lose 10% of their birth weight, then quickly gain about an ounce a day once they start eating (about their third day of life). This is sure to cause you anxiety, particularly if you are breastfeeding. For details, see the "infant calorie and nutrition needs" section in Chapter 5, "Nutrition and Growth."

Q. When is the hearing screen done?

The American Academy of Pediatrics recommends hearing screening for *all* newborns. The reason? Congenital hearing loss occurs in 3 per 1000 newborns. Early detection can make a considerable difference for a child's language development. The simple, non-invasive screening test is done before your baby goes home from the hospital. Some birthing centers are able to offer this screening, but if not, your pediatrician can advise you on getting it done elsewhere. *(AAP)*

Q. What is the newborn screening test?

The first newborn screening test dates to 1961, when Dr. Robert Guthrie discovered a way to diagnose a newborn with a genetic metabolic disorder called phenylketonuria (PKU) using a little dried blood on some filter paper.

This was a huge deal because babies with PKU weren't ordinarily diagnosed until at least six months of age . . . after they were permanently neurologically impaired.

Newborn screening has come a long way since then. Every state in the U.S. now requires an extensive panel of blood tests on every newborn—done with just a few drops of blood on filter paper.

Most of the tests detect "inborn errors of metabolism." Translation: these are diseases caused by a failure of the body to break down (metabolize) certain products. If these products are not broken down, they start to build up in the body and create problems—heart enlargement, intellectual disability, and even death. Other tests screen for hormone abnormalities, blood disorders, and cystic fibrosis.

Q. Do all babies get tested for metabolic diseases?

Yes. Every state in the U.S. performs a panel of blood tests on every newborn. All states test for at least 31-35 standard "core" disorders in the recommended uniform screening panel.

There are also tests for 26 additional disorders. Whether or not you are required to do these tests varies by state. These 26 other diseases are very rare and there's no treatment, even if a diagnosis is made in the first weeks of life. That's why some states don't require these tests. To find information on required screenings in your state, go to Baby's First Test (BabysFirstTest.org).

Q. Are there more newborn metabolic screening tests available other than those required by the state?

Yes. If you live in a state that only tests for core disorders, you can get your baby tested for many more disorders on your own dime. Private laboratories and academic institutions offer a low-cost expanded test that screens for over 60 metabolic disorders.

When blood is drawn for the state-mandated screening test (shortly after birth or at the two-week well check), additional blood can be used for these optional tests. The cost varies, but it is usually about $50-100. You probably spent at least that much on a diaper bag. For more information on supplemental newborn screening, check out this helpful grassroots advocacy organization, Hunter's Hope (HuntersHope.org).

Keep in mind that disorders tested for in the optional screen are quite rare (about 1 in 56,000). That's why some states weigh the cost of testing, the low number of abnormal results, and lack of treatment and opt to test only for the more common disorders.

Our opinion: in an ideal world, there would be one NATIONAL standard for newborn screenings. But that just isn't reality today.

 BOTTOM LINE: Although most metabolic diseases are rare, early detection is very important.

Q. Will my baby's blood type be tested?

Sometimes. Blood types are not routinely tested in the hospital. This might worry some parents, who are concerned that not knowing their baby's blood type immediately is dangerous. You should know that any person with a medical emergency (such as a car accident) that requires a blood transfusion gets type O negative blood regardless of their blood type. O negative blood is compatible with ALL blood types. For less urgent situations that require a blood transfusion, a person's blood type is tested to find a donor blood match.

Your baby's blood type will be tested if Mommy has O blood type because blood type incompatibility (i.e. baby is A or B) can lead to problems with jaundice. See jaundice (**ABO INCOMPATIBILITY**) information in "The 411 on Jaundice" section later in this chapter.

Q. I am Group B Strep positive, does my baby need to be tested?

Mothers are routinely screened at the 35th to 37th week of their pregnancy for the presence of a bacteria that lives harmlessly in the genitals and intestines of some healthy women. This bacteria, called Group B Strep, can infect a newborn as they pass through the birth canal.

Moms who are carriers for Group B Strep get intravenous (IV) antibiotics during labor to suppress the growth of this bacteria. If Moms who go into labor before 37 weeks, has water broken for more than 18 hours or has a fever greater than 100.4 degrees, also gets IV antibiotics because of the risk of Group B Strep infection. (If you have a C-section before going into labor

 BEHIND THE SCENES: MORE ON OPTIONAL SCREENS

Although most metabolic diseases are rare, early detection is critical to the health of an affected baby. Many states have expanded the number of government-subsidized tests. However, some states still only offer a bare bones minimum. If your state is one of those, you can pay for additional testing on your own. FYI: If you choose to bank your baby's cord blood, you may get a "free" supplemental newborn screen to go with it. For more information, here are some groups you can contact:

1. **Perkin Elmer.** PerkinElmer.com (866) 463-6436
2. **Mayo Clinic.** mayomedicallaboratories.com (800)-533-1710

you don't have to worry about this stuff).

Doctors get worked up about Group B Strep because it can cause blood infection (bacteremia), pneumonia, and meningitis in newborns. All newborns are watched closely, but those babies with moms who test positive for Group B Strep are watched even more closely.

It is standard protocol to get a complete blood count and blood culture on a newborn *if:*

◆ Mom is Group B Strep positive and didn't get pretreated with at least one dose of antibiotics at least four hours prior to delivery
◆ Mom appears to have a womb infection (chorioamnionitis)
◆ Or if a baby starts misbehaving (temperature instability, labored breathing, etc.). (*CDC*)

Reality Check

Don't be too alarmed if you carry Group B Strep. This does not mean you are Typhoid Mary. Most babies with Group B Strep positive mothers do not get sick— they are just at a slightly higher risk.

Q. Are there any vaccinations given to the baby at the hospital?

The Hepatitis B vaccine is recommended for all newborns as part of the universal immunization series. Infants usually get the first of three doses between birth and two months of age. It is ESSENTIAL to get the first dose at birth if Mom tests positive for Hepatitis B to prevent infection in the newborn. For more information see Chapter 12, "Vaccines."

This wasn't in the birth plan!

While most full-term deliveries and post-partum days go smoothly, your newborn may throw you a curve ball. While we don't mean to freak you out, here are some of the more common complications that might happen:

◆ *Group B Strep.* As we discussed in the section above, your baby may have blood tests done in certain situations to look for infection.

◆ *Blood sugar testing.* If your baby is very large (over eight pounds), very small (under five pounds), feeding poorly, jittery, cold, or very sleepy, they will have blood sugars tested to be sure that the level is high enough (usually that magic number is three consecutive pre-feeding levels greater than 50 mg/dl in the first forty-eight hours of life). Blood sugar is also routinely tested in babies whose mothers have diabetes or gestational diabetes. Be aware that some hospitals will test at-risk babies several times in the first couple of days. If your baby's blood sugar is low, you may need to supplement with sugar gel or formula for a day or two, even if breastfeeding is your long-term plan.

◆ *Meconium.* Babies who are stressed prior to or at delivery may pass their first poop before they leave the womb. That poop can be seen in the amniotic fluid. If the meconium enters the baby's lungs, it can cause inflammation and problems breathing. So, it's important to clear the baby's airway before they take their first breath. If your water breaks and your OB sees the meconium, a neonatal team is called to attend the delivery. Yes, even more people get to see you naked—you won't care at that point, trust us.

◆ *Labored breathing.* Babies who are delivered by C-section don't get their fetal fluid squeezed out of their lungs because they don't squeeze through the birth canal. As a result, some babies may have temporary labored breathing for the first few hours after delivery (called Transient Tachypnea of the Newborn, or TTN). Occasionally, babies delivered vaginally will have this too. If your baby has TTN, the medical staff monitors them for a little while in the nursery before they get their first snuggles with you.

◆ *Fever.* Your baby's body temperature will be watched closely during the first two days. If your baby runs a fever of 100.4 (taken rectally), they will have lab tests done to rule out infection. Occasionally, a baby will have an elevated body temperature (in the 100 to 100.3 range) if they are dehydrated. If your breastfed baby has lost close to 10% of their birth weight and their body temperature is rising, you may need to supplement with formula to avoid extensive testing for infection.

◆ *Jaundice:* See the next section in this chapter for details.

The 411 on Jaundice

Q. Why is my baby turning yellow? What is jaundice?

Here's the 411 on jaundice. While it sounds scary, there are two types of jaundice when it comes to newborns: NORMAL jaundice and ABNORMAL jaundice. Yes, you read it right—there is a form of jaundice that is NORMAL in newborns.

So what is jaundice? Short answer: it's body garbage that hasn't been eliminated yet. Long answer: humans make body garbage called bilirubin. Bilirubin breaks down in our livers and comes out in our poop. The problem: a newborn's liver is not working at full speed yet, nor are their intestines.

So, for most newborns, the body garbage (bilirubin) will start to collect in the skin. This is normal jaundice. Bilirubin has a yellow pigment, causing the whites of the eyes and skin to yellow. The level of yellow (jaundice) correlates with how far down the yellow gets on the body (increasing from head to toe.) The level will continue to rise until baby is eating and pooping regularly (day four to five). You will notice that the poop changes from black to a yellow/green/brown color at that time.

Again, by day four or five of life, bilirubin *normally* comes out in the poop and no longer collects in the skin. For **LATE PRETERM INFANTS** (born at 34 to 36 6/7 weeks gestation; see more on this in the "Preemie Primer" section later in this chapter), it is no longer an issue by day five to seven of life.

What about abnormal jaundice? See the following red flags.

RED FLAGS: Abnormal Jaundice.

These are signs for ABNORMAL jaundice (see the previous discussion of normal versus abnormal jaundice):

◆   Jaundice is seen in the first 24 hours of life
◆   Jaundice persists more than five days of life

◆   Level of jaundice descends below the belly button

Q. What happens if my baby has ABNORMAL jaundice?

In most cases of jaundice, doctors check bilirubin levels with a blood test on a daily basis until the level plateaus or drops, and the baby is eating and pooping well.

There is a graph based on gestational age and number of days old (called a *nomogram;* see below) that doctors use to predict how high the bilirubin level is likely to rise. So, for instance, your doc might be concerned about a full-term baby who has a bilirubin level of ten at two days of life, but not concerned at all if it is ten at five days of life. That's because on day two, that baby's bilirubin level is just beginning to rise. On day five, it's unlikely that the bilirubin will go anywhere but down as the baby's body metabolizes and eliminates it properly.

If the blood bilirubin level continues to rise and could potentially reach a point that might result in **BILIRUBIN-INDUCED NEUROLOGIC DYSFUNCTION (BIND)**, doctors intervene and help the baby break down the bilirubin until he is capable of doing it himself.

Some babies either have a delay in eliminating bilirubin, or produce higher levels than their bodies can eliminate effectively. Those reasons include: being a late-preterm infant, having a traumatic delivery (see **CEPHALHEMATOMA**), or having a blood type incompatibility with mom (see ABO incompatibility below). These babies are more likely to need help for a few days to get rid of the bilirubin.

Bottom line: Your baby may need their blood drawn every day to monitor their bilirubin level until the doctor gives the "all clear." If the level is significantly high, they may need treatment to bring it down.

Factoid: ABO Incompatibility: What is it? When mom and baby's blood types are different (mom is O and baby is A or B). Mom's blood can potentially mount a response that destroys some of baby's red blood cells. This leaves the baby with even more bilirubin to break down than your average newborn. If Mom's blood type is O, a blood test called a **COOMBS TEST** or a direct antiglobulin test (DAT) is done to see if mom mounted a response to her baby's

YELLOW BABY 411: JAUNDICE

Although most newborns turn a little bit yellow, pediatricians monitor all babies closely for a rare, but preventable form of brain damage (see **BILIRUBIN-INDUCED NEUROLOGIC DYSFUNCTION (BIND)** caused by excessive bilirubin levels. Levels of bilirubin (see **JAUNDICE**) start to rise just as babies go home from the hospital at 48 hours of life. The levels usually peak between 3-5 days of life. Breastfeeding can be a risk factor for jaundice if the baby is not feeding at least eight times a day or there is a delay in mother's milk coming in.

The American Academy of Pediatrics wants to improve identification of any babies at risk for brain damage. The AAP recommends that parents ROUTINELY schedule an appointment with their baby's medical provider at three to five days of life—even if that means an appointment on a weekend! And if your baby starts to look like a pumpkin, don't wait to call your doctor.

? ?

BIRTH DAY

blood. If the test is positive, the baby routinely gets a bilirubin level check at 24 hours of life since we know that baby is at risk to have abnormal jaundice.

Q. How is jaundice treated?

One or more of the following interventions are used to reduce the bilirubin load:

1. Supplementation with formula until Mom's milk comes in. Remember the more your baby eats, the more they will poop, and the more they will get rid of their bilirubin. If your mature milk isn't in yet, this is a justifiable health reason to supplement with formula.

2. Phototherapy. This technique uses blue light to breakdown the bilirubin. Babies either rest with a lighted blanket around them or under a bank of lights similar to a tanning booth. If your baby is jaundiced while at the hospital, either method may be used. If your baby needs treatment after you've been discharged home, you can rent a "bili blanket" or a "bili bed" from a home health agency or medical supply company.

What are the risks of phototherapy? The short-term risks are potential for dehydration and interference with parental bonding. The possible long-term risks include an increased risk of seizures, autism, and some childhood cancers. But the key word here is *possible*. For each concern, only one observational study suggested an association. No other studies have found similar results, which would obviously make the concerns more valid.

Bottom line: currently the risk of untreated jaundice is far greater than the theoretical risk of the treatment. *(Wickremasinghe), (WU), (Newman), Auger)*

3. Intravenous fluid. Dehydrated babies have more trouble with jaundice. In rare cases, a baby might need an IV to get fluid and nutrients.

Jaundice: which babies are at highest risk?

BIRTH DAY

? ?

BOTTOM LINE: If you are nursing, the first line of treatment is to supplement with expressed breast milk and formula. If your baby needs more aggressive intervention and you are already at home, a phototherapy blanket/bed can be rented temporarily. Your doctor will check bilirubin levels everyday and continue therapy until the levels drop significantly. Another warning: that drop could take a day or two or it could take up to a week! Be patient.

If the bilirubin level is extremely high, or it's not dropping enough with home phototherapy, or your baby is severely dehydrated, they may need to be readmitted to the hospital for additional treatment.

FYI: It is NOT recommended that you lay out poolside with your newborn, or place them by a sunny window to treat jaundice. It's not that effective and can overheat them. Yes, everyone will tell you to try this, but it's not a good idea.

Optional Procedures: Cord Blood Banking, Circumcision

These are decisions you'll want to make before your baby is born. So, we are hoping you read this chapter ahead of D-Day (Delivery Day). Why the rush on these decisions?

If you decide to privately store your baby's cord blood, you need to contact the cord blood bank *before* delivery so you have the supplies necessary for your obstetrician to collect the blood.

If you decide you want to have your son circumcised, you will want to find out if your obstetrician performs this procedure or if you need to make arrangements with a different healthcare provider. (And, if you are planning a ritual bris, it is good to have a mohel lined up to call once your baby is born.)

If neither of these situations applies to you, skip to the next section!

Cord Blood Banking

Q. What exactly is cord blood banking anyway?

The era of modern medicine has given us the opportunity to collect and store the blood and tissue from your baby's umbilical cord.

Why is this a cool idea? Well, that blood is loaded with the "seeds" (hematopoietic stem cells) that later grow into white and red blood cells. These very special cells are also found in the bone marrow of all humans.

As a result, the umbilical cord blood/tissue can be used like a bone marrow transplant. These cells are currently used to treat some genetic and blood disorders and certain types of cancer. One of the advantages of using a cord blood transplant as opposed to bone marrow transplant is that you don't have to have a perfect genetic match to the recipient and there may be less transplant rejection.

Q. Does cord blood contain "embryonic stem cells"?

No.

The cells in cord blood come from your baby's blood after birth, not from an embryo. The only similarity here is that both cord blood cells and embryonic cells are considered "stem" cells because they can develop into mature cells. Stem cells from cord blood are considered "hematopoietic" (blood) stem cells because they can become white and red blood cells and other specialized types of cells. To make things even more confusing, umbilical cord *tissue* contains "mesenchymal" stem cells that have the ability to grow into other cell types, raising the possibility of additional medical uses. The placenta is also rich in stem cells, which is why some private cord blood banks offer placental storage options.

Q. What can cord blood be used for?

Cord blood transplants are now used for several diseases, and there are more potential therapeutic uses in the pipeline.

Note: your baby may not be able to use their own stem cells for certain diseases, though. For example, if your baby ends up having leukemia, their frozen stem cells cannot be used to treat it. Those stem cells may already have pre-cancerous changes in them.

But here is the good news: your healthy baby's stem cells could be used for another family member (sibling, parent, etc.) who has a disease treatable with cord blood.

Q. Are there options for storing the cord blood?

Yes. There are basically two options for banking your baby's cord blood: private and public.

With a private, or "family" bank, you pay a company to store your baby's cord blood for potential personal use. If you bank your blood privately, only your family or loved ones who need it and are an acceptable match can use it.

Public banks are donation programs, where families contribute cord blood for use by the general public. If you donate cord blood to the public bank, anyone who needs it can use it. Every day, 6000 patients worldwide are looking for a match in the national donor registry to treat their leukemia, lymphoma, or other disease with a bone marrow or cord blood transplant.

A limited number of U.S. hospitals participate in the public cord donation program. But it is possible to collect the blood and have it shipped to a regional, centralized public banking facility. For more information go to the National Marrow Donor website at BeTheMatch.org.

If you want your baby's cord blood to go to the public donor program, you just need to pass some screening questions before the program accepts the donation. You should contact these folks before 34 weeks gestation if you want to donate. We'll discuss private cord blood banking next.

Insider Secret

If you have twins (or more) you cannot donate to the National Donor Program. The reason? With two or more umbilical cords, there is a potential to mix up the blood, making it too risky.

Q. Is it worth the money to privately store cord blood?

And you thought selecting a crib was a major decision…

Here's some information to help you decide if you want to open an account at the local blood bank:

What are the odds your or a family member will need to use the cord blood? The estimates vary from 1 in 400 to 1 in 200,000. (*AAP, Pasquini*) The odds are a bit of a moving target because no one can look into a crystal ball and predict the potential uses of umbilical cord blood in the future. If you already have a family member with a disease known to be treatable with cord blood, obviously the likelihood of ever needing it goes way up. (*AAP, Pasquini*)

DR B'S OPINION

"Don't let potentially life-saving cells go to waste. Donate them if possible."

The stem cells may have great potential to treat many diseases, but many of the treatments are experimental at this point. The chance you'll use it will depend on a variety of factors, like scientific advances and if the blood specimen is still viable when you are 70. At this moment, these potential uses are being tested in the research labs of academic medical centers and pharmaceutical companies. If your family has a genetic disorder, banking might be worth it for you.

Here are the costs: there is an initial enrollment fee ranging from about $1700 to $2200. Then there is a storage fee of $130 to $200 per year. Those fees are just for cord blood; there are additional fees to store umbilical cord and placenta tissue, both of which have promise to treat medical disorders in the future.

Some banks charge a one-time, lump sum fee to store the cord blood "forever." (With current technology, banks can freeze and utilize cord blood for at least 20 years.)

Reality Check

◆ Be sure to use a company that processes and stores cord blood in their own facility. Why does that matter? Because some companies subcontract the storage to another company.

◆ If a company you're interested in does other lab work besides cord blood banking, make sure their storage facilities are intended for long-term use. Special cryogenic techniques are required to make sure the blood is stored properly.

◆ Ask about the bank's storage method. Studies show that cord blood can be preserved and used for at least 20 years. Virtually all American cord blood banks store the blood in multi-compartmental bags to prevent contamination.

◆ Most obstetricians are experienced in cord blood collection. It is imperative that the blood be collected quickly (within ten minutes) and that enough blood is collected (at least 40 ml). Obviously, if you don't get enough cord blood, the specimen cannot be stored. Multiple births and low birth weight reduce the chance of getting enough blood. Most companies offer training resources for doctors. Obstetricians will charge a fee ($100 or more) to collect the cord blood even if it is for donation. Be sure to find out this cost in advance.

Q. If I want to privately bank my baby's cord blood, which company should I choose?

An excellent non-profit web site with advice on evaluating cord banks is ParentsGuideCord Blood.com. The site is run by an astrophysicist who lost her daughter to leukemia.

? ?

BIRTH DAY

Q. What happens to cord blood if it isn't saved or banked?

It clots in the umbilical cord and gets sent to the pathology lab with the placenta. Ultimately, it gets disposed of in a biohazard bag. If you don't authorize it to be publicly or privately banked, the blood is discarded.

Circumcision

Before we delve into this hot topic, we have a major disclaimer. Discussing circumcision is like a "friendly" discussion on abortion—this is a topic that provokes very strong reactions in some people. And like other parenting decisions, the pendulum swings back and forth.

We realize no matter how "fair and balanced" we are, some readers will NOT be happy (believe us, we've tried). Even a discussion of "pros and cons" of circumcision is considered blasphemy—anti-circumcision groups believe circumcision should not be an option at all. They also complain that the studies showing medical benefits of circumcision are flawed and biased.

Our goal for this section is to let parents hear both sides of the argument so you can make an informed decision on your own. Honestly, we don't have an agenda here (beyond providing a balanced look at the subject)—what you decide to do with your son's penis is your decision (or your son's).

Q. What is a circumcision anyway?

Circumcision is the surgical removal of the foreskin of the penis. It's been done as a religious ritual for centuries.

The practice of circumcision (surgical removal of foreskin) became common in the United States in the late 1800's for hygienic reasons as well as a proposed way to reduce masturbation (ha—didn't work, did it?). It has continued to be a popular choice for many American boys . . . and the subject of much controversy.

Q. When do I need to make this decision?

Before your son is born, you should decide whether or not you want a circumcision. That's because doctors typically perform the procedure before a baby goes home from the hospital, or within the first week or two of life in the doctor's office. When a circumcision is part of a Jewish religious ceremony (a "Brit milah" or "bris" for short), it is done at eight days of life.

Alternatively, you could wait and let them decide later in life, but it is a much bigger ordeal to go through circumcision as an adult. If you feel weird thinking about the future of your son's penis, join the club.

Q. What are the arguments FOR circumcision?

In a nutshell, lower risk of HIV, sexually transmitted infections, hygiene problems, and risk of cancer.

1. **Reduced risk of HIV.** Why? In uncircumcised men, the area under the foreskin makes a nice spot for the HIV virus to set up shop. A landmark study in South Africa found that circumcised men were 60% less likely to acquire HIV from infected female partners. (*Quinn*). (But, practically speaking, just using a condom with all sexual encounters would go a long way to reducing HIV risk.)

2. **Reduced risk of sexually transmitted infections.** Besides HIV, circumcised men are also 30-45% less likely to become infected with nasty little germs like genital herpes (HSV-2). (*Centers for Disease Control*) (Again, routine condom use alone would also lower the risk of sexually transmitted infections.)

3. **Better hygiene.** Compared with a circumcised penis, it can be more challenging to keep the uncircumcised penis clean. The foreskin can get infected and swell (see **BALANITIS**). Although balanitis doesn't occur often, it really hurts. The foreskin can also get stuck in a pulled back position (see **PARAPHIMOSIS**)—OUCH!

4. **Fewer bladder infections.** Bladder infections (see **URINARY TRACT INFECTION-UTI**) occur more frequently in girls. However, boys who are uncircumcised have a three to 12 times greater risk of infection than their circumcised friends. In general, uncircumcised boys have about a 1% risk of getting a bladder infection. Circumcised boys have a 0.1% risk. This risk is greatest in the first six months of life. This again is due to hygiene reasons.

5. **Less risk of cancer.** Again, the foreskin of an uncircumcised penis can harbor germs. When it comes to cancer risk, the issue here is a virus called **HUMAN PAPILLOMAVIRUS—HPV.** HPV infection can lead to cancer of the penis, anus, throat, and cervix. (Note: oral, vaginal, and anal intercourse allows HPV virus to spread to these areas.) Circumcised men have a 30% lower risk of being infected with cancer-causing strains of HPV. They have a lower risk of developing cancer of the penis, and their female partners may have a lower risk of developing cervical cancer. (*Centers for Disease Control*).

Reality Check

Since the HPV vaccine is recommended for both young women and men, your daughters and sons can reduce their risk of HPV-related cancer by being vaccinated—making that last argument for circumcision less relevant.

Q. What are the arguments AGAINST circumcision?

Like any surgical procedure, circumcision has risks:

1. **The risk of surgery.** Circumcision involves cutting the foreskin away from the head of the penis. As with any surgical procedure, there is a small chance of bleeding (1 in 3000 risk) or infection (1 in 1000 risk).

2. **Penile adhesions.** Occasionally, the skin between the shaft and the head of the penis will get stuck together due to a collection of sticky, cream cheesy stuff called smegma. The penis will look like it is uncircumcised. Minor adhesions will resolve on their own. But if the adhesions are really tight, they may need to be treated by using steroid cream, having a doctor pull the skin back, or having another surgical procedure ("circumcision revision"). For more details, see Chapter 4, Hygiene, and **PENILE ADHESIONS**).

3. **The hidden penis.** It sounds like a concealed weapon, doesn't it? Chubby baby boys have a fat roll above their genitals. It causes the circumcised penis to get sucked inwards. The penis looks normal as the boys grow up, but it's always concerning to parents.

4. **Reduced sexual pleasure.** Some concerns have been raised about the removal of sensitive nerve fibers in the foreskin when a male is circumcised. Anti-circumcision groups contend that circumcision is genital mutilation. So what's the latest science on this subject? Studies that address this question report conflicting results. Some studies show a decrease in sexual pleasure; others show heightened sensitivity and orgasm after circumcision. The data is based on men who were circumcised as adults who subjectively rated their sexual pleasure before and after circumcision. (*Collins, Masood, Kim*)

Q. What do the experts say about circumcision?

What's the right thing to do? Let's see how the experts weigh in.

None of the major medical organizations have updated or modified their position on circumcision in the past decade. The American Academy of Pediatrics, American Urological Association, and the Centers for Disease Control feel the procedure should be presented as an option to families so that parents, teenage boys, and men can make an informed choice. In short, healthcare providers should explain the risks and benefits…like we just did here.

Ultimately, *you* have to make the call.

Q. Who performs the circumcision?

Most often, your obstetrician performs the circumcision procedure just before your baby leaves the hospital. But family practitioners or pediatricians may also do it. As long as the person has been trained to do the procedure, it does not matter what the doctor's specialty is.

Why the obstetrician? Many pediatricians, like me, do not perform any surgical procedures—for good reason. You wouldn't want to see the way I slice my Thanksgiving turkey! Obstetricians have surgical training and are already at the hospital taking care of Mommy. Ask your OB first what the usual protocol is. Urologists can also perform a circumcision on your baby. This requires special arrangements, however. Urologists do not generally come to the hospital to perform routine circumcisions. You'll need to do some homework if you choose this option.

What if you decide to circumcise your son after you leave the hospital? That's fine, but there is one caveat: some insurance providers will NOT cover the cost of the procedure once baby goes home.

Circumcision is performed as a religious ritual for some families. The person performing the procedure is called a mohel. Families pay out of pocket for this service.

Q. Is any pain medication used during the circumcision?

Most of the time, yes. Every doctor has their own approach. You can ask your doctor what they feel comfortable doing. Here are the options:

1. Injecting numbing medicine directly into the area (nerve block).
2. Applying topical numbing cream one hour before the procedure.
3. Giving the baby sugar water just prior to the procedure.

Q. How do I care for the area once the procedure is done?

You will need two things to make a dressing for the wound: gauze pads (2"x2" or preferably 3"x3") and a big tube of petroleum jelly (Vaseline).

The goal: keep the scab on the wound from sticking to a diaper and pulling off with each diaper change (that sounds excruciating and we don't even have male parts!). And one cautionary note: the yellowish stuff stuck to the penis is the scab, NOT pus. Do not try to brush or scrub it off!

At all poopy diaper changes and whenever else the need arises, remove the dressing and gently clean the penis with gauze soaked in warm water. Because urine is sterile, you don't have to change the dressing just for a wet diaper. Once the penis is completely healed, you can use diaper wipes.

Put a big glob of petroleum jelly in the center of the gauze pad and place it over the penis. Fold the gauze in half over the penis so it looks like an envelope. You will "seal" the ends of the gauze with all that petroleum jelly squishing out. Voila.

Continue to apply a dressing until the skin of the penis is covered with new skin. That's usually three to five days after the procedure.

If your doctor used a "plastibell" for the procedure, the plastic ring falls off around one week later.

DR B'S OPINION:
CIRCUMCISION

While there are some medical benefits to circumcision, the benefits are not clear enough for every medical group to advocate for the procedure. If everyone engaged in safe sexual behavior, there would be fewer sexually transmitted infections, including HIV. I think it is a very personal decision, without a right or wrong answer. And while it is hard to assess how circumcision affects sexual pleasure, I don't think either group of men is complaining.

Once the penis is completely healed (usually seven to 14 days later), make sure you can always see the head (glans) of the penis distinctly from the shaft. It should look like a helmet with a rim. Pull back at the base of the penis at your son's diaper changes so you can specifically clean that area. If you don't, your son will end up with a circumcised penis that develops adhesions and looks somewhere between circumcised and uncircumcised. Avoid this, obviously!

We realize this care sounds a bit daunting, if you are a first-time parent. Ask your baby's doc for more advice or if you need help.

Check out Chapter 4, Hygiene, for more details on circumcision care after the initial healing is over.

Red Flags: Circumcision Complications

◆ Excessive bleeding.
◆ Pus draining from circumcision site.
◆ Fever of 100.4 F or above.
◆ Extreme lethargy more than four hours after procedure

Bottom Line

The whole procedure is relatively brief. Yes, it hurts—but pain medication minimizes most of the discomfort. Most babies will go to sleep afterwards as a stress response and wake up happy to see you.

The Baby 411 Two-Week Survival Guide
a.k.a. What Do I do NOW?

Okay, now you are ready to take your baby home. Without the luxury of the nursery nurses right down the hall, you are probably scared to death.

Hopefully, this book will be helpful in answering all those questions you have. But remember, your pediatrician or family practitioner is only a phone call away. We've covered the basics in this section, but each chapter in this book has information pertinent to newborns. We'll refer you to those sections for more details.

Q. When will I need to use a car seat?

Every time you take your baby with you in the car! This includes your trip home from the hospital. It's the law, folks. Here's what you need to know:

◆ All 50 states require that infants under one year of age be restrained in an approved car seat. Laws vary from state to state beyond a year of age. However, the American Academy of Pediatrics advises that children be in a safety restraint (convertible car seat and then a booster seat) until they are 4'9" tall.
◆ Infants should ride rear-facing until they are at least two years of age, as long as they do not exceed the seat's height and weight limits.

- Kids under age 13 should be in the back seat of your vehicle. Front air bags deploy right at the level of a child's head, which can be fatal.

- So what do you need to buy now? Newborns can sit in either an infant car seat (birth to 30+ pounds) or a convertible car seat (birth to 40 or 65 pounds). To save money, you can conceivably use only a convertible car seat from birth. But most parents choose the more expensive option of getting the infant car seat (knowing they'll have to get the convertible car seat after their baby outgrows the infant seat) because it's more portable. When your baby falls asleep in the car, you'll find it's worth the investment.

- Practice using the car seat *before* game day so you don't feel foolish. In fact, the hospital staff will only let you take your baby home by car in a properly installed car seat (and no, they will not install it for you!) You may need an engineering degree to figure out how your particular car seat works, especially if you bought a fancy Swedish one. Our advice: get your seat safety-checked BEFORE the baby is born to make sure it is correctly installed.

- Where to get help: The National Highway Transportation Safety Administration is the government entity that regulates car seat restraints. Check out their extremely helpful website at NHTSA.gov/equipment/car-seats-and-booster-seats. There, you can determine which car seat your baby needs, watch videos on proper installation, and even find a car seat inspector nearest your home.

- Car seat test: hospitals test premature and small babies in their car seats to be sure they can breathe properly while restrained. Ask your healthcare provider about this simple test if your baby is born before 37 weeks or weighs under six pounds.

Insider Secret

Shopping for a car seat can be pretty overwhelming. Check out our sister book/website Baby Bargains (babybargains.com) for recommendations of infant car seats.

BOTTOM LINE

According to researchers at Oregon Health and Science University, newborns are at risk from poor car seat installation. They found 84% of new parents make at least one critical safety error when installing the car seat or securing their newborn in it. Most often, parents install the car seat too loosely, install it at an improper angle, or forget to lock the seat belt. And up to 70% of parents do not adjust the harness tightly enough to keep their baby secure. Take the time to properly install your child's car seat. Get help from experts if you need it. *(Hoffman B)*

Q. When can I take my baby outside?

It is perfectly fine to go outside with your baby at any age. Dress them in the same layers you would wear.

However, I recommend avoiding crowded restaurants, grocery stores, and airplanes until your baby is four weeks old (if possible). This minimizes exposure to COVID-19, as well as common cold and flu viruses that are spread from respiratory droplets (coughs and sneezes). For details, see Chapter 13, "Common Infections."

Next: our detailed two-week survival guide. We've divided this advice into five areas: breathing, feeding, elimination, sleep and skin. Let's go:

1 BREATHING. As adults, we breathe about 12 times per minute at an even rate. As we discussed earlier in this chapter, newborns breathe 30 to 40 times per minute and have episodes of *periodic breathing*. This means that your baby may breathe rapidly several times, p-a-u-s-e, then breathe again. This pause can last several seconds (less than ten seconds). This is normal, but is bound to freak you out.

Nasal congestion is normal in the first several weeks of life. Use saline nose drops to flush the secretions.

RED FLAGS: Breathing
◆ When a pause between breaths lasts 15 to 20 seconds.
◆ If your baby is panting, or breathing over 50 to 60 times per minute.
◆ If your baby's rib cage sucks in (*retractions*), nostrils flare, or they make grunting noises.

OLD WIVES TALE
My baby will catch pneumonia if they get cold.
Pneumonia is an infectious disease. It does not infect people who are cold; pneumonia infects people who *have* a cold. Here are two more old wives tales:

◆ *Baby will catch pneumonia if they are out in cold weather.* FALSE!
◆ *Baby will get an ear infection if the wind blows in their ears.* FALSE! Wind blows into the outer ear canal. Ear infections are due to pus behind the eardrum, where the wind cannot reach anyway.

Q. My baby has a snotty nose. What can I do about it?

All newborns have nasal congestion for four to six weeks after birth. It's not a cold. And it's not an allergy to your cat.

Some congested babies are extraordinarily loud. They may snort, snore, cough, and sneeze. That's all normal. If the congestion interferes with feedings or sleep, use saline nose drops to clear the mucous.

Saline is just salt water (1/2 tsp salt to 8 oz. water). You can make it or buy it. It is impossible to overdose and can be used any time your baby has thick mucous or congestion. Shoot several drops in each nostril before feedings. *You do NOT need to suck it out with a bulb syringe or a Nose Frida "Snot Sucker"* (yes, this is a real product).

The saline will either make your baby sneeze or loosen the mucous enough for the baby to swallow it.

BOTTOM LINE
Leave the bulb syringe at the hospital!
Bulb syringes can irritate a baby's nostrils to the point of nosebleeds. And if you don't evacuate the air in the bulb before sucking out the snot, you may get some

unpleasant results. One family I know tried this…the baby was shocked and held its breath. The parents were shocked and called 911. Saline drops are a more effective and less traumatic way to deal with baby snot.

2 **FEEDING.** Whether you breast or bottle-feed, your newborn will be very sleepy for the first few days. The result? They may fall asleep during a feeding, sometimes after only a few minutes. Encourage your baby to stay awake by rubbing their head, playing with their feet, or unwrapping and placing them away from your warm body. If breastfeeding, you can try compressing your breast during a feeding to spurt some milk into their mouth—which often encourages them to wake up and have a drink.

How often does a newborn eat?

◆ A breast-fed baby usually eats every two to three hours (at least eight times in 24 hours).

◆ A formula-fed baby eats about two to three ounces every three to four hours (six to eight times in 24 hours).

Either way, your baby should wake up spontaneously and eat frequently. In the first two weeks of life, *do not let your newborn go more than FOUR hours without eating*. You need to wake baby up to feed them if this occurs. (Note: after two weeks of age, if your baby wants to sleep longer *at night* and is gaining weight appropriately—let them!)

Mom's mature breast milk usually arrives on the baby's third to fourth day of life. Until then, the baby gets antibody rich (but lower in calorie and volume) colostrum when they nurse. This is all your baby needs right now.

Spitting up some milk is normal. It can look fresh or curdled. Both are normal. Vomiting up large volumes at every feeding is not normal.

RED FLAGS: Feeding

◆ You consistently have to awaken your baby to eat.

◆ Your baby is consistently vomiting large volumes of milk (i.e. the whole feeding)

◆ If nursing, your milk has not come in after three or four days.

Insider Tip: Vitamin D

Your baby will need to take a daily Vitamin D supplement regardless of whether they are breast milk or formula fed. It's not urgent, so you don't need to order it on Amazon right this second! But, your pediatrician will recommend it at one of your first office visits. See Chapter 5, "Nutrition", for a full discussion on vitamin supplements.

Q. Can I put my newborn on a feeding schedule?

Nope. You need to let go of being in charge for a little while.

Newborns are learning how life works outside the womb. Before birth, they had a 24/7 all-you-can-eat buffet coming through the umbilical cord. Now your newborn feels hungry (and will tell you about it) when their body needs energy. They will eat better when is they are hungry than when you decide it is time for them to eat. That is why experts advise feeding on demand.

Newborns need to eat about eight to 12 times in a 24-hour day. This may be every 1 1/2 hours for a few cycles, then four hours later, then two hours, etc. Most babies manage to eat at least eight feedings a day—without any prodding from their parents. Obviously everyone would like their baby to have "cluster feeding" of every 1 1/2 hours during the day and a nice four hour stretch at night. But trying to control the feeding behavior of a newborn will backfire. Trust us, let it go for now. And sleep when you can.

For more information on this topic, check out Chapter 5, Nutrition and Growth, Chapter 6, Liquids and Chapter 8, The Other End. See the end of this section for a handy guide to keep track of feedings.

Q. My baby has the hiccups all the time. Is this a problem?

Nope, not a problem.

Hiccups are result of the diaphragm muscle under the rib cage that is spasming. Newborns have very immature nervous systems and often hiccup when they are overstimulated. It doesn't take

NEW PARENT 411: GERM-O-PHOBIA

Many new parents have a mortal fear of germs, especially after enduring a pandemic. And we can understand that. As a doctor, I recommend your newborn avoids crowd scenes and social gatherings for the first four weeks of life (or longer, depending on surges in COVID-19 cases in your community). Why? If your baby catches a bug and develops a fever of 100.4 or more during the first 28 days of life, they must be admitted to a hospital and endure lots of unpleasant tests. Yes, even if it is just a cold.

Of course, that doesn't mean you must live in fear and never have contact with the outside world! Here is a Q&A with some practical suggestions to limit your newborn's exposure to germs.

◆ *Can your newborn go for a stroll around the neighborhood?* Yes.
◆ *Can a few family members and friends come over to your house and hold the newborn?* Yes. But require them to wash hands first and not visit if they are sick. And in our pandemic era, you may also ask them to wear a mask and make sure their vaccinations for COVID-19, flu, and whooping cough are up-to-date. (You can always say your baby's pediatrician made this request!)
◆ *Can you hold your newborn if you are sick?* Yes, but wash hands wear a mask if you have a respiratory infection like COVID-19 or a common cold virus. If your spouse can take over the baby chores, go for it. Yes, you can and should continue breastfeeding.
◆ *Can your newborn be around other children?* Yes, as long as they are not sick. You can have a rule that the children can touch baby's head or feet, but not their hands or mouth. It is absolutely appropriate to ask that children wear masks and ensure their vaccinations are up-to-date before visiting. Again, you can blame your crazy pediatrician! We really don't mind.

much to overstimulate a baby. They are eating and then they're not. They are sleeping and then wake up. Just give them some snuggles and walk around for a bit and the hiccups will go away.

3 **ELIMINATION**. Your newborn's body is just learning how things work initially. In the first 24 hours of life, they may pee (urinate) and poop (stool) only once. When they really begin to take food in, things should start to come out. This is a good way to tell if your infant is eating enough, particularly if you are nursing. Your hospital may give you a diary to keep track of intake and output. Or, use an app (like Glow Baby) on your smartphone to tally those feedings and diapers.

Urine: By the fourth day of life, your baby should pee at least four times a day. By one week of age, six to 12 wet diapers a day is normal.

Stool: The first few poops are called **MECONIUM** and are black and *tarry* looking. The poop will change to a dark green color on Day of life 2-3, and then a yellow, seedy, watery texture (if breastfed) or a lighter green and pasty texture (if formula fed) on Day of life 3-5.

RED FLAGS: Elimination

◆ Your baby is not urinating at least every six hours by the fourth day of life.
◆ Your baby's poop looks red, mucousy, or does not change from the black meconium.
◆ Your baby's poop looks like yours.

For more information, check out Chapter 8, The Other End as well as our website at Baby411.com for pictures!

4 **SLEEP.** Your baby sleeps 17 to 20 hours a day, but rarely more than four to five hours at a time. They may be very hard to console initially and force you to walk with them or rock them to sleep. *You can't spoil a newborn.* Do what it takes to get them to sleep. Bad habits happen AFTER two months of age.

Yes, you can swaddle your newborn with a light receiving blanket (see details on the "baby burrito wrap" in Chapter 9, Sleep). Just be sure to wrap the legs loosely so your baby can move their hips around.

RED FLAGS: Sleep

◆ Your baby consistently needs to be awakened to eat.
◆ Your baby is completely inconsolable for over three hours straight. *For more information, check out Chapter 9, Sleep.*

NEW PARENT 411: THE NEWBORN HOLD

If you have never held a newborn, keep reading. Newborns have poor control of their neck muscles, and thus, cannot hold their relatively large heads up. If possible, hold your newborn with two hands, one supporting the body, and one supporting the head. If you don't have two free hands, cradle their head in the crook of your arm (kind of like a football). With a little practice, you'll be an old pro in no time.

5 **SKIN.** Your newborn may have a few bruises from delivery that will fade with time. They may also have a few rashes—also normal.

◆ *Jaundice*, is often normal, but is something that should be followed. Your baby's liver is just starting its job of breaking down a body waste called bilirubin. Until this happens, the skin on the face may be a little yellow as a result of the bilirubin's pigment. That's okay. What is NOT normal: if you see this in the first 24 hours of life, or if the yellow color descends below your baby's waistline.

◆ *The umbilical cord* takes one to four weeks to fall off. Until then, the stump is gooey. This is normal. If the skin around the cord is getting infected (see **OMPHALITIS**), the area is red, tender, and foul smelling.

RED FLAGS: Skin

◆ Jaundice occurs in the first 24 hours of life or below the waistline once you get home.

◆ Redness of the skin around the umbilical cord, or pus draining from it. *See Chapter 4, Hygiene and the glossary for more information.*

6 **FEVERS.** We'll discuss fevers in-depth in Chapter 15, First Aid. For now, read the red flags below for the basics.

RED FLAGS: Fever

From birth to three months of age, *any* fever can be a sign of a serious infection. You need to call your doctor immediately if your baby has a temperature greater than 100.3 F taken *rectally*. (See the section how to take a rectal temp in Chapter 15, "First Aid").

Ear thermometers tend to be unreliable and since a fever in an infant is so concerning, these are not recommended for use. Fever medications should not be used for infants under three months of age unless recommended by your doctor (for example, when your baby is vaccinated).

NEW PARENT 411: DR. BROWN'S STOOL RULES

1. Once your baby starts to eat, their poop will change colors and texture.
2. Breastfed babies often have yellow, watery, seedy poop. Seeing this color and texture of poop reassures you that your baby is eating mature breast milk.
3. Formula fed babies often have green, pasty strained-peas or pesto poop.
4. Any shade of yellow, green, or brown is normal.
5. Stool frequency can vary from once every feeding to once a week. The frequency is not an indication of constipation—the texture is. However, in the first two weeks, frequency of stool is a reassuring sign that your baby is getting enough to eat.
6. All babies (not just yours!) turn red and grunt when they poop.

Q. My mother/mother-in-law will be helping me for the first couple of weeks at home. Do you have any suggestions to keep my sanity?

Some people get along with their parents and in-laws better than others. But even if you have a terrific relationship, a newborn makes things more stressful. New moms are sleep deprived, healing from childbirth, and off-the-charts hormonally. Throw in a well-meaning grandmother who wants to share their sage advice—which often is interpreted as criticism—and it takes you over the edge.

So, before the fireworks start, think about *how* you and your mother (or mother-in-law) will spend time together. A few suggestions:

NEW PARTNER 411: 4 TIPS

Hello partners and spouses! Yes, we know you read baby books too—so let's go over a few specific tips to help out in those first days.

1. BYOW. That is, Bring Your Own Wipes. Surprise! You will be doing most of the diaper changes at the hospital—especially if your partner had a C-section. But as we discussed earlier, those first poops will not be pretty (meconium, that black, tar-like stuff). Now, the hospital will probably give you gauze pads and water for this task . . . and that frankly won't be up to the job. Our advice: bring in your own baby wipes. If for some reason your baby's skin is super sensitive, you can go back to the gauze if necessary.

2. Pay attention to the lactation consultant (LC). If your partner is breastfeeding, you will need to watch how the baby latches on to the breast (that's where a LC works their magic). After the LC departs, you may need to help position the baby's mouth on mom's nipple (it sometimes takes four hands to maneuver this in the early days). *You* will be the lactation consultant at home, so take notes!

3. Sleep when you can. The first few days of your baby's life is so exciting. Well-wishers are calling and visiting you throughout the day. Guess what—that's when your baby is sleeping! You will then be up all night with the little rugrat. So, take advantage of daylight hours to catch a nap and encourage your partner to do the same. Turn off all electronic devices for the duration of the nap!

4. Smile, nod and be supportive. Your partner will be on a hormonal roller coaster after delivery. That will equate to laughter one moment and tears another. Be on the lookout for something above and beyond normal emotions. (See the discussion on baby blues and postpartum depression on the next page.)

? ?

BIRTH DAY

◆ *Baby chores.* If you are breastfeeding, put grandma in charge of everything else baby: diaper changes, rocking, bathing. It will be her pleasure.

◆ *Household chores.* Don't be a control freak. Let her cook, clean, or even run a few errands.

◆ *Ask for advice on small matters.* "How did you swaddle your babies?" It will make them feel important—and that their opinion is valued.

◆ *Avoid conflict.* If you run into conflicting parenting approaches, feel free to quote your pediatrician's advice (feel free to blame any controversial decision on your baby's doc).

Nearby is a useful chart to help you track your newborn's pee and poop for the first seven days. After day eight, you can probably stop this tracking madness if your baby is eating, pooping, and peeing numerous times daily. Of course, there are also iPhone and Android apps that do this as well!

2 week survival guide

BABY BLUES

Here is a newsflash for you...your life will never be the same. I know, everyone has told you this during your entire pregnancy. But by now reality has hit you like a sledge-hammer. Becoming a parent is the most amazing experience of your life—so why are you crying right now?!!

Let's see. Your physical body feels like it was run over by a truck. Your hormone levels are off the charts. You haven't had a good night's sleep since the baby was born. You understand why sleep deprivation is used as a form of torture in POW camps. You find it difficult to make rational decisions, or any decisions for that matter.

Here's another newsflash for you . . . you are normal. No matter how wonderful it is to become a parent, it takes time for your body and mind to adjust to it.

 ### RED FLAGS: When Mom has Postpartum Depression

The Baby Blues are short-term feelings of sadness that subside after a few much needed breaks provided by supportive family and friends. Postpartum depression doesn't go away that easily. Here are the clues that professional help is needed:

1. Frequent episodes of crying or weepiness.
2. Lack of enthusiasm for living (big clue: Mom doesn't smile anymore).
3. Lack of interest in the family or the baby.
4. Loss of appetite.
5. Difficulty sleeping. (This is a big clue since new moms sleep whenever they can!)

Mothers who experience postpartum depression often don't recognize the clues. If a family member expresses concerns about you, be smart and let them get you some help!

BIRTH DAY

? ?

Handy Feeding & Elimination Table: The First 7 Days

Instructions: Circle the hour your baby nurses.
Circle W for wet diaper (urine). Circle S for soiled diaper (poop).

Day 1
Goal 6-8 feedings
Diapers: 1 wet, 1 soiled

12am 1 2 3 4 5 6 7 8 9 10 11 12pm 1 2 3 4 5 6 7 8 9 10 11

W   S   (black, tarry)

Day 2
Goal 8-12 feedings
2 wet   2 soiled

12m 1a 2 3 4 5 6 7 8 9 10 11 12pm 1 2 3 4 5 6 7 8 9 10 11

W W   S S   (black/brown)

Day 3
Goal 8-12 feedings
2 wet   2 soiled

12m 1a 2 3 4 5 6 7 8 9 10 11 12pm 1 2 3 4 5 6 7 8 9 10 11

W W   S S   (green, yellow)

Day 4
Goal 8-12 feedings
4 wet   3 soiled

12m 1a 2 3 4 5 6 7 8 9 10 11 12pm 1 2 3 4 5 6 7 8 9 10 11

W W W W   S S S (yellow)

Day 5
Goal 8-12 feedings
5 wet   3 soiled

12m 1a 2 3 4 5 6 7 8 9 10 11 12pm 1 2 3 4 5 6 7 8 9 10 11

W W W W W   S S S (yellow)

Day 6
Goal 8-12 feedings
6 wet   4 soiled

12m 1a 2 3 4 5 6 7 8 9 10 11 12pm 1 2 3 4 5 6 7 8 9 10 11

W W W W W W   S S S S

BIRTH DAY

Day 7

Goal 8-12 feedings
6 wet   4 soiled

Special Situations: Preterm Babies

Premature babies (before 37 weeks gestation) make up 12.5% of all babies born in the United States each year. (*Hovert*) While this is certainly not in the master plan for any pregnancy, it could become reality with little notice.

Instead of that special bonding time with your newborn post-delivery, your baby may be whisked away to a neonatal intensive care unit (NICU). Scary? Yep. What a way to be initiated as a new parent! Keep your chin up—most parents graduate from the NICU with healthy babies . . . it just may take a while.

Key point: Babies born between 34 weeks and 36 6/7 weeks are considered premature. They are called **LATE PRETERM INFANTS (LPI).** In fact, late-preterm infants make up 70% of all preemies. These little peanuts account for most of the surge in preterm deliveries in the past decade. Although they don't have many of the major medical complications that more pre-mature babies do, they still need to be treated with more care than their full-term friends. Here's some more advice on LPI's.

Q. My baby is a late preterm infant. Is there anything special I need to look out for?

Yes. Just like babies are not little adults, late preterm infants are not little versions of full-term babies. Your baby is immature. Here is a list of their unique issues:

◆ **Neurologic:** About one-third of a baby's brain volume grows in the last eight weeks of gestation, so it's no surprise that your newborn will be neurologically immature. What does that really mean? Well, they'll probably be very sleepy and need to be awakened for feedings. They may have a poor ability to suck, which can make feedings (especially breastfeeding) a real challenge. They may be cranky, startle or get over-stimulated easily, and have difficulty being soothed (don't get too discouraged). They may also not be great at regulating their body temperature yet (in addition to having very little body fat to retain heat). All of these things resolve, they just take a little time until your baby's brain and body matures.

And because long-term studies show that late preterm infants are at risk for mild learning disabilities in the school years, you should watch your little one extra carefully for developmental delays.

◆ **Respiratory**: Your baby is being born just about the time their lungs are fully mature. If you baby is on the younger end of the spectrum of LPI's (34-35 weeks), it's still possible that they will have respiratory distress and need temporary breathing support because of immature lungs. Due to neurologic immaturity, your baby is also at risk for forgetting to breathe (also known as **APNEA OF PREMATURITY** or AOP). Obviously, your baby won't be allowed to go home from the hospital until they remember to breathe! You also need to take extra care when hold ing your newborn upright, as they have very poor head control and can collapse their airway.

◆ **Infectious Diseases:** Being born early is considered a risk factor for newborn blood-stream infection (sepsis). So although the chance of this is very small, your baby may have lab work and tests to rule it out.

◆ **Gastrointestinal:** Your baby will be a pokey eater (more on that below) and as such, they also won't be pooping very much. That, and an immature liver, make your baby more at risk of developing jaundice than their full-term peers. And while term newborns may encounter jaundice for the first four to five days of life, late preterm infants may have jaundice issues for the first five to seven days.

◆ **Growth/Nutrition:** This is a major issue with late preterm infants. They are notoriously difficult feeders. They are sleepy. They don't wake up on their own for feedings. They tire easily and fall asleep feeding. And their sucking ability, to put it bluntly, sucks. So your baby is at risk for excessive weight loss or poor weight gain—both of which can lead to dehydration. To complicate matters even further, your baby is also at risk for low blood sugar in the first 24

FEEDBACK FROM THE REAL WORLD: TWINS!

Meet Agustina, mom of twins, who'll give you some great real world tips throughout this book:

"When my twins, Malena and Gael, were born, I wanted everything to be perfect. It is natural for expectant moms to over-prepare (i.e., overspend) to meet the challenges and demands of raising infant twins. Hopefully some of my tips and strategies, which I learned from experience, will save you time and money.

Tired, dazed and confused summarizes my first six months of motherhood with twins. Call on family and friends for support, or hire a night nanny—well worth the money if it is within your means.

My head was spinning between pumping milk, feeding babies, changing diapers and cleaning all the equipment every two or three hours. Once the cycle was complete, it was time to go at it again. I found feeding logs from the hospital very helpful to keep track of feeding times and amounts, diaper changes and medicines.

One of our twins was born with a congenital heart defect while the other one was born at a low birth weight, so keeping track of their calorie consumption and medicine was very important. With little sleep, it was hard for me to see through the fog. At times I couldn't remember whose diaper I had changed or who I had fed! The log sheet was also a great way of communicating with my night nanny. At one glance, I could see a quick overview of the night.

The log sheet also helped me understand my twins' natural tendencies of awake/sleep time and the amount of calories consumed during the day. I came to realize that their calorie consumption during the day was a good predictor of how the night would go. The logs were a systematic and organized way of keeping track and also proved pivotal in putting them on a schedule."

hours of life—which would prevent just about anyone from having the energy to eat. Don't worry—we have lots of tips below to help with all these problems.

So, here are some top tips to navigate your baby's special challenges. More feeding tips are covered in the breastfeeding section in Chapter 6:

◆ **Temperature regulation:** Swaddle your baby with two or three receiving blankets and have them wear a hat for those first days after birth.

◆ **Feedings:** Aim for eight feedings a day. Wake your baby up if they don't wake on their own. Maximum feeding time should be 40 minutes because your baby will tire easily. If you are breastfeeding, use a nipple shield if your baby has a poor latch and be sure to get some help from a certified lactation consultant. (See more details on this in the breastfeeding section in Chapter 6, Liquids). Don't be discouraged. Your baby may also temporarily need sugar gel or formula supplements if their blood sugar is low.

◆ **Late discharge:** Your baby is not ready for primetime. Don't head out the door for home until they are ready to go. That means 48 hours in the hospital at the very least! Here are the criteria established by the American Academy of Pediatrics for Late Preterm Infant discharge: stable vital signs (body temperature, blood pressure, heart rate, and respiratory rate) for at least twelve hours before discharge, 24 hours of successful feedings with coordinated sucking/swallowing/breathing, formal breastfeeding assessment by a trained caregiver, at least one spontaneous poop, dehydration assessment if baby loses over 3% of their birth weight per day or more than 7% during hospitalization, jaundice assessment, and a plan for follow up with pediatrician in 24 to 48 hours. (*AAP Clinical Report*)

◆ **Car seat test:** Your baby should have a formal car seat test done by the hospital staff before you go home (see details in this chapter). But here are some specific tips: Your car seat should have a weight limit of less than five pounds. It should have a five-point harness, with multiple shoulder slots with the lowest slot less than ten inches from the seat bottom, and multiple crotch slots with the closest slot less than 5.5 inches from the seat back.

◆ **Jaundice:** Remember that your baby's peak jaundice issues will occur between five to seven days of life. If your baby looks yellow at home, take them back to your baby's doctor to check it out.

◆ **Watch development:** While your baby does not necessarily need a special evaluation with a developmental specialist, keep your eyes out for any delays in developmental milestones and mention them to your baby's doc. Be sure to give your baby lots of tummy time when they are awake. With a floppy head and increased sleep needs, they are more at risk for developing a flat head. (*AAP*)

Q. My baby was born before 34 weeks. What should I be prepared for?

Well, that really is a book in and of itself. But the basic concept is this: your baby needs to mature outside the womb and will not go home until they are ready to face the world. Discharge Day usually equates to near or at their actual due date. Hopefully, that path to maturity goes smoothly, but there can be some unpredictable bumps along the road.

While we don't have enough room in this book to go over all the medical issues you may face with a premature baby, there are two books we'd recommend for further reading: *Preemies: The Essential Guide for Parents of Premature Babies*, by Dana Linden and *The Preemie Primer*, by Dr. Jennifer Gunter.

Once you are ready to head home with your preemie graduate, here are some key issues. You'll also find more preemie advice scattered throughout the rest of this book. (*Sturgeon*)

Neurologic/Developmental
Intraventricular hemorrhage

If your baby was born before 32 weeks gestation or less than three pounds, they've probably had at least one ultrasound to rule out bleeding in the brain (**INTRAVENTRICULAR HEMORRHAGE** or **IVH**). If an abnormality was detected, you will need to follow up with a pediatric neurologist.

Eye exams

If your baby was born before 32 weeks gestation or weighed less than three pounds, a pediatric ophthalmologist has already done an initial consultation exam at the hospital, looking for immaturity of the eyes (**RETINOPATHY OF PREMATURITY OR ROP**). Premature babies are also at risk for **AMBLYOPIA, STRABISMUS**, and **REFRACTIVE ERRORS** (see Chapter 14, "Diseases" in the eye section for details). Your baby will need to have their vision checked periodically by the eye doctor once you go home.

Hearing tests

A routine hearing screen is done on all newborns. Babies who are born prematurely have a ten to 20 times greater risk of hearing loss than full term babies. If an abnormality is detected or concerns arise later, you should follow up with an ear, nose, and throat specialist and an audiologist.

Developmental assessment and therapy

Babies who are born prematurely are developmentally delayed compared to their peers who are the same age. To know where your child's milestones should be tracking, subtract the number of months missed in pregnancy from the baby's current age to determine the "adjusted age." For example, your four-month-old baby who was born two months early will be expected to have the milestones of a two-month-old. Preemies should catch up on their milestones by two years of age. However, very low birth weight babies (under three pounds), are at risk for the following delays: communication (including autism), large and small muscle group, and learning. All premature babies should be assessed by developmental assessment program (often referred to as "Early Childhood Intervention") in your community.

Respiratory
Apnea of prematurity

If your baby has trouble remembering to breathe (**APNEA OF PREMATURITY OR AOP**), your doctor may prescribe medication (caffeine) and a breathing monitor. Most NICU's will not discharge a baby home until they have outgrown this issue. But occasionally, a baby goes home with a monitor. Parents will need to download data from the monitor periodically and review those findings with a lung specialist.

Chronic lung disease

If your baby has chronic lung disease (**BRONCHOPULMONARY DYSPLASIA OR BPD**), you will also need to consult with a lung specialist.

Infectious Diseases

After being a NICU veteran, you have learned the art and science of good hand washing. Keep up the good work at home. No doubt the NICU nurses have instilled the fear of God in you when it comes to infections (especially **RSV**—see below).

RSV/Synagis injections

Depending on the time of year and the age of your baby, they may get an injection of Synagis, a medication that contains antibodies to a virus called **RESPIRATORY SYNCYTIAL VIRUS** or **RSV**. Your baby will need to continue to get Synagis injections on a monthly basis during the peak time RSV hits your community (usually the fall/winter/early spring). You may need a referral to a community resource that administers this injection—many pediatric offices do not routinely stock it. For more information on Synagis, see the Medications section in the Appendix A.

Flu vaccine

If you are bringing baby home during flu season, be sure your entire household has received a flu vaccine.

COVID-19 and Whooping Cough Vaccines

Everyone in the household who is eligible should be up-to-date on their COVID-19 and Whooping cough vaccine.

Other vaccinations

Babies who weigh under 4.5 pounds under one month of age do not routinely get their first Hepatitis B vaccine because they do not mount an adequate immune response. This first dose may be given at one month of age, as long as the baby is medically stable. If your baby spends their two-month birthday in the NICU, they can get their other first shots there before heading home.

Gastrointestinal
Gastroesophageal reflux

If your premature baby has **GASTROESOPHAGEAL REFLUX** (**GERD**), they may be on a prescription medicine even after you come home. The therapeutic dose of that medication is based on their weight. Since they'll be growing like a weed, be sure to ask your pediatrician to re-calculate the dose based on their weight each time you visit the doctor.

BIRTH DAY

? ?

Growth/Nutrition

Catch up growth

Your baby will be doing catch up growth for several months. Full-term newborns gain 3/4 to one ounce a day. Ideally, your baby should grow about one ounce a day for the first four months of life. Consider buying or renting an infant scale to weigh your baby once a week for at least the first four to six weeks. Alternatively, you can pop in and borrow your doctor's scale. For information about preemie growth, see the special growth chart for premature babies at the back of this book.

Breastfeeding a preemie

Many preemie grads go home on a diet of both breast milk and high-calorie premature formula (which has 22 calories per ounce).

If you are breastfeeding, you'll probably find that your little one gets tired out long before their tummy is full. And since your baby is small or weak, they may not be able to rev up your breast milk supply with their demand. Therefore, it's a good idea to pump after nursing sessions to improve your milk production. You may be doing a combination of feeding at the breast, and supplementing with expressed breast milk from a bottle. Our advice: it's wise to meet with a lactation consultant to make sure breastfeeding is successful. If you are exclusively breastfeeding, your baby may need "human milk fortifier" added to expressed milk to increase their calcium, phosphorous, and caloric intake. We have several more tips on breastfeeding a preemie in Chapter 6, Liquids.

Babies who were less than 3 lbs. at birth (very low birth weight or VLBW) and those who had poor growth in the NICU should probably get at least two bottles of high-calorie premature formula a day. This should continue until the baby is nine months old (adjusted age) to improve bone growth. (*Abrams*)

Premature formula

Whether you are breastfeeding and adding human milk fortifier, breastfeeding and supplementing with high-calorie premature formula, or exclusively formula feeding with high-calorie formula, there is no magic age or weight at which you can discontinue fortifying or switch to the regular (and cheaper) formula. As we discussed above, very low birth-weight babies (under three pounds at birth) should probably remain on the premature formula until nine months adjusted age. For bigger preemie grads, there's less consensus on when to make the switch. (*Shaheed*)

Vitamin supplements

Premature babies may benefit from a daily multivitamin and iron supplement, depending on what they are eating (breast milk/formula). If your baby is sent home from the NICU on these supplements, you can continue them for the first year of life.

Feeding schedules

Your baby was probably on a rigid feeding schedule of every three hours in the NICU. Once you are home, if your baby sticks with that routine, great. Depending on how old your baby is when they leave the NICU and how they are growing, you may be able to relax that schedule a bit, and even let them sleep at night if they want to—be sure you have the green light to do this from your doc, however.

Dental

Premature babies are at increased risk of poor development of tooth enamel (**ENAMEL HYPOPLASIA**) as well as cavities. Be aware of these potential problems. You should visit a dentist at your baby's first birthday.

Sleep

You may still need to wake your baby up at night for feedings, depending on their age and growth.

But even if your doc gives you their blessing to let your baby sleep through the night, your baby may have their own ideas. As you will see in our chapter on sleep, the ability to sleep through the night is based on a baby's neurological maturity. So, if your baby is six months old, but was born three months early, they're really only three months old (brain-wise) ... don't expect miracles.

Safety

You may not be able to use a standard infant car seat to transport your child home from the hospital. Why? Infant car seats do not fully recline so you may find your baby's head plops forward when placed in the car seat causing a blocked airway. For situations like this, you can purchase a car bed, a seat that allows your child to lay flat but still be protected in case of a crash. FYI: your child will be given a car seat test before leaving the NICU to be sure you have the appropriate safety seat.

Another tip: parents and caretakers should all take an infant CPR course before going home.

So, let's sum up your to-do list with a preemie:
- ◆ Follow-up eye exam.
- ◆ Assessment by developmental assessment program (often called Early Childhood Intervention).
- ◆ Monthly Synagis injections.
- ◆ Flu, COVID-19, and whooping cough vaccines for the entire household.
- ◆ Rent/buy infant scale or weigh regularly with pediatrician.
- ◆ Get help with breastfeeding. Use human milk fortifier.
- ◆ Feed or supplement with high-calorie formula made for premature babies.
- ◆ Continue multivitamin and iron supplement, if prescribed.
- ◆ Do car seat test before checkout.
- ◆ CPR Class for parents and any other caregivers.

Special Situations: Adoption

Having a child is quite an exciting experience, no less so for parents who choose to adopt. In their case, there's more to it than just picking up their new baby and heading on home. Here are some topics for adoptive parents to consider while you're waiting to adopt.

Q. I plan on adopting a baby. Is there anything special I should know?

It depends on the age of the baby at the time of adoption, and from whom you are adopting the baby (for example, international adoption). Here are some considerations:

1. If you are adopting the baby in infancy, adoptive mothers can try to stimulate their breast milk production with a prescription medication. If this is something you are interested in, contact your doctor.

2. It is helpful to know the medical history of the birth parents (if possible). Parental drug use and high-risk sexual activity are important to find out. For all babies, screening tests for HIV, Hepatitis B and syphilis are encouraged.

3. For infants adopted internationally, additional testing is suggested including the following:

◆ Stool culture for intestinal parasites (especially adoptions from Russia, Eastern Europe, China).
◆ Complete blood count.
◆ Hepatitis A screening.
◆ Hepatitis C screening (especially adoptions from Russia, Eastern Europe, Southeast Asia, China).
◆ TB (tuberculosis) screening test.
◆ Tests routinely done in U.S. on state metabolic screens (thyroid, phenylketonuria, sickle cell disease, etc.). You can also opt for the expanded metabolic screening.

4. Vision, hearing, nutrition status, anemia testing, and developmental milestones can be assessed when your baby meets the pediatrician.

5. If the baby's immunization status is unknown, they are presumed NOT to be immunized and will start the series at the beginning. (*AAP, Centers for Disease Control*) If there is any doubt about the quality of the country's vaccine supply, it is better to err on the side of repeating the entire vaccination series.

For more information, check out the Centers for Disease Control website at CDC.gov.

Q. Are there special doctors who care for children who are adopted?

Because adoption is an increasingly common choice for families, most pediatricians and family practice doctors feel comfortable taking care of these children.

Whew. Congratulations on your newborn and getting through this very large chapter! Up next, getting to know your baby's doc.

You & Your Baby's Doc

Insider Tips & Advice

Chapter 2

"There is no such thing as fun for the whole family."
~ Jerry Seinfeld

What's in this Chapter

◆ Finding a doc
◆ The schedule of well baby checkups
◆ How and why to schedule a sick visit appointment
◆ The difference between a sick visit and a consultation
◆ Insider tips for booking appointments
◆ What to do in the evening and on weekends
◆ Getting in touch with your doc

Welcome to your baby's second home—the doctor's office. Since you will be spending some quality time with your child's pediatrician, it's important to select someone you like and trust! Ideally, you will want to make that decision before you deliver, since that doc will see your newborn at the hospital or at the first office visit between 3-5 days of life. We'll give you insider tips on how to meet potential healthcare providers and find a medical home for your little one.

Once you've picked the person you want to be your baby's doctor, it's important to understand how their office works—and the insider tips and tricks to making your time here as smooth as possible. We'll take a walk around to familiarize you with the place.

Selecting a Doctor

Q. Do I need to select a pediatrician before the baby is born? If so, why?

Yes. It's helpful to meet a pediatrician (at a prenatal consultation or meet and greet event) before the baby is born. Here are three reasons:

1. **It gives the pediatrician a chance to review any medical problems** during your pregnancy or with your family members that could affect the baby. (The doctor appreciates being prepared.)
2. **You can get advice** regarding medical decisions you'll be making in the first few days of your baby's life. (You'll appreciate being prepared.)

3. **You will be more relaxed** knowing who is examining and advising you in those first days after your baby is born—yes, your pediatrician's job begins after delivery. (More details in Chapter 1, Birth Day.)

Q. So, how do I pick a pediatrician?

Ask your OB-GYN for a recommendation or consult with friends, relatives or other parents. Then, schedule a "prenatal consultation" visit or attend a meet and greet session with each candidate (keep the list short to maintain your sanity). While doctors consider this meeting a consultation, it's really a job interview—you are considering hiring this doctor to take care of your baby, from birth to college. Consider your prenatal consultation as parent-doctor bonding time.

Q. When should I schedule a prenatal consultation?

Hopefully, you are reading this book and this chapter before you have the baby. Ideally, it is best to schedule a consult in your third trimester of pregnancy. Why so early? Two reasons: first, to get some help making the medical decisions you need to make about your newborn. Second, because your pregnancy and due date are unpredictable—your baby could be early. You don't want to be shopping for a pediatrician while you are recovering from labor!

If you are reading this chapter after you have the baby, the best way to meet a pediatrician is to schedule an appointment for your baby and see how it goes!

Q. Do pediatricians charge a fee for prenatal consultations?

Some do, some don't.

Pediatricians are about the only physician specialists who routinely schedule "meet the doctor" visits. Such visits aren't just for the parent's benefit—it helps give the doctor a heads up about any potential medical problems the baby may have. Don't be offended if you get a bill—it is perfectly kosher. Pediatricians are offering their time to answer parenting questions— and some parents come in with lots of questions! A smart move: when you schedule the appointment, ask if there is a charge for the prenatal visit.

If you have already delivered, most pediatric practices will ask that you schedule a real appointment for the baby at which time you have a chance to meet the provider. "Meet and greet" visits are typically only offered to expectant parents.

Q. What general questions should I ask at a prenatal consultation?

Just about every pregnancy guide has a list of questions to ask at your prenatal visit. Here is some advice: ignore those cookie-cutter lists and make your own, based on the issues that are important to you. This could include:

1. **Ask questions about topics you are wondering about.** You may be so overwhelmed, you can't come up with specifics and that's okay—just pick the topic and we can fill in the details. Example: allergies. You might discuss how to avoid food allergies or the history of allergies in your family.

2. **Ask open-ended questions.** You definitely want to get a feel for how you and the doc communicate. Questions with "yes" or "no" responses don't lead to conversation.

3. **Ask questions about how the practice flows.** There is more to your office experience than your doctor. You need to be an informed consumer. Medical care has changed dramatically since you were a kid. We'll discuss more details on this next.

BOTTOM LINE: You don't have to ask *every* question that you have in your first meeting with your pediatrician.

Q. Okay, what smart questions SHOULD parents ask of a pediatrician?

Let us walk you through a typical prenatal visit and tell you what parents USUALLY ask . . . and what questions parents SHOULD ask instead. (Note: at the end of this section, we'll organize all these questions you should ask in one handy list).

Parent asks: What is your training?
A better question: How did you decide on pediatrics?

All pediatricians have about the same training. Just look on the wall. We spent a lot of time and money to get all those degrees. Our parents would kill us if we didn't get them framed and hung up in our office. Pediatricians complete four years of medical school and then three more years of a residency program focused only on children's medical care. Family Practitioners complete four years of medical school and then three to four years of residency that includes child and adult health care. Regardless of where a doctor trained, we all take a Board Certification Exam to prove we learned our stuff. Look for the letters F.A.A.P. or F.A.A.F.P. after our names. The "F" stands for Fellow, a distinguished title doctors get for passing our boards in either pediatrics or family practice. All pediatricians take continuing medical education courses annually and periodically go through a recertification process to make sure we are keeping up with current trends in medicine. Ask why the doctor chose pediatrics for a career, instead of say, urology. It's a more open-ended question. You'll likely hear the credentials in the answer, but you'll get a better idea of whom this person is.

Parent asks: Do you divide the sick and well waiting rooms?
A better question: How long will I be sitting in your waiting room?

Even if the practice's waiting room is divided into sick and well areas, don't expect the entire doctor's office to be germ free. But in the pandemic era, pediatric practices have made extraordinary efforts to keep sick children away from other patients. Some practices avoid using the waiting room entirely. Feel free to ask about it.

I'd also want know how long I have to entertain my child before the doctor sees us. You'll get an idea by how late the doctor is for the prenatal visit. We all try to be as punctual as possible, but unexpected things happen. A practice that flows well should get you and the doctor face to face within 30 minutes of your scheduled appointment.

BABY'S DOC

? ?

Insider Secrets

Be prepared for your doctor to be running behind. Bring extra entertainment for you and your child and even snacks. Another tip: if you are sitting in the office and are not called within 20 minutes of your appointment time, it's time to find out what's going on—ask the front desk for an update on the doctor's situation. Don't add to your stress—never schedule another appointment or meeting immediately after your doctor appointment. Doing so (and then running late) will only add to the frustration.

Let's talk about acceptable wait times to see your baby's doctor. Some parents wait as little as ten or 15 minutes while others report average wait times of an hour or more. You can decide what is "acceptable," but know that some practices are more efficient than others and better at managing the schedule for the day. However, there are several things that usually conspire to make a doctor run late. And it is not because they are shooting the breeze over a latte with other doctors!

See the box,"Behind the Scenes" for more on this.

Parent asks: How do I schedule well child visits/sick visits?
A better question: How does your daily schedule flow? How much time is allotted for visits?

Most practices schedule well child checks in advance. A smart tip: in a busy practice, schedule the next well child visit when you are in the office having one. The office staff can advise you when another well child visit is needed.

BEHIND THE SCENES: WHY IS MY DOCTOR SO LATE?

Do you ever wonder why your doctor is late? I'll let you in on the secrets behind the waiting room door. Let's look at a typical morning at my practice:

◆ "Dr. Brown, your 8 am well child appointment is stuck in traffic, can you see them at 8:20 am?" (Answer—"Yes.") That patient actually arrives at 8:25 am and is brought to an exam room at 8:30 am.

◆ My 8:15 am well-child appointment is brought back to a room at 8:35 am because they had new insurance that needed to be verified first (HINT: Always bring your insurance card to every office visit—especially if your insurance has changed.)

◆ My 8:30 am sick child with the flu also has asthma and needs a breathing treatment. I need to go back and examine them a second time after my nurse administers a treatment.

◆ "Dr. Brown, your 8:45 am sick visit has a sister who is sick, too. Do you have time to see both kids?" (Answer—"Yes," . . . but now I am double booked at 8:45 am.)

Sick visits are usually scheduled on the same day you call. Obviously, you can't predict when your child will get sick and you won't settle for waiting until tomorrow to be seen. This is probably different than what you are used to with your own doctor. I once tried to see my doctor for a sick visit and was told I could have an appointment a week later. I told the receptionist, "Thank you. I could be dead by then." But I digress.

What you really want to know is how much time you will spend with the pediatrician. Every practice varies, but well checks usually get more time than sick visits. A typical well check may be a 15-minute appointment. A sick visit may be ten minutes. If there is a chronic problem (e.g. headaches, constipation, school problem, behavior problem), we may schedule consultation appointments which are 30 minutes or longer. You'll note these time guidelines are never published or posted in a doctor's office. Why? Because doctors will take as long as needed to address the issues at hand—even if this means making other patients wait (which leads us back to the earlier discussion of why it takes so long to see a doctor). Remember appointment slots are just a framework for a doctor's day.

BOTTOM LINE

Sick visits are "problem oriented." Be prepared to ask all your questions up front. If you have numerous issues or chronic issues to discuss, schedule a separate consultation. Doctors expect your list of burning questions at *well check* appointments, not sick visits. You can always call or utilize a patient portal (if the practice offers one), for questions that come up between visits.

So, at 8:35 am, I have five patients in four exam rooms that all need to be seen.

By 9 am, I'm already 20 minutes behind and will need to play catch up. It's about this time I'm dreaming of sitting on a beach somewhere with a drink adorned with a cute umbrella.

All hope is not lost. Some sick visits are simple and will take less time than the appointment slot (i.e. rashes, ear infection rechecks). Some days, there are only sick kids that are "sicker than billed" and parents that need extra handholding. I will be behind all morning.

Reality check: doctors are notoriously behind schedule because we try to address the needs of each patient, no matter how long it takes. It helps if we can anticipate those needs. If you want to discuss your child's school problems during an appointment for a sore throat, tell the appointments person. Otherwise, it's likely your doctor will ask you to schedule another appointment so there is more time to talk.

Finally, another point to remember with the after-hours and urgent care clinics popping up everywhere. There is still value in having a medical home, continuity of care, and healthcare provider you know and trust. It's not just about convenience.

Parent asks: What is your philosophy? (This one must be on some parenting website because everyone asks it.)

Better questions to ask: How do you approach the doctor-parent relationship? How do you feel about complementary therapies? How do you feel about vaccinations?

Doctor-parent relationships have changed since you were a child. When you went to the doctor, they told your mother what to do to make you feel better. Your mother said "thank you" and followed the doctor's instructions. There was no debate . . . and no "complementary therapies" mom could look up online. Doctors still wistfully reminisce about these days like a retired hall-of-famer recalls the '64 World Series.

When some parents ask about "philosophy," they really want to know about what type of medicine the doctor practices. An M.D. (medical doctor) educated in the United States is almost exclusively trained in traditional medicine. They learn how the body works and malfunctions and how to fix the body with medicine or surgery. Doctors also learn how scientific research is done and how to read medical studies critically. As a rule, doctors are skeptical of new therapies unless they see data and good science to support the treatment.

If you want to integrate complementary therapies into your child's healthcare, consider a medical provider who is on the same page so you will have a good fit. And if you have significant vaccination concerns, now is the time to speak up. It's good to get honest, reliable advice from your baby's potential doc *before* it's time for all those shots. (See Chapter 12, Vaccines to read up on this subject)

Parent asks: Do you accept our health insurance?

A better question: Do you have a list of health insurance plans you accept?

Both big and small businesses switch insurance plans as frequently as the weather changes. The result: doctors lose patients when they change insurance. There is a reasonable chance that the doctor you select now may not perform your baby's college physical. Watching your child grow is one of the most rewarding parts of any pediatrician's job. So losing a family to another practice due to insurance change is something most doctors try hard to avoid. A smart practice tries to negotiate reasonable contracts with *several* insurance plans.

Parent asks: Are you on staff at my delivery hospital?

Better questions to ask: Who cares for my child after delivery, if he needs to go to the emergency room, or if he needs later hospitalization?

The answers to these questions will vary significantly depending on where you live. Gone

NEW PARENT 411: WELL-CHILD VERSUS SICK VISITS

Doctors divide their visits with your baby into two categories: well-child and sick visits. Well-child visits are what you might think of as a routine check-up—these are scheduled at regular intervals to check your child's general health, do vaccinations, etc. Sick child visits are when your child is, well, sick. FYI: Each of these visits is scheduled differently by most doctors.

are the days of the "Do It All Doctor" unless you live in a rural area.

Although continuity of patient care is important, doctors realize they only have so many hours in a day. The current trend in medicine is to divide outpatient care (office-based primary care practice) and in-patient care (hospital-based practice). Our patients get more specialized care and we experience less career burn-out. So, this is how many practices work:

1. **An office-based pediatrician may or may not go to the hospital to examine newborns.** If your pediatrician does not make hospital rounds, a hospital-based pediatrician will care for your newborn until they go home. And if there is a problem with the baby at the time of delivery, there is likely to be a hospital-based pediatrician or neonatologist to handle emergencies.

2. **An office-based pediatrician is available by phone ("on-call") in emergency situations.** But if a visit is warranted at an emergency room or urgent care center, an emergency room physician who works at that facility will evaluate and treat your child. Back in the day, that doctor used to call your doctor to discuss a plan. This still happens if there is a serious problem. But these days, you need to request the ER or urgent care center send a copy of your child's visit to your primary care doctor.

3. **An office-based pediatrician will refer a child to be admitted to the hospital.** But a hospital-based pediatrician ("hospitalist") will be responsible for your child's care while they stay in the hospital overnight (an admission). Your pediatrician should be notified at the time of discharge so they know what happened and what follow-up might be necessary.

BOTTOM LINE: You may not see your own doctor if you have an emergency or a hospital stay.

Parent asks: How are phone calls handled?
Better questions to ask:
1. What is the best way to reach the office during the day?
2. What is the best way to reach the office in an emergency at night/weekends?
3. What is the expected waiting time for a response from the office?

Most pediatric practices still rely on the good old telephone to discuss urgent medical concerns and schedule appointments. Unless you are instructed otherwise, it is always best to call the office if you need immediate assistance.

In some practices, a nurse will screen and answer all phone calls. On the other extreme, the doctor will answer all calls (a rarity now, as most doctors are busy seeing patients). Most practices fall somewhere in the middle. In general, most practices will have a nurse who can answer routine calls efficiently and hand the more complicated calls over to the doctor.

Some practices offer online scheduling. Other practices offer health privacy compliant patient e-mail portals where, yes, you can actually email your doctor. While this is obviously convenient for all of us living in the digital age, this communication is best reserved for non-urgent or behavioral/developmental concerns. Your doc may only check portal e-mail during regular business hours. You don't want to wait a day or two for a reply about a potentially serious or emergency health issue.

A few practices will even offer health privacy secure text messaging, which offers direct access to your healthcare provider (awesome) but often at a premium. (By the way, sending your doc a note on Twitter or Instagram or by regular e-mail is a no-no. Your doc would violate federal health privacy laws by responding.)

After the office is closed, there is usually a recorded message with instructions on how to reach the after–hours answering service or "on-call" doctor. The on-call doctor is usually (but not always) an associate in the practice. You will likely see or speak to all of your doctor's partners at some point in your child's life. Some practices utilize a nurse call center after hours to handle routine calls. Call centers use strict protocols to manage every type of emergency imaginable. Even with a call center, the on-call doctor is still available for questions.

Here are more questions to ask about reaching the office:

1. *What is the name of the nurse who handles phone calls?* You two will be on a first name basis soon, so ask now.

2. *If you want to speak to the doctor, can you?* You should never feel that there is a fortress built around your doctor. You have every right to talk to your doctor directly. If it's not an urgent call, it may take until the end of the business day to get back with you . . . but it should be an option.

3. *How long does it take for the nurse or doctor to return calls, portal messages, or texts?* If you don't hear from us in a "reasonable" amount of time you should try again.

4. *Do you charge for calls, texts, or portal message consultations?* Many (but not all) doctors charge a nominal fee for medical advice dispensed in any format. Other practices charge an annual fee or concierge membership fee that includes periodic communications with the healthcare providers. It's wise to know this up front!

Insider Secret

If your pediatric practice offers a patient portal, utilize it for *non-urgent* issues. It's great if you want to touch base on how toilet training is going, for instance. But if your baby has a potential health emergency such as a fever, breathing problems, or a head injury, always call the office or after hours line.

BOTTOM LINE: THE 13 QUESTIONS YOU SHOULD ASK

Okay, let's sum it up again. Here are the 13 questions we suggest you ask any potential pediatrician. (See earlier in this chapter for an explanation of why we think these questions are important—and some good answers you should hear from the doctor).

BEHIND THE SCENES: CALLING YOUR DOC AT 3AM

When doctors are on call at night, we are not sitting in our offices waiting for your call. We go to sleep at home with our cell phones at our bedside table. So if you talk to us at 3 am and we sound sleepy . . . we are. In our residency training (the medical equivalent of boot camp), doctors become experts at answering questions while sleep deprived. I'm not gonna lie. Don't expect us to schedule appointments or be excited about discussing diaper rash creams at 3 am. Be a friend and save those calls for office hours.

1. How did you decide on pediatrics?
2. How long will I be sitting in your waiting room?
3. How does your daily schedule flow?
4. How much time is allotted for visits?
5. How do you approach the doctor-parent relationship?
6. How do you feel about complementary therapies? Vaccines?
7. Do you have a list of health insurance plans you accept?
8. Who will care for my newborn during my hospital stay?
9. Who cares for my child in an emergency hospital visit, or hospitalization?
10. What is the best way to reach the office during the day/night/weekends?
11. Who answers emergency calls at night?
12. What is the expected waiting time for a response from the office?
13. Does your practice offer a patient portal or electronic communications with the office?

Q. How do I decide which doctor is right for my child?

Go with your gut instincts. Think to yourself, "Will I feel comfortable asking this person some really embarrassing questions?" If the answer is yes, go for it.

Pediatricians develop a relationship with you and your child. Doctors enjoy being a part of your family and watching your child grow with you. Unless you move or change insurance, your doctor will see your child until they move out of your house. That means you will probably see your pediatrician more than any other medical provider until you get your AARP card and senior discounts at the movies.

Welcome to your baby's medical home

Sometimes you want to go where everybody knows your name. No worries. With the number of trips to your child's pediatrician, you will be on a first name basis with the entire staff. Welcome!

Q. Does my baby need to be seen by a doctor regularly?

Yes. The very first office visit occurs at three to five days of life. Then, there are many well-child visits that follow.

Bringing your child in at regular intervals is an important part of their health care. These visits let your doctor evaluate your child's health, growth, and development. It lets you address issues that concern you. Smart advice: make a list of questions to discuss at each appointment. At the first few visits, your list may be quite lengthy (up to several pages!). But by the one-year well check, your list will probably fit on a sticky note. That's when you know you have graduated to professional parenthood.

Q. Is there a standard well child visit?

Yes. Most pediatric practices follow the guidelines of the American Academy of Pediatrics

(AAP) for routine well child checks. At every visit, we examine your child head to toe. Some visits involve screening tests and immunizations. Below is a standard well child visit schedule up to age five. Note: the immunization schedule has some variability, but this gives you a rough idea of what to expect.

Age at visit	Screening Tests	Immunizations*
Birth	Metabolic screen, hearing	Hep B
2 weeks	Metabolic screen	
2 months		DTaP, IPV, Hep B, HIB, Prevnar, Rotavirus
4 months		DTaP, IPV, HIB, Prevnar, Rotavirus
6 months		DTaP, IPV, Hep B, HIB, Prevnar, Rotavirus
9 months	Hematocrit, Lead screen	
12 months	First dental visit	MMR, Prevnar, Hep A
15 months		DTaP, HIB, Varicella
18 months	Lead screen, Developmental/Autism screen	Hep A
2 years	Body Mass Index (BMI), Cholesterol screen Developmental/Autism screen	
2.5 years	Developmental/Autism screen, BMI	
3 years	Blood pressure, BMI	
4-5 years	Hearing, vision, BMI	DTaP, IPV, MMR, Varicella

* What the heck is a DTaP? IPV? HIB? Yes, the world of immunizations has a language all its own. We'll explore the topic of immunizations (and decipher these codes) in Chapter 12, Vaccines.

Screening Tests

◆ **Metabolic Screen.** This is a blood test performed at 24 hours of life and repeated at two weeks of age. The number of tests varies by state, but at the minimum includes screens for (big words alert) phenylketonuria, congenital hypothyroidism, galactosemia, sickle cell disease, and adrenal gland insufficiency. (See Chapter 1, Birth Day and the glossary.)

◆ **Hearing Screen.** The AAP recommends all newborns have a hearing test before leaving the hospital. This simple test identifies children with congenital deafness (Again, see Chapter 1, Birth Day and BAERS in glossary). A hearing screen is often repeated before starting kindergarten.

◆ **Hematocrit.** This is a blood test performed at nine months or one year of age to determine if your child is anemic. This test may be repeated as necessary.

◆ **Body Mass Index.** This calculation (which compares the height and the weight) measures the risk of health-related consequences due to overweight and obesity. It is measured annually at each well child visit, starting at two years of age.

BABY'S DOC

◆ *Urinalysis.* A urine sample is no longer done as a routine screening test. It may be done as needed to evaluate for infection, diabetes, or kidney function.

◆ *Vision screen.* A formal vision test is performed at age four to five and may be repeated as necessary. If your school district screens annually, this may be omitted from your child's physical exam. Some practices offer a high-tech device to assess lazy eye and refractive errors as young as one year of age, but many insurance plans do not cover the cost of this cutting edge screening test (yet).

◆ *Lead Screen.* This blood test demonstrates exposure to lead. High levels can cause anemia and neurological problems. A child is screened for potential exposure with a series of questions asked at nine, 12, and 18 months old. Routine testing is performed in high-risk areas. If you live in a house built before 1978 that has peeling paint or has been renovated, notify your baby's doctor. If you have other concerns about potential lead exposure, your child can have a blood lead level tested at any time.

◆ *Developmental/Autism Screen.* Parents fill out a standardized questionnaire at the 18 month and two year well check to assess for autism.

◆ *Immunizations.* This is a whole chapter unto itself, literally. (See Chapter 12, "Vaccines.")

Q. What kind of appointment do I make if my baby is sick?

A sick visit. This is a problem-focused appointment. Your child has a problem (fever, ear ache, rash) that needs to be evaluated. Your doctor will focus on the issue and likely do a physical exam limited to the problem. We point this out so you can appreciate the difference in appointments.

BEHIND THE SCENES: Who is the American Academy of Pediatrics (AAP)?

Just who is the AAP? And why are their "policy statements" so important? The AAP is an organization of 67,000+ pediatricians who are "dedicated to the health, safety, and well being of infants, children and adolescents in North, Central, and South America."

This active group makes recommendations (called policy statements) that allow doctors to maintain the highest standard of care for their patients. The policies are reviewed and updated frequently. You can check the AAP's policy statements online at aap.org.

Doctors who bear the letters, F.A.A.P. after their names are pediatricians who are Fellows of the American Academy of Pediatrics. Fellowship is granted after passing a standardized board certification exam and learning the secret handshake (just kidding on that last one). Look for the FAAP designation from your pediatrician. This means your doctor is not only trained in pediatrics, but also has proof of competency.

BABY'S DOC

? ?

Reality Check

Your baby can get vaccinations at his well child visit even if they are sick. Many families cancel a well child visit if their baby wakes up ill on the day of their appointment. This causes delays in getting the baby immunized. Unless your baby has a fever of 102 degrees or greater, they can still get their shots. There are also lots of other things to do at a well baby check besides shots. Bottom line: keep your well child appointments!

Q. What kind of appointment do I schedule if I have several/chronic issues I want to discuss?

See if your doctor schedules consultations.

Many doctors offer longer office visits for patients with chronic medical problems or several involved issues. Typically these concerns are behavioral issues, sleep problems, school problems, or medical problems that have been occurring for more than three or four weeks. If the appointment is scheduled this way, your doctor can provide ample time to assess these problems.

Insider Tips: How To Make Friends With The Office Staff

Bringing cookies is helpful. Just kidding! Seriously, here are five tips to make a nice impression in the doctor's office:

1. **Bring your insurance card.** Most doctors' staffs verify proof of insurance at *every* office visit.
2. **When you come for your first office visit, arrive 20 minutes before your appointment time.** You'll need to fill out a lot of paperwork and the office staff needs to verify your insurance. The same is true if you have changed insurance plans. If the practice posts their new patient forms online or via encrypted text, take advantage of the convenience. Fill them out ahead of time!
3. **If you are an established patient, come a few minutes early for well child visits.** You will soon understand why. You will need to completely undress your baby to take measurements. This itself can be an event. Then, inevitably, the baby will either poop or pee on the measuring scale, which then further delays the measurements being taken. Multiply this experience by two if you have twins.
4. **If you have more than one child that needs to be evaluated by the doctor, schedule an appointment for each of them.** It shows that you respect your

NEW PARENT 411: WHEN DOES MY CHILD STOP GOING TO THE PEDIATRICIAN?

It depends on the child. Some teenagers wouldn't be caught dead in their pediatrician's waiting room. Other teenagers never want to leave the nest. Most pediatricians feel comfortable seeing their patients until the age of 18-21 years, if they still want to see us. (My pediatrician kicked me out after he performed my physical examination for medical school.)

Family practice physicians are comfortable seeing teenagers. Internal medicine physicians (internists) are not. They often limit their practice to age 18 and up.

BABY'S DOC

DR B'S OPINION: WELL CHECKS

Don't try to squeeze in a well-child visit when you come in for a sick visit. Busy families frequently bring their baby in for a sick visit and ask, "So, can't you do a well check today since we are here?" I usually say no, unless my schedule is light. I need time to do a complete exam and evaluation. Doing a quick once-over isn't doing justice to the importance of a well-child visit.

doctor's time. If everyone would follow this mantra, there's no doubt that wait times to see your doctor would decline.

5. **If you are running late for an appointment, call your doctor.** Most medical offices can modify their schedule if they know when you are coming.

Insider Tips: The Best Time To Schedule Appointments

Let's make an analogy to an airport. Your baby's doctor's office is a bit like La Guardia. When is the best time to fly? In the early morning, before delays pile up. When is the worst time to fly? Monday mornings, Friday afternoons, and national holidays. Now let's look at some trends in the doctor's office. Because many doctors' offices are closed on the weekends, parents tend to bring their sick kids in either before the weekend or after enduring a long weekend with them. Translation: *peak volume days are Mondays and Fridays.*

Seasons also cause volume trends. Cold and flu season (October through April) is the highest patient volume all year. Christmas Eve is always busy because no good parent will allow their child to be ill on Christmas. National holidays are popular times to visit because many parents have the day off from work.

In the summer (June through August), our older patients keep us busy with well child visits because they don't have to miss school. They also need camp or sports physicals. May and September are the slowest months of the year (that's when I usually take a vacation!)

If you want to visit your doctor when the office is quieter (or running less behind) here are some tips:

1. *Schedule well checks on Tuesdays, Wednesdays, or Thursdays.*
2. *Try to get the first appointment of the morning or afternoon to avoid delays.*
3. *Schedule well baby visits that occur in the winter months far in advance.* There are often fewer well child visits offered to make room for the sick visits.
4. *If you want to avoid the rush for school or camp physicals, consider booking in May or September.*
5. *See if your doctor offers weekend hours. Then you can avoid the Monday/Friday crunch.*

Insider Tips: How To Save Money

With medical care costs soaring, how can you save on your baby's healthcare? Follow these tips to save hundreds of dollars:

Insurance

◆ **If you don't have insurance for your kids, apply for CHIP** (Children's Health Insurance Program). Administered by your local state health department, CHIP is intended for working parents or those between jobs. More folks can qualify for CHIP than Medicaid because the income requirements are not as strict.

◆ If you don't have health insurance or have a restrictive plan that doesn't cover the cost of shots, **consider the Vaccines For Children program (VFC).** While the program includes all public health clinics, many private practices also participate. The government supplies doctors with free vaccines. Ask your doctor about it. There should be no reason that your baby gets behind on his shots.

Medications

◆ **Ask your doctor or pharmacist for a generic medication**, if one is available. Good news: almost all routine oral antibiotics for kids are now available in generic form.

◆ **If the prescription is a brand name medication, ask your pharmacist if there are any coupons.** Many pharmaceutical companies provide online coupons to that defray or eliminate the co-pay of a medication. So as a patient, it pays to speak up.

◆ **Ask for samples.** Again, don't be shy. As a doc, I try to give samples out as much as possible. I'm happy to give them to families—especially those who are uninsured or paying out of pocket.

◆ **Make your own.** Two obvious examples: saline and Pedialyte. Saline is just salt water that can be made at home (1/2 tsp salt in 8 oz water). Pedialyte is 4 cups water, 1/2 tsp salt, 2 Tbsp sugar, 1/2 tsp instant Jello powder for flavor.

Avoid unnecessary appointments

◆ **If you are on the fence about whether your child really needs to be seen for that cough or cold, call the nurse/doctor before booking your appointment.** You may be able to wait it out a day or two and if so, things may clear up without an appointment.

◆ **Avoid going to the emergency room**. Some visits are impossible to avoid, but you may be able to make it until morning for others (like an earache, which is not an emergency). Consider using a pediatric after-hours or pediatric urgent care center instead of the ER. Find out your doctor's office hours—some offer extended and weekend hours.

◆ **Get a home nebulizer if your child has asthma.** This will save you office visits, ER visits, and maybe even a hospitalization. Insurance companies know this and some cover the cost of purchasing the machine.

◆ **Use this book and our website's rash-o-rama.** We give a guarantee that we'll save you at least one co-pay if you take the time to read about your child's symptoms. What's worri-

BABY'S DOC

BEHIND THE SCENES: CONFIDING IN YOUR BABY'S DOC

If you found yourself struggling with depression after your baby is born, who would you turn to for help? A doctor? Friends? TikTok?

A recent study looked at mothers of young children and whether or not they felt comfortable discussing their "emotional health" with their pediatrician. Although pediatricians could be a resource for help, many moms said that discussing stress with their pediatrician would be admitting failure. (Hello? Isn't stress part of the job description?) Moms relied on breastfeeding groups, postpartum groups, playgroups, and the Internet as sources of support. Yet, over 50% of pediatricians feel it is their responsibility to recognize postpartum depression.

Bottom line: it's okay to confide in your baby's doctor. They might just steer you in the right direction.

some? And what's not? You'll find all the answers here. Common rashes like yeast diaper rash do not require an appointment (and can usually be treated over-the-counter).

Q. Who will I meet in the doctor's office?

Let me introduce you to the office staff. Practices vary a great deal, but these are the usual folks that you will encounter.

◆ *The medical provider or "primary care provider:"* This is the person responsible for your child's medical care. This may be a pediatrician or family practice doctor, depending on whom you select. Their initial medical school training is through a certified medical school (M.D.) or a school of osteopathic medicine (D.O.). Their specialty training is either in children's healthcare (pediatrics) or a combination of both adult and children's healthcare (family practice). When all is said and done, either type of provider will have at least seven years of training beyond college before they have their own office.

◆ *Advanced Practice Providers:* These people have been popular additions to busy offices. Nurse practitioners (NP's) and physician assistants (PA's) help with straightforward sick visits and well child visits. They can evaluate patients, make decisions, and treat patients with the supervision of a medical provider. Nurse practitioners have at least two years of training beyond their bachelor's degree in nursing (B.S.N.). Physician assistants complete a two-year master's program after completing college.

◆ *Nursing staff:* The staff may have a variety of degrees. The head nurse may have either a R.N. (registered nurse) or L.V.N. (licensed vocational nurse) degree. Many pediatric offices utilize medical assistants who are trained to administer shots and perform screening tests.

Q. What do I do if my baby gets sick in the evening or on the weekend?

It is Murphy's Law: your baby will only get sick when the office is closed.

Be prepared for this and have a game plan. Some offices offer limited evening and weekend hours. Find out the specifics for your doctor's office.

If the office is closed, the next option is a minor care center or an emergency department of your local hospital. Ask your office for their recommendation. The most convenient location may not be the best place to go. Look for some practical tips on navigating the ER in Chapter 15, First Aid.

BOTTOM LINE: Always call your doctor first before you go running anywhere. What may seem like an emergency to you may not be. Your phone call might save you a trip in the middle of the night.

Q. What is the best way to contact my doctor's office?

Ah, the age of technology. So many options—email, text message, etc.

Despite the digital age, the most effective way to contact the office is by picking up the phone. Doctors' offices anticipate numerous calls during office hours and have systems in place to answer the calls efficiently.

Some progressive offices answer questions online via a health privacy secure patient portal. However, most offices still rely on the telephone to communicate with patients. Why are docs resistant to change? The law protecting medical information (HIPAA) is rather onerous, with stiff fines for knowingly or unknowingly violating a patient's privacy. As a result, medical offices cannot transmit medical records via unencrypted email or text message—or leave medically sensitive information on answering machines or voicemail. Although this may seem like a hassle, these restrictions are meant to protect you.

Reality Check

You should feel comfortable talking to your child's pediatrician about any topic that might impact their health and development. Any pediatrician worth their salt will be honest and provide scientifically sound advice. In other words, your pediatrician may not agree with all of your parenting approaches if they may be hazardous to your baby's health (cue up discussions about making DIY baby formula!). View your conversations as a chance to learn from an expert! That's why they are there for you and your baby.

PARENTHOOD

Chapter 3

"When choosing between two evils, always choose the one you haven't tried yet."
~ Mae West

WHAT'S IN THIS CHAPTER

◆ **PICKING A PARENTING STYLE**

◆ **CHILDCARE OPTIONS**

Yes, your job as a parent begins the moment your baby is conceived. You will find yourself instinctively making decisions from a parent's viewpoint. Maybe it's the hormones. Or, maybe for the first time in your life, you have a sense of responsibility to a helpless little urchin inside of you. Yes, YOU are now a GROWN-UP.

This sense of responsibility will cause you to ponder the questions that all parents ponder.

1. Will I be a good parent?
(Babysitting and pet ownership are helpful job experiences.)

2. Can I be as good a parent as my parents were?
(Yes. You've learned from their mistakes!)

3. Will I handle discipline dilemmas better than my friends do? (Maybe. It's very easy to be critical when you aren't yet a parent.)

4. Will I make the right decisions for my child's health? (That's why we're here—to help point the way to the best choices for you and your child).

As you enter parenthood, it's helpful to have a game plan. If you are doing this solo, you decide what style and approach you want to take. If you are co-parenting, you'll need to have a united front with your partner. It's important to have one consistent parenting style for the household that guides your decisions. We'll explain the four basic parenting styles and how those styles can impact your child's development and self-esteem.

We'll also tackle that endless debate of parenthood: child-

PARENTHOOD

? ?

care. Is it better to stay at home with your baby or can you work outside the home and be guilt-free? We'll discuss the latest research and give our perspective as real-life moms. What are the options for childcare? We'll discuss the choices. Our advice: try to mull over this issue before or shortly after baby is born—that's because other expectant parents are already putting their names on waiting lists for the hottest day care options in your community.

Finally, we will give you some insider tips on how to balance work and family life.

First and foremost is determining your team's parenting style.

Welcome to Parenthood

Everyone will warn you, but there is no way you will completely understand how life-changing it is to become a parent. You suddenly have an enormous responsibility to a little human who needs your constant attention! And with that, other things like household tasks, self-care, and relationships with friends/family/partner often fall to the wayside. We caution you to remember that all those other things and people (including yourself) are still very important. Don't lose sight of that. You may feel very inadequate— so give yourself some grace, accept help, and remember that a happy parent is a better parent.

Q. How do I pick a parenting style?

Remember Dorothy in the Wizard of Oz? She always wore the shoes to get back home, but didn't realize it. You, New Parent, are wearing the shoes. You have the skills and instincts to be a great parent. TRUST YOURSELF.

Your style reflects your approach to certain situations. Note: there are parenting decisions (such as opting to use environmentally friendly diapers) and then there are healthcare decisions

---

Baby 411 Decision Timeline

DECISION	WHEN IT NEEDS TO HAPPEN
Childbirth classes	28-34 weeks (of pregnancy)
Breastfeeding class	32-38 weeks
Infant CPR class	Ideally, before delivery
Recommended tests	First 20 weeks
Cord blood banking	Anytime before delivery
Circumcision decision	32-36 weeks
Expanded newborn screen	Before delivery
Hire a doula	Start interviews at 28 weeks
Select a pediatrician	28-34 weeks
Find lactation consultant	Ideally, before delivery
Work/childcare options	Ideally, before delivery
Make a will	Now

This spent cat off

(following the standard recommended vaccination schedule). Sometimes parents blur the lines between these decisions and then feel like their healthcare provider is judging their parenting choices. (We're not. We are just guiding you to make wise healthcare decisions!)

Every generation of parents faces trendy choices, but honestly, there are really just a few child-rearing philosophies and the pendulum has been swinging back and forth for years.

In the 1960's, developmental psychologist Dr. Diana Baumrind defined three types of parenting styles. Baumrind found a clear association between these styles and the behaviors of children from preschool age to adulthood.

The styles differ in parents' responsiveness and expectations of their kids. Parenting styles influence early decisions such as feeding schedules, sleep routines, and managing naughty behavior (like throwing food or yanking the dog's tail for fun). But they also impact the big picture because a healthy parent-child relationship is key to nurturing a child's self-esteem. No pressure here!

Whichever approach you choose, the hallmarks of good parenting are fairness, consistency, and parent-child relationships based on mutual love and respect.

Here are the basic schools of thought:

1 **AUTHORITATIVE PARENTING (TRENDY NAME ALERTS: POSITIVE PARENTING, GENTLE PARENTING, ATTACHMENT PARENTING).** This household is run like a democracy. Authoritative parents set up rules and expect their children to follow them. These rules and limits guide children's behavior. Although there are clear expectations, these parents are willing to listen to their children's perspective and problem-solve together. The basic gist is to teach and model empathy, personal responsibility, and emotional regulation in an age-appropriate way. Of course, there are a variety of approaches and flavors to this category. Kids who grow up in these households turn out to be pretty independent and have high self-esteem.

2 **AUTHORITARIAN PARENTING (TRENDY NAME: TIGER PARENTING).** This is a dictatorship. Parents know best. Authoritarian parents have firm rules and high expectations and do not want to hear the child's opinion. These households are more parent-centered than child-centered and resort to punishment instead of teaching as a form of discipline. Children who grow up in these households are more likely to have poor self-esteem and rebel later in life. This parenting style is less popular today, but some families still choose it based on their personal values.

3 **PERMISSIVE PARENTING (TRENDY NAME: FREE RANGE PARENTING).** Welcome to anarchy. Permissive parents are very responsive to their children, but they don't set up limits, rules, or expectations. In these households, parents are friends with their kids, but not leaders or advisors. As you might expect, the result is usually chaos.

4 **UNINVOLVED OR NEGLECTFUL PARENTING.** This is also a form of anarchy. The difference here is that parents are not focused on parenting at all. They may be struggling with mental health or other life stressors that take priority over parenting. Children are left to care for themselves. The result is also usually chaos. These children have higher rates of substance abuse, delinquency, and suicide.

You will find that some parents (and experts) can be very passionate about these camps. Don't let friends, family, or random TikTok creators dictate how you raise your child.

PARENTHOOD

? ?

We all come to parenthood with the experience of being children ourselves (and the baggage we carry from our parents). We want to emulate what they did right and avoid the child-rearing practices that irritated us, or worse, keep us up at night with post-traumatic stress nightmares.

You and your partner will need to discuss these issues and come to terms that are agreeable to both. You both need to be happy about your strategy. This can be modified once you really have a baby to care for, but it helps to have some of the ground rules in place. Remember you are a team and you need to support each other! You will not win every parenting Battle Royale. If you are struggling to find common ground, find a professional therapist or parenting coach who can help.

Be flexible—sometimes the best parenting style is a combination of approaches, mixing a bit of this and some of that. Your style may change over time as well. Your child's temperament (see Chapter 11, Temperament and Soothing) may also influence your natural parenting inclinations—one size does not fit all here. And yes, your parenting style will change out of sheer necessity when you have more than one child. You will be more confident in your skills, and you won't have time to sweat the small stuff. That's why children have certain personality traits based on their birth order.

Remember, you are giving your child roots and wings—a solid foundation that fosters their independence.

Finally, federal law requires us to warn you of the following: you may not agree with some parts of this book. . . especially if you feel strongly about one parenting school of thought.

We don't mean to be flip, but we didn't write this book to advance a political agenda. Instead, our goal is to be pro-science. We want to arm you with the best and latest research and medical information. Then you decide how to raise your baby.

Yep, we realize folks feel passionately about certain healthcare issues (just take a look at the debate on circumcision in Chapter 1). So take the parts of this book that work for you and combine them with other parenting advice to create your own parenting style. There are lots of ways to be a terrific parent.

Childcare

It's probably safe to assume that you have been working outside the home before becoming a parent.

Raising a family is one of life's major crossroads that makes you ponder which path to take.

Should you drop your current career and make raising your child your new career? Can you carve out some creative combination of working part-time and staying at home with your little one? Or, will you return to the daily grind and make the most of your family time when you are able? These decisions weigh heavily on the minds of working parents, and for some, choosing to stay at home is not an option because their salary is paying the bills.

For those who have a choice whether or not to work, this decision can be very stressful and laden with guilt.

Our advice? Make your decision and then make the best of it. You can always re-assess down the road and change your mind.

We give you this advice based on scientific data. Research shows that quality time is more important than the sheer number of hours you spend with your child. Kids do best when their parents focus their attention, engage, and respond to them. (Huston)

Q. When do I need to start thinking about childcare?

Now.

It's best to begin the process before you even become a parent. Yes, it IS that competitive. The best daycares and preschools in town will have your baby's due date (instead of birth date) listed on the waiting list application.

Q. Why is my selection for childcare so important?

That seems like an obvious one—your baby is the most precious gift in the world to you. And you want to give your baby the best childcare you can find. Here are some things you should think about:

Studies have consistently shown that the first three years of life are critical times in your child's development. This is when your baby learns to trust others, function independently, problem solve, and learn the boundaries of acceptable behavior. The person/people you choose to care for your baby are incredibly important. Of course, there are economic decisions as well. Consider what your family can afford.

> **DR B'S OPINION**
>
> *"If you decide to be a stay-at-home parent, enjoy your new identity and don't look back. You will never regret being there to watch your baby grow."*

Reality Check

Your child's illness may cost you a lost workday, and the price of co-payments and deductibles when you visit the doctor.

Q. So what are my options for childcare?

Your baby stays at home with someone, goes to someone else's home, or goes to a licensed childcare facility. Let's go over these options so you can get moving on this one.

1 **PARENT AT HOME.** Your childcare cost is the loss of one parent's salary—which may be significant unless you already have a single-earner household. Think of your parenting job as a career change. Full time parenting is hard work, and an admirable profession. (I have great respect for stay at home parents! My job at work is much easier than my job at home.)

Reality Check

First babies in the household rarely get sick from birth to one year. They spend their days playing on the living room floor with their own toys. When playgroups get together (a good sanity break), the infants play independently of each other. When children start playing with each other and sharing toys (12 to 24 months), they start

? ?

PARENTHOOD

sharing germs. Firstborn babies who stay at home don't get sick that often.

However, your second child will get *much* sicker in the first year of life. Why? Big brother or sister brings illnesses home from preschool, the drop-off childcare at your gym, etc. Second babies also get dragged around to more family activities. It's almost guaranteed that you'll have more trips to the doctor with each subsequent child.

2 **FAMILY CARETAKER.** This is when a grandparent or some other willing family member cares for your baby while you go to work.

It is a great alternative if you have someone who is able and willing. It lets you pay the bills while your baby is at home with someone you can trust. Not only is family childcare free, but your child develops a special relationship with a family member.

Your child's frequency of illness is the same as if a parent stays at home.

Reality Check

Be sure you have a healthy grandparent! Infants require lots of lifting and time on the floor to play.

3 **NANNY/AU PAIR.** You hire someone to parent your child in your home. This may be a professional, or someone who just enjoys taking care of kids.

This is a great way to have a consistent caregiver. Your child will have a special relationship with another caring adult. Because you are paying this person and they aren't your mother-in-law, you can set up the parenting guidelines you have in mind. If your child gets sick, you don't need to miss work. You'll only have a problem if your provider gets sick, needs to take a vacation or (yes, it happens) quits.

And it is the most expensive form of childcare. Some parents fear that they cannot trust someone (other than a family member) alone with their child. This option requires good instincts of both the parents and the provider.

DR B'S OPINION

"You won't be able to call all the shots on childrearing. It's difficult to tell your mother-in-law what to do! Set up a consistent parenting plan with your caretaker before differences in parenting styles arise. Otherwise, it could get ugly!"

Reality Check

You won't need a Nest or home surveillance system to check on your caregiver, although many parents use one. An infant will tell you if they are uncomfortable with someone—they won't be happy to see that person. Obviously, you need to do an extensive background check on a nanny BEFORE you hire them. See our other book, Baby Bargains (see the back of this book for details), for tips and advice on how to do a background check on potential caregivers.

Tips for finding a nanny

There are various ways to find a childcare provider who will come to your home. If you use Care.com or put an ad on Craigslist, you'll need to rely on your first impression to make a decision. If you go through a nanny or au pair placement service, you can pay huge sums of money to them to screen candidates for you. (They will do a police, credit, and reference background check.) Our advice: we'd recommend a trial day with your prospective provider to see how it goes before hiring them.

4 **IN HOME DAY CARE.** A parent has a license to care for a few children (in addition to their own kids) in their home.

This is a way to hire a mother for your child. It can be great. Your child will be around different ages of children. Often, older kids enjoy playing with the little ones. Your child may get lots of love and attention and may also see these kids as role models. Sick child policies with in-home daycare tend to be less rigid than those in licensed daycare facilities. So, you can go to work occasionally, even if your child is ill. The cost is moderate but if your child gets sick, you may need to take off work.

Reality Check

As discussed in the stay-at-home scenario, second kids always get more illnesses. You will be adding your child to an existing household of children, so expect the same result. Also, those older kids may not be great role models. You might want to interview both the provider *and* the children she cares for before you make any decisions.

Tips for finding in-home daycare

To find these hidden gems, you'll need to start asking friends, neighbors, and co-workers for possible leads of in-home daycare providers. It's definitely a word-of-mouth kind of option.

5 **LICENSED DAY CARE FACILITY (CENTER CARE).** This is a popular option for many parents, so I'll spend a bit more time talking about it. If you plan to have your child in daycare, you should already have done some homework. If not, put this book down right now and start!

COSTS: CHILD CARE OPTIONS

CHILD CARE	COST	MORE INFO
Au Pair	$9750-$10,825 annual program fee plus $250 per week	AuPairAmerica.com or AuPairCare.com
Nanny	$40,000 per year	Nanny.org or $770 per week
Day Care	$15,000 to $24,000 per year	Naeyc.org or $300 to $600 per week

PARENTHOOD

? ?

Tips for finding a good daycare facility

Here are some quick tips on finding a good center care facility:

◆ *Look for a program that is NAEYC (National Association for the Education of Young Children; naeyc.org) approved.* This organization sets high standards for childcare facilities. If a program has been accredited, you are more likely to be in good hands. Check their website for helpful guidance on your childcare search.

◆ *Look up your potential program's last inspection.* Most states now post childcare facility inspections, citations, and complaint investigations online. Unfortunately, the amount of info can vary dramatically from state to state. And some inspections only happen once every three years—so the information may not be totally up to date.

◆ *Talk to parents whose kids are in the program.*

◆ *Find out how approachable the teachers and director are.* Are modifications made if there is a problem?

◆ *Spend some time observing in the classroom.*

◆ *How do the teachers manage discipline?*

◆ *Do the teachers get down on the floor and play with the kids?*

◆ *Are both the children and the adults having fun?*

◆ *What are the program's policies regarding infection control (sick child policy)?* Some programs are so strict that they require a doctor's note for your child to get back in. Many programs modified their policies due to the pandemic, so find out the most updated rules.

Center care is the most popular form of childcare in the United States. Parents have a sense of security knowing that the providers are licensed professionals. You can always check up on them. Also, good news—many daycares are trending towards a "preschool" format. Translated, they emphasize a more structured environment and learning through play.

Center daycare is relatively inexpensive as far as childcare goes. But there are hidden costs: you will have to factor in several missed workdays and doctor bills into the price tag.

GOOD NEWS FOR WORKING PARENTS: QUALITY TIME IS KEY

You can have a nurtured, well-adjusted child even if you and your partner both work outside the home. A study in the journal *Child Development* proved that "quality time" is more important than the sheer number of hours parents spend with their young children. (*Huston*)

Reality Check

Hopefully, you are sitting down for the following statistic: *young children have an average of eight to ten viral infections per year.* (*Celedon*) Infants are at highest risk of getting respiratory infections in the first several months of daycare attendance. In fact, six-month-olds who are day-care attendees have a 79% greater risk of being admitted to the hospital for an acute respiratory infection than their stay-at-home friends (who don't have siblings). (*Kamper-Jorgensen*) Your child will be asked to leave daycare every time they get sick and asked not to return until they are fever free for 24 hours. With each illness, expect your child to be contagious for the first two to four days of the illness.

The Monster Virus from Venus

As parents (we, the Fields) of a new baby, we got a quick lesson on daycare sickness—and it wasn't pretty. Our oldest son, Ben, was about two years old when he started a part-time program at a local daycare center. When the MONSTER VIRUS FROM VENUS struck, we didn't see it coming.

See, as parents who worked at home, the most human contact we had was with the UPS guy. And as long as they weren't coughing on us when they made a package delivery, we were fine. Then our son started at the day care center. About a month into the adventure, he came home with a new friend—we called it the monster virus. Sure, he had a slight fever and stuffy nose—one day later, he was fine. But not Mom and Dad. Somehow, this little virus mutated and by the time it hit us it had become a cross between Ebola and the Black Plague. We were so sick, we couldn't get out of bed for three days and had to call in the emergency parent response team (that is, grandma).

The lesson: be prepared to be struck by all sorts of bizarre diseases if your baby starts daycare. And it won't only be your baby that will suffer . . . everyone in your family is going to have to deal with this!

 Feedback from the Real World

There's nothing more vexing than searching for the right childcare for your child. And the "answer" is always a moving target—your childcare needs will change as your child grows. We asked our readers how they made sense of all the childcare options out there. Here are their tips on finding the best childcare:

◆ *Look for a referral service.* MK Krum of Ohio points out that many local YMCAs "offer a free or low-cost referral service. You tell them what kind of daycare you are interested in (center, provider's home, your home, etc) and they match it up to you by zip code." Each year the providers are required to resubmit their info along with letters of recommendation. "It gave us several options both close to work and home."

◆ *Evaluate your commute.* You may find it makes more sense to use a day care close to your home or work, depending on the circumstance.

◆ *Look for red flags when you visit a childcare facility.* Do children seem unattached to their caregivers? Or vice versa?

PARENTHOOD

? ?

◆ *Consider going slow to ease the transition.* Instead of dropping your child in to a new childcare situation cold turkey, take it slow. "Bring them for a few hours one day while you're with them," said one mom we interviewed. Or do a new program part-time for a week or more to ease the transition.

◆ *Don't make any firm decisions about childcare until AFTER your baby is born.* Now that sounds like a contradiction with the previous tip, but it isn't—getting on a waiting list for a popular childcare alternative in your town does NOT mean you have to take the spot. Meanwhile, many parents advise waiting until after baby is born before you make your decision about whether to go back to work. Deb Steenhagen, Muskegon, MI emailed her advice: "You may feel completely differently once the baby is born. Give yourself as much time for maternity leave as possible, it helps to bond with the baby strongly before you go back to work and then you'll have those memories to hold onto after you do go back."

◆ *"If you can find one, go with an in-home provider,"* emailed E. White of Maple Grove, MN. "They are much cheaper. The different centers I looked at cost twice as much as in-home daycares."

◆ *"Talk to friends and co-workers about what they did.* You might stumble upon a great nanny referral or a nanny share option. My co-worker turned me on to a great service (non-profit organization) in our area that links parents to home daycare providers. While I was leery of home daycare providers (because they have no standards governing their behavior), these particular providers are subject to rules and regulations set by the non-profit organization. Now our son is being watched after by a wonderful woman and we could not be happier!" T. Ross, Arlington, Virginia.

◆ *"In Texas, some of the best center care to be found is provided by churches, which don't advertise heavily like private day care centers*. Ask around, visit lots of places, and ask the tough questions." L. Alvarado, Houston.

◆ *Consider an au pair.* Au pairs are authorized cultural exchanges—a young woman in her 20's comes to live with you to do childcare. Pros: you have one person who takes care of your baby in your home and the au pair becomes part of your family instead of just hired help. Downsides: you have to have a separate bedroom because you have a new family member and they must leave after two years. For more info, go to AuPairAmerica.com.

◆ *Accept the fact that your babysitter or nanny will do things differently than you do.* As long as your child is content and healthy, that is just fine. Don't try to micromanage day care.

◆ Laura L. of Hot Springs, AR says *getting some help cleaning your house was critical to her sanity*: "Hiring a housekeeper, even one that comes every two weeks, is worth every penny you pay. Amazing how much more time it gives you with your baby and family to have that help, even if your budget is already strained!"

Feedback from the Real World

If you plan on returning to work after your baby is born, be prepared for a fine balancing act. I suggest you strongly consider how your life will "work."

Just getting out the door in the morning may be more stressful than any board meeting you've attended. Getting yourself ready is the easy part. If you use out-of-the-home childcare, you will have to get your baby ready and fed, plus pack up their food for the day. This can take awhile because your baby has no idea what your schedule is, nor do they care. They also won't care if they spit up on your silk blouse or suit jacket.

Another point: be prepared for that phone call from childcare telling you that your baby is sick and needs to be sent home.

Balancing Act: Juggling work and family

How do you balance family, career—and your sanity? While the ideal situation would be to be at home for your baby 24/7, some parents find they want to work outside the home at least some of the time. For others, it is a necessity.

So, let's take a look at how parents do the seemingly impossible—juggling baby, career, marriage/significant other relationships and more. How do they do it all?

Real talk: it's not a cake walk, people. Be prepared for some tension and arguments as you adapt to your "new normal". We will avoid pontificating about the shared domestic burden and the true mental load of parenthood. But we would be remiss if we did not include this topic in a book about your baby's first year.

It's your first year, too, and you have lots to learn about your own personal growth. The best advice we can give you is to have periodic honest, open discussions with your partner about everyone's role and division of labor—and KEEP THOSE COMMUNICATION LINES OPEN!

Marital satisfaction often goes down once a baby enters the picture, mostly because partners are exhausted (and then, resentful) and are too afraid to speak up about their own needs. Don't be a martyr and lose your identity (and/or your partner).

We also asked our online community to share their wisdom. Here are their tips and tricks on juggling family and a career.

Tips for Balancing Work & Baby

1 **FORGET BALANCE.** When we say "balance" work and family, this implies some kind of happy equilibrium. Forget it—the best you can hope for is OCCASIONAL peaceful coexistence between your family and job. Something will always be working to upset the balance, however . . . a childcare situation, sickness, job demands, etc.

2 **DO THE MATH.** Sit down with a piece of paper and do a serious cost/benefit analysis before returning to work. Kelly Anderson of San Diego, CA suggests: "Most people would be shocked to see how all the hidden costs of working outside the home add up (dry cleaning, taxes, eating out, gas, plus the fact that someone else will be essentially raising your child for you). For many people, the benefits just don't outweigh the costs." Good point: even if you have a good job with excellent pay, the cost of childcare and other hidden expenses may wipe out a good part of the earnings.

3 DUAL CAREERS, DUAL SACRIFICE. Both you and your partner must make sacrifices for this to work. While nothing in life or relationships is always 50/50, both parents must help to make the schedule work.

Decide what is truly important to you as a family and how—as a couple—you will accomplish those goals.

4 MEET THE NEW BOSS—YOUR BABY. That means your old boss at work must adjust to your new life. "You don't want to work for a boss who does not put family first," says reader Tricia Gagnon. If your boss doesn't understand why you need to take a day off to care for a sick child, you need to find a new job.

5 AVOID THE GUILT TRIPS. Whatever you decide for your baby, get ready for second-guessing from friends, relatives and complete strangers. E. Moeller, Boulder, CO, wrote in to stress this important point: A happy parent makes for a happy baby. "If you are fulfilled and enjoying your work and have made good childcare choices, your baby will thrive."

6 WILL IT MATTER NEXT MONTH? OR NEXT YEAR? When you have to decide whether to work late or another weekend, ask yourself: "How important is my job as a _____ compared to my job as a parent. Will this project matter next month, year or in five years?" Your child will.

Day-to-Day: Tricks for Juggling Family & Career

Sometimes it is the small details that make the difference—here are some great tricks, courtesy of our online community:

◆ *The routine is KING.* Reader Wendy Stough suggests: "Create one that works for you and do your best to stick to it, to some degree. It cuts down on the chaos of little things like lost keys and forgotten diaper bags and allows us, as parents, to take advantage of those special moments when our children need us most. Even when chaos reigns, you'll still know where the keys are!"

◆ *Make up snacks in advance.* Reader MK Krum of Toledo, Ohio makes up snacks and even sippy cups for snack-time a week in advance. "In the morning, just grab what you need and stick it in the diaper bag and go!"

◆ *Don't be afraid to ask for help.* When you feel overwhelmed, ask friends and relatives to pitch in.

◆ *Look for a local "Parents Day Out" program* to get a break once in a while. Laurie Galbreath of San Antonio gave us this tip: "Many churches (and YMCA's) offer this and you don't have to be a member! It is also very reasonable."

◆ *Create shortcuts to make your life easier.* Example: use white boards in each room of your house to write down needed supplies. This tip was sent in by Debby Moro of Cumming, GA. "I stuck a small write on/wipe off board on the back of every door in the house. When I was in a particular room and noticed I was getting low on some supply, I jotted it down then and there. Before I hit the store, I walked through the house, made out the list, and avoided forgetting something."

◆ *Use tech.* Delivery services like Amazon and Instacart are your friend. It's less stressful than going to the store with your baby in tow, and less expensive than paying for a babysitter if you want to go without company. And always consider the value of your time—it may be better to shop online and save a trip.

◆ *Pack the diaper bag the night before.* Avoid forgetting something during morning rush by packing that diaper bag and leaving it by the door the night before.

◆ *When you cook, double the quantity*—then freeze the extra portion for a quick meal later in the week.

◆ *Get up a bit earlier.* This will give you a jump-start on the day—many parents find they can get some chores done in the 30 minutes or so before baby wakes up.

◆ *Have a "two stop" rule.* We found our children would get very cranky/hungry/(fill in blank) when we tried to do more than two errand stops. While it is tempting to try to sync errands together by stopping at X, Y and Z after work, we found there was a limit to our children's patience—usually more than two stops would make life less than pleasant for all.

◆ *Know your employer's sick leave policy.* The Family Medical Leave Act (FMLA) allows parents to stay at home with a sick child without penalty (except for lost wages).

◆ *Schedule fun time.* One parent takes ten minutes out of every morning to jump on the bed or read stories with their toddler. A few stolen moments like that can make the difference.

◆ *Cook on the weekend for the rest of the week.* "That way we always have home-cooked meals that are healthy and tasty ready to pack for lunches or to re-heat at dinner time," noted Lori Lankey of Woodbury MN. "It saves time and energy during the week, not to mention calories and money if we ended up eating out instead."

◆ *Have a backup sitter plan.* And then get a backup for the backup. That way, if an emergency strikes, you have a plan B. And plan C.

So, let's sum it up. Here are the Top Tips to Balancing Work & Family:

1. Be organized.
2. Trust your instincts.

3. Prioritize.
4. Stick to the routine.
5. But be flexible too.
6. Ask for help when you need it.
7. Lower your expectations.
8. Control freaks need not apply.
9. Laugh! Keeping a sense of humor about EVERYTHING is key.
10. Schedule a little "me" time.

Now that we've covered the important highlights of establishing care with a medical provider, creating a parenthood plan, finding childcare, and juggling your new life, let's move on to taking care of your little one. Next up: hygiene!

Section 2

Care & Feeding

HYGIENE

THE SPA TREATMENT

Chapter 4

"Ray! You take that diaper off your head, you put it back onto your sister!"
~ Raising Arizona

WHAT'S IN THIS CHAPTER

- ◆ THE FIRST MANICURE
- ◆ YES, IT'S OKAY TO USE DIAPER WIPES
- ◆ HOW MANY LAYERS OF CLOTHING YOUR BABY REALLY NEEDS
- ◆ WHAT TO DO ABOUT DIAPER RASHES
- ◆ BELLY BUTTON/CORD CARE
- ◆ SOAPS, CREMES, AND DETERGENTS
- ◆ NATURAL SKIN CARE
- ◆ CRADLE CAP
- ◆ ECZEMA
- ◆ SUNSCREEN AND INSECT REPELLENTS
- ◆ THE BOY PARTS
- ◆ THE GIRL PARTS
- ◆ THRUSH, DENTAL CARE, AND DROOL

You survived nine months of pregnancy, Birth Day and the hospital food after your baby was born. Now the fun begins—it's time to take baby home.

Due to budget cutbacks at the federal government, babies are no longer sent home with personal butlers or detailed care instructions on cleaning and hygiene. Just kidding! They never used to do that. You are expected to know about this stuff on your own. Consider this chapter your baby care primer.

Warning: we'll talk candidly about diaper rash. No it isn't pretty, but there are several steps you can take to stop it. Next, it's on to belly button care. Also, we'll discuss the topic of dressing your baby as well as tips on cradle cap, sunscreen, dental care and more. And let's talk about your baby's private parts—you've got questions and we've got the answers!

Q. When can I clip my newborn's nails?

Around three to four weeks of life.

The fingertip and nail are stuck together for the first few weeks. Attempts to use a nail clipper will result in drawing blood. For now, you can use a nail file and give your baby a manicure.

Helpful Hint
You can place socks on your baby's hands if they are scratching their face and you want nice pictures. Or just use a filter app!

Q. When can I use diaper wipes?

Now.

Most hospital nurseries use gauze pads soaked in water for diaper cleanups. This is done to prevent potential skin irritation. If nurseries don't use wipes, should you? Short answer: yes. Wipes are safe—98% of babies have no problem with typical diaper wipes. Diaper wipes do contain a preservative called methylchloroisothiazolinone (MCI), which can be irritating to about 2% of the population. *(Chang WU)* If your baby develops a rash, just switch back to gauze pads.

Note: In 2017, both the Honest Company and Babyganics recalled their preservative-free organic baby wipes after mold was discovered growing in the boxes. That's why most diaper wipes contain preservatives!

DR B'S OPINION

"Bring your own diaper wipes to the hospital. If your baby's skin gets irritated, then you can use water and gauze pads. After your first diaper change cleaning meconium, you will understand why I recommend using diaper wipes."

Helpful Hint

Some parents like to keep alcohol-based hand sanitizer at the changing table (for mom and dad's hands). It's not a bad idea, since you need to keep your hands and your eyes on your baby.

Q. How many layers of clothing should my baby wear?

As many as you do.

Babies live at the same body temperature as we all do. They will be comfortable in the same number of clothes as you are. It is true that your baby loses heat a little more quickly than you, so keep an eye on them in cooler weather.

If you have a late preterm newborn (34 to 36 6/7 weeks gestation), you'll want to wrap them up in an extra receiving blanket or two in the first several days of life. But once they have their temperature regulation under control and a little meat on their bones, the same rules apply as with full-term newborns.

Reality Check

Parents often dress their babies for an arctic freeze in July. Then they wonder why their baby has a heat rash.

Q. How often do I clean the belly button?

While the idea of cleaning your baby's belly button may seem a no-brainer, there is actually quite a bit of debate about it. According to the American Academy of Pediatrics, "no single method of umbilical cord care has proved to be superior in preventing…disease (that is, infection of the belly button)." (*AAP*).

So what do you do with the umbilical cord stump once you get home? Well you can't just pretend it's not there and ignore it! Check on it at diaper changes, and clean it if it seems icky

HYGIENE

TREATING DIAPER RASH: 5 TIPS & TRICKS

There are basically two kinds of diaper rashes:

Irritated skin. Flat red rash caused when poop and pee break down the skin, causing redness and irritation.

Yeast infection. Raised, pimply rash surrounds an area that looks like raw meat. (Yeast likes the diaper area because it is dark, warm, and moist.)

Curious to see exactly what these different rashes look like? Check out our web site at Baby411.com (click on Bonus Material). For basic skin irritation, creating a barrier to protect the skin from further insults is key. Here are our tips:

1. **Use petroleum jelly** (Vaseline) **or zinc oxide** (store brand: Balmex, Desitin) at every diaper change. Pastes and ointments are more effective than cremes. Avoid powders—baby can inhale the powder into his lungs when it is poured out.

2. **Let your baby "air dry."** If you are feeling brave, let your baby go bare bottomed for a while. For the less ambitious types, use a blow dryer on a cool setting and dry the diaper area after cleaning.

3. **For more severe rashes,** try Dr. Smith's Diaper Ointment, Triple Paste, or Boudreaux's Butt Paste. These products are a little thicker and more protective.

4. **Use lanolin.** Many women use this for cracked nipples caused by breastfeeding. It's very expensive to recommend as a first line of defense against diaper rash, but if you have it in the house, use it. If you want save some cash, order some Corona Ointment on Amazon.com. Yes, it's designed for horses—but the active ingredient, lanolin, is the same!

5. **If the rash looks like yeast, try an over-the-counter antifungal** (e.g. Lotrimin AF or Triple Paste AF)—the package will say it's for jock itch and athlete's foot. Don't be alarmed. Apply twice daily for a week.

If none of these tricks work, check in with your doctor. Most docs have additional tips for stopping diaper rash.

(for example, oozing or dried blood, poop explosion event). Keep an eye out for infection too. Infection clues: redness and swelling around the cord, constant bleeding, yellowish pus and/or foul smelling discharge from the area.

How should you clean the belly button? You have two choices: sterile water or rubbing alcohol. The time-honored method is alcohol. But we now know that using rubbing alcohol does not prevent infection or make the cord fall off any faster. The only benefit to using alcohol on the cord stump is to keep the belly button from getting stinky. Alcohol should be applied to the BASE of the belly button, where the gooey stuff is—exactly where you are afraid to go. *(Zupan)*

The alternative: you can spot clean the cord with sterile water on a gauze pad if it gets dirty. Whichever method you choose, just make sure the cord stump stays clean.

RED FLAG: Belly Buttons

A foul smelling belly button with pus draining from it and surrounded by red skin indicates infection (see **OMPHALITIS**). You need to call your doctor immediately.

Q. When will my newborn get their first bath?

Your baby will get cleaned up shortly after delivery. Most hospitals will sponge bathe newborns and recommend parents do the same at home until the umbilical cord falls off. Babies don't get that dirty and sponge bathing minimizes heat loss.

Sponge-bathing also keeps the umbilical cord dry until it falls off. You can sponge bath your baby with soap, water, and a washcloth every few days. Once the cord falls off, you can give them their first real bath.

Q. I heard in my childbirth class that it's better NOT to bathe your newborn in the first 24 hours of life. Is this true?

Let's go over the usual hospital protocol first. After you give birth in a delivery room, you spend about the next hour getting to know your newborn and having your first nursing session. (That's assuming you are nursing, your baby is full term, and has no immediate medical issues to deal with.)

Then, you get cleaned up and transferred to your postpartum room, and your baby heads to the nursery to be examined, monitored, and bathed. While this is the norm, it does have a couple of disadvantages. Occasionally, the baby gets cold after their bath and then has to stick around the nursery under warming lights until their body temperature rises. This delays getting the baby back to you.

The other issue with the first bath is that it usually washes off the baby's **VERNIX** (that white cheesy stuff that protects the fetus' skin from getting pruny in the amniotic fluid). Vernix also fights off germs so it's not a bad idea to let it stay a little while longer. In fact, the World Health Organization recommends waiting on that first bath until six hours after birth. (*World Health Organization*)

But here's a little reality check and the downside to delaying a bath: your baby isn't just covered with vernix. They are also covered in your blood and vaginal secretions after delivery. If you choose to wait and give baby their first bath after 24 hours (or even later, at home), anyone handling your newborn (healthcare providers, grandparents, other well wishers) will need to wear protective gear and gloves. This avoids any handling of bodily fluids that are caked all over your baby's skin.

Bottom line: If you deliver at a birthing center, or at home and no one is going to be handling your baby but you, do whatever you like. If you deliver at a hospital, get a good nursing session in and some skin-to-skin bonding time—then let them get cleaned up. Waiting beyond six hours of life makes handling baby a hassle and doesn't have any major health advantages.

Q. How often should I bathe my baby?

As often as you wish.

You can bathe your baby every day if you like. Many parents and babies enjoy the time together. On the other hand, your baby does not make body odor or play in the sandbox yet. You can bathe as infrequently as two to three times per week.

Q. What soap products should I use on my baby?

We like Dove (bar soap) or Cetaphil soap, because they are perfume and dye free. Plus, they contain a moisturizer (particularly good for babies with eczema). Johnson's hypoallergenic baby shampoo or the generic off-brand is fine for most babies (although most of them are slightly scented).

Helpful Hint
A good rule for baby products—if it smells good or has a color, don't use it on your baby.

Q. Can I put lotion on my baby's dry skin?

Sure. Just be sure it is perfume-free and dye-free.

Most newborns have dry skin from swimming around in water (technical term: amniotic fluid) for nine months and they are just exfoliating. But, if you really feel compelled to do something, we personally recommend hydrated petroleum jelly (Eucerin or Cerave are examples of brand name products). When it comes to dry skin, the greasier the better.

Q. I'd prefer to use natural, non-petroleum based products on my baby's skin. Any suggestions?

Parents preferring non-petroleum based products often gravitate to skin lotions and creams

BATHING BABY 411: THE 10 STEP METHOD

Never bathed a baby before? Relax. Here is your 10 step how-to guide for a sponge bath:

1. **Get everything ready first.** Have two baby towels, washcloth, a bowl of warm soapy water and a bowl of warm water for rinsing, baby comb, shampoo, fresh diaper, and clean outfit.
2. **Place a towel in the infant tub** (you won't be filling the tub with water).
3. **Put naked baby onto the towel in the tub.** Cover all body parts not being cleaned at the moment.
4. **Expose one body part at a time (starting head to toe) and wash with soapy water except eye areas.** Rinse.
5. **Take the other towel and dry the area that has been cleaned.**
6. **Be sure to get into the creases,** especially under the chin/neck.
7. **Shampoo hair, rinse, and dry quickly.**
8. **Move baby from the towel they are sitting in and dry them completely with the other towel.**
9. **Diaper and dress.**
10. **Clean up mess later.**

using food products.

Warning: products claiming to be "hypoallergenic" or "natural" can contain food products that are highly ALLERGENIC. Avoid skin care products that contain milk, almonds or peanuts (also referred to as arachis oil) in their ingredients. And think twice about using coconut oil-based products. For some people, the active ingredient in coconut oil, cocamidopropyl betaine (CAPB), can actually irritate the skin!

There is emerging research to suggest that introducing food proteins through cracked skin can actually increase the chances of developing a food allergy to that food. The theory is that the body is more tolerant of potentially allergenic food proteins when introduced to them through the gut.

The take home message: read those labels! And, remember this mantra: just because it is natural, does not mean it is safe and harmless.

Q. My baby has acne. Should I buy some zit medicine?

No. Do nothing and it goes away by eight weeks of life.

Acne develops from your baby's rapidly changing body hormones. It is the worst from age four to eight weeks. Putting creams and lotions on the skin only makes it worse. Most importantly, your baby is not bothered by it.

Q. What laundry detergent do I use to clean baby's clothes? Do I really need to wash everything before I use it?

It depends on the baby.

Stick with the perfume-free and dye-free rule, especially for babies with sensitive skin. But, that does NOT necessarily mean that your baby's laundry needs to be washed separately with his own expensive detergent. The whole family's laundry can be done with a product like ALL Free and Clear or Seventh Generation Free and Clear.

For the baby with sensitive skin, pre-wash items before use. It may also be helpful to double rinse the laundry. And remember to avoid dryer sheets (they all contain perfume).

Helpful Hint

Have a spray bottle of stain remover next to baby's laundry basket. You'll probably need it for the shoulders on all of your shirts, too.

Q. What is the scaly stuff in my baby's hair?

It's called cradle cap, although you might be tempted to call it cradle crap because it is kind of icky.

Cradle cap (see **SEBORRHEA**) is caused by baby's hormonal changes and possibly yeast. It causes dry, flaking patches on the scalp, eyebrow and behind the ear. It can last for several months and sometimes, even years.

Because it is similar to dandruff, it can be treated the same way. Anti-dandruff shampoos (Head and Shoulders, Selsun Blue, Sebulex) work well if used two or three times a week. You can also massage vegetable oil into the areas and lift the scales up with an old toothbrush. You can use an anti-yeast product like Nizoral AD shampoo (over the counter) for resilient cases.

Eyebrows can be treated with 1% Hydrocortisone cream (over the counter) twice daily for a week.

Reality Check: Cradle cap may bother you, but it doesn't bother baby.

Q. Does my baby need a waxing?

Nope. We know you may find your baby's ear or back hair cosmetically undesirable, but it's not permanent.

Q. When can my baby start using sunscreen?

Now. Sunscreen can be applied to babies under six months of age, although staying out of the direct sun (especially during peak hours of 10am to 4pm) is a better choice to avoid sun damage and sunburn. Per the American Academy of Pediatrics, use sunscreen "on small areas of the body, such as the face, if protective clothing and shade are not available." (AAP) We advise limited use because of the potential for skin irritation as well as the possibility for the product to be absorbed through the skin.

But you can liberally apply sunscreen on older babies and kids. The risk of skin cancer (1 in

ECZEMA: ADVICE ON DEALING WITH DRY SKIN

About 15% of babies develop dry, scaly patches on the skin (see **eczema**). It gets worse when the skin is dry. The key to keeping it in check is using a moisturizing soap and frequent applications of moisturizing cream. For some reason our family (the Fields) has been unlucky enough to be plagued by eczema. Perhaps it's thanks to the ultra-dry climate here in Colorado, where the relative humidity is often measured in single digits. Mom, Dad and both boys have had it, including one child with severe, chronic eczema. Here are our tips for living with this itchy-scratchy skin condition:

1. **Baths:** Avoid bubble baths, oils, perfumes, dyes, and detergents. Try Dove bar soap (not the liquid), Cetaphil, Aveeno, or Cal-Ben's Seafoam liquid soap (available online or at natural food stores).
2. **Moisturize constantly.** As a side benefit, this is a great way to bond with your baby when you massage ointments or creams into thier skin frequently. A room humidifier will help introduce moisture as well. Insider tip: if your baby's skin does not feel greasy, you need to apply more moisturizer/emollient.
3. **Use "clear" detergents.** For laundry, use perfume-free and dye-free detergents such as All Clear Free.
4. **Observe** whether severe eczema shows up when you start adding new foods to baby's diet. Eliminating the offending food will obviously help. And if it happens frequently, you should consider seeing a food allergy specialist.
5. **Don't be afraid** to get a referral to a dermatologist if your baby's eczema gets really bad. Dermatologists are skin experts with knowledge of the newest treatments.

75 over a lifetime) is a legitimate concern. Sunscreen is critical because sun damage and sunburn at an early age is correlated with a higher risk of skin cancer later in life. Translation: use the sunscreen on your baby.

Select a sunscreen with a SPF of 30 to 50. FYI: Avoid sunscreens with the chemical PABA—sunscreens with PABA are more likely to cause skin irritation than PABA-free sunscreen.

Other tips: apply sunscreen liberally (at least a half ounce each time) and reapply frequently (every two hours and after swimming or sweating). If possible, convince your baby to wear a three-inch wide brimmed hat and 99% UV-protection youth sunglasses. Good luck on that!

Both UVA and UVB sunrays can cause skin damage and cancer. Buy products that have "broad spectrum" coverage for both UVA and UVB protection. Titanium dioxide and zinc oxide containing products are very effective and safe to use on babies. If possible, limit or avoid products containing the active ingredient, oxybenzone, due to the potential for estrogen hormone exposure. *(Witorsch RJ), (Baron ED)*

The key to preventing sunburn is to RE-APPLY the sunscreen frequently.

Old Wives Tale
Dark skinned people do not need to wear sunblock.

All humans who have skin need to wear sunscreen. While it is true that darker-pigmented people have less risk of skin cancer, there is still a risk. Sunscreen also prevents premature aging of the skin.

Q. My spouse and I are both black and our newborn looks white! Is this normal?

Yes. The skin pigmentation, called melanin, develops as the baby grows. Babies born with light skin may get significantly darker with time.

Q. When should I apply insect repellent on my baby?

Apply it when your baby (of any age) is hanging out in the great outdoors, especially at dawn or dusk in the summer months.

Mosquitoes and ticks are known carriers of illness. The most notable diseases spread by these bugs are Zika Virus (mosquitoes), West Nile Virus (mosquitoes), and Lyme Disease (deer ticks). The safest option to avoid mosquitoes is to stay inside at dawn and at dusk, when they are out in greatest numbers. If you go out and about, have your baby wear light colored clothing, long sleeves, and long pants. And you can get insect netting to cover little ones who are just sitting in their infant carriers or strollers.

As far as insect repellents go, the most effective products contain DEET, picaridin/KBR 3023 (sold as Cutter Advanced or Off Skintastic), or Oil of Lemon Eucalyptus. But the age of your child limits your options. Picaridin based products are the only ones approved for use in babies from birth to two months of age. DEET based products are considered safe for babies *over* two months of age. And Oil of Lemon Eucalyptus is only recommended for kids over three years of age (because even small doses in young children have led to serious side effects—like coma and seizures).

Many parents want to avoid using harsh chemicals on their child's skin and have turned to citronella-based repellents. However, products containing citronella repel mosquitoes for a mere 9.6 minutes, while 23% DEET will repel mosquitoes for five *hours*. (*Fradin*) Picaridin is the most effective non-DEET alternative for kids zero to age 3.

The problem with DEET is that it can be absorbed into the body via the skin and cause "neurotoxic effects" like dizziness (and rare, more serious adverse effects in massive doses). Therefore, you should wash the DEET repellent off once returning indoors. Here are some additional safety tips for using insect repellents on your baby: (*Wall Street Journal*)

1. **Young children should not apply repellent themselves**–that's your job.
2. **Don't apply repellent under clothing or to wounds. It goes on exposed skin**–yes, that means ALL exposed skin areas, not just the arms or legs.
3. **Don't put any repellent near children's mouths or eyes**–and avoid getting it on their hands.
4. **Insect repellents come in several forms**–the liquids, sprays, washcloths, and lotions are effective. Exception: The DEET wristbands don't work.
5. **When you come back inside, WASH your baby's skin.**
6. **DEET products with a concentration of 30% are as safe as those with 10%.** 30% DEET lasts for five hours, 10% just two hours.
7. **How much DEET should you use?** That depends on how long you plan to be out-doors–10% is fine for less than two hours, etc.
8. **DEET should only be applied once a day.** Picaridin based products should be re-applied every 3-4 hours.

The Boy Parts

Q. When can I stop using gauze around my newborn's circumcision?

Once a scab starts to form (around four days after circumcision).

This question usually comes up at the two-week well baby check–but you can stop long before that! The nurses at the hospital will show you how to apply a gauze dressing and petroleum jelly (Vaseline). I tell parents to place a big dollop of jelly in the center of the gauze, position the penis right where the jelly is, fold over the gauze, and seal it like an envelope (the petroleum jelly will allow it to stick together).

You'll want to change that dressing at least three times a day and every time your son poops. Since urine is sterile (germ-free), you don't necessarily have to change the dressing with every wet (urine) diaper.

The skin starts to heal around three or four days after a circumcision procedure is done. It starts to look gross with a yellowish scab. You will think it looks infected, but it's not. When it looks like that, it no longer needs gauze to protect it.

Helpful Hint

A parent remarked to me, "You need to tell me the endpoint for certain things. Otherwise I'll think I'm just supposed to keep doing it." If you are still putting gauze on your six month old, you have gone above and beyond the call of duty! Bottom Line: If you don't know when to stop, ask your doctor. It will save you a lot of time and labor.

Q. How do I care for my son's circumcised penis in the long term?

Make sure you always see a definite separation between the head (technical term: glans) and the shaft of the penis. In the first week after the circumcision, you won't see this separation due to swelling from the healing process. But once it is completely healed, you should see what we are talking about—the head of the penis should look like a helmet, with a defined rim.

When you change your baby's diaper, gently pull down at the base of the penis and clean the area where the head meets the shaft. This area collects dead skin (this is called smegma; memo to Seattle-area musicians, this would be a great band name). If the smegma remains there, it can cause the head and shaft to adhere together (see **PENILE ADHESION;** second memo to Seattle bands—this is NOT a good name).

Be sure to follow these instructions and ask your baby's doc for help if you are uncertain. Over the past decade, there has been a steady rise in the number of re-do circumcisions to remove adhesions.

Q. My son's circumcised penis is stuck and I can't see the head. Now what do I do?

There are a few options to "Free Willy" (a patient's father gets the credit for coining this term). If the skin on the shaft is stuck to the head of the penis (see **PENILE ADHESION**), it can be unstuck. The options: applying a prescription steroid cream, manually pulling it apart, or having a surgical procedure to correct it. Check in with your doctor to decide on the best plan. If the adhesion is minor, it may even un-stick on its own.

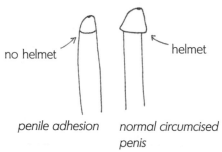

no helmet   helmet

penile adhesion   normal circumcised penis

 Reality Check

Often, a boy with a penile adhesion is also one with a hidden penis (we also discuss this in the circumcision section of Chapter 1, Birth Day). These thriving little boys have fat rolls above their genital area, which allows the penis to naturally sit in a sucked in, or concealed position. Bring that penis out (by pulling down at the base) for a cleaning at diaper changes, or you'll be dealing with a penile adhesion later. No, you won't still be doing this when your son is a teenager. It's usually not an issue after your son is about two years old.

Q. How do I care for my son's uncircumcised penis?

Here are four rules:

1. Do NOT forcefully pull the foreskin back to clean the penis.
2. Dead skin (smegma) collects under the foreskin and will come out on its own.
3. Once the foreskin pulls back on its own (usually by age five years), clean under the foreskin one or two times per week with water. Always push the foreskin back down after pulling it up to clean it.
4. Teenagers need to clean under the foreskin daily.

? ?

HYGIENE

The foreskin is attached to the shaft of the penis with tight tissue called adhesions. Most of the time, these adhesions loosen up by the age of five. Some boys, however, may have adhesions into their teen years and this is still okay (but check it out with your doctor).

Rarely, the foreskin remains tight and hard to pull back (see **PHIMOSIS**). The foreskin can also get pulled back and unable to be manually brought back down (see **PARAPHIMOSIS**).

BOTTOM LINE

If your son has a red, swollen penis, or an abnormal stream of urine, call your doctor.

The Girl Parts

Q. How do I clean my daughter's private parts?

Front to back, and in every crease. Parents—time to pay attention.

Poop has bugs in it (bacteria). Pee (urine) does not. If the poop ends up in the opening to the bladder (urethra), the bacteria will climb in and grow there (see **BLADDER INFECTION/UTI**). This is a bad thing.

Look at your daughter's private parts. Gently separate the lips (labia). You will see two holes. The top hole is the urethra; the bottom hole is the vagina. These areas, including the lips, need to be poop-free zones. Wipe from the top of the genitals, down to the anus. Never go backwards and use several wipes if you need to.

BOTTOM LINE

Don't ever hesitate to change your daughter's poopy diaper, even if it isn't your turn. Delay can lead to a bladder infection.

Q. When can I get my daughter's ears pierced?

Although ear piercing is a safe procedure for your infant, there is no consensus on the right time to do it. Here are some things to consider:

◆ *Infection*: Inserting a needle through the skin carries a small risk of infection. You might want to wait until your baby is at least four months old.

◆ *Allergy*: Some people are allergic or sensitive to the metal in the posts or backing. Use either surgical steel or 14k gold products.

◆ *Scarring*: Some people have poor wound healing where a thickened area of skin forms at the break in the skin. These are called keloids. If a family member has this problem, it's better to pierce the ears before 11 years of age, or not at all.

◆ *Cosmetic result*: Babies can be moving targets. Be sure the person performing the procedure is comfortable with infants or you could end up with uneven results!

Mouth Care

Q. Why is my baby's mouth coated in white? Is that milk?

It is either milk or thrush (a yeast infection in the mouth).

When babies are toothless, their mouths don't have many bacteria (germs) living there. Teeth provide a home for bacteria (that's what plaque is). Remember the yeast diaper rash? Yeast likes dark, warm, wet places that don't have other germs around. A newborn's mouth is a perfect locale.

How do you tell the difference between milk and thrush? Milk wipes off and is only on the tongue. Thrush collects on the gums and inner cheeks and can't be wiped off. Thrush requires a prescription anti-fungal mouthwash to be treated. Call your doctor.

Helpful Hint

If your baby gets thrush, you need to sterilize any products that go in baby's mouth (rubber nipples, pacifiers), as yeast will continue to grow on these items. Breastfeeding moms frequently develop a yeast infection on their nipples when their baby has thrush. See Chapter 6, Liquids, in the breastfeeding troubleshooting section for top tips to treat yeast infections with nursing moms.

Q. When do baby's teeth come in?

Around six to 12 months old. There are some kids whose teeth come in earlier or later, though. Universally, the first tooth to erupt is a bottom, middle one. The rest come in randomly. See the chart on the next page for more info on which teeth come in when.

Q. How many teeth should my baby have at their one-year birthday?

When it comes to one-year olds, teething varies widely.

Some babies have several teeth at their one-year birthdays, others may just have one. Don't worry if your child only has one tooth at their first birthday and their other friends have more than that.

Your baby's doc is looking for at least one tooth that is in the midst of eruption or has already erupted by the first birthday. That means your baby's tooth development is okay.

If there are more teeth than that, terrific. If not, no worries.

Reality Check

Drool is not a reliable indicator of teething. All four-month-olds are drooling and usually toothless. Why? The salivary glands are getting revved up at this age to start digesting solid foods. Yes, a baby may drool more when they are teething, but they may just drool a lot with or without a tooth coming in.

Q. How can I tell if my baby is teething?

Babies who are teething have a lower coping threshold and trouble settling down. But, they usually forget the pain of throbbing gums when they are busy playing.

As a doc, I think I have heard it all when it comes to symptoms blamed on teething—from red rosy cheeks, runny nose, diarrhea, and fever, to sleep disruption. *Teething pretty much gets blamed for everything and is usually responsible for nothing.* Your baby is allowed to have a cold virus AND teething . . . or acid reflux AND teething. It's a good idea to check things out and not just blame every problem on teething.

First-year molars come in somewhere between 12 to 18 months, even if the more central teeth are not in yet. And yes, these do hurt more than the others when they start to erupt. Don't be fooled when your baby starts pulling on his ears—it's most likely not an ear infection. Look in their mouth. It's often the jaw pain from the molars that causes the ear pulling. It will save you a trip to the doctor.

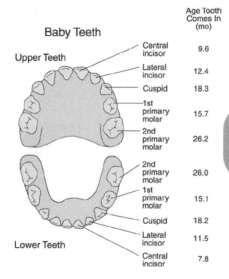

Baby Teeth		Age Tooth Comes In (mo)
Upper Teeth	Central incisor	9.6
	Lateral incisor	12.4
	Cuspid	18.3
	1st primary molar	15.7
	2nd primary molar	26.2
	2nd primary molar	26.0
	1st primary molar	15.1
	Cuspid	18.2
	Lateral incisor	11.5
Lower Teeth	Central incisor	7.8

Old Wives Tales:

Teething causes a fever. False. Teething causes diarrhea. False.
Teething causes a runny nose. False. Teething causes rosy cheeks. False.

Q. There's something purple in my one year old's mouth. Is this an emergency?

Nope, it's just a one-year molar trying to break through.

When teeth are trying to erupt through the gums, they sometimes form a bruise or blood blister in the surrounding gum area. It looks swollen and purple or blue. This is particularly true for molars, but can happen with other teeth as well. It's called an **ERUPTION HEMATOMA.** No worries. It doesn't hurt and it goes away on its own once the tooth erupts. If you see the hematoma, the tooth will be coming through in about two or three weeks.

Feedback from the Real World

When your baby/toddler is cutting molars, let your little one gnaw on frozen celery. Thanks, Mr. Silber, for your helpful tip.

Helpful Hint

Acetaminophen (Tylenol) is the safest and most effective medication choice for teething pain at bedtime. Ibuprofen (Motrin, Advil) is also fine for babies who are at least six months of age. For daytime, try frozen mini-bagels or a cold teething ring to gnaw on. Teething gels (Numzit, Orange) can have adverse health effects and the FDA warns against using them.

We also discourage use of homeopathic teething tablets, which previously contained trace amounts of belladonna (a toxin) and caffeine. The FDA does not regulate homeopathic products and dispatched a warning about them in 2017 due to reports of infant deaths.

New Parent 411: Teething Necklaces

Another product to avoid: amber teething necklaces. Sellers claim these necklaces offer a "natural" remedy of succinic acid that gets absorbed through the skin while wearing this nifty accessory. But makers also warn that the product is NOT intended for children under three years of age or children who are sleeping. Hmmm. That pretty much eliminates the target market for teething!

Q. When do I start cleaning baby's teeth?

Pediatric dentists often advise wiping your baby's mouth with a soft cloth after every feeding even before they have teeth, according to Steven Adair, DDS, MS, Professor and Chair of Pediatric Dentistry at the Medical College of Georgia.

But if you don't get around to that, you should definitely start regular tooth care when your baby's first tooth comes in. Use a wet washcloth or soft bristle brush to wipe the teeth, at least twice daily. Both dentists and pediatricians advise using a rice-sized amount of fluoride-containing toothpaste to cleanse the teeth. Yes, your baby will swallow it and that's okay.

Here is a key point: you absolutely need to clean your baby's teeth AFTER the last feeding of the night, before baby goes to sleep. Yes, that means you may be waking up a baby who has fallen asleep while feeding. If you don't, you will be asking for cavities (aka, **NURSING CARIES**).

Parents fall into the routine of feeding/nursing their babies to sleep (and back to sleep throughout the night)—and then don't know when to stop doing it. If your baby is old enough to have teeth, I guarantee they are old enough to fall asleep on their own and sleep through the night without a feeding. The alternative is poor sleep habits, reliance upon sucking/eating to fall asleep, and high dental bills. Remember, we'll cover the sleep routine issues in depth in Chapter 9, Sleep.

Fluoride is a whole topic unto itself. You'll find that in Chapter 5, Nutrition and Growth in the vitamin supplements section.

Q. When is the first trip to the dentist?

Both the American Academy of Pediatrics and the American Academy of Pediatric Dentistry recommend a first dental visit at one year of age.

Which babies are at greatest risk for tooth problems? Those include kids:

- ◆ Whose mothers have cavities.
- ◆ With special medical needs.
- ◆ With teeth, who fall asleep with a formula bottle/sleep with a formula bottle. Or with teeth who breastfeed throughout the night (and don't brush after each nursing).
- ◆ With plaque buildup on their teeth.

However, even if your baby doesn't fall into a high-risk category, it is a good idea for ALL kids to have an initial dental visit around their first birthday so you can establish a "dental home." You'll then have a point person if you have questions or a dental emergency. Your child can visit the dentist every six months after that. While a professional cleaning may not happen until your child is two years old, these early visits can provide guidance and direction.

FYI: Tooth decay is contagious. Plaque is bacteria that can be passed from person to person. So parents should NOT share food utensils or clean pacifiers by using saliva (that's gross if you think about it, anyway)! (*AAP*)

NUTRITION & GROWTH

Chapter 5

"A baby is an inestimable blessing and bother."
~ Mark Twain

WHAT'S IN THIS CHAPTER

◆ **WHAT GROWTH CHARTS MEAN**
◆ **HOW INFANTS GROW (HEIGHT, HEAD SIZE, WEIGHT)**
◆ **FLAT HEATS & TUMMY TIME**
◆ **TEETH**
◆ **CALORIES & NUTRITION FOR THE FIRST YEAR**
◆ **FEEDING SCHEDULES, OR LACK THEREOF**
◆ **VITAMIN SUPPLEMENTS**
◆ **CAM BABIES EAT TOO MUCH?**
◆ **CALCIUM, FIBER, & IRON**
◆ **ONCE YOUR CHILD TURNS ONE**

Welcome to the world of food. This section of *Baby 411* is dedicated to growth and nutrition—first, we'll look at the general questions you might have about your baby's growth, like what those ominous-looking growth charts really mean. We'll also discuss HOW your baby will grow (height, head size, weight), as well as the needed calorie and nutrition for the first year. Should you put your baby on a feeding schedule? We'll hit that hot-button issue here, as well as discuss vitamin supplements, obesity and your baby's needs for calcium, fiber and iron.

The next two chapters (six and seven) will get into the nuts and bolts of nutrition, as we discuss liquids (breast milk, formula, juice) and solids (baby and table foods). But first things first—let's talk about your baby's amazing growth!

Infant Growth

Q. At my baby's well checks, my doctor charts her growth on a chart. What's this for?

Growth charts help your doctor follow the trends of your child's growth.

Your baby's height, weight, and head size are checked at every well child visit. (Weight is usually checked at sick visits too, to assess the severity of an illness—for example, dehydration—and in case medication needs to be prescribed).

Most doctors use the World Health Organization (WHO) growth charts for children under two years of age and U.S.

Centers for Disease Control (CDC) growth charts for kids age two and up. The WHO charts compare your child to other children the same age and gender across the globe and reflect how a breastfed baby grows. For example, a boy in the 75th percentile for height is taller than 75% of boys their age. Note: if you are formula feeding, your baby may look slightly heavier on the WHO charts.

See Appendix E to find the WHO growth charts. Once a child turns two, doctors use the CDC charts to assess a child's growth compared to American kids.

The key issue: is your baby's growth consistent? In other words, if your child is at the 50th percentile for height at three months, they should roughly be at the 50th percentile at six months. What if your child's height and weight percentiles are significantly different? We'll address the issue with a discussion of this later in the chapter. Also later: what if you child's head size is growing too fast or too slow? We'll cover that too.

Q. How much weight can I expect my baby to gain in their first year?

Here are some general guidelines. Babies double their birth weight by four to five months of age. They triple their birth weight by one year, and quadruple their birth weight by age 2. After age 2, kids gain about four pounds a year until they hit puberty.

For example: A seven-pound newborn should weigh about 14 pounds at five months and 21 pounds at one year. (*Behrman*)

Q. How tall will my baby grow in their first year?

Babies will grow ten inches in their first year (about an inch a month for the first six months and 1/2 inch per month from seven to twelve months). They'll grow another four inches from age one to two. After that, they'll grow three inches a year from ages three to five, then two inches a year until their growth spurt at puberty (rule of thumb is 10-4-3-3-2 inches per year). For example: A 20-inch tall newborn should be about 30 inches tall at one year.

Q. Can you predict how tall my baby will be?

For boys: Add five inches to Mom's height and average that number with Dad's height.
For girls: Subtract five inches from Dad's height and average that number with Mom's height.
This number is your baby's growth potential. Of course, some people exceed their poten-

PREEMIES & CATCH-UP GROWTH

Babies born prematurely experience a phenomenon called catch-up growth. Most preemies catch up to their peers by the age of two, but some continue to play catch up until age seven. Your baby's measurements can be plotted on the full term baby growth chart both by *chronological age* (determined by birth date) and by *adjusted age* (determined by due date).

The head catches up the fastest, followed by weight, then height. (*Bernbaum*) That's why doctors continue to adjust for their age for 18 months for head size, 24 months for weight, and 40 months for height.

? ?

NUTRITION

tials and some people never reach their potentials.

The first fairly accurate height predictor is the measurement taken at age two years. Kids have established their growth curves by then. A good rule of thumb is that kids are half of their adult height at 24 to 30 months old.

Q. Why do you measure my baby's head size?

Because your baby's brain is also growing at a tremendous rate. Most of this growth occurs in the first two years of life. Their brain weight doubles, just in the first six months. We want to make sure this is happening, and that the skull is providing enough room for this to happen (see **CRANIOSYNOSTOSIS**).

Some babies have huge heads (see **MACROCEPHALY**) and some babies have tiny heads (see **MICROCEPHALY**). Most of the time, this is thanks to their gene pool. The apple doesn't fall far from the tree. A baby's head size percentile may be completely different than their height or weight percentiles—and that's okay.

The average newborn head size is 35 cm. It grows 12 cm. in the first year, and then only 10 cm. more for an entire lifetime!

Q. My baby has a flat head. Will they need to wear a helmet?

Unlikely.

Changes in infant sleep position recommendations have done wonders to reduce the risk of sudden infant death syndrome (SIDS) by 50%. (See Chapter 9, Sleep in the sleep safety tips section for more discussion of SIDS.) However, many babies have flat heads (official name: **POSITIONAL PLAGIOCEPHALY**) as a result of being placed to sleep on their backs. In most cases, the head shape improves once babies begin to move and reposition themselves during sleep. But this means babies should be free to move around in their sleep space by two months of age (no swaddling, no Snoo swaddle feature, no Magic Merlin sleep suits—more on this later!) Helmets are recommended as one of a few treatment options for severe flattening, and only effective if used between four and 12 months of age. *(AAP)*

A recent study compared children at two years of age who had mild to moderate flat heads as infants. Examiners could not tell the difference between kids who wore helmets and those who did not. Bottom line: unless your baby has a severely flat head, skip the helmet! *(Van Wijk)*

See the nearby section later in this chapter for more on flat heads and tummy time.

Q. When does the soft spot (anterior fontanelle) close?

Anywhere between nine to 18 months. The anterior fontanelle gives the brain the growing room it needs.

Pediatricians rely on that soft spot to provide clues for fluid status (dehydration), infection (meningitis), and problems inside the skull (brain tumors, hydrocephalus).

Q. When will my baby's teeth come in?

Anytime between six and 12 months.

Teeth may erupt as early as two months, but that is a rare event. As discussed in Chapter 4, teething is variable. A baby might have several teeth at his one-year birthday, another may just have one. Don't worry either way.

As a rule, the first teeth to erupt are the bottom middle teeth (medial incisors). After that, it's anyone's guess. There is no order to further eruptions. Frequently, a baby's one-year molars will come in before the middle or eye teeth (incisors/canines).

By the way, once the teeth arrive, you need to clean them! See Chapter 4, Hygiene section on dental care for teeth cleaning tips and a handy visual aid to explain which teeth are which.

Flat heads and tummy time!

Why do some babies wear helmets? Why is it important for babies to have tummy time? And what the heck is tummy time, anyway?

Before we answer that, here's a quick 411 on your baby's skull: newborns have skull bones with soft tissue between them (sutures) and a couple of bigger gaps or soft spots (anterior and posterior fontanelles). This skull structure allows the baby's head to squeeze through the birth canal and the brain to grow rapidly in the first two years of life.

By the time the child is two years old, their skull has hardened and those gaps and sutures have closed.

A newborn's malleable skull can put their head at risk for some really odd shapes after delivery. Later if a baby spends much time on their back (or in one position), the skull may flatten. While most newborn heads will eventually round out and look normal, here are some things to be watching for:

◆ *Molding.* Some newborns look like they have a "cone head" because the skull compresses as it goes through the birth canal (more common in vaginal deliveries than C-sections). Babies who have had vacuum- or forceps-assisted deliveries may have pretty dramatic molding or even a large bruise (**CEPHALHEMATOMA**) that can harden and leave a lump on the skull for several weeks. These irregular head shapes are present at birth and resolve by six to eight weeks of life.

◆ *Positional Plagiocephaly.* Yes, we know this is a mouthful—it literally means "oblique (flat) head." A baby who spends significant time lying on their back or leaning their head back (sleeping, sitting in a car seat, lounger, recliner, or in an infant swing) is at risk for a flat head. This odd head shape becomes noticeable after eight weeks of life. In most cases, the flattening is mild or moderate, and rounds out over the first year. You can try to avoid this problem by following the tips at the end of this section.

◆ *Torticollis.* A tightening, shortening, or bruising of a neck muscle when baby's head favors in one position for a long time. This becomes a vicious cycle, because the baby then develops a preference for turning their head to one particular side. The result? The skull flattens on one side and the facial structure starts to look asymmetric. **TORTICOLLIS** can be present at birth or begin during infancy. Aggressive neck stretching exercises are required to fix this problem.

◆ *Craniosynostosis.* This is a premature closure of one of the suture lines that sits between the skull bones. Unlike some of these other problems, **CRANIOSYNOSTOSIS** is not something that is

? ?

NUTRITION

preventable—it's an uncommon disorder that just happens to some kids. Early closure not only causes a funny looking head shape, but also interferes with the brain's ability to grow. If untreated, these babies can be at risk for vision defects and increased pressure within the skull. Surgery is required to fix this problem.

Now you know how your newborn's skull will change and what problems to look for. But let's look at the most common cause for head-shape problems: sleep position.

Ever since safety advocates recommended infants sleep on their backs, babies have spent an increasing amount of time in that position. Add in time spent in car seats, recliners, loungers, and swings—and you can understand why positional plagiocephaly (flat head) is an increasing concern. Of course, there is a simple answer: tummy time.

So, what is tummy time? Simply put, tummy time is an opportunity for your baby to lie on their belly while awake and practice lifting up their head. This will develop neck and other muscles for head control and rolling over. Tummy time also keeps the pressure OFF the back of baby's head by altering their position.

Here are some simple guidelines for tummy time. Do tummy time exercises as often as you do diaper changes. For babies under two months of age, aim for two or three minutes about ten times daily. An easy way to remember: Try tummy time on the changing table after each diaper change. For older babies (two months and up), gradually increase the length of time your baby is doing their "cobra" or "upward facing dog" yoga poses. Stop when they tell you they are no longer enjoying the experience.

What if your baby hates tummy time? One idea: have them lie on your chest and they will work to lift up their head. Or get on the floor with baby so it doesn't seem so lonely down there. To help baby lift up their head, you can use a rolled-up receiving blanket under the chest.

What else can you do to prevent a flat head?

◆ Alternate which direction you do diaper changes so your baby has to turn their head both ways to look at you.

◆ Alternate turning your baby's head from left to right on their back when they are sleeping.

◆ Play "airplane" with your baby and let them lift their head to look at you.

What to do once your baby has a flat head or torticollis:

1. Aggressively work on **neck stretching exercises** at home. See Chapter 14, Common Diseases, in the muscles/bones section for specific advice on exercises you can do.

2. Hire a personal trainer (okay, really it's a **physical therapist**) to help with neck exercises.

3. **Encourage your baby to spend more time holding their head up**—see the tummy time tips above.

4. **Check in with your doctor** every month so they can monitor your baby's progress.

5. If the head is significantly misshapen and not improving with exercise, **consult with a neurosurgeon or a craniofacial surgeon** and consider a helmet. Again, your doctor should be able to give some guidance. (*Nield, Persing*)

Infant Calorie and Nutrition Needs

Q. How quickly will my newborn grow on a day-to-day basis?

Faster than you want them to.

After you look at the following stats, you will never buy newborn clothes as baby gifts again. You can also understand why babies need to eat all the time. It takes a lot of caloric energy to grow that much.

On a day-to-day basis, here is what you can expect:

◆ *Birth to four days old:* A weight LOSS of 5-10%. As we discussed earlier, babies are born with extra baggage for the trip out into the world.

◆ *Four days to three months:* A weight GAIN of about 2/3 to one ounce a day (1/2 lb. a week). Note: newborns should be back to birth weight by their second week doctor visit.

◆ *Three months to six months:* A weight gain of about 1/2 to 2/3 ounce a day (1/2 lb. every 2 weeks).

◆ *Six months to 12 months:* A weight gain of about 1/4 to 1/2 ounce a day (3/4 to 1 lb. per month).

Q. How many calories does my baby need to eat?

It depends on their age. Another factor: babies born very small . . . or very big.

The calculations are listed on the next page, but please don't get too wound up about these numbers. Do NOT do calorie counts on your baby. As you can see, your baby's calorie needs will increase as they grow.

COMMON CONVERSIONS

For the mathematically challenged (that is, us writers) and for those who have forgotten the metric system, here are the common conversions you'll need to digest this chapter:

cc (cubic centimeter) or ml (milliliter) are ways of measuring fluid volumes.
1cc = 1ml
5cc or 5ml = 1 teaspoon
15cc or 15 ml = 1 tablespoon
3 teaspoons = 1 tablespoon
There are 30cc per ounce, or 2 tablespoons per ounce (oz).
There are 16 ounces (oz) in 1 pound (lb).
There are 2.2 pounds in 1 kilogram (kg).

There will be a quiz on this next Tuesday.

Real world tip: baby's appetite can vary from day to day. This advice also applies to older children. Focus on what your child eats over the space of a week, not every meal. Let's put this in bold: *Obsessing over every ounce of milk/formula or bite of food isn't healthy for you or your baby.*

That said, here's how many calories a baby typically needs to eat per day (given your baby's weight in kilograms):

◆ Babies birth to two months consume 90-110 calories per kilogram in 24 hours.
◆ Babies three to five months consume 80-95 calories per kg in 24 hours.
◆ Babies six to 12 months need 80-85 calories per kg in 24 hours.

Don't know your baby's weight in kilos? To convert pounds to kilograms, divide the weight in pounds by 2.2. For example, a baby weighing seven pounds would weigh 3.2 kilograms.

Now that we have all the formulas, let's figure out how many calories your average seven pound newborn will need each day to grow normally. Realize this is a ballpark figure because each person has individual energy (calorie) needs. Your little 3.2 kg bundle of joy needs between 288–352 calories per day (3.2 x 90 or 110). Breast milk and formula have 20 calories per ounce. So divide 288 or 352 by 20 calories per ounce and you'll find that your baby needs to consume about 14 to 18 ounces a day. But, once again, obsessing over every ounce will only give you an overwhelming need for Tums.

A word on preemies: Premature babies have higher calorie needs to catch up on their growth. Some babies go home from the Neonatal Intensive Care Unit (NICU) with a higher calorie diet requirement. This is achieved with either a higher-calorie formula or a special human-milk fortifier that is added to expressed (pumped) breast milk.

A word on big babies: The calorie calculations we've made here are accurate for average sized babies. All babies gradually increase their daily breast milk/formula intake and eventually max out at *about 30 to 40 oz. a day.* Average-sized babies get to that point at four to six months of age. A ten-pound newborn may reach that maximum before their friends do and will just stick to that volume. We point this out so you don't try to give them 50 or 60 oz. at six months of age.

Q. Can you show me how a baby's calorie needs change for the first year of life?

Okay, here is an example . . . but remember these are *ballpark figures.* Fair warning: we get many messages from worried readers who think their babies aren't reaching these numbers. Again, there is no reason to obsess over these figures.

So, on the following page, here are the numbers for a 7 lb. newborn: (*AAP Committee on Nutrition*)

Age	Weight (lbs)	Weight (kg)	Calories per day	Breast milk or formula per day
Newborn	7 lbs	3.2 kg	288-352	14-18 oz
1 month	8 lbs 4 oz	3.75 kg	338-412	17-21 oz
2 months	10 lbs 2 oz	4.6 kg	414-506	21-25 oz
3 months	12 lbs	5.5 kg	440-522	22-26 oz
4 months	13 lbs 14 oz	6.3 kg	504-598	25-30 oz liquid + solid food (0-4 oz)
6 months	16 lbs 8 oz	7.5 kg	600-638	24-32 oz liquid + solid food (4 oz or more)
9 months	19 lbs 8 oz	8.9 kg	712-756	liquid (~24-36 oz) + solid food (6-14 oz)
1 year	21 lbs	9.5 kg	760-807	liquid (~20-30 oz) + solid food (10-18 oz)

Insider Secret

A simpler (but less accurate calculation): Babies from two weeks to three months of age need to eat approximately 2.5 oz. per pound of body weight. *(West)*

BOTTOM LINE

Do NOT calculate your baby's dietary needs at every moment. You will drive yourself, your spouse (and your doctor) nuts. This is especially challenging to do if you are breastfeeding and can't see the volume. It's just helpful information to help you gauge things.

It's also helpful if you are planning to return to work and need to estimate how much expressed (pumped) breast milk to leave behind for your baby's meals. In general, three to six month olds will need 25-30 oz a day and six to twelve month olds need 20-30 oz a day* (depending on amount of solid food intake). And, some of that volume will also come from nursing when you are home.

The Big Picture: Nutrition For The First Year

The details will become clearer to you as you read through the next couple of chapters, but here is the big picture:

1. **Babies need either formula or breast milk exclusively for the first four to six months of life.**
2. **Some babies are ready to eat solid food (a.k.a. "complementary food") at four months old, and others aren't.** The right time to start offering solid foods mostly depends on when a baby knows what to do with food in their mouth.

NEW PARENT 411: GROWTH SPURTS

Babies will have growth spurts and their appetites may seem insatiable at times. These episodes usually occur at three weeks, six weeks, and occasionally later in the first year. They may last a couple of days or a week. If you are breastfeeding, do not be alarmed that you can't satisfy your baby. Their appetite will ramp up your milk supply.

However, allergists, nutritionists, and pediatricians all agree that there is no need to start before four months of age. Breast milk and formula are the *main source* of nutrition and solid food is complementary. (For details see Chapter 7, Solids).

3. **From six to nine months of age,** a baby drinks less liquid nutrition (breast milk or formula) as they eat more solid food nutrition.
4. **From nine to twelve months of age, a baby usually eats three solid meals a day** and takes 20 to 30 oz of breast milk or formula.
5. **After a year of age, a toddler can drink breast milk or whole or 2% milk,** with a goal of 16 oz. or dairy serving equivalent a day. Formula is no longer needed. The norm: three solid meals and one to two snacks per day. Toddlers can continue breastfeeding, but they need additional sources of nutrition.

Reality Check

When it's your first baby, you can't wait to start solid food. When it's your second or third child, you'll avoid it as long as possible! Why? Solid food becomes yet one more chore you have to do—and it's really not that much fun.

We'll go into further detail on how liquid and solid nutrition divide up in Chapter 6, Liquids and Chapter 7, Solids.

See later in this chapter for information on calcium and dairy requirements at one year of age. For a more detailed chart of liquids and solids, see Chapter 7 in the section titled "The Big Picture on Liquids and Solids."

Reality Check

Babies have "off" days and growth spurts. So, your baby may not be as predictable as you would like when it comes to meals. Occasionally, they will be less interested in feedings. And sometimes, they will seem like they haven't eaten in days.

Feeding Schedules

Q. I've heard about putting my newborn on a feeding schedule. How do I do it?

You don't. Your baby does it for you. Watch your baby, not the clock.

The phrase "newborn feeding schedule" is an oxymoron. Newborns are learning how life works outside the womb. Before birth, they were on a 24/7 feeding schedule. Now, your newborn will have to rely on their innate sense of being hungry when their body needs energy. However, it's unlikely to be a neat and tidy schedule.

Newborns need to eat about eight to 12 times in a 24-hour day. This may be every 1 1/2 hours for a few cycles, then four hours later, then two hours, etc. Somehow, in 24 hours, they do it. This is called "ad lib" or feeding on demand. Ideally, parents (and their doctors) would like their baby to have "'cluster feeding'" of every 1 1/2 hours during the day and a nice four hour stretch at night. But, short of divine intervention, there is little that can be done to *make* this happen.

For parents of preemies: Premature babies *really* need those feedings frequently. Their smaller tummies, and need for catch-up growth often require feedings every two to three

NUTRITION

? ?

hours until they are at least four months old. (That is, four months from the original due date, not the actual birth—their so-called adjusted age).

BOTTOM LINE

Although newborns can't be put on a schedule, by four months of age, your baby WILL BE capable of regular feeding and sleeping patterns. Some lucky moms and dads will have a baby that falls into a predictable feeding/sleeping pattern by two months old.

Q. My six-week-old seemed to have somewhat of a feeding schedule . . . but now seems insatiable. Is my milk drying up?

No. Babies often have growth spurts at three weeks and six weeks of age. They will have feeding frenzies during those periods of time. As your baby's demands increase, so will your milk supply. (We have a comprehensive breastfeeding chapter ahead in Chapter 6, Liquids.) If your baby continues to act this way, it's time to check in with your doc and make sure you are making enough milk and your baby is appropriately gaining weight.

Old Wives Tale

Adding rice cereal to formula or expressed breast milk will make your baby sleep through the night.

The truth: Only if your baby has heartburn. Let's think about this in a scientific way. Formula has 20 calories per ounce. If your baby is taking a six oz. bottle, they get 120 calories. A teaspoon of rice cereal flakes has about five calories. It's not providing any calories to fill them up. But it is heavier. If your baby has acid reflux, they may be happier but they still won't sleep through the night! (We will explain more about acid reflux in Chapter 8, The Other End.)

Special Concerns

Q. My 6 month old has dropped their weight percentiles from 75% to 25% since their four-month visit. What happened?

Did your baby start solid food? Solid foods contain *significantly* fewer calories than formula

DR B'S OPINION:
FEEDING SCHEDULES?

The AAP advises parents that "newborns should be nursed whenever they show signs of hunger, such as increased alertness or activity, mouthing, or rooting... newborns should be nursed approximately eight to 12 times every 24 hours until satiety." This is termed "ad lib" or "on demand" feedings. And that's pretty much the way it should be for the first eight weeks with your newborn.

Here's the take-home message: lower your expectations. Yes, your baby IS in charge of your house right now. That'll change in about 18 years. Or 26.

or breast milk. When babies are given solid foods before their milk, it reduces the amount of formula or breast milk they drink. Don't get carried away with feeding your baby solid foods until they can take two to four ounces—not spoonfuls—of solid food at a sitting. What many parents don't realize is that your baby will tell you when they want more. If your little one is finished, you'll know it. And until they are asking for more, don't push the solid food. (We cover solid foods in-depth in Chapter 7.)

If you are still nursing, you may want to make sure your milk supply has not dropped (by doing a pre-feeding and post-feeding weigh in with your baby's doc or doing a pumping session to see how much milk you produce). Most of the time your baby will tell you this is the problem, though, because they are unsatisfied when they get a snack instead of a full meal.

Q. My nine month old seems to be dropping on their growth percentiles. Is this a problem?

Probably not.

Babies these days are born much bigger than they used to be (good for them, bad for Mom's pelvis)—thanks to good prenatal care. But not all babies turn out to be sumo wrestlers. Their genetic makeup (i.e. Mom and Dad) determines their ultimate size. Big babies that have more average sized parents start to plateau, showing their truer growth curves as they approach a year of age.

Your doctor will check for iron deficiency anemia at this age, as this can also be a cause of poor growth (a drop in growth percentiles). If your baby is dropping off the growth charts, your doctor should perform a thorough evaluation to figure out what's going on.

Q. My baby has dropped off the growth charts for weight. What is wrong?

The official term for this problem is **FAILURE TO THRIVE.**

Babies whose weight percentiles start off fine, then plateau or fall below the third percentile need to be evaluated. The causes are various and include: poor feeding routines, incorrect formula preparation, gastroesophageal reflux, malabsorption of food from intestinal problems, kidney disease, metabolic disease, hypothyroidism, and anemia.

An extensive medical evaluation is usually performed, unless a cause is found easily. If no cause is identified, a higher calorie diet is initiated and baby's weight is checked frequently.

Vitamin Supplements

Q. Does my baby need a Vitamin D supplement?

Probably. But bear with us—the answer is confusing.

Babies from 0-1 years of age need 400 IU (International Units) of Vitamin D a day to prevent **RICKETS,** a bone malformation (see glossary). Vitamin D may have other health benefits as well but the data on this is less conclusive.

While Vitamin D is present in some foods (cod liver oil, salmon, sardines, fortified milk), we get most of our Vitamin D from the sun's rays. Our bodies are supposed to produce Vitamin D in our skin after sun exposure. Mother Nature didn't plan on humans creating sunscreen.

Yes, it prevents skin cancer but it also blocks UVB rays—an essential component of Vitamin D synthesis. (*Gartner, Taylor*)

Because it is impossible to determine the amount of sunlight every baby needs to make enough Vitamin D (skin color, sun block, and your home's latitude complicate the equation), the American Academy of Pediatrics and the National Institutes of Health recommend Vitamin D supplements for all babies. (*AAP Committee on Nutrition*)

Before we list the specific guidelines, here are few comments:

◆ Breast milk is perfect nutrition with one caveat. Often, there is not enough Vitamin D in breast milk for your baby's growth (even if mom is taking a Vitamin D supplement herself). It makes sense to have a breastfeeding mom take a Vitamin D supplement for her and her baby's health, right? The problem: one needs to take TEN times the recommended adult daily intake (not a typo) 6400 IU of Vitamin D daily to ensure adequate amounts in breast milk. The maximum daily limit is 4000 IU daily. (*Hollis*)

◆ One formula, Enfamil Premium "Newborn" formula (it has a big "N" on the label) contains higher concentrations of Vitamin D, allowing a 0-3 month old to get 400 IU of Vitamin D by drinking 27 oz/day.

Here are the Vitamin D supplement guidelines from the AAP. Vitamin D supplements of 400 IU per day are recommended beginning after birth for:

1. Babies who are exclusively breastfed.
2. Babies who are primarily breastfed or exclusively formula fed and drink less than 32 oz of standard infant formula daily.
3. Babies who drink less than 27 oz of Enfamil Newborn formula daily.
4. After twelve months of age, children and adults need 600 IU of Vitamin D daily. Since that would require drinking SIX cups of milk or consuming other Vitamin D rich foods (salmon, or a daily dose of cod liver oil) on a daily basis, most people need to take a Vitamin D supplement. Yes, that means you, too.

FYI: Babies who are at the greatest risk of Vitamin D deficiency rickets are those with darkly pigmented skin living above latitude 40 degrees (that's Iowa and north). However, breastfed babies in Texas and Georgia have been found to have rickets too.

Factoid: The peak incidence of rickets is between three and 18 months of age. But all people need Vitamin D for their bone health. While there are plenty of studies looking at the potential benefit of Vitamin D in preventing autoimmune disease, cancer, and heart disease, there is no convincing data at this point to prove it. (*Institute of Medicine*)

DR B'S OPINION:
SUPPLEMENTS

I have no brand preference for Vitamin D drops. The goal is 400 IU Vitamin D daily for babies. I do like BioGaia ProTectis if you want to give your baby both Vitamin D and probiotics. All these supplements are available over the counter.

Q. Does my baby need an iron supplement?

There are a few kids who will need this.

Here's the 411 on iron. Our bodies need iron to carry oxygen on red blood cells. Iron deficiency causes **ANEMIA** (see glossary). Anemia causes fatigue, poor weight gain, and poor intellectual functioning.

Newborns have a large iron bank, thanks to Mom. They fill up that bank while in the womb during in the third trimester (which is one reason why babies born prematurely are more prone to iron deficiency). As withdrawals are made from the bank, the supply needs to be replenished via baby's nutritional intake. By six to nine months, the original iron stores are gone and baby is on their own.

Formula-fed babies get an appropriate amount of iron in their iron-fortified formula. However, nutrition experts caution that breastfed babies need an additional source of iron at four months of age to prevent anemia. (*AAP Committee on Nutrition*) Some breastfeeding experts disagree with this position. We point this out because you may hear conflicting advice on this topic.

Here are the latest AAP guidelines on iron:

◆ Babies who are born full term and are fed with an iron-containing formula do NOT need iron vitamin supplements. Babies should eat iron-rich foods whenever they start solid foods. (See the list later in this chapter in the "Calcium, Fiber, Zinc, and Iron" section for food ideas!)

◆ Babies who are exclusively breastfed or primarily breastfed (supplemented with only a small percentage of formula) have two options beginning at four months of age. Option 1: They can start eating iron-rich solid foods like pureed meats and fortified cereals daily. Option 2: They can take a daily vitamin supplement such as Poly-Vi-Sol with Iron from four to six months of age until they begin eating iron-rich solid food.

◆ Babies who are born prematurely (under 37 weeks) DO need an iron supplement (2mg/kg of weight—your baby's doc can give you the dosing) starting by one month of age. Breastfed preemies need that iron supplement until they are weaned to formula or they begin eating iron-containing solid foods . . . although some docs may recommend an iron supplement be continued until age one.

◆ Babies from 6-12 months of age should get about 11 mg per day of iron in their diets. While there are several iron-containing foods, our bodies absorb iron from meat food sources more readily than non-meat sources.

◆ Toddlers from 1-3 years of age need 7 mg per day of iron in their diets. (If you have a toddler who definitely does not eat iron-containing foods—we know, toddlers can be picky—consider a vitamin supplement like Poly-Vi-Sol with Iron.)

◆ All children should be screened for iron deficiency anemia at 12 months of age. Many docs screen their patients at either the nine-month or one-year-old well child visit. A child needs an iron supplement if they are anemic.

BOTTOM LINE

Many babies get the iron they need, but make a concerted effort to offer iron rich foods once your baby starts eating solid foods. And if you have a preemie or you are exclusively breastfeeding, be sure to ask your child's doc about iron supplements. Now you can see one of the key reasons to start solid food at four to six months of age: to get more iron into your baby's diet. (*Baker*)

Helpful Hint

If your doctor prescribes an iron supplement for your baby, do not give it with a dairy product (e.g. breast milk, formula, whole milk). The calcium and iron compete for absorption in the digestive tract and will decrease the amount of iron that the body gets.

Q. Does my baby need a multivitamin?

Babies do NOT need multivitamin *if* they born at full-term, are growing appropriately on breast milk or formula and have a relatively "balanced" diet once they start eating solid foods. So, no, we don't routinely recommend iron or multivitamins for all babies.

Q. Does my baby need to take probiotics?

No, but it might be helpful. Newborns come into the world essentially germ-free. Over the first several months of life, good germs move into their guts and assist in digestion. Until that happens naturally, there is growing evidence that taking daily probiotics (specifically Lactobacillus reuteri and Bifidobacteria infantis) in the first three months of life may reduce discomfort from gas, colic, and acid reflux. As Dr Bryan Vartabedian, pediatric gastroenterologist and author of *Looking Out for Number Two* says, "I am a strong believer in the power and potential of healthy bugs."

Probiotics are not recommended for babies with weak immune systems or serious illness. Ask your baby's doc before using probiotics if your baby was born prematurely or has any other health issues.

The most popular brands are Biogaia Protectis, Gerber Soothe, and Evivo.

Q. Does my baby need DHA/fish oil supplements?

Docohexaenoic acid (DHA) is an Omega-3 fatty acid used in our bodies to make nerve tissue, hormones, and cell membranes. Found in fish oil among other foods, DHA promotes brain and vision development in infancy. But are there lifelong health benefits to daily DHA intake?

Here's a reality check: there is no long-term data that shows DHA has a significant health impact. The most compelling studies, however, show some protection against heart disease and high cholesterol.

Foods that contain DHA naturally are human breast milk, fatty fish (salmon, herring, tuna, rainbow trout, whitefish), and organ meats. Most commercial infant formulas contain DHA. Some foods, including commercial baby foods, are now "fortified with DHA."

? ?

NUTRITION

But here's the rub: the fortified foods do NOT have nearly the same amount of DHA that you can find in fish. Example: a three-ounce serving of Atlantic salmon has 1825 mg of DHA. An eight ounce cup of Horizon Organic milk fortified with DHA has 30 mg.

While there is no official recommendation about adding fish oil supplements to your child's diet, the AAP does recommend that nursing moms have 200-300 mg of daily DHA. (*AAP*) FYI: Adults with heart disease should have 1000mg of DHA per day. There are no such nutritional guidelines for kids.

Bottom line: if you want your child to get DHA in his diet (beyond what they get in breast milk or formula), offer fish on a regular basis.

Q. I've heard about fluoride supplements. Does my baby need this?

Well, it's complicated. Here's the key point: babies *under* six months don't need fluoride, babies over six months do. Both breast and formula-fed babies should drink fluoride-containing water on a daily basis starting at six months of life. The dose for fluoride intake is in milligrams or "mg". And babies need 0.25mg fluoride daily.

The long answer is below.

Fluoride prevents tooth decay. The process of adding fluoride to water supplies that do not contain it naturally is one of the top public health achievements of the twentieth century. Despite the overwhelming evidence of benefit, there are a few vocal skeptics who think this is a government conspiracy to hurt children. I'll respectfully disagree on that one.

However, kids need the *right amount* of fluoride. Too little, and you risk tooth decay. Too much, and you risk fluorosis (a permanent stain on tooth enamel). Fluorosis occurs only in teeth that are developing under the gums—the teeth are not at risk once they have erupted. So, the greatest risk of fluorosis is in kids under three years of age.

So, how much fluoride is the right amount? This is ridiculously complicated so stick with us here. Fluoride is measured in parts per million or "ppm." The U.S. government says that the maximum fluoride level in drinking water should be 0.7 ppm. You can contact your local water department or public works agency to find out the fluoride level in your local tap water.

So, exactly how much water (containing 0.7 ppm fluoride) should baby drink to get the recommended 0.25mg dose? Well, there's no easy answer. That's because your child gets fluoride from sources other than drinking water. Fluoride is not only found in your tap water, but also in foods you prepare with water, and commercially produced beverages, etc. Since the American Dental Association (ADA) doesn't specify volumes, I'll conservatively suggest four to six ounces of fluoridated water a day.

Because striking the right balance for fluoride intake is key in babies, the American Dental Association (ADA) has some very specific advice:

◆ **Breastfed babies.** Breastfed babies should drink fluoride-containing water (tap or bottled water that has 0.7 ppm fluoride) daily starting at six months of life.

◆ **Formula-fed babies.** Warning: mind-numbing content ahead.
Always prepare formula (powder or liquid concentrate) with low-fluoride water for the entire first year, but offer drinking water with fluoride (0.7ppm) starting at six months of age. For formula preparation, use bottled water specifically labeled "purified, demineralized, deion-

ized, distilled or reverse osmosis filtered." *(ADA)* Reverse osmosis filters are home water treatment systems that remove fluoride from your tap water.

FYI: Just to make your life difficult, bottled water companies are *not* required by the government to label fluoride content. That's why it's easier to go with the type of bottled water the ADA recommends.

Reality Check

Call your water supplier and find out how much fluoride is in your water.

Insider Tip

Once your baby has teeth, the ADA recommends using a rice-sized amount of fluoride containing toothpaste to clean the teeth daily. Yes, your baby will swallow the toothpaste since they will not know how to spit it out. That may be enough daily fluoride to avoid an additional supplement! Ask your baby's doc for their opinion.

Q. I've heard that fluoride can cause cancer. Is this true?

No. This and many other myths about fluoride, including adverse effects on IQ, have been solidly debunked by numerous scientific studies. Just browse the website, ILikeMyTeeth.org, to get the facts regarding fluoride safety concerns. That website is the word of the American Academy of Pediatrics and their message is clear: Life is better with teeth!

There have been debates about fluoride ever since communities began adding it to their water supplies seventy years ago. Fluoride is very safe as well as very effective in preventing cavities. The only problem with fluoride is when a child gets way too much of it.

Can Babies Eat Too Much?

Q. I am concerned that I am overfeeding my baby. Is that possible?

It is unlikely, but it can happen in rare cases.

Let's look at this rationally. Most infants do not think, "I'm full, but that dessert looks pretty good." That is a *learned* behavior in our society. Most infants self-regulate. In other words, they will eat until their tummies are full and stop. If they do overindulge, they usually just throw up.

But, it is a good idea to learn your child's cues. Some new parents think their baby needs to eat every time they cry. This becomes a set up for obesity.

Key point: if you are bottle feeding (formula or expressed breast milk), hold the bottle as horizontally as possible without allowing air into the nipple. This is called paced bottle feeding. It makes the baby work a little bit to eat, simulating what it is like to nurse at the breast, and slows down the feeding.

If you hold the bottle upright with a slight angle as most parents instinctively do, the baby will guzzle the milk like they are drinking from the tap and may take more than they really need to because it is pouring into their mouth.

Bottom line: your baby gets weighed in at every well child visit with their doctor. That's when you will see if your baby is eating enough or too much

Q. Is it possible for my baby to be overweight? Their weight percentile is off the charts!

Yes, but that does not mean they need to join Weight Watchers.

A landmark study found that 32% of American babies were already overweight at *nine months* of age and 44% of those babies were still overweight at age two. Boys and those of Latino heritage are most at risk.

If your baby fits into this category, your baby's healthcare provider may chat with you about appropriate baby-sized serving sizes of solid foods, daily intake of breast milk/formula, and discontinuing night-feedings if they were born full-term and over five months of age.

Q. Is there anything I can do while my baby is an infant to prevent obesity later in life?

Yes. Here are three things you can do.

1 START A HEALTHY DIET AND LIFESTYLE FOR YOU AND YOUR CHILD FROM DAY 1. Before parenthood, maybe you didn't work out as much as you should have . . . or ate too much take-out food. It's time to change those habits. Your baby looks to you as a role model—so be a good one. They also look to you to put food on the table for the next 18 years—so make it good, healthy food.

2 BREASTFEED FOR AT LEAST FOUR MONTHS. Breastfeeding for at least the first four months lowers the odds of childhood obesity. Breastfed babies (no matter when they begin eating solid food) have only a one in 14 chance of being obese as a preschooler.

3 START SOLID FOODS AT FOUR MONTHS OF LIFE OR LATER. Introducing solid food at four to six months of life seems to reduce childhood obesity rates. One study showed that formula-fed babies who started solid food *before* four months of age had a one in four chance of being obese at three years of age. Those who indulged in solid food at four to five months of age had only one in 20 odds. (*Huh*)

Q. How can I find out if my child is overweight?

For babies under two years of age, we compare the weight-for-length ratio. For kids ages two and up, there is a calculation called the **BODY MASS INDEX (BMI)** that compares your child's height to his weight. The formula is applicable to children ages 2-20 years of age. The ranges vary for gender and age (because the BMI varies as kids grow). While the BMI is certainly not a perfect way to diagnose obesity, it is a starting point to help identify children potentially at risk.

Here's the formula:

$$\frac{\text{Weight in lbs.}}{(\text{height in inches}) \times (\text{height in inches})} \times 703 = \text{BMI}$$

For children, the risk for obesity is a BMI of 85-95%. An overweight child has a BMI of 95% or higher. To check your child's BMI, go to http://bit.ly/bmicalculatortool.

For more information on body mass indexes for both children and adults, check out the Centers for Disease Control's website at: cdc. gov/nccdphp/dnpa/growthcharts/bmi_tools.htm

Calcium, Fiber, Zinc, And Iron

Q. Are there any nutrients that children eat too little of?

Calcium, fiber, zinc, and iron. Let's take a look at each.

1 CALCIUM. Calcium is a key nutrient for healthy bones. The requirements change as children grow. Babies from birth to 12 months get enough calcium from breast milk or formula. For ages one to three years, children need 500 milligrams per day (mg/day). If your child has a milk intolerance or allergy, try plant-based calcium fortified beverages, broccoli, rhubarb, or tofu as alternative calcium sources.

Calcium Content Of Foods

Food	Calcium content (mg)
8 oz cup of milk	250 mg
1 slice of cheese	200 mg
1 cup of ice cream	175 mg
4 oz cup of yogurt	200 mg
3 oz salmon	200 mg
1/2 cup tofu	200 mg
1/2 cup white beans	80 mg
1/2 cup broccoli	30 mg
1/2 cup collards	130 mg
8 oz cup calcium plant-based drink*	300 mg

Note: As you can see, milk is the most efficient way of getting calcium.

But don't lose sleep if your child has a milk allergy. Calcium fortified beverages have comparable absorption to dairy products (depending on the product) and the calcium in green leafy vegetables is absorbed better than milk (that is, if you can get your kid to eat kale or collards).

2 FIBER. Not only does fiber make your child a regular guy or gal, it also has potential benefits including reducing heart disease. So, make it a little family project to increase everyone's fiber intake.

The fiber requirement for children is calculated by: Age in years + 5 = Number of fiber grams/day. Example: a two-year old needs seven grams of fiber day. However, there are no established guidelines for children under one year of age. So, you and your baby's healthcare provider will have to tinker with how much fiber to offer if your baby gets constipated! Adults need 25–30 grams of fiber per day. The average American diet doesn't come anywhere close to our daily needs.

So, how do you get a baby to eat high fiber foods? Try whole grain cereals and breads, prunes and other fruits, beans, and green leafy vegetables. If you are laughing at the prospect of convincing your baby to eat kale, see the section Solid Food Equals Solid Poop in Chapter 8, "The Other End" for our tricks.

Reality Check

Many parents don't realize that the source of fiber in many fruits is the skin, which usually gets peeled off before a child gets to the fruit.

3 ZINC. Zinc is necessary for immune function, cell growth and repair. Babies from birth to six months need 2 mg per day and babies from seven months to age three need 3 mg per day of zinc.

Zinc is in both breast milk and formula. However, babies need an additional source of zinc in their food, starting around six months of age. This is especially important for babies who were born prematurely and are growing faster than their peers.

The best and most practical source for zinc is meat. Lentils are another great option. Fortified cereals for infants also contain zinc, but this is less effective (it is harder for the body to absorb this type of zinc). Less baby friendly sources of zinc include oysters, beef liver, and crab.

4 IRON. We have already chatted about this one. It's important for babies six to 12 months old to have a daily intake (11 mg/day) for growth and brain function.

Here are some good sources of iron:

Meat, poultry, fish, bread, enriched pasta, dark green vegetables (spinach, broccoli, kale), legumes (dried beans, soybeans, lentils), eggs, nuts/seeds, peanut sauce and butter, dried fruits (raisins, etc)*, cereals (infant as well as grown up breakfast cereals are iron fortified). *Note: Eating iron in combination with Vitamin C (orange juice, etc), helps the body absorb iron.*

Because of risk of choking, hold off on these foods until after three years of age.

Happy Birthday, You're Turning One!

Yes, your child is turning one! How exciting, no? Remember that food pyramid we learned about in science class? Yeah, well that doesn't exist anymore. The following servings should help you determine the proper diet for your child.

Food Guidelines for a One Year Old

The serving size is listed beside the food item.
The average calorie intake for a one year old is 900 calories. Two to three year olds consume 1000-1400 calories a day

Breads/Grains	**4-6 servings/day**
Whole wheat bread	1/2 slice
Cooked cereal, rice, pasta	1/4 cup
Cold cereal	1/2 cup

Fruits/Vegetables	**4 servings/day**
	(1 Vitamin A/ 1 Vitamin C)
Vitamin C	
Citrus, berries, melons,	1/4 cup
Tomatoes, broccoli, potatoes,cauliflower	

(Continued on next page)	
Vitamin A	
Peaches, carrots, peas,	2 Tbsp
Green beans, melons, apricots	
Other	2 Tbsp

Milk/Dairy	**4 servings/day**
Whole or 2% milk	1/2 cup
Cheese slice	1 slice (1 oz)
Yogurt	4 oz
Ice Cream	1/2 cup

Meat/Protein	**2 servings/day**
Beef, chicken fish, pork	2 Tbsp
Egg	1 egg
Beans	1/4 cup

| **Fats** | **3 servings/day** |
| Butter, mayo, ranch dressing | 1 tsp |

Q. My one year old is on a hunger strike. Help!

Very few one year olds have a world cause they support that passionately!

The *toddler diet* appears as your baby approaches one year old. The typical toddler eats well once every three days or eats one good meal in 24 hours. The food that is loved for seven straight days will be refused shortly thereafter. A good strategy is to offer three food choices in a meal. Pick one that is sure to be a hit—the others are trial offerings. If your child refuses everything, *do not make another meal for them.* Mealtime is over. Don't worry, your child will eat at the next opportunity.

All humans have both a hunger and thirst drive that compels us to fulfill our calorie and fluid needs. Your toddler is regulating their food needs. Embrace it.

Now that you have the big picture on your baby's nutrition, let's get specific: next up is a discussion of both liquids (breast milk, formula, milk) and solid foods. We'll start with the liquids.

LIQUIDS

Chapter 6

"In short, breastfeeding occurs above the eyebrows as much as or more than it occurs in the mammary glands."

~ Judithe A. Thompson

WHAT'S IN THIS CHAPTER

BREAST MILK
◆ **THE ADVANTAGES OF BREAST MILK**
◆ **GETTING STARTED**
◆ **TROUBLESHOOTING**
◆ **WHERE TO GET HELP**
◆ **HOW TO PUMP AND STORE BREAST MILK**
◆ **REAL TALK (DIET, GOING BACK TO WORK)**
◆ **INTRODUCING A BOTTLE**
◆ **SPECIAL SITUATIONS**
◆ **WEANING**
◆ **BIG PICTURE FOR THE YEAR**

FORMULA
◆ **FORMULA OPTIONS**
◆ **BOTTLE MANAGEMENT**

OTHER LIQUIDS
◆ **WATER, JUICE, MILK**

For about the first six months of your baby's life, you only have one decision to make about her nutrition: breast milk or formula. You can guarantee that decision won't occur in a vacuum: friends, neighbors, relatives and complete strangers at the grocery store will want to weigh in on what's "best." But you are the only one who can make that decision for your baby.

This chapter will offer you the pros and cons of both breast milk and formula. We promise we won't make judgments about your choice. But like every medical organization on this planet, we agree that human breast milk is the perfect nutrition for human babies. No matter how much formula companies tinker with their products, formula will only be a close approximation to the real thing. Breast milk has living ingredients (including all those antibodies you've been making your entire life)…and you just can't package this stuff and sell it in the grocery store.

So, we will do our best to convince you to breastfeed and to stick with it—with lots of tips and handholding along the way. However, we won't make you feel guilty if you decide on formula or can't make a go of breastfeeding. We just hope you give breastfeeding your best effort, because any breast milk you feed your baby is a gift.

If you decide to go with infant formula or need to supplement your breast milk supply, this chapter explains what you need to know about formula options.

Besides breast milk and formula, you'll be addressing the question of what other liquids to serve your child. These include water, juice and cow's milk. We'll discuss these other liquids in this chapter as well.

Breast Milk

Q. I have heard that breastfeeding is best for babies, but what are the real advantages?

There are advantages for both baby and mom. Let's take a look at each:

Breastfeeding Advantages for Baby:
Mother's milk:
1. **Has the ideal ingredients for a human body.** Breast milk is living food.
2. **Carries the mother's antibodies to protect baby** from various infections.
3. **Reduces the severity of certain infections**, like stomach viruses and the common cold.
4. **Is hypoallergenic.** It is rare to be allergic to human milk.
5. **Is a gut builder.** Breast milk naturally contains good germs (bifidobacteria) and nutrients (oligosaccharides, IgA) that encourage those microbes to grow, promoting healthy digestion and immunity. In short: breast milk builds the baby biome. *(Mueller)*
6. **Reduces risk of obesity, diabetes, inflammatory bowel disease, asthma, and some forms of cancer later in life.**
7. **Reduces a baby's risk of Sudden Infant Death Syndrome (SIDS).** *(Vennemann)*

Breastfeeding Advantages for Mom:
1. **It may be the easiest way to lose those pregnancy pounds** and still eat like you are a professional wrestler.
2. **It is always ready to serve, at the perfect temperature.**
3. **It's free. Formula can cost $1200 or more for the entire first year of life.**
4. **It reduces a woman's risk of breast cancer.** Any amount or duration of breast-feeding lowers your risk of developing breast cancer before menopause. Currently, one in eight women will get breast cancer.
5. **It may reduce a woman's risk of ovarian and endometrial cancer.**
6. **It may lower a woman's risk** of osteoporosis, diabetes, high blood pressure, heart disease, and rheumatoid arthritis. You can lower your risk of many of these disorders by nursing for at least a year of your life (not necessarily with just one baby). You can lower your risk of having a heart attack or stroke after menopause by 10% if you nurse for at least one month.
7. **It can be a form of birth control, but don't rely on it exclusively** (unless you want a toddler and a newborn in the house!)

BOTTOM LINE: Breastfeeding is worth the effort it takes to learn how to do it.

Q. How long should I breastfeed my baby?

The American Academy of Pediatrics recommends breastfeeding for at least the first year of life. The latest statistics show that 83% of American babies go home from the hospital

ENCOURAGING BREASTFEEDING

How can both doctors and parents ensure that breastfeeding is successful? Here are the AAP's guidelines:

◆ Encourage "rooming-in" with your newborn at the hospital to learn baby's cues.
◆ Trained caregivers should formally evaluate breastfeeding (latch, position, etc) at least twice daily while newborns are at the hospital. (If that doesn't happen, speak up!)
◆ Supplements (water, sugar water, formula) should not be given to a breastfed newborn unless ordered by the baby's doctor for a medical reason.
◆ Pacifiers are discouraged until breastfeeding is going well.
◆ Breastfed babies should see their healthcare provider at three to five days of life and again at two weeks of age to assess breastfeeding.
◆ "Complementary foods" (solid food) should be introduced from four to six months of life.
◆ Babies should sleep in close proximity to their moms to encourage breastfeeding. (Note the word choices here—the AAP is not recommending a family bed).

breastfed. But only 58% are still breastfed at six months of life. The numbers are even lower for babies who are breastfed until one year of age. *(CDC)*

Q. If breast milk is recommended for the first year of life, why do most American families stop before then?

That's a great question. We'll give you general idea here and then more details throughout this chapter.

Most women stop nursing because breastfeeding can be a real pain (literally and figuratively) for the first couple of weeks. Some lack support to overcome the initial challenges. Others stop when they return to work, when they find it nearly impossible to balance their work-life and nursing-life.

Here are the five key reasons why moms stop nursing before their baby's first birthday and our solutions:

1 IT HURTS. *The Problem*: Breastfeeding is a learned process. It's not as natural as you might think. Babies know how to suck, and Mom's body knows how to make milk. But the technique of getting the baby latched on correctly requires a great deal of patience and sometimes *four* hands. Throw in a hormonal roller coaster after delivery and you'll understand why many women give up. Then comes **ENGORGEMENT**. This is what happens when the milk actually comes in. Your breasts may be more impressive than your neighbor's boob job. Your spouse will want to take pictures. *You* will wish that it is a bad dream and hope that your old breasts will be back when you wake up—engorgement often means tenderness, pain, sore nipples and more.

The Solution: Get professional help to learn how to get the baby latched on appropriately.

Know that engorgement will pass. And check out our troubleshooting guide later in this section.

2 **YOU'RE EXHAUSTED AND LACK SUPPORT.** *The Problem:* You are the only one who can feed your baby for the first few weeks while you establish your milk supply to meet your baby's demands. That means you never get a stretch of sleep longer than three hours at a time . . . at the same time you are recovering from childbirth.

The Solution: Sleep when your baby sleeps (don't try to do laundry or catch up on Instagram). After a few weeks, you can start pumping (expressing) your breast milk. Then your partner (and anyone else who is willing) can take a turn feeding your baby with a bottle of expressed breast milk. Put any other friends and family to work cooking dinner, changing diapers, and soothing your baby. And this will give you the freedom to concentrate on breastfeeding your baby.

3 **YOU DON'T HAVE ENOUGH MILK.** *The Problem:* It doesn't happen that often, but some women cannot produce enough milk to meet the demands of their baby. Trying to rev up mom's supply takes a lot of effort, medication, and persistence. And even then, the milk might not come in for some moms. The reasons: advanced maternal age (over 35), some types of breast surgery, or hormonal issues. Watching a hungry baby scream at the breast 24/7 can make any mom want to throw in the towel.

The Solution: You may be able to increase your milk supply by nursing often, pumping between nursing sessions, and taking medication to increase milk production. And remember, every ounce of breast milk counts—even if you don't breastfeed exclusively. Your baby still reaps the benefits from breast milk. See our troubleshooting guide to follow for details.

4 **YOU RETURN TO WORK.** *The Problem:* Working moms, in general, have trouble finding time to pump. To completely keep up with your baby's demands, you need to pump every three hours (nearly impossible, right?). But remember, pumping *some* breast milk is better than none at all. This is not an "all or nothing" situation.

The Solution: Figure out what works for you. Some moms can only pump once while at work, and continue to nurse while at home. Your body can adjust to many different feeding patterns . . . which means you can continue some level of breastfeeding even after you head back to work.

5 **YOUR BABY HAS A PROBLEM THAT MAKES BREASTFEEDING DIFFICULT.** *The Problem:* If your baby was born prematurely (before 37 weeks), has acid reflux (GERD), or a significant food allergy, it may be even more challenging to breastfeed successfully.

The Solution: Get professional help from a lactation consultant and your baby's doctor regarding pumping, supplementing, or eliminating foods in your own diet to accommodate for your baby's dietary issues. See the section on "Special Situations" later in this chapter for our tips.

Q. If I have trouble breastfeeding, whom should I turn to for help?

A poignant comment from one nursing mom we interviewed: "If everyone would just leave the baby and I alone, we could figure it out!" Truer words were never spoken. However, if

The Facts of Life—a.k.a. Science of Breastfeeding

Keep in mind these four tips on the "science" of nursing your baby:

◆ Breast milk production is a supply and demand phenomenon. Most women have no trouble making enough milk if the demand is there. Nursing at least eight times in 24 hours promotes a good supply.

◆ Colostrum, the first milk, is all your baby needs for the first few days of life. Mature milk, the high fat stuff, arrives when your baby needs it—around the fourth day of life.

◆ ALL babies are exhausted by the birth process and are not very interested in eating for the first 48 hours. They latch on, get cozy…and fall asleep after five minutes. This behavior will change (at almost the same moment you leave the hospital!)

◆ Babies are born with 10% extra baggage to carry them through the first few days of life. They will lose 5-10% of their birth weight—expect that. Do not think you are failing at breastfeeding because your baby is losing weight.

you are at wit's end, utilize your pediatrician and a lactation consultant. Lactation specialists (IBCLC's) are medical personnel certified to handle breastfeeding challenges. We suggest you ask your obstetrician or pediatrician for a recommendation. Lactation consultants who have an established relationship with your doctor are best. It is helpful to have everyone working towards the same goal: your success!

Q. What do I need to know about my baby's first few days of breastfeeding?

Let's break this down, day by day…

(Note: the rundown of breastfeeding for the entire first year is at the end of the breastfeeding section of this chapter.)

First Day of Life (0–24 hours old):

1. Nurse your baby for the first time within an hour or so of birth. They will be awake, alert, and interested.
2. At two hours of life, they will be exhausted and hard to arouse for several (three to four) hours. Don't get too worked up about trying to nurse right now. Take a nap yourself. Or, place your newborn skin to skin with you and relax together.
3. Frequency goal: six to eight feedings in the first 24 hours of life.
4. Your baby will probably fall asleep at the breast after a few minutes of nursing. An acceptable feeding session for today is five to ten minutes per breast.

Second Day of Life (24–48 hours old):

DR B'S OPINION

"Despite all these challenges, it is well worth the effort to make breastfeeding successful. Breastfeeding is like running a race, with the hardest hurdles up front. Many moms don't realize that they will be coasting the rest of the way if they just make it past the first mile."

BREASTFEEDING MOJO: LINDA'S TIPS

Before we delve into our breastfeeding tips, we'd like to give a special shout out to a special expert here at Baby 411: Linda Hill. Linda is a registered nurse and a certified lactation consultant (IBCLC). Linda and Dr. Brown have worked together for 20 years. We appreciate her sharing her thoughts and advice. Look for "Linda's Tips" throughout this chapter.

1. Today's goal is working on your technique. It may take a second set of hands to position the baby while you hold your breast. You will fly solo eventually. See tips to survive the first two weeks later in this chapter.
2. Frequency goal: eight feedings in 24 hours. Do not let your baby sleep more than three hours during the day or four hours at night or you will have trouble meeting this goal.
3. Length of feedings goal: at least five to ten minutes per breast. Do not take baby off the breast at ten minutes if they are still actively sucking.
4. If your nipples are cracked and bleeding, you need help with your technique.

Third Day of Life (48–72 hours old):
1. Your baby is suddenly awake and sometimes, insatiable. You will likely have a VERY LONG night. As long as your baby has lost less than 10% of their birth weight (and has no other risk factors—see below), keep your chin up and resist the temptation to supplement with formula. Your baby's demand is precisely what your body needs to create the supply of milk.
2. Make sure your technique is okay and you are comfortable when your baby latches on.
3. Frequency goal: eight feedings in 24 hours (it should be an easy goal to reach today!)
4. Length of feedings goal: at least ten minutes per breast.
5. You may feel that your baby is on your breast non-stop. If that is the case and your nipples are sore, take a break if you have nursed for more than 45 minutes. Let someone else have a chance to soothe your baby. (Letting baby suck on someone's finger may be helpful.)

Fourth Day of Life (72–96 hours old):
1. Hello milk! There is usually little question of whether or not your milk has arrived. How will you know? Your breasts will be much larger, heavier, and tender. You should feel full before you nurse, and softer after you nurse. You should also see milk when you burp your baby (and sometimes when you shower). The change in your baby's poop will also tell you the milkman has arrived. See the section Newborn Poop in Chapter 8 "The Other End" for more.
2. If your breasts are rock hard and your areola (the darker colored ring around your nipple) are flattened against them, you are officially engorged. This lasts for a day or two. See troubleshooting tips below.
3. Frequency goal: eight feedings in 24 hours. Do not let your baby sleep for more than 3.5 hours during the day or a four hour stretch at night.

LIQUIDS

4.   Length of feedings goal: at least ten to 15 minutes per breast. Once your milk supply is well established (around four weeks of life), some women prefer to nurse with one breast per feeding. For now, use both at each feeding as it stimulates your milk production.

NEW PARENT 411: BREASTFEEDING LINGO

Breastfeeding has a language all its own. Here is a quick overview:

◆ **Colostrum.** The first milk that your breasts produce. Some women start making (and leaking) it before the baby is even born. It is a high-protein drink, filled with mom's antibodies that boost the immunity of a newborn. It has fewer calories than mature milk because of a lower fat content.

◆ **Mature Milk.** The milk that arrives on the third or fourth day after birth. It is about 50% fat.

◆ **Foremilk.** The milk that comes out in the first several minutes of feeding. In general, it contains slightly less fat. Babies who "snack" end up getting mostly foremilk, leading to more frequent feedings (and possibly, fussiness).

◆ **Hindmilk.** The milk that comes out in the later part of a feeding. It is slightly higher in fat than foremilk. Babies who drain a whole breast in a feeding tend to be more satisfied, for good reason.

◆ **Let down.** When your milk rushes into the milk ducts as your baby suckles or as you pump. Most women feel this "let-down."

◆ **Engorgement.** In the first days when you make mature milk, your breasts may feel full, tender, lumpy, and hard.

◆ **Plugged ducts.** An area of the breast has obstructed milk flow, creating a hard, tender lumpy area. These areas are at risk of getting infected (mastitis—ouch!). See tips below for more info.

◆ **Inverted nipples.** Your nipples have an indentation in the center. It can make it more difficult for your baby to latch on.

◆ **Flat nipples.** Your nipples are flush against your breast tissue. Like inverted nipples, flat nipples can make it difficult for baby to latch.

◆ **Breast shells.** Plastic devices that pull out inverted nipples. They can also be worn to protect sore nipples from rubbing against your bra.

◆ **Nipple shields.** Plastic devices that protect sore or cracked nipples. These are also used for moms with flat or inverted nipples. Unfortunately, they can sometimes limit the amount of milk that flows to the baby's mouth.

◆ **Lanolin.** A thick emollient that helps heal cracked nipples. Brand names: Lansinoh, Pur-lan. Available at breastfeeding boutiques and even Wal-Mart.

◆ **Compression.** Squeezing breast tissue during nursing to improve milk flow and encourage baby to drink. It can also be done while pumping to express more milk.

◆ **Paced Bottle Feeding.** Holding a baby upright and holding a bottle of expressed breast milk/formula horizontally to simulate a feeding session at the breast. This technique makes baby less frustrated when they resume nursing.

You should be on your way now. Your baby should be gaining about an ounce a day.

Days 5–14

1. Breastfed newborns eat about every 2-3 hours (or 8-12 times) in a 24-hour day. They may cluster feed as often as every 90 minutes (that's from the beginning of one feeding to the beginning of the next). They usually eat about 2-3 ounces at each feeding.
2. Babies who try to nurse more frequently than every 90 minutes are either nursing for comfort or not getting enough milk. So, if it has been less than 90 minutes since the beginning of the last feeding, try using your finger to let them suck. Your breasts will thank you.
3. If your baby is truly nursing non-stop, go get your baby weighed. Make sure you have enough milk supply to meet your baby's demand.
4. On the other hand, do not let your baby go for more than 3.5 hours during the day or more than 4 hours at night without nursing. Frequent feedings improve your milk production and give your baby what they need to grow.

Two Weeks

If your full term baby is at or above birth weight at their check up, you have my blessing to let your baby sleep as long as they want at night.

The One Month Mark

Your baby should be more efficient at feeding sessions. And nursing is (hopefully!) on auto-pilot.

NEW PARENT 411: ANXIETY HEADING HOME

You will go home from the hospital with a shrinking baby and no "mature" milk in your breasts. Understandably, this often creates great anxiety for new parents. Your baby will do just fine with colostrum as long as your breast milk comes in around the fourth day. The circumstances that interfere with this perfect plan are:

1. Jaundice (elevated bilirubin).
2. Prematurity or small gestational age (small for dates).
3. Loss of more than 10% of birth weight.
4. Delay in milk's arrival.

The AAP recommends follow-up appointments for babies at the third to fifth day of life to make sure things are heading in the right direction.

It's a good idea to keep a breastfeeding diary (see our handy two week survival guide earlier in Chapter 1) that tracks both feeding and elimination for the first two weeks. Or try an app like Glow Baby for iPhone or Android. If the milk is going in, it will come out the other end. If you are still uncertain of how things are going, schedule an appointment!

See the section called The Big Picture: Breastfeeding for the First Year, later in this chapter for a nice summary of what lies ahead this year.

Helpful Hints

◆ When you are told that babies feed every two to three hours, time is measured from the BEGINNING of one feeding until the beginning of the next. If the feeding session itself lasts 45 minutes or an hour, that may leave less than an hour before it's time to nurse again.

◆ Your goal is to nurse at least EIGHT TIMES a day. This may be every two to three hours or

TOP 10 SURVIVAL TIPS FOR THE FIRST TWO WEEKS

And now, from the home office here in Austin, TX, our top 10 list of advice for breastfeeding success in the first two weeks:

1. Make sure your baby is latched on to your areola and not just the tip of your nipple.
2. If it hurts for more than a few seconds, take your baby off your breast and reposition them. Do not be a martyr.
3. If the position you are using is not working, try another one. See more tips on positions in this chapter.
4. Have a spouse or willing volunteer get the baby's open mouth to your breast while you hold your breast. Have this person pull down your baby's chin gently with their finger.
5. Ask for a nipple shield (a plastic covering with a hole) if your nipples are too tender or cracked to nurse comfortably. This is a controversial option because the volume of fluid coming to baby is reduced. But it may make the difference for some women if used for a day or two. If you choose this option, schedule a follow-up appointment with a lactation consultant.
6. One word: LANOLIN. Various brands of this ointment (such as Lansinoh) are available. Any product with this active ingredient provides comfort to healing nipples. (It's also great for baby's bad diaper rashes.) If your nipples are really in dire straits, you can buy a wound dressing (brand names: Elastogel, Comfort Gel Pads, or Soothies Gel Pads). Your doctor can also prescribe an antibiotic cream if necessary.
7. Use both breasts during each feeding to stimulate milk production. Once your milk supply is established at four weeks, it is fine to nurse on one breast per feeding if your baby consistently refuses the second breast and is gaining weight. One exception: veteran moms may have plenty of milk to accomplish this sooner.
8. Sleep when your baby sleeps. Your baby should not sleep more than a four-hour stretch in the first two weeks.
9. Don't be afraid to ask for help.
10. Don't give up. The first two weeks can be rough, but then it will all be worth it!

LIQUIDS

? ?

it may be a series of cluster feedings every 90 minutes, followed by a four-hour stretch. As long as the number of feedings add up to eight in a 24-hour period, it is fine. And, some babies nurse 11-13 times a day. Look at your baby and not at the clock.

◆ Remember this word: COMPRESSION. Just because your baby is at the breast, it does not mean they are drinking. If your baby seems to be doing more sleeping than swallowing, try the following trick. Encircle your breast with your hand and gently squeeze the breast tissue with your thumb. Do not stroke or massage the tissue, just squeeze and hold it down briefly. It gets the colostrum/milk flowing and will encourage your baby to have a drink.

Old Wives Tale
"My doctor told me I didn't have enough milk."

The truth: Fifty years ago, doctors thought breast milk was supposed to come in immediately after birth—and hence when it didn't appear in day one or two, panic bells went off. We now know that it is Nature's Way to have colostrum first and mature milk later. This is one of the reasons why our grandmothers did not breastfeed.

BOTTOM LINE: Be prepared for the 72 hour Colostrum Zone. Your mature milk will arrive soon enough.

RED FLAGS
Check in with your baby's doctor if:
1. You don't have a dramatic change in your breasts by the fifth day of life.
2. You don't hear your baby swallowing ("cuh" sound) when they are at the breast.
3. Your baby's poops have not changed from black tar (meconium) to a greenish-yellowish color by the fourth day.
4. Your baby does not have at least four wet diapers on the fourth day.
5. Your baby is sleepy and hard to arouse for feedings.
6. Your baby is nursing non-stop.

Q. Is it okay for me to take pain medication when I am nursing?

Yes.

The medications that your OB prescribes for discomfort after delivery are safe to take while you are breastfeeding. It's true that a tiny amount of these medicines end up in your breast milk, so it's important to watch your baby for extreme lethargy (for example, not waking up for feedings).

Breastfeeding positions

◆ *Cradle hold:* Baby's head rests on Mom's forearm with their belly next to Mom's (that is, left arm holding baby for feeding at the left breast).

◆ *Football hold:* Baby's head rests on Mom's hand with their body coming underneath Mom's armpit. (Good for after a C-section, large breasted moms, preemies, and twins.)

◆ *Side-lying:* Baby and Mom lie on their sides and face each other, tummy to tummy. (Popular at night feedings) (*Danner*)

◆ *Cross cradle hold (not pictured):* The baby's neck and upper back are supported by the opposing hand (that is, left hand cradles the baby's head to the right breast and right hand holds right breast). This is a good position to start with as it gives you more control. When the latch is comfortable, you can switch to the cradle hold.

Linda's Tips: Positioning

- ◆ Mom should be comfortable with arms and back supported.
- ◆ Mom should not lean over the baby. Instead, use a breastfeeding pillow—a firm pillow that wraps around Mom's waist and allows baby to rest supported. Linda's favorite brand is called (don't laugh at the name) My Brest Friend because it provides more support than the competing brands on the market.
- ◆ Baby should directly face the breast without having to turn their head.
- ◆ Baby's stomach should be pulled in close to Mom, tummy to tummy. Using a footstool may be helpful to bring baby closer to mom.
- ◆ Baby's ear, shoulder, and hip should be in a straight line.

The other critical issue is making sure your baby's bottom lip latches onto the pigmented area (areola) and not at the base of the nipple.

Linda's Tips for a comfortable latch

- ◆ Position your baby at the breast so that their nose is directly across from your nipple.
- ◆ Aim your nipple up with your thumb so that it is pointing to the roof of their mouth when opened.
- ◆ Touch their lips with your breast and they will look up to the nipple as your baby opens their mouth.
- ◆ Have their bottom lip latch onto the pigmented tissue (areola) beneath the nipple. Push your nipple into their mouth as you pull your baby into you.
- ◆ If it hurts more than 10-20 seconds beyond the initial latch, break the suction seal (see below), reposition, and try again. DO NOT NURSE IF IT HURTS BEYOND THE INITIAL LATCH. It's normal to feel a tugging sensation. It's not normal to feel pinching, burning, or stinging. You are not doing yourself or your baby a favor by suffering. Pain means you don't have a good latch—or you are paying for previous damage you've already done.
- ◆ You should hear gulping ("cuh") noises. Take your baby off if you hear a clicking sound.
- ◆ Signs of a bad latch: Your nipple looks like a tube of lipstick or you see a white line across the nipple that eventually leads to cracks, bleeds, and scabs.

breastfeeding

LIQUIDS

? ?

 Helpful Hint

To take your baby off of your nipple without causing excruciating pain, place one of your fingers into the corner of their mouth and break the suction seal. If the seal doesn't break, slip your finger deeper into their mouth to relax the jaw.

Insider Secret

We recommend two great online resources for evidence-based breastfeeding help:

◆ Ibconline.ca: created by Dr. Jack Newman, Canadian pediatrician/lactation consultant.
◆ Kellymom.com: created by Kelly Bonyata, BS, IBCLC, American certified lactation consultant.

Infant Feeding Behaviors

Newborns can be divided into five types of feeding styles. Identifying what type your baby is may help you understand how to help him feed better. The types listed below were characterized by a study done in the 1950's, but are still relevant today:

1. **The Barracuda.** This little one attacks the breast and gets down to business. Mom's nipples sometimes pay the price for this style in the beginning weeks.
2. **The Excited Ineffective.** Yes, this is the baby who is so excited to eat that they lose their latch. Calming, then reattempting to latch helps until baby figures out the routine.
3. **The Procrastinator.** The baby who waits until the milk lets down to bother with eating. There is no rush. Be patient and keep trying.
4. **The Gourmet.** They must mouth the nipple, have a taste test, then begin the meal. Again, there is no need to rush. Let them do their thing.
5. **The Rester** (similar to a cow who grazes). They take their own sweet time. This baby eats for a few minutes, rests, then continues. They will eventually finish the meal and eat well but you can encourage them by rubbing their back or head. (*Barnes*)

Q. Is it okay to supplement with formula until my mature milk comes in?

Yes, it's okay, but it's usually not necessary.

Mother Nature has an elaborate plan for babies and breast milk. Newborns arrive with some extra nutritional baggage to carry them through the first few days of life. That's good because they'd rather sleep than eat. It's also good because your body is making early milk (**COLOSTRUM**) that is antibody-rich, but calorie-poor (it has fewer calories in it than mature milk, which shows up around day three or four).

In fact, we pediatricians expect most newborns to *lose* about 10% of their birth weight by the third or fourth day. That's supposed to happen.

At about 48 hours of life (at precisely the moment most of you are heading home from the hospital), your baby suddenly says, "Hey, I'm starving, what have you got to eat around here?!" They'll act completely differently than the first two days and want to nurse non-stop. That demand drives your milk supply up. Although that can be pretty nerve-wracking for about 24 hours or so, it's what gets your milk production going.

BOTTOM LINE: You don't need to tinker with Mother Nature's grand scheme by offering formula. Unless there is a medical reason to give formula (see below), let nature take its course.

Top 6 reasons why you SHOULD supplement with formula

Women who are certain they want to breastfeed are often devastated if they need to temporarily supplement with formula.

The key point to remember: you are not a failure. And it isn't the end of the world. There are some key medical reasons why it's necessary. And offering formula for a short time won't sabotage breastfeeding success.

1 PREMATURE NEWBORN. If your baby is born between 24 to 34 weeks gestation, they probably won't be able to breastfeed initially. Depending on how premature your baby is, they might not even eat by mouth at first. You'll need to start pumping to stimulate your milk production. When your baby can get their nutrition by mouth, they can either drink your pumped (expressed) breast milk through a feeding tube or take it from a bottle. Most likely, they'll also need some formula made especially for premature babies to fulfill their nutritional needs.

2 LATE PRETERM NEWBORN. Babies born between 34 to 36 6/7 weeks gestation tend to be very sleepy, lazy, and inept at efficient suckling at the breast. So, until your baby gets the hang of it, you may need to offer the breast and then some pumped breast milk in a bottle after each nursing session to fulfill their nutritional needs. If you don't have enough milk, formula will work. You can nurse exclusively once your baby's skill and energy level improves, they are gaining weight appropriately and you are making at least 3 oz. of milk combined from both breasts for each feeding. This is usually for a week or two, or until your baby reaches the day they were *supposed* to deliver.

Linda's Tip: In the first month, be sure to pump for ten minutes every time you "top your baby off with a bottle." This rule applies even if you already breastfed and even if nothing is coming out. It's very important for the stimulation to equal the baby's demand when you are establishing your milk supply.

3 LOW BLOOD SUGAR (HYPOGLYCEMIA). Some newborns have trouble maintaining an adequate blood sugar level. Low blood sugar can become a vicious cycle. Babies with low blood sugars lack the energy to eat, which leads to persistently low blood sugar. Besides its negative impact on feeding, sustained low blood sugars can lead to brain injury and seizures. Hence, the temporary solution is to offer sugar gel in addition to nursing until your baby maintains normal blood sugar levels. For a full term baby, born between 37 to 40 weeks, this may be for a feeding or two, or a day or two at most.

4 EXCESSIVE WEIGHT LOSS. A newborn that loses more than 10% of their birth weight usually needs both breast milk and formula until they start to gain weight. As we mentioned earlier, it is normal and expected for your baby to lose 10% of their weight at birth. But more than 10% means that your baby is dehydrated. Dehydrated babies are not happy babies. They lack energy to eat (another vicious cycle) and so they lose more weight, end up with low blood sugar, and develop jaundice (more on this next). Don't let your baby become a martyr in the name of breastfeeding. If they are dehydrated and your mature milk hasn't arrived yet, supplement with formula. It prevents them from having other medical issues. Remember, this is temporary until your baby gains weight and your mature milk is plentiful enough.

5 SIGNIFICANT JAUNDICE. Let's talk about poop for a minute. Humans clear out a waste product (called **BILIRUBIN**) in their poop. Bilirubin has a yellow pigment to it. In the first few days of life, a newborn doesn't clear out much bilirubin because their liver (which breaks it down) doesn't function at 100% and they aren't pooping very much (since they aren't eating much). As a result, all newborns temporarily collect some bilirubin in their skin, causing a yellowish glow (called *physiologic jaundice*). This resolves on its own around three to five days of life once they eat a lot, poop a lot, and have fully functioning livers.

For a variety of reasons, some newborns get significantly jaundiced. If there is more bilirubin than the skin can handle, it collects in the brain and can cause permanent brain damage (called *bilirubin induced neurologic dysfunction or BIND*). It goes without saying that everyone wants to avoid this! There are several ways to prevent BIND, but the first and simplest thing to do is to get a newborn to eat and poop more. The more baby eats, the more baby poops, the more they get rid of their bilirubin load. For a breastfed baby, that means supplementing with formula for a few days.

Once you see the poop turn from black to dark green to yellow (that yellow pigmented bilirubin makes it change color) and your mature breast milk is in, the bilirubin levels will drop and you'll be able to resume nursing exclusively.

6 MATERNAL REASON. Sometimes a mom intends to nurse, but encounters a medical problem that prevents nursing at first. Those problems include: postpartum bleeding, high blood pressure, etc. If this happens to you, don't let it get you down. Nurse as much as your OB doctor allows and let your baby have some formula until you have recuperated. Your baby will be fine. You need to be healthy to be able to make milk. If you can, pump to protect your milk supply.

Insider Secret

Here is another important breastfeeding term: PACED BOTTLE FEEDING. If you have to supplement with expressed breast milk or formula, hold your baby in an *upright* position and hold the bottle in a *horizontal* position. This position forces the baby to work a little bit to get the milk, more like the flow at the breast. Most people instinctively recline the baby and tilt the bottle, allowing the baby to chug the milk. If your baby chugs breast milk or formula with a bottle, they are likely to become very impatient when they go back to the breast.

LIQUIDS

Top 3 reasons why women end up supplementing (but don't need to)

◆ **Exhaustion.** Delivering a baby is an exhausting experience. After many hours of labor, you'll just want someone to tuck you in for a long night's sleep. No such luck for a breastfeeding mom. You might get about four to five hours of sleep after delivery (the "honeymoon" period while your exhausted newborn sleeps too). Then, the party is over. You'll need to feed your baby at least EIGHT times every 24 hours—yes, that's every three hours on average.

To get your milk production up to speed, you shouldn't go any longer than four hours between feedings. With that pace, it's no wonder new parents want to give bottle of formula and get some shut-eye. If this is the deal breaker for whether or not you will continue breastfeeding, okay, take a break. But we don't recommend it. Once you start on this road, you're more likely to give up nursing altogether. If you can get through these early days, we promise it gets easier!

breastfeeding

THE LOW DOWN ON BREAST PUMPS

You can rent a hospital grade pump, purchase an electric pump, or purchase a manual pump. Insurance companies usually cover the cost of a breast pump. A smart move: call your insurance company before you deliver so you can get your pump, familiarize yourself with it, wash the parts and be ready to go.

A popular model is the Spectra S2 Pump, available at large retail stores for about $150. Nursing moms report that it is quieter, more efficient, and more comfortable than other more expensive pumps. And, good news, many insurance companies cover the cost for this particular pump.

Alternatively, you can also rent a pump when you go home from the hospital. Renting lets you figure out whether you need a pump long term, without making a financial commitment. Most hospitals offer rentals.

Moms who are returning to work but still want to pump have two options: rent a pump for an extended period of time or buy a pump. Either way we recommend a professional-grade dual electric pump. You can control the speed and pressure, which less expensive models don't allow. For working moms, efficiency is key. You can pump both breasts simultaneously in 15 minutes. A Medela rental pump will cost $45-75 per month to rent. It pumps 50 cycles per minute (baby sucks about 60 times/minute) at a comfortable pressure.

Insider tip: Invest in a $15 Haakaa milk collector/manual breast pump. It passively collects let down or leaking milk on the non-nursing breast and provides a gentle suction to draw excess milk from the breast. It's cheap and easy peasy.

FYI: For an in-depth discussion on buying a breast pump (including brand name reviews) as well as the best milk storage options, check out our other book *Baby Bargains* (see back of this book for details).

◆ *Pain.* If you start off with poor technique, each breastfeeding session is incredibly painful. The thought of bringing the baby to the breast can bring some moms to tears. Hopefully, our tips will prevent this situation from happening. But if you find yourself in this place and need to take a break from nursing for a few feedings or 24 hours until your nipples can heal, so be it. You need to continue removing milk from your breasts for every feeding, though. Pump and offer that expressed milk to your little one. You can also temporarily use nipple shields while nursing. You are more likely to continue nursing if you can forge ahead (with proper technique going forward, of course).

◆   *Fear.* Parents mistakenly fear that their baby is not getting enough to eat when they are producing early milk (**COLOSTRUM**). They see their baby losing weight and get worried. Don't worry! If your baby has no medical issues and your pediatrician does not feel you need to supplement with formula, you don't need to supplement with formula! If you start supplementing when you don't need to, your baby will fill up. You need baby's hunger drive to get your breast milk production going. Don't mess with Mother Nature.

Nursing: Concerns & Questions

At the two-week mark, nursing should be fairly routine and comfortable (if not, read the next section on troubleshooting). Take a look at the Big Picture summary at the end of this section to see how your baby begins to take larger quantities of breast milk at each feeding. But in general, expect that your baby will continue to eat about every two to three hours during the day and start eating less often (and sleeping more) at night after the first two months of life. Here are some common breastfeeding concerns and questions.

Q. Can my baby use a pacifier if I am nursing?

Yes. Babies are soothed by sucking. In the first two months of life, sucking on a pacifier may be the only thing that reliably settles your baby. Despite what you may hear, binkies and breastfeeding can mix.

Experts used to believe that pacifiers shortened the length of time that moms continued to nurse. So it was almost taboo to offer a binky to a breastfed baby. Research suggests otherwise. Pacifiers don't make a baby or mom stop breastfeeding. Parents who use a binky choose to discontinue nursing for a variety of other reasons. (*O'Connor*)

In our opinion, breastfeeding and pacifiers are not mutually exclusive—pacifiers are NOT evil. But it is wise to wait on introducing a pacifier until your baby is a confident breastfeeder (between one and four weeks old) because babies suck pacifiers differently than the breast. Plus, frequent suckling at the breast helps establish mom's milk supply in the early weeks.

We like the Philips Avent Soothie brand (green with a long nipple) as it is more similar to the human nipple than other brands. A reasonable alternative to the pacifier is a parent's finger. The other obvious alternative is to offer your breast for comfort nursing. This may or may not be for you.

Note: as we'll discuss in the section on Sleep Safety Tips in Chapter 9, Sleep, pacifiers have been shown to reduce the risk of SIDS in babies under six months.

LIQUIDS

BOTTOM LINE

If you opt to use a pacifier, we suggest getting it out of your baby's life by six months of age when they no longer need to be soothed by sucking. For more information, see the section on Soothing a New Baby in Chapter 11, "Discipline."

Q. My baby prefers one of my breasts to the other. Is that ok?

Yes. Why does this happen? One of your breasts may produce more milk than the other, flow differently or be easier to latch onto. And your baby will figure that out and may develop a preference for the better-producing breast. Some babies will even refuse the breast that has slower flow or less volume.

If your baby doesn't get too frustrated, offer the slower flow breast first because they will nurse more aggressively at the beginning and that helps increase your supply. When baby becomes frustrated, switch to the other breast. And try pumping the lower-producing breast after nursing to improve production.

No worries if your baby completely refuses one breast. It's possible to make enough milk from one breast to completely satisfy your baby. (I've even had a patient whose mom had a mastectomy and successfully nursed on the remaining breast!). Nutrition is not the issue. You will just start to look rather lopsided if you nurse on only one side!

Q. My baby fills up after taking just one breast. Can I nurse alternate breasts at each nursing session?

Yes. Once breastfeeding is well established and your milk supply is stable, it's fine to alternate breasts for each feeding. For first time moms, that's about 3-4 weeks after delivery. For seasoned moms, their milk supply is fairly stable after two weeks.

Insider Tip

Some moms place a safety pin on the bra cup of the breast they used at the last feeding. (Sleep deprivation takes a toll on the memory!)

Q. I am exhausted after several weeks of every-two-hour nursing sessions 24/7. Will I get more sleep if I supplement with formula?

Nope. A recent study compared a mother's level of sleep deprivation (and ability to function) after living with a newborn (between 2–12 weeks old) to what the baby ate—exclusively breast milk, exclusively formula, or a combination of breast milk and formula. The answer? There was absolutely no statistical difference . . . all the mothers were walking zombies! (*Montgomery-Downs*)

Although what you feed your baby doesn't make a bit of difference, you are certainly entitled to a few hours of uninterrupted shut-eye for your physical and mental health. After 2–4 weeks, you can pump (express) some breast milk and let your partner take a turn doing an evening feeding. Getting a four or five hour stretch of sleep will feel like an amazing night's sleep!

LIQUIDS

? ?

INSIDER SECRETS: TOP 8 BREASTFEEDING

Sure, you know that breastfeeding is best for your baby . . . but if something goes wrong? Don't give up! Here are the top eight breastfeeding problems and how to solve them.

PROBLEM	SOLUTIONS
#1 Underproduction ◆ *Newborn*: less than three poops a day by Day 3 of life, poop not yellow/seedy by Day 5 of life, less than six wet diapers a day by Day 4 of life, no weight gain by Day 5 of life, birth weight not regained by Day 14. ◆ *Day 5-4 Months:* weight gain less than 5 oz/week. ◆ *4 Months-1 Year*: weight gain less than 3 oz/week.	◆ *Discuss options to increase milk production with healthcare provider* ◆ *After nursing, feed baby with expressed breast milk or formula (see Paced Bottle Feeding earlier in this chapter)* ◆ *Check baby's ability to get milk at the breast (milk transfer) with a certified lactation consultant.*
#2 Overproduction ◆ *Baby*: coughs or chokes while nursing, excessive weight gain, green frothy poops. ◆ *Mom*: always feels full, milk shoots out forcefully.	◆ *Nurse on one breast per feeding and return to that same breast if baby wants to nurse within two hours.* ◆ *Manually express, pump off for a minute, or use a Haakaa to collect milk before having the baby latch on (don't overdo it, or you will have even more milk production!)* ◆ *Lean back while nursing to reduce the flow.*
#3 Engorgement ◆ *Baby*: has trouble latching on. ◆ *Mom*: has severe fullness and pain, nipples are flattened.	◆ *Increase milk removal by nursing more often or pumping.* ◆ *Cold packs for 10-15 minutes after feedings.* ◆ *Ibuprofen.* ◆ *Should get better in 1-2 days, if not, visit a lactation consultant.*
#4 Nipple Pain ◆ *Mom*: nipples/areola are red, cracked or bleeding, look like a tube of lipstick after nursing, look blanched after nursing, or have blebs (white cysts).	◆ *Check baby's mouth and chin (tongue tie or a recessed chin can cause a latch problem).* ◆ *Have a lactation professional assess how baby is latching on.* ◆ *Have a lactation professional assess mom for a nipple infection.*

LIQUIDS

PROBLEMS . . . . . . AND SOLUTIONS!

#5 Nipple Bacterial Infection
◆ *Mom*: nipples are cracked, painful during latching, draining pus or has golden crust.

◆ *Mom's doctor can prescribe an antibiotic cream until nipples are healed.*

#6 Plugged Duct
◆ *Mom*: localized area of a breast is painful, red, and tender usually before nursing, decreased milk production, fever free or temperature below 101.3F.

◆ *Breastfeed frequently, always starting on the affected breast.*
◆ *Position baby with chin pointing towards the affected area.*
◆ *Massage the area while nursing or pumping. Apply heat before and ice after feedings.*
◆ *See a lactation consultant for more help.*

#7 Mastitis
◆ *Mom*: Fever, body aches, redness or red streak on breast(s), decreased milk production

◆ *Milk is safe to use. Nurse frequently on the affected breast.*
◆ *Use a hot pack on the breast for four minutes before each feeding (if breast is not feeling hot).*
◆ *Alternatively, if the breast feels hot, use ice pack before and after feedings.*
◆ *Mom's doctor can prescribe an oral antibiotic that's ok to use while nursing.*
◆ *Mom can take probiotics while taking antibiotics to prevent a yeast infection.*

#8 Yeast infection
◆ *Baby*: may be symptom free, or may have white adherent plaques on the tongue, inside of cheek, inner lip, and gum line.
◆ *Mom*: may be symptom free or may have sharp/shooting/burning pain while nursing, shiny/red areola, cracked/ easily bleeding nipples, painful or itchy nipples/breasts throughout the day.

◆ *Mom and baby should be treated for infection, even if only one party has symptoms.*
◆ *Baby: doctor can prescribe oral antifungal medication.*
◆ *Mom: can use over-the-counter antifungal cream on nipples or doctor can prescribe oral antifungal if pain is deep. Take probiotic supplement.*
◆ *Sterilize all pacifiers, teething toys, pump parts, breast shells, bottle nipples daily.*
◆ *Good hand washing before and after breastfeeding. (West)*

This chart is adapted with permission from Physician's Breastfeeding Triage Tool Kit, developed by Diana West, IBCLC, for International Lactation Consultant Association, Copyright 2007.

breastfeeding

DR B'S OPINION

"Babies will get what they need from breast milk, at the expense of Mom's body. I recommend continuing your prenatal vitamins if you are nursing."

Q. My four month old still nurses every two to three hours at night. Is this really necessary or is it just a habit?

Four-month old babies who were born full-term, don't have acid reflux (GERD), and are gaining weight appropriately should be able to sleep at least six hours without needing to eat. Five-month olds can go at least nine hours. And six-month olds can go up to twelve hours! Bottom line: your baby should have at least one, long sleep stretch a night. Then it may be mealtime every two to three hours after that. If our baby awakens after six hours, asks to eat and actually EATS, then assume they are hungry and continue to follow their cues.

But if they fuss and fall asleep at the breast without actually eating much, that is your clue that they don't really need to be fed. Next time just try patting them back to sleep. That will help begin the process of lengthening that "long stretch" of sleep.

However, even if your baby is sleeping longer, you may have to get up and pump. Some moms need to pump after six hours, otherwise their milk supply vanishes. Moms who struggle to make enough milk often have to follow this rule: *aim for at least six to eight stimulations a day (whether pumping or breastfeeding) and take no longer than one six hour break of no stimulation.*

Reality Check

Babies continue to eat about every two to three hours during the day for a very long time. Even preschoolers eat three meals and two snacks a day (eating about every three hours). Do not try to increase the time interval between meals during the day—just aim for spacing them out at night.

Q. I need to leave my baby for a few days. Do you have any tips?

Leaving your nursing baby can be anxiety producing for both mom and baby. Some ideas to make life easier are:

- ◆ Start stockpiling expressed breast milk in the freezer a few weeks before the trip. Try pumping after feedings as often as you can.
- ◆ Take an electric breast pump and a hand held one if you have a long flight.
- ◆ Offer breast milk in a bottle once daily before your travel begins.
- ◆ Take a picture of baby with you to inspire you to let down.
- ◆ Leave your slept-in nightie or another clothing item with your scent on it for your baby.
- ◆ Know that your baby will be just fine while you are away and happy to see you when you return.

Linda's tip: Fresh breast milk is always better for your baby than frozen. Freezing/warming destroys certain properties in your milk like some vitamins and antibodies. So, while this thawed breast milk is still better for your baby than formula, it is better to pump for the next day's supply

---

DIETARY RESTRICTIONS FOR CERTAIN CIRCUMSTANCES

Two and a half percent of all newborns have a hypersensitivity to cow's milk. Occasionally, babies with a milk allergy can have problems if their breastfeeding moms have milk products in their diet (see "I Give Up" story later in this chapter). For more information on food allergies, see Chapter 7, Solid Nutrition. (*Sampson*)

---

and only have an emergency stash of frozen milk in the freezer. If you are going to be away from your baby for a few days, then stockpiling in the freezer is the way to go!

Trouble Shooting

When breastfeeding goes wrong, these are the usual suspects:

- ◆ **Underproduction (low milk supply) or insufficient milk transfer to the baby.**
- ◆ **Overproduction.**
- ◆ **Engorgement.**
- ◆ **Nipple pain.**
- ◆ **Nipple bacterial infection.**
- ◆ **Plugged duct.**
- ◆ **Mastitis.**
- ◆ **Yeast overgrowth/infection.**

Here is our discussion on these problems and solutions in full detail. See the handy summary table of survival tips earlier in this chapter.

UNDERPRODUCTION (LOW MILK SUPPLY) OR INSUFFICIENT MILK TRANSFER TO THE BABY.

Q. My milk supply is low. Can I do anything to improve my production?

Milk supply is based on demand. So if your baby is not stimulating you enough (premature babies and late preterm infants are often at fault for this), use a breast pump to rev up the supply. Pump a few minutes after each feeding session.

And yes, some women do not make enough breast milk to feed their baby. Here are some suggestions to pump up the volume:

1. Try pumping with a high-efficiency breast pump AFTER nursing sessions. An empty breast signals the body to make more milk.
2. Eat and sleep more. Your milk production depends on you taking good care of yourself.
3. Try eating a combo carbohydrate/protein snack just before or during nursing. This increases your prolactin hormone level, which in turn, increases milk supply.
4. Try herbal supplements. There are several popular herbs that may improve milk sup-

ply (the official term is 'galactogogues') although current studies show mixed results. More on herbs below.

5. Power Pump. Once or twice a day, try to pump for 10 minutes, rest for 10 minutes, pump for 10 minutes, rest for 10 minutes, and pump once more for 10 minutes.

Herbs are not regulated by the FDA, even if they are being used for medicinal purposes. So, if you buy a random supplement it is hard to know what quality or quantity of herb you are actually taking.

With those caveats, many lactation consultants recommend trying malunggay (derived from the Moringa oleifera plant), blessed thistle, fennel, goat's rue, and nettle leaf. Note: malunggay can cause blood sugar to drop so diabetic nursing moms should consult with their doctor before use. *(Bazzano 2016)*

Our lactation consultant advisors for this book recommend these trusted herbalists who pride themselves on quality products and sourcing: Motherlove.com, Golacta.com, and Legendairymilk.com.

Linda's tip For Low Milk Supply: It's important to do these suggestions to give your body the best possible opportunity to increase milk production. I recommend moms try all of the above for at least a couple of weeks. If you see very little improvement, you probably have *insufficient glandular tissue* or IGT. Your breasts must have enough glandular tissue to make milk and some women simply do not have enough tissue. Do not beat yourself up about it! You tried everything. Everyone is going to be okay. Do what you can for as long as you can as breastmilk is "medicine" that your baby cannot get in infant formula. Remember, it doesn't have to be all or nothing. Even just an ounce or two of breastmilk a day is helpful. But if nursing/pumping is causing you emotional stress, it is time to stop.

Q. My pediatrician thinks there is a milk transfer issue. What does this mean?

Simply put, you are making plenty of milk but the baby is not effectively getting it from the breast. Sometimes the problem lies with the baby, and not with the mother. This is called *insufficient milk transfer*. This may happen with late preterm babies, babies with medical issues (for example: heart, neurologic problems, etc.), and babies with mouth abnormalities like a

**DR B'S OPINION:
TRAINED NIGHT FEEDERS**

Some parents opt for a more relaxed approach to feedings and schedules. Keep doing what you are doing if you enjoy night nursing and do not need/desire a schedule. But, please know that if your healthy, thriving baby is over six months of age and nursing every two to three hours at night, they are officially a "trained night feeder." That behavior can be easily changed. Read Chapter 9, Sleep so you can all get more sleep! I just want you to know what your baby is capable of so you can make an informed decision.

? ?

LIQUIDS

tongue-tie (see more on this below).

Milk transfer issues can also occur when mom uses a nipple shield as some of the milk gets caught in the shield.

Depending on the problem, there are a variety of solutions. The key is to protect mom's milk supply (usually by pumping, expressing breast milk, and giving it to the baby) until the milk transfer issue resolves.

2 OVERPRODUCTION.

Q. Holy cow! I have to change my shirt before I start nursing! I have so much milk, what do I do?

Some women naturally make an overabundance of milk. We're not talking just in the first couple of weeks, when your supply and your baby's demand are trying to sync. We are talking several weeks down the road, you still look like Dolly Parton, and your milk shoots out across the room. If this describes your situation, your baby may be unhappy (and even upset). They may feel like they're treading water in the ocean with the excessive flow. And as a result, baby may choke, cough, and arch while nursing.

If you have this issue, try nursing at just one breast per feeding. Lean back or lie flat while you nurse to slow down the velocity of that milk stream!

Linda's tip: Remove your baby from your breast after the first several gulps. Use a Haakaa breast milk collector to catch the milk let down. When the stream slows, put the baby back to the breast. Repeat with each let down or gulping phase. And, save that milk! It's mostly foremilk, but you can add it to any pumped milk and store it.

3 ENGORGEMENT.

Q. My breasts look like I have had implants and my baby can't get latched on. Help!

Welcome to engorgement. Don't worry, this is only a two or three day experience at most.

DR B'S OPINION:
MEDICATIONS AND BREASTFEEDING

Mothers frequently call me about medications they are taking and if they are okay to use while breastfeeding. Although I sound smart knowing all the answers on the phone, I find the answers in a book called *Medications and Mother's Milk* by Thomas Hale, Ph.D. If you are planning on nursing for the long haul, or have a chronic medical condition, it may be worth buying the iPhone app, Infant Risk HCP. (Find more info at infantrisk.com or 806-352-2519).

When your body first starts making milk, it sometimes gets carried away. This also happens if your baby takes less volume or suddenly starts sleeping through the night. Here are some ways to feel better:

1. **Pump or manually express for a few minutes before getting baby latched on.** Your nipple will stand more upright, be soft, and compressible.

2. **Pump or manually express only to soften the breast.** Pump off after feedings only if your baby is unsuccessful in nursing. Otherwise it can create an even greater supply of milk.

3. **Wear a bra 24 hours a day for support.** No underwires, ladies.

4. **Take a hot shower and massage breasts to encourage let down.**

5. **Cabbage leaves.** Yes, they can help. Try this: wear washed, chilled, crushed cabbage leaves in your bra. Replace wilted leaves every fifteen minutes for a total 45 minute experience, three times daily. Reality check: your baby may refuse the breast due to the cabbage flavor, so try to keep the cabbage away from your nipples.

6. **Put a bag of frozen vegetables** on your breasts for ten to 20 minutes before nursing if your breasts are hard and not leaking. Some feel better using ice packs after nursing, too.

7. **Encourage your baby to nurse at least ten minutes on each breast.** This is the time nursing moms usually get desperate and wake their babies up to relieve their own discomfort.

8. **Take some ibuprofen (Motrin).** Yes, it's safe to use while breastfeeding. (*Huggins*)

4 NIPPLE PAIN.

Q. Ouch! My nipples hurt! Any suggestions?

There are several reasons why your nipples may hurt during or after nursing. Solving this mystery, and fixing the problem will make breastfeeding much more pleasant and enjoyable. And in turn, it will enable you to successfully continue nursing!

◆ **Poor position.** There are several positions that keep you and your baby comfortable. If one is not working, try another one. See the recommendations below and the graphics earlier in this chapter.

◆ **Poor latch.** You should hear your baby swallowing/gulping. Clicking is NOT a sound you should hear. Get your baby to open wide, with lips curled out. Make sure their nose and chin are next to your breast. Don't let go of your breast until your baby is securely latched on. Poor latch leads to sore nipples. If your nipple looks like a new tube of lipstick after nursing, you have a problem (see picture). When your nipple returns from the lipstick shape to the normal shape after a few minutes, you may see a bruised line (called a **compression stripe**) down the center of your nipple. With continued shallow latches, that bruise will turn into a more significant injury, where the skin will start to split, bleed and scab. If all of this describes your nipples, seek professional help, try different positions so that the nipple isn't always being injured in the same place, and start "moist wound healing" to prevent scabbing (use lanolin and gel pads on your nipples). Bottom line: cracks and open wounds are a dead giveaway for a latch issue (ouch!)

Normal nipple

◆ **Houston, we have a nipple problem.** Flat and inverted nipples pose a challenge. The football hold may help get baby latched on. Stimulating inverted nipples to stand out prior to nursing may help. Breast shells (see Breastfeeding Lingo box earlier in this chapter) also help inverted nipples. Lactation consultants are very helpful for this situation.

Lipstick nipple

◆ **Mouth problem.** Babies with tongue thrusting and tongue-tie can have poor technique. See more about tongue-tie below. Babies who thrust their tongues forward while nursing can be taught how to suck correctly (with a lot of patience and professional help).

◆ **Tongue-tie.** Sometimes a baby has a poor sucking technique because they have a tongue-tie (**ANKYLOGLOSSIA**). This leads to cracked, painful nipples in Mom and poor intake because baby has trouble compressing the nipple.

There are four types of tongue-tie. Two types (1 and 2) are usually detected on the newborn exam because the tip of the tongue is forked and the tongue cannot extend out. Type 3 ("anterior tongue tie") is often missed on exam because the tongue moves outward normally. For types 1, 2 and 3 experts agree that the tongue cannot reach the roof of the mouth, which is an issue with breastfeeding as well as with speech later in life.

If you think this may be a problem, let your pediatrician know about it. For an anterior tongue tie, the thin piece of tissue causing the problem can be easily clipped before you leave the hospital or in an office setting in the first couple of weeks of life. This procedure is called a **FRENULECTOMY**. It takes just a minute or two to perform the procedure and the improvement in latch is usually immediate.

So what is Type 4? Well, this is pretty controversial. Most pediatricians and ear, nose, and

---

FLAT AND INVERTED NIPPLES

When people get physically cold, it's normal for nipples to harden and stick out. If this doesn't happen to you, you might have flat or inverted nipples.

Flat nipples: Is your breast perfectly smooth? Try pinching the pigmented area (**AREOLA**) just beneath the nipple to help your baby find it. Avoid baby bottles and pacifiers in the beginning, as your baby will prefer them since they are easier to latch on to.

Inverted nipples: Do you see an indentation in the center of your nipple? Try pinching your nipple. Does it stick out or go in? If it goes in, pull your nipple out before offering it to your baby. If it "hides," then you may want to wear *nipple shells* during your pregnancy. You can also use a breast pump after you deliver to help bring out your nipple. *Nipple shields* are useful if the baby can pull the nipple into the shield.

throat experts think Type 4 does not exist. Some babies just have very short tongues. Lactation consultants disagree. They feel that some babies have Type 4, a "posterior tongue tie", which limits tongue mobility and interferes with nursing success. And yes, there are a handful of practitioners (usually dentists) across the country, willing to perform a laser procedure to cut into the muscle of the tongue in hopes of improving suckling. The procedure is more involved and so is the recovery.

Consider using a nipple shield for your own protection until the tongue-tie can be clipped. Getting the procedure done sooner rather than later prevents your baby from developing bad sucking habits. If your lactation consultant feels your baby has a posterior tongue tie, you'll want to go over the treatment options with your baby's healthcare provider.

Factoid: Tongue-tie often runs in families.

DR B'S OPINION: TONGUE TIES

For a posterior tongue tie, the risks of the procedure outweigh the benefits. Some babies just have short tongues and will not be able to successfully nurse at the breast. Thank goodness we have bottles and breast pumps.

Q. My nipples are already cracked and it's only my second day of nursing! My nurse offered me some nipple shields. Are these okay to use?

Yes, temporarily.

As we've discussed, a nipple shield is a piece of thin plastic that you place on top of your nipple and surrounding tissue (**AREOLA**) while you nurse. It has four holes that allow most of your breast milk to pass to your baby. They can be a real lifesaver for you if your nipples/areolas are raw, cracked, or bleeding because they keep your baby from being able to do any more damage and give you some time to heal.

Another suggestion: Lansinoh Soothies or Ameda Comfort Gel Pads—a lifesaver for sore nipples!

Of course, these are only temporary solutions. The long-term goal is to have good nursing technique so you don't have repeated injuries!

Get help from an IBCLC certified lactation consultant.

Q. My nipples are really sore. What can I do to get some relief?

Linda has several tips to help your nipples heal:

◆ *Get out some shot glasses.* While you might consider doing some tequila shots to ease your pain, we have something else in mind. Place a mixture of one teaspoon of Epsom salts to one cup water in the glasses and soak your nipples in them twice daily for two to five minutes.

LIQUIDS

◆ *Go topless.* Let your nipples air dry for a few minutes twice a day. You can also expose them to sunlight through a sunny window for additional comfort.

◆ *Lube up.* Before you nurse or pump, apply a tiny amount of pure lanolin ointment or olive oil to the wound(s). The lubrication will protect the tender skin from further insults.

◆ *Get rid of germs.* After you nurse or pump, apply antibiotic cream—either over the counter polysporin or prescription mupiricin (Bactroban)—to the wound(s).

◆ *Two words—Gel Pads.* These are basically bandaids for boobs. You can buy these gel pads just about anywhere. Place the gel pad over the wounded area (and over the antibiotic cream if you are using it) *after* you have nursed or pumped.

◆ *Pump it up (and out).* If you are in complete agony, try pumping and offering your milk through a bottle occasionally. But to maintain your milk supply, you'll need to pump each time your baby gets a bottle. If you do bottle feed your nursing baby, keep the bottle in a horizontal position so they have to work to get the milk like they do at the breast.

Linda's Tip: Cracked Nipples. Your body can heal itself. Squeeze out some breast milk and place it on your nipples after every feeding. And if your nipples are painful from pumping, try putting some olive oil on them beforehand.

5 **NIPPLE BACTERIAL INFECTION.** If your nipples are already cracked and bleeding, you are at risk for getting a bacterial infection. If you notice redness, draining pus, or golden crust, call your OB doc for a prescription antibiotic cream. Wash your nipples daily with soap and water and wipe off any excess antibiotic cream before getting your baby latched on to nurse.

6 **PLUGGED DUCT.** Equate this to a clogged pipe. The milk backs up and causes a hard, lumpy, tender area. Massage these areas while you nurse. Use moist heat before feedings and ice afterwards. Nurse or pump frequently (at least every three hours). Beware of any redness on the skin or fever. Plugged ducts are the precursor for a breast infection called mastitis (see later in the chapter for more info).

Linda's Tip: Try nursing your baby with his chin pointing to the plugged duct—the suckling motion will massage the area and perhaps help unplug the duct. You can also try the "Haakaa Hack." Place three tablespoons of warm water plus one tablespoon of Epsom salts in a Haakaa collector. Place the Haakaa on the affected breast over the nipple and squeeze to suction it on. The nipple should be in the solution and it can often pull out the plug. It is okay to repeat two or three times daily.

7 **MASTITIS.**

Q. So, what is mastitis?

A breast infection due to raw nipples and germs from your baby's mouth.

New mothers often have trouble with their baby's latch initially, leading to raw and cracked nipples. This lets baby's mouth germs enter Mom's breast. Symptoms include fever, chills (like you have the flu), pain/swelling/ redness of the breast. Nursing moms are usually afflicted with

LIQUIDS

? ?

this one to four weeks after delivery.

Treatment requires antibiotics (you need to call your OB for this) and continued elimination of breast milk from the breasts. Yes, you either need to continue nursing or pumping through this unpleasant experience. Your baby will not be harmed—it's *their* germs that did this to you!

If you take antibiotics, we suggest you also take probiotics (also known as acidophilus or lactobacillus). These are good germs (found naturally in yogurt) that will help prevent you from getting a yeast infection on top of everything else!

What causes mastitis?

1. Cracked nipples (mostly from poor latch technique)
2. Plugged milk ducts (from incomplete emptying at a feeding, tight clothes)
3. Missed feedings (lack of nursing or pumping for several hours)
4. Stress and exhaustion
5. Rapid weaning (lack of nursing)

If you notice that you have a tender, painful area on your breast—do something about it ASAP. Massage the area while you nurse or pump to unclog the duct. Apply a warm compress to the area. Try the Haakaa Hack as discussed earlier. Nurse or pump every two to three hours. And get some sleep! (*Lawrence*) If your symptoms persist or worsen, call your OB.

8 YEAST OVERGROWTH/INFECTION

Q. My nipples are burning every time I nurse. Why?

This is likely to be a yeast infection.

Pediatricians try to stay out of Mom's medical care, but parents often ask their opinion. Yeast infections also come from your little one's mouth. Babies (who are toothless) have some bacteria in their mouths, but not nearly as much as we do (because plaque goes along with teeth). Yeast likes dark, warm, moist, low bacteria places. So, newborns often get yeast or **THRUSH** infections in their mouths. It looks like curdled milk that can't be wiped off the gums, cheek lining, and roof of their mouth.

If your nipples burn or itch and you experience shooting pains every time your baby nurses, check your baby's mouth, and check with both your obstetrician and pediatrician. A family practitioner should be able to handle both of these problems.

Your baby can get an antifungal mouthwash and you can get an antifungal cream or oral medication.

There is evidence to show that the yeast clears more quickly if both mother and baby are treated, even if only one party is showing symptoms of infection. And some yeast infections get passed back and forth for what seems like forever. If that is your situation, see below.

Linda's Tips: Top 10 Tips to Beat Yeast

◆ Wash hands with hot, soapy water and dry with paper towels before and after nursing, toileting, and changing baby's diaper.

◆ Wash laundry in hottest water possible. Add a cup of white distilled vinegar to final rinse.

- If you have intercourse, use condoms to prevent cross-infection.
- Sterilize all pacifiers, bottle nipples, pump flanges daily.
- Do not freeze breast milk while being treated. But it is OK to nurse and pump for daily use.
- Use non-disposable breast pads and change as soon as they become moist. (Disposable pads have a plastic lining that traps moisture at the breast.)
- Wear a clean bra each day.
- Get help from an IBCLC certified lactation consultant.
- Take probiotics daily.
- Decrease your consumption of refined sugars. Increase your veggie and garlic intake.
- Wash nipples with a mixture of vinegar and water (1/4 cup vinegar to 1 cup water) after each feeding. Apply over-the-counter antifungal cream (like clotrimazole) to your nipples afterwards. Gently wipe off any excess prior to the next feeding.

Whew! That's a lot of things that can go wrong! We sum up the Top 8 breastfeeding problems and solutions with the chart earlier in the chapter.

Breastfeeding Books

Among the best is *The Nursing Mother's Companion* by Kathleen Huggins, R.N. It will hold your hand and give you 25 different ways to relieve engorgement. Also good: *The Womanly Art of Breastfeeding* by La Leche League.

Expressing Milk

Q. Why would I express breast milk (that is, pump)?

Many mothers pump to survive engorgement. You can pump off the excess milk to get more comfortable and baby can have an easier time getting latched on. For parents working outside the home, it's essential to pump to maintain breast milk supply. For stay-at-home parents, it allows you to escape your house for a little while.

Q. How do I pump and store my milk?

Here's what you need to know:

- Wash your hands.
- Clean all breast pump apparatus thoroughly.
- Freshly pumped breast milk will last eight hours at room temperature and 24 hours in a cooler with blue ice.
- Fresh breast milk retains more of the antibodies and vitamins than breast milk that has been frozen and then thawed/warmed. So limit the amount of breast milk that is frozen and stored.
- Yes, you can combine expressed milk from different pumping sessions together in one container. Just keep it going for a full day, then divide the milk up into individual

? ?

LIQUIDS

servings.

◆ Most people use disposable, leak-proof milk storage bags to store individual servings.

◆ Start with three oz. servings of milk to freeze. Store four to six oz. servings when your baby starts taking more at a feeding. Leave room in the container; fluids expand when frozen. Squeeze out the excess air and press the seal to close it.

◆ Lay the bags flat to freeze for easy storage. Write the date and amount on the top label of the bag. Use the oldest milk first.

◆ Milk storage bags fit nicely in a 24-count soda cardboard box. Just cut out the top and stick the bags in. Add new bags to the back and pull from the front to use.

◆ Newly expressed breast milk can sit out at room temperature for up to six to eight hours. So you can take freshly pumped milk with you when you are out and about without keeping it on ice. (*Human Milk Banking Association of North America*)

See the handy chart later in this section for details on how long expressed milk can safely be refrigerated or frozen.

Reality Check

Plastic disposable bottle bags are very convenient. You can pour the milk directly into them and freeze. For use, immerse the bag in a bowl of warm water to thaw it out.

Another reality check: Breast milk can be different colors (white, yellow, blue, brown, black) and that's okay. Once it is frozen, it can smell kind of like soap. If it smells rancid, it has spoiled and needs to be tossed. If you notice this rancid smell with freshly expressed milk, try Linda's tips below to salvage your liquid gold.

Linda's Tip: More on Sour Milk. Does your refrigerated milk or thawed frozen milk smell soapy, metallic, rancid, fishy, or like vomit?? Your baby can still drink this milk but is likely to refuse it (and who can blame them?!). It may be due to excess lipase (an enzyme) in your breast milk or an oxidation issue sometimes related to a nursing mom's diet.

Troubleshoot by doing a science experiment in your kitchen. Try scalding the milk by heating a small sample on the stove until bubbles form around the rim of the pot, then cool quickly in ice water. (This deactivates the immune function of the milk but may salvage your precious breast milk.)

If this trick does not work, reduce oxidizing agents in your diet (tap water, anchovies, sardines, nuts, seeds, fish, seed oils, and oysters), freeze breast milk immediately to slow oxidation, and store in a container that blocks out light in the freezer.

Q. How do I serve my expressed breast milk?

Warmed and gently shaken. Some tips:

1. Thaw frozen milk in the refrigerator overnight.
2. Warm it up by placing the bottle into warm water.
3. Do not microwave it! It may lead to hot spots that can burn baby's mouth.
4. The milk will separate into water and fat. Mix the bottle up before serving.

5. Once the milk has been thawed, it will last in the refrigerator for up to 24 hours.
6. Thawed (defrosted) milk is good for one hour at room temperature.

An unfinished (fresh, not defrosted) breast milk bottle can be placed back in the refrigerator and used within four hours. It's okay to reheat it.

To maintain the most nutritional value of expressed breast milk and offer it safely, here is a chart with the optimal time frames for use. If a baby drinks all breast milk from a bottle or if they are premature or immune deficient, use milk within the "optimal" time frame. If your baby gets most of their nutrition directly from the breast, then the longer time frame is considered "acceptable".

TIMEFRAMES FOR USE:	OPTIMAL	ACCEPTABLE
Freshly expressed, at room temp (up to 77 F) *never frozen*	4 hours	6-8 hours
Feeding begun, *refrigerate leftover**	4 hours	
Refrigerator (39 F)	3 days	5-8 days
Standard Freezer (0 F)	3 months	6 months
Deep Freezer (-4 F)	6 months	12 months
Previously frozen, *thawed in refrigerator but not warmed**	4 hours	24 hours
Previously frozen, *brought to room temperature**	1 hour, then discard	
Infant has started feeding *Fresh milk, never frozen*	4 hours refrigerated	

*Do not refreeze
(*Source*: Human Milk Banking Association of North America)

Reality Check

Good news: The Affordable Care Act requires insurance plans to cover the costs of lactation services and breast pumps. Bad news: insurance companies may have their own interpretation of these laws. Check with your insurer to get details and read the fine print. At the very least, breast pumps and breastfeeding supplies are currently tax deductible. Stay tuned for updates from the U.S. Department of Health and Human Services at hrsa.gov/womensguidelines/.

Q. When can I introduce a bottle?

Ideally, introduce one bottle a day of expressed (pumped) breast milk at two to four weeks of age. Why?

◆ The non-nursing parent gets involved.

◆ The nursing parent can go out to get a hair cut (remember you are nursing every 2-3 hours).
◆ Baby learns that food comes in different packages.

A common mistake is waiting until the end of maternity leave or when you want a date with your spouse to try a bottle. Once a baby is in the breast-only mode, they are less flexible about change.

Linda's Tip: Introducing a Bottle. Do paced bottle feedings. Keep the bottle more horizontal, keeping the nipple half full of milk when you are bottle feeding a breastfed baby. Using a "vented" bottle also helps. That way, the baby has to actively remove milk from the bottle, just like at the breast. Don't let them chug it or they may not want to work at the breast. A key tip: it is very important to maintain a bottle a day in your baby's routine, so that they don't "forget" how to take a bottle. Many parents get their babies to take a bottle but then don't offer one for a couple of weeks. Then, surprise, baby won't accept a bottle anymore!

DR B'S OPINION

"It is very healthy for your marriage to leave your baby at home with a loving family member or friend! I frequently prescribe this form of mental health therapy to my families. Dinner or a movie (you won't have time for both) is much cheaper than marital counseling."

Q. My baby is refusing to take a bottle. Help!

Babies are smarter than you give them credit for. They can see and smell Mom if they are anywhere in sight. Get out of the house and let someone else feed your baby the bottle.

Babies have thirst and hunger drives. No matter how stubborn your baby is, they will eventually accept a bottle of your breast milk if they are not given an option.

This is not cruel or unusual punishment. It's also a good excuse for you to spend a day at the spa.

Linda's Tips for Bottle Refusal: First of all, do not go out and buy twenty different bottles! Here are a few tried and true strategies:

1. Increase the flow. If your baby used to take a bottle and is now refusing, try increasing the nipple flow. From 0-3 months of age, slow flow nipples work well. But 3-6 month olds are usually ready for medium flow. Some babies move on to fast flow nipples, but many just keep using the medium flow.
2. Sweeten the deal. It's okay to sweeten the deal—temporarily. Make a simple syrup solution to dab on the bottle nipple for enticement. (It's also great in cocktails, by the way.) In a medium low heat pot, add two parts white sugar and one part water and heat until mixture becomes clear. Seal tightly in a container and store in the refrigerator for up to one month of use.
3. Try daily. Do not give up. If your baby gets angry, stop the feeding and calm them. Walk around the room or outside for added distraction. Try the bottle again, once your baby is calm.

Final tip: if there is lots of drama with bottle refusal, be sure to wait at least thirty minutes before offering the breast.

LIQUIDS

Considerations for Mom

Q. I have small breasts. Will I make enough milk?

Probably. Size doesn't matter. It's what's inside that counts.

You should have enough milk if you have normal breast tissue (milk ducts, nipples), make hormones that trigger milk production, and have enough stimulation from your baby suckling or using a breast pump.

Q. I have very large breasts/nipples. Is this good for nursing?

Sometimes yes, sometimes no.

If you have large, pendulous breasts, you may have more difficulty getting your baby correctly latched. You may want to try the "football hold" or lying on your side while nursing so you don't have to hold up the weight of your breast.

You can also try a nursing pillow (or a rolled up receiving blanket or burp cloth under your breast) that supports both your breast and your baby.

If your nipples are too large for your baby, you may need to pump and bottle feed until their mouth gets bigger. Real talk: all nursing moms think their nipples are too big for their tiny babies. It is rarely a problem.

Q. I've had a breast reduction. Will this be a problem?

Possibly.

Certain types of breast reduction surgery disrupt the milk duct super-highway. This may mean you do not have enough milk to breastfeed exclusively. You may not even make more than a drop or two at each nursing session. In this scenario, formula feeding is the most reasonable choice for your baby.

However, no one can predict whether you will be able to nurse or not before you try. And even if you cannot nurse for the long haul, it's great to offer your first milk (**COLOSTRUM**) to your newborn. Work with a lactation consultant to get help with your situation.

Q. I have implants. Can I still nurse?

Yes.

However, certain types of reconstructive surgery may interfere with your ability to breast-feed exclusively. Key point: it is important to experience breast growth during pregnancy. Growth indicates that there is sufficient glandular tissue (that is responsible for milk production) within the breast tissue. If there hasn't been any growth, size A breasts will still be size A breasts, even if you are a size D with implants. Make sense? If you have concerns, consider professional help from a lactation consultant.

Q. I've heard I need to restrict my diet while I am breastfeeding. Is this true?

Not really.

Human milk is remarkably uniform despite differences in women's diets. It is always a good idea to eat healthfully for both you and your baby, though. There are actually very few restrictions. Here are the recommendations, according to the Institute of Medicine:

1. Avoid diets that promise rapid weight loss.
2. Eat a wide variety of foods including breads/grains, fruits, vegetables, dairy products, meats or meat alternatives daily.
3. At least three servings of milk (dairy) products daily.* But see below for details on milk protein allergies in babies.
4. Specifically eat Vitamin A rich foods: carrots, spinach, greens, sweet potatoes, cantaloupe.
5. Drink water when you are thirsty.
6. Caffeine-containing products (cola, coffee) are suggested in moderation (300mg or less per day). A standard 12 oz cup of coffee has about 200mg of caffeine. The caffeine enters the breast milk—so nurse first, and then have your coffee. Preterm babies and newborns may metabolize caffeine at a slower pace and be a bit more sensitive to it—so take that into consideration.
7. Avoid eating shark, swordfish, king mackerel, and tilefish because they may contain high levels of methyl mercury which can interfere with neurological development. (*Suitor*)
8. It's okay to eat 12 ounces or less of shellfish, canned fish, small ocean fish, or farm-raised fish (and less than six ounces of canned tuna) per week. (*Suitor*)

*If you drink cow's milk or eat dairy products, some of the cow milk protein ends up in your human breast milk. And some babies who are sensitive to this protein end up extremely gassy and fussy. Babies with true milk protein allergies who are consistently exposed to cow's milk protein end up having blood-streaked or mucousy/stringy poop, or diarrhea. Hint: if your baby's poop looks like snot, let your doctor know.

If your baby has a true milk protein allergy, you'll have to cut out ALL milk and dairy products from your diet (more on this below). If your baby just seems sensitive, you can try eating dairy products that have been cooked or fermented (yogurt, cheese) and avoiding milk for the first six months of breastfeeding. Why? Milk contains unprocessed cow milk protein, which seems to be more problematic for allergic babies than protein that's been processed in other dairy products.

For more details on food allergies in general, flip over to the section on food allergies in Chapter 7, Solids.

Feedback from the Real World: Cow milk allergy and breastfeeding

One of our readers sent us a note, in desperation, regarding her baby's problems. The mom had been exclusively breastfeeding her baby. She wrote, "it breaks my heart to hear her scream all the time... to have your child be so obviously unhappy and/or in pain all the time is the worst feeling in the world...I think it's time for me to give up (breastfeeding) because nothing else I've tried seems to work." A milk protein allergy was ultimately diagnosed.

Our response: You are not alone. Babies who suffer from this problem leave both baby and parents in misery. But do not fear—your child will not be like this forever. Some babies outgrow this problem by six months of age, and over 80% outgrow it by age five. Babies who are breastfed and have a cow milk protein allergy can still have problems because mom's milk/dairy intake can end up in the breast milk. If you want to continue breastfeeding, you need to avoid ALL products containing milk or dairy. There are often hidden dairy sources, so it's not only the obvious dairy products you need to avoid. Check out the web site FoodAllergy.org or InfantProctocolitis.org for more information.

When your doctor gives you the green light to reintroduce dairy into your diet how will you accomplish this? After all, you don't want to start drinking a half-gallon of milk a day with extra-cheese pizzas and such. Here is a reasonable approach to introducing dairy gradually:

◆ Step 1: Start with small amounts of hard cheeses (cheddar, Swiss) or yogurt for the first week.

◆ Step 2: If baby does well, try soft cheeses (gouda, cottage, cream, American) for week two.

◆ Step 3: If baby does well, try butter, ice cream, and cooked dairy products for week three.

◆ Step 4: If baby does well, have a glass of milk.

Of course, if your baby shows allergy symptoms again, it's back to the dairy free diet for you.

Old Wives Tale
You need to drink excessive amounts of water when you are nursing.
The Truth: Your body will increase its thirst drive to accommodate for your fluid needs. You don't need to go overboard.

FYI: Your daily caloric needs will be higher if you are breastfeeding. The average recommended daily allowance for non-pregnant women is 2100 calories. With breastfeeding, the recommendation is 2700 calories. (*Lawrence*) Don't bother counting calories, though, unless you are losing too much weight or having a problem producing enough milk.

Old Wives Tale
You need to avoid gassy foods like beans because they will make the baby gassy.
The truth: You may want to avoid gassy foods because other people might not want to be around you. Your baby is unaffected by this food choice.

Q. Is there any truth that some foods in my diet will make my baby fussy?

Yes, but there is no reason to restrict your diet unless you identify a problem. Foods that *might* cause a problem: cabbage, turnips, broccoli, rhubarb, apricots, prunes, melons, and peaches. (*Lawrence*)

Linda's Tip: Funky food, fussy baby? Is your baby fussy because of something you ate before nursing? Remember it takes anywhere from four to 24 hours to notice the effect. So if your baby is acting unusually fussy, think about what you ate in the past day. Since the oils from the foods you eat transfer into breast milk, your baby may not like the "taste" of something you ate.

Q. Can I smoke/vape nicotine if I am nursing?

No.

If you are nursing, don't smoke. (We don't recommend it for formula-fed babies either, by the way). Besides the health reasons, you won't get much sleep. Nicotine passes into breast milk and nicotine exposed babies sleep about 30% less than their non-exposed friends. If you want more sleep, quit smoking! That's just one of the many good reasons to kick the habit.

Q. Can I use marijuana while nursing?

The party line consensus amongst experts is no. This is mostly based on the concern the active ingredient, THC, could be passed through the breast milk to the baby. One study estimates that babies get about 2.5% of the mom's dose if their nursing mom is a regular cannabis user. THC exposure in breast milk has been associated with sleepiness and slowed weight gain in babies. Although there are no studies that demonstrate a clear connection, we know that THC can impact brain cells, and we know that a baby's brain is growing at a tremendous rate in the first few months of life—hence the precaution.

Sidebar: smoking cannabis in the household (by anyone) is also a risk factor for Sudden Infant Death Syndrome (SIDS), so please refrain from doing so. *(LactMed)*

Q. Should I take DHA (Omega 3 fatty acids) supplements while I am nursing?

Not necessarily. DHA is an essential fatty acid found in fish oils and may promote brain and vision development in infants (although this data is lacking for DHA supplements in infant formula). Breast milk typically has adequate levels of DHA in it, but the amount varies depending on the nursing mother's diet. So, it is a good idea for a nursing mom to eat a diet rich in DHA (salmon, flax seeds, walnuts, soy beans) for both mom and baby. If a nursing mom doesn't have a diet rich in DHA, they can take 200-300 mg a day of DHA supplements.

Q. Can I eat sushi while I am nursing?

Yes. Just be aware that consumption of raw fish (whether you are nursing or not) carries a slight risk of food-borne infection. And the FDA recommends that you eat less than 6 oz a week of tuna. So, order less toro and more unagi.

Q. Can I eat peanuts and peanut butter while I am nursing?

Yes! With the increase in people with peanut allergies, there has been quite a bit of research on this subject. A landmark study in the *New England Journal of Medicine (NEJM)* looked at the diets of breastfeeding women and later development of food allergies in infants. The results: there was no association or prevention of peanut allergy even if mom avoided these foods in her diet. And more recent studies have found the same results. *(Sicherer)*

LIQUIDS

Q. Can I drink any alcoholic beverages while I am nursing?

Yes, in limited amounts.

Alcohol enters the bloodstream and the breast milk anywhere from 30-90 minutes after inges-tion. The levels in the milk drop quickly. Each individual's metabolism is slightly different. So, a good rule of thumb is to avoid nursing for at least two hours after drinking. And don't nurse if you feel tipsy!

I'd suggest you limit your intake to one alcoholic beverage, sporadically, if you are nursing.

Old Wives Tale
Drinking alcohol improves your milk supply.
The truth: Drinking alcohol may help relax an over-stressed mother, but it does not improve breast milk volumes or let-down reflexes.

Q. Should I get the COVID-19 vaccine while I am nursing? Is it safe? Will it protect my baby?

Yes. Yes. Yes.

As we go to print, this is an evolving situation with advice based on the most current data. If you are due to get a COVID-19 vaccine and you are nursing, by all means get it. The safety data for you and for your baby are pretty well established now by the research studies and after millions and millions of doses have been given.

Regarding protection, the most recent study to date demonstrated that COVID-19 anti-bodies are still detected in human breast milk up to six months after a nursing mom receives the vaccine. *(Perez).* The big question is, how much breast milk is needed to offer protection? We know that "passive immunity" from antibodies transferred from mom to baby are like giv-ing a daily dose of medication to a baby. It's not like giving a vaccine directly to a baby, which offers immunity for a more extended period of time (or may even be lifelong, in some cases). That said, babies benefit the most from this passive immunity when they are exclusively breast-fed on a daily basis. Sorry, but giving an ounce or two to your toddler every day is not going to be very helpful.

Q. Are there any medications to avoid while I am nursing?

Yes, lots of them.

The short answer to this question is, always inform your doctor that you are breastfeeding. That way, a medication choice for you can be made safely. You can always call your child's doc-tor, or your pharmacist to double check.

See Appendix A, "Medications" or InfantRisk.com for more information.

Q. I love exercising. Any problems with that while I am breastfeeding?

If you exercise vigorously then nurse, your milk may have a sour taste that your baby may not like. Exercise produces lactic acid in your body, which goes into your breast milk. It's not harmful, it just tastes funny. There have also been anecdotal reports of infant fussiness up to six hours after Mom's exercise/nursing session. Here are some suggestions:

? ?

LIQUIDS

◆ Pump or express for a minute or two before nursing.

◆ If your baby gives you a strange look, use some stored breast milk for that feeding!

Reality Check

While we are on the subject of sour tasting milk…your breast milk may change flavors during your period (if you have one). And it may not be a flavor your baby likes, according to lactation expert Dr. Ruth Lawrence.

Q. I am going back to work after my maternity leave. How am I going to make this breastfeeding thing work?

Setting aside time, having a progressive workplace, and being committed.

Some women are able to go back to work AND provide breast milk to feed their babies. It may take some trial and error to figure out what works for you, but here are some ideas.

1. Leave for work a little early and pump BEFORE you start working. Or, nurse before childcare/work.

2. Invest in a high-powered, double pump. You can successfully pump in 15 minutes with one of these models.

3. Let your boss/co-workers know of your intentions. You may be surprised at how understanding people are.

4. Think about where you will be able to pump and how often.

5. Think about where you will *store* your expressed milk until you get home. It can sit in a cooler with ice packs if you don't have access to a refrigerator.

6. Start stockpiling expressed milk BEFORE maternity leave is over. See "Linda's tip" regarding stockpiling earlier in this chapter.

7. Be prepared for being exhausted the first few weeks. It does get better.

If you don't have enough breast milk for the whole time you are away, supplementing with formula is okay. Your baby will benefit from any milk you can provide. Every ounce counts!

Reality Check

The percentage of fat, protein, and sugar in breast milk not only varies from the beginning let down (foremilk) to the latter part (hindmilk) of the nursing session, but also in the time of day. If you notice your baby seems more satisfied with your evening nursing sessions more than morning ones, it may be because your breast milk has more fat in it during that time of day!

Q. I have a fever, can I still nurse?

Absolutely!

Your body is producing antibodies to whatever infection your body is fighting. Those antibodies are going directly to your baby. This includes COVID-19 infection. If you have a cold or upper respiratory infection, not breathing on your baby would be helpful! Yes, you can wear a mask.

Contact your doctor (obstetrician, preferably) if you have a fever shortly after the birth of your baby. You could have a bladder infection, womb infection, or mastitis.

LIQUIDS

Special situations

Q. I am adopting a baby. I have heard that I can take a medicine to stimulate my milk supply. Is this true?

Yes. While there are natural remedies to stimulate milk production, there is no scientific data on how effective these are. A good web source for info on this topic is AskLenore.info.

Q. I am unable to breastfeed, but I want my baby to receive breast milk. Can I buy breast milk?

Yes. There are several programs across the country called Mother's Milk Banks that sell breast milk, primarily to ill, premature babies. The donors are rigorously tested to be certain they are free of infectious diseases like Hepatitis B and HIV. And the breast milk is pasteurized. If a bank has excess supply, they will sell it to healthy newborns. It's quite pricey ($4.25 per oz). Check with your area hospital's lactation services or visit the Human Milk Banking Association of North America's website at hmbana.org.

On the flip side, if you have more milk than your freezer can handle, consider making a donation!

Reality Check

Certified milk banks check donors and their milk rigorously for infection before the milk is sold. It is becoming trendy for moms to purchase breast milk from neighbors, friends, and even wet nurses online. Let the buyer beware—this is probably not the safest idea for your baby.

Q. I have twins and want to breastfeed. How do I make it work?

The key is getting both babies fed at the same time. Otherwise, it will be a challenge to get any sleep. Start this routine from day one and you will have more success.

When it comes to multiples, you will do a little more scheduling and a little less feeding "on demand." If you are able to get some hired or volunteered help around the house, things may be less chaotic for you.

The football hold and/or the cradle hold work well for simultaneous feeding sessions. It's probably wise not to have one breast exclusively designated for one baby. That way, they will accept either breast in the long run. And, just in case one breast produces more milk than the other, one baby won't get short-changed.

Q. I have a baby who was born prematurely. Anything special I need to know about breastfeeding?

Yes—it's even more important to breastfeed these little ones. Here are some special considerations:

1. Many premature babies get tired easily while nursing. If you no longer hear your baby swallowing, take them off the breast and burp them. Then return to feeding.

2. Many premature babies have poor technique (sucking, latching). Get professional help (from a lactation consultant) if you are having trouble.

3. You may be supplementing with formula or expressed breast milk for a while. Don't give up.

4. Rent a hospital grade pump for the first month because you will need to pump eight times daily to protect your milk supply until your baby is feeding well at the breast. A rental pump is the fastest, easiest option when pumping this often.

5. Weigh your baby once or twice weekly to make sure they are gaining, ideally, an ounce a day. Eventually you can stop doing this—check with your doctor. You can usually stop the weekly weight checks when you reach your baby's actual due date.

6. The football hold works well for little preemies. That way you have better control of positioning and latch.

7. Give baby skin to skin time. This stimulates your milk production (and promotes bonding!)

8. Most babies born 37 weeks gestation or younger do better at the breast with a nipple shield, as this helps stimulate their sucking reflex.

9. Because it is often difficult to tell if your baby is actually eating at the breast versus pacifying, it is helpful to do the following:

   ◆ Limit breastfeeding to about ten minutes per side in the beginning weeks when your baby is falling asleep at the breast.

   ◆ Pump for ten minutes after all daytime feedings and at least once during the night.

   ◆ Supplement the baby with 15-30 ml (1/2 to 1 ounce) of expressed breast milk after breastfeeding to guarantee he is getting enough calories.

10. When you are supplementing, you may notice that your baby is getting lazier at the breast in anticipation of taking the easier bottle. If that is the case, then supplement BEFORE offering the breast.

As your premature baby gets closer to their real due date, they will have more energy and be able to stay awake longer. At that point, you can start experimenting with getting baby off of the nipple shield and taking away the supplemental feedings and pumpings.

Q. My baby was born at 35 1/2 weeks gestation. Should I treat them like a full-term baby when it comes to breastfeeding?

No. You have a "late preterm infant" who may have more difficulty with nursing because they may not have the skills or the energy to suck effectively. Here are some specific tips to make breastfeeding successful:

◆ Aim for at least eight feedings a day.

◆ Wake your baby up if: they don't wake up on their own, it has been more than three hours between feedings during the day, or four hours at night until they reach their real due date.

◆ Feeding time should be 40 minutes, tops. After that, your baby will be exhausted.

◆ Use a nipple shield if your baby has a poor latch—most late preterm infants do!

? ?

LIQUIDS

◆ Use a "supplemental nursing system" to offer expressed milk or formula while your baby is at your breast. You can use a tube with a bottle reservoir that attaches to either your nipple or your finger. Offer 5-10 ml (1-2 tsp) per feed on Day 1, 10-20 ml (1/2 oz) per feed on Day 2, and 20-30 ml (up to one oz) per feed on Day 3. The nurses or lactation consultant at the hospital can show you how to use these supplemental nursing systems.

◆ Pump after each feeding to stimulate your milk production, because your newborn won't.

◆ Have a lactation consultant check to make sure your milk is successfully being transferred to your baby when they are at the breast.

Don't be discouraged. Do weight checks every week until your baby reaches their actual due date.

Reality Check

American Red Cross makes an infant scale that is accurate, user friendly, and moderately priced at Walmart or Amazon.com for about $50. Here is one, for example: http://j.mp/scaleredcross

Q. I have a baby with acid reflux (GERD). Is there anything differently I should do when I am nursing?

We'll tackle gastroesophageal reflux (GERD) in depth in Chapter 8, The Other End. But yes, nursing a reflux baby presents special challenges.

First problem: Positioning. Reflux babies do better when they are more upright with feedings. Unless you are a Cirque de Soleil performer, it's physically impossible to nurse your baby upright. However, if you keep them at a 45-degree angle with their bottom down more towards your lap, they may fare better. Also, avoid the side-lying position.

Next problem: what do you do when you've just completed a nursing session, your baby spits it all back at you, and then wants to eat again? You won't have much milk left at your breast to offer. But you can still put them back to the breast. Why? Breast milk is made as your baby sucks. And that richer, heavier hindmilk is more likely to stay down.

If that doesn't work, you may have to offer a bottle stashed away in your freezer.

Breastfeeding moms quickly realize they need to have a stash of expressed milk, just in case the entire feeding comes back up.

Other breastfeeding moms offer expressed milk in a bottle (instead of direct nursing at the breast) for one or more feedings. This enables you to feed your baby in an upright position. You can also discuss thickening the expressed breast milk with xantham gum or carob bean gum (similar to adding corn starch to thicken gravy) to help it stay in the stomach. Heavier milk uses gravity to help it stay down and not come back up.

Here are the take-home tips for nursing a baby with acid reflux:

◆ Read your baby's cues and adjust their feedings accordingly.

◆ Burp them more frequently.

◆ Don't sit them up to burp—that creates too much pressure on the tummy.

◆ Let them rest between breasts.

LIQUIDS

? ?

◆   Make sure your "let down" of milk isn't too fast, causing them to gulp down a lot of air while nursing.

Weaning

Q. When should I wean my baby off of breast milk?

When one or both of you is ready.

The American Academy of Pediatrics recommends breastfeeding for at least a year, with the addition of "complementary" solid food by six months. Hopefully, both you and your baby will enjoy nursing for at least that long. Some nursing teams (mother and baby) opt to continue even after one year.

So, the right time to wean is when one or both of you thinks it is time to stop. That time may be when your baby refuses the breast, when you decide you want your body to yourself, or when your ten-year-old asks for your breast by name. It is really a personal decision.

Reality Check

Americans tend to nurse their babies for less time than many other cultures. In some cultures, women nurse one child until the next one arrives. These same women have lower rates of breast cancer. Food for thought.

Q. I am planning to wean my baby. How do I do it?

Slowly and methodically.

If you stop breastfeeding abruptly, your body will be unhappy with you. Milk ducts get clogged (and infected). With that said, here is a typical strategy:

1.   Create a timetable for the projected target date of nursing completion.
2.   Eliminate one nursing session every 3-4 days, 2-3 weeks before your target date. The length of time for the entire weaning process depends on how many times a day you are currently nursing.
3.   If you are weaning prior to one year of age, replace that feeding with either previously expressed breast milk or formula.
4.   Eliminate the first morning and last evening feeding at the end of the weaning process.
5.   Once you have completely stopped nursing, you may continue to leak milk for a week or two.
6.   Wear an old bra (non-nursing), even though it is a little binding.
7.   If your breasts feel so full that they are going to explode, pump or manually express just enough milk to get comfortable.
8.   Taking pseudoephedrine (Sudafed) during the day, diphenhydramine (Benadryl) at night, and/or drinking three cups/day of sage tea may also help.

Q. I want to continue breastfeeding, but my nine-month old seems to be weaning on their own. Is that okay?

Yes, but you may gently encourage them to continue. Babies go on strike (from formula or bottles, too) for various reasons.

◆ Some babies get distracted during feeding sessions when they realize the world is pretty interesting. Nurse in a boring, dark, quiet place. Or nurse while they are drowsy or almost sleeping.

◆ Some babies don't want to suck if they are teething. Try using acetaminophen to relieve teething discomfort.

◆ Ear infections and nasal congestion can also discourage a baby from nursing. Check in with your doctor.

If none of the advice above helps, transition to formula in a bottle or a cup (depending on your baby's age and skills). Transition to whole milk if your baby is over a year of age. (*Lawrence*)

Linda's tip: You will need to protect your milk supply during this time of breast refusal by pumping and offering your milk in a bottle or cup. Try to get your baby back to the breast by offering it when they are almost asleep or drowsy. Don't let the breast become a battleground. These strikes can last up to a week sometimes. Be patient. Skin-to-skin time in the bathtub together can often work wonders!

Insider Tip

Sometimes babies are less interested in nursing because mom's milk supply has dropped off. That may be rectified by using some of the supply-enhancing tips discussed earlier in this chapter.

Q. If I stop breastfeeding before my baby is one year old, what do I offer instead?

Commercial-brand formula is the acceptable substitute for breast milk in the first year of life.

Note: cow's milk, soymilk, goat's milk, and rice milk are NOT substitutes for breast milk in the first year of life.

The Big Picture: Breastfeeding for the First Year

Okay, let's sum up this breastfeeding section with an overview of nursing for your baby's first year:

Birth to 2 weeks: (14-20 ounces/day)

Breastfed newborns tend to eat every two or three hours. That adds up to eight to 12 times in a 24-hour day. They may cluster feed as frequently as every 1 1/2 hours (that's from the beginning of one feeding to the beginning of the next). If you are expressing breast milk and feeding via a bottle, your baby will probably take two or three ounces at a feeding.

Babies who try to nurse more frequently than every 90 minutes are usually nursing for comfort. Babies have no other way of consoling themselves. They can't just pull it together and settle

LIQUIDS

? ?

down. Sucking is extremely soothing. So, if it has been less than 90 minutes since the beginning of the last feeding, try using your finger to let him suck. Your breasts will thank you. **Note: If your baby is truly nursing non-stop, have your baby weighed to ensure proper weight gain. Make sure you have enough milk supply.**

On the flip side, your baby may take a four-hour stretch before feeding again. In the first two weeks of life, do not let your baby go more than four hours without feeding. Why?

◆ Breast milk is a supply and demand phenomenon. To get your supply established, the demand must be there.

◆ Your breasts will feel like they are going to explode. If that four-hour stretch is during daylight hours, you are in for a long night of cluster feedings.

2 weeks to 2 months: (17-25 ounces/day)

Once your baby is two weeks old, you can relax a bit. Your milk supply will be better established and your baby will have regained their birth weight. If they sleep through the night, let them! You may need to pump to get comfortable during the night, but don't wake a sleeping baby. By the way, this is unlikely to happen. If it does, don't tell your friends about it. They will hate you.

This feeding "pattern" goes on for at least the first two months of life. While this seems a bit erratic, it is normal for a newborn to be irregular with their feeding (and sleep patterns).

2 to 4 months: (21-30 ounces/day)

Your baby will start to have some regularity! They will have more predictable wakeful periods and sleep periods. Hopefully, you will be down to one or two night feedings. If you are returning to work and pumping, plan on four ounces per feeding at two months of age and up to eight ounces per feeding at four months. **Babies usually max out at 40 oz per day at four months of age.**

4 to 6 months: (25-32 ounces/day)

You can look forward to five or six breast feedings a day. You should be able to get an evening stretch of six hours without nursing. Six hours is considered "sleeping through the night", although this is probably not your definition.

You may begin offering complementary solid food between 4-6 months of age. While there are some differing opinions, the American Academy of Pediatrics recommends your exclusively breastfed baby receive an iron supplement from 4-6 months if you wait to offer infant iron-fortified cereal until six months of age.

Initially, solid food is dessert. Your baby needs the same volume of breast milk until they take large volumes of solid foods.

6 to 9 months: (24-36 ounces/day)

Your baby will nurse four or five times per day. You should be done with night feedings. If you are not, do some problem solving with your doctor. You may enjoy those cuddly moments nursing in the middle of the night, but these are not a necessity. Your baby is comforted and used to feeding at night. Frequently, so is Mommy. If both of you are enjoying this situation, keep doing it. If one of you (Mom) is not enjoying it and wants more sleep, read Chapter 9, Sleep.

Solid foods should be in full swing at this point (see the next chapter on solid nutrition). You'll probably see your baby eat more and drink less between 7-9 months of age.

9 to 12 months: (20-30 ounces/day)

Babies are well into solid foods and start to wean—that is, their volume and frequency of nursing decline. Your baby may nurse three or four times per day.

By one year of age, babies wean to 16 to 24 oz per day. At this point, you deserve a gold medal of honor. If you and baby are ready, you can stop breastfeeding.

We recommend switching to whole or 2% milk with Vitamin D added at one year of age. The goal is two cups of milk per day (or dairy serving equivalents). Remember, breast milk is low in Vitamin D and iron. So, if you want to go beyond a year of nursing, find other nutritional sources for these nutrients.

Now that you've learned all you wanted to know about breastfeeding, let's talk about formula.

Before we get into the nitty gritty details of baby formulas, we need to give a shout out to Bridget Young, PhD, CLC, Research Assistant Professor of Pediatrics at the University of Rochester School of Medicine and Dentistry for reviewing this section. Her expertise and passion for perinatal nutrition goes well beyond the scope of this book, so if you need more help you can find her online at BabyFormulaExpert.com!

Formula

Q. Is it okay to feed formula to my newborn?

Yes.

Your baby will be fine if they are formula-fed. Here are the key advantages to formula:

◆ It's about as close as it gets to human milk. Formulas are specially prepared to contain the appropriate amount of fat, protein, carbohydrates, and other nutrients that growing babies need.

◆ It's convenient. You can take a formula bottle anywhere you go. And yes, there are portable bottle warmers for picky babies. (It's somewhat less convenient at 2am when your baby is screaming while you frantically have to warm up a bottle.)

◆ It isn't mom-dependent. Yes, any willing and able-bodied person can feed a baby a bottle of formula anytime during the day or night.

◆ There are options. While not all babies can tolerate cow, soy or goat milk-based formula, there are several alternatives for babies with food allergies.

◆ But formula is also very expensive. Expect to pay $550+ for a year if your baby tolerates the least expensive cow's milk based powdered formula (that's a generic brand formula bought in bulk from a warehouse club). Name brand powered formula is about $1200 a year. Hypoallergenic formula could run $2000 to $6000 or more.

Q. I have chosen to feed my baby formula. What formula do you recommend?

The American Academy of Pediatrics (AAP) advises using a cow or goat milk protein based

LIQUIDS

? ?

formula with iron for healthy babies 0-12 months of age. That's it. Easy, right? But with 90 infant formulas on the market, it may feel like a very difficult decision!

Here's the thing—the FDA requires all U.S. made infant formulas to resemble human milk, with 30 essential nutrients. So, your baby will get their nutritional needs met regardless of which product you select. But, we do encourage you to be a label reader and decide what is most important to you. See the AAP guidelines for choosing a baby formula here: https://bit.ly/AAPFormulaAdvice

Like human milk, all infant formulas contain macronutrients (protein, fat, sugar), and micronutrients (vitamins and minerals). While not FDA required, some formulas also contain probiotics, prebiotics, and omega-3 fatty acids (DHA) in an effort to be more similar to human milk. And, a few infant formulas are certified organic and/or use non-GMO products for families who desire it.

Let the buyer beware: while the World Health Organization has strict marketing rules regarding baby formula, US manufacturers uniformly ignore those guidelines. Ignore claims that a particular infant formula is "closest to mother's milk."

The most important difference between formulas is the protein. Formula manufacturers tinker with the protein base (cow milk, soy, goat milk, non-dairy/non-soy amino acids), the ratio of whey to casein proteins, and whether the proteins are intact or partially predigested ("hydrolyzed" or "hydrolysated"). Protein, especially casein, is the key ingredient that can cause tummy aches, constipation, and food allergy. Human milk protein is a combo of 60% whey and 40% casein (hence a 60:40 ratio). The higher percentage of whey is what makes it move through the gut more quickly and makes breast milk easier to digest. Cow milk straight from the cow is 20% whey and 80% casein, so formula manufacturers have to modify it to make it more like human milk.

Many standard cow milk protein-based formulas have about a 60:40 whey:casein ratio. Goat milk protein-based formulas, which are popular in Europe and Asia, and recently introduced in

THE HISTORY OF BABY FORMULA

1700's: "Wet nurses" were paid to breastfeed infants who could not be fed by their mother.

1800's: Milk from other animals (cow, sheep, mare, goat) was used as a substitute.

1700's

1800's

1838: The ingredients of animal milk and human milk were analyzed. We learned that cow's milk had a higher protein and lower sugar content which could cause problems for infants trying to digest it. This led to the first chemical "formula" that was added to cow's milk.

1870's: Nestle made the first infant formula that only required water to be added. It was very expensive and therefore quite unpopular.

The inventions of evaporated milk (1883), pasteurization (1890), and the refrigerator (1910) allowed parents to make infant formula in the comfort of their own home.

WHAT ARE DHA AND ARA? LIPIDS?

DHA stands for Docosahexaenoic Acid. ARA stands for Arachidonic Acid. DHA and ARA are also called "lipids." Walk into your grocery store and you'll see lots of formula cans hyping their added lipids. So, what is this stuff? Lipids (DHA/ARA) are polyunsaturated fats that occur naturally in breast milk. They are also found in fish oils, egg yolks, and algae/fungal oil.

There has been a fair amount of research done on these fatty acids because they are present in nerve tissue and the eyes. Some earlier studies showed improved vision and scoring on infant developmental testing when babies have DHA and ARA in their diets. (Chandran). But several other studies have proven no benefit in adding these lipids to infant formulas. (Jasani)

Although there is no benefit, most major brand-name and generic formulas jumped on the lipid train a while ago, adding lipids to their products. It won't make your baby smarter or have x-ray vision either way.

formula

the U.S., also have a 60:40 whey:casein ratio. Soy protein-based formulas are available for babies with health problems or for vegetarian families who seek a non-dairy formula. Fully hydrolyzed and amino acid protein-based formulas are designed for babies with cow milk protein allergies. The size of the proteins in partially pre-digested (partially hydrolyzed) protein formulas is in between the large proteins of standard formulas, and the tiny proteins of truly hypoallergenic formulas. These partially predigested (hydrolysated) protein formulas are probably a little easier to digest, which begs the question, why aren't all baby formulas hydrolysated? Cost.

Dr. Young's tip: If you prefer a baby formula with a whey:casein ratio more like human milk

1940-1960: Parents made infant formula out of evaporated milk, water, and corn syrup or sugar. The elaborate process of making formula daily provides much of the basis for the Old Wives Tales you hear about formula today.

1900's   **PRESENT DAY**

1960's: Commercial formulas become popular due to a reduction in cost and ease of preparation. Breastfeeding rates drop sharply.

1970's: Only 25% of newborns left the hospital breastfeeding. As a result, the parents of this generation are the most formula fed babies in recorded history.

1980's and 90's: New studies tout the benefits of breastfeeding, spur renaissance in nursing.

2020: 84% of babies go home from the hospital breastfeeding, but only 58% are still breastfeeding at six months.

??

DIFFERENCES BETWEEN BREAST MILK & FORMULA

To understand the differences, you need a brief chemistry lesson here. Milk contains fat, protein, and sugar, known collectively as macronutrients. Vitamins and minerals are called micronutrients. Use the following table as a reference:

	Human Milk	Cow Or Goat Milk Formula	Soy Formula	Fully hydrolyzed protein
Calories	20 cals/oz	20 cals/oz	20 cals/oz	20 cals/oz
Protein % **of calories**	5%	10% Cow/goat milk, whey	10% soy protein	10% of calories casein hydrolysate or whey
Fat % **of calories**	54%	50% Vegetable oil	50% Vegetable oil	50% of calories Vegetable oil
Carbohydrate **% of calorie**	41% Lactose	40% Lactose (+/- corn sugar)	40% Corn syrup/ Sucrose	40% of calories Corn syrup/ Sucrose
Live cells **Antibodies**	Yes	No	No	No
DHA, ARA	Yes	Yes	Yes	Yes

Special notes:
1. Human milk has lactose sugar, so it makes sense to opt for lactose-based formula.
2. Soy formulas contain soy protein.
3. Fully hydrolyzed protein formulas are hypoallergenic because the protein is pre-digested.
4. All U.S. made formulas contain the recommended daily iron requirement for babies. European infant formulas contain less iron.
5. Note that 50% of the calorie intake comes from fat.

(in the 60:40 range), look for whey to be listed near the top of the ingredient list.

So, which of the 90 infant formulas is right for your baby? It boils down to three important questions:

1. What does your baby like?
2. What do you like?
3. What does your wallet like?

Decision tree for what your baby likes:

Healthy baby –> standard cow or goat milk-based protein based formula (basically, "standard" formula). (Enfamil Infant,

DR B'S OPINION

"Although we encourage you to breastfeed your baby for obvious benefits, your baby will be fine if they are formula fed."

Neuropro, or Enspire, Similac Advance, Pro-Advance, or 360 Total Care, Gerber Goodstart Gentle, Earth's Best, Burt's Bees, Kirkland, Kabrita and others)

Dr. Young's tip: Store brand versions of these formulas are a great option at a cheaper price.

Extraordinarily fussy or constipated baby –> Goat milk-based infant formula,100% whey cow milk protein (all Gerber formulas) or predigested (partially hydrolyzed or "gentle" or "comfort") cow milk protein based formula. (Enfamil Gentlease and Reguline, Similac Total Comfort, Gerber Goodstart Soothe, Burt's Bees Ultra Gentle)

*Cow milk-protein allergic baby –> extensively hydrolyzed protein based formula (Nutramigen, Similac Alimentum, Gerber Extensive HA, and other store brands)

*Cow milk-protein allergic baby who cannot tolerate extensively hydrolyzed formula –> amino acid protein based formula (Neocate, Elecare, PurAmino)

*A baby with a true cow milk protein allergy—usually diagnosed by slimy, mucus-containing poo (with microscopic blood in it) and/or eczema, needs an uber-expensive infant formula that has no trace of cow milk, goat milk or soy in it. Many babies with a cow milk protein allergy may be able to tolerate the trace amounts found in less expensive (but still pricey) hypoallergenic extensively hydrolyzed formula, so doctors often try it first.

Insider Tip
Special formulas are expensive. Some insurance companies will partially cover the cost for "medical foods," so be sure to inquire about it.

Reality Check
Amino acid based/hypoallergenic formulas taste pretty bad. It's okay to add a drop or two of vanilla extract if your baby refuses to drink it!

Decision tree for what you like:

If you have strong opinions about organic food, GMO's, and other particular ingredients, that may factor into your decision-making process. From a scientific standpoint, none of these popular concerns have strong evidence to sway our advice. And no infant formula is 100% organic because all of them must add synthetic vitamins and minerals. We will share this information with you to help you make an informed decision.

Sugar: Human milk contains lactose.
Because lactose is the main sugar in human milk, it makes sense to opt for lactose-containing infant formulas over formulas that use corn syrup solids. We agree that lactose is the preferred choice since that is what is in human milk and babies digest it just fine (it is RARE to be born lactose-intolerant). But corn syrup solids, maltodextrin, and brown rice syrup are still safe to use.

◆ **Lactose sugar based formula** –> Most standard formulas are 100% lactose now.
Dr. Young's tip: To be sure, look on the list of ingredients. If you DO see the word

ENFAMIL

Enfamil Premium Infant	Cow milk and whey	lactose
Enfamil Gentlease	Partially hydrolyzed cow/whey	lactose, corn syrup
Enfamil Enspire	Cow milk	lactose
Enfamil Reguline	Partially hydrolyzed cow	lactose, corn syrup
Enfamil AR	Cow milk	lactose, maltodextrin, rice
Enfamil ProSobee	Soy	corn syrup solids
Nutramigen	Fully hydrolyzed casein	corn syrup solids

SIMILAC

Similac Pro-Advance	Cow milk and whey	lactose
Similac Pro-Sensitive, +Non-GMO	Cow milk	lactose, maltodextrin, sug
Pure Bliss	Cow milk and whey	lactose
Similac Organic	Organic cow milk	lactose
Similac Total Comfort, +Non-GMO	Partially hydrolyzed whey	corn syrup, sugar
Similac Soy Isomil	Soy	corn syrup solids
Similac Spit Up, +non-GMO	Cow milk	rice starch, sugar
Similac Alimentum	Hypoallergenic cow	sugar/maltodextrin

GERBER

Goodstart Gentle Pro (also soy, hypoallergenic)	Partially hydrolyzed whey	lactose, maltodextrin

OTHER BRANDS   (each may have various options that include 100% lactose and reduced-lactose formula

EARTH'S BEST (also soy and sensitive)	Organic cow milk	organic lactose
WALMART: Parents' Choice Organic	Organic cow milk	corn syrup solids, lactose
COSTCO: Kirkland	Cow milk	lactose
TARGET: Up and Up	Cow milk	lactose, various

EUROPEAN

HIPP Stage 1 (not approved for US)	Organic cow milk	lactose
Holle Stage 1 (not approved for US)	Organic cow milk	lactose, maltodextrin
Lebenswert Stage 1 (not approved for US)	Organic cow milk	lactose
Topfer Stage 1 (not approved for US)	Organic cow milk	lactose, maltodextrin
Kabrita Infant	Goat milk	lactose

HYPOALLERGENIC

Neocate	Amino Acid based	corn syrup solids
Elecare	Amino Acid based	corn syrup solids

BREAST MILK

	HUMAN MILK	lactose

Protein	Fat with Palm Oil	DHA	Probiotics	Prebiotics	Non-GMO
60% whey	✔	✔		✔	✔
Partially hydrolyzed 60% whey	✔	✔		✔	✔
60% whey	✔	✔		✔	✔
Partially hydrolyzed 60% whey	✔	✔		✔	
20% whey	✔	✔		✔	
soy protein	✔	✔			
hydrolyzed casein	✔	✔	✔		
50% whey		✔		✔	✔
20% whey		✔		✔	✔
50% whey		✔		✔	✔
20% whey		✔		✔	
Partially hydrolyzed whey		✔		✔	✔
soy protein		✔		✔	
20% whey		✔		✔	✔
hydrolyzed casein		✔		✔	
Partially hydrolyzed whey	✔	✔	✔	✔	✔
30% whey	✔	DHA option		✔	✔
whey + casein	✔	✔		some	✔
whey + casein		✔		✔	✔
whey + casein	✔	✔		some	✔
whey + casein	✔	✔	✔	✔	
whey + casein		✔			✔
whey + casein	✔				✔
whey + casein	✔	✔	✔		✔
whey + casein		✔		✔	✔
amino acids		✔			
amino acids		✔			
whey:casein 60:40	Fat blend	✔	✔	✔	

LIQUIDS

"lactose" and do you NOT see any corn syrup, brown rice syrup, glucose syrup, maltodextrin or sucrose, then you know the formula sugar is 100% lactose.

Fat: Human milk contains palmitic acid.

Many infant formulas try to mimic human milk by using vegetable palm olein or palm oil. You may hear that palm olein/palm oil causes constipation. We agree that palm oil is less soluble than other fatty acids but most babies do just fine with it.

As Bridget Young, PhD, perinatal nutrition expert, and founder of BabyFormulaExpert.com points out, some formula companies are now starting to use a newer form of palm oil (High 2 Palmitic Oil) that is less likely to cause hard poo. Other vegetable oils like safflower/sunflower (oleic) oil, soy oil, and coconut oils are also very safe.

◆   *Non-palm oil formula* –> Similac, Kirkland, Kabrita

Omega 3 Fatty Acids,

Because DHA and ARA are found in human milk, most major U.S. infant formulas add DHA. But studies show this supplement makes absolutely no difference with brain and vision development.

◆   *DHA-free formula* –> Earth's Best No Added DHA/ARA formula (in the green can)

Note: Lutein, another vision promoting ingredient in human milk, is added to some infant formulas.

Organic Formulas.

These are the certified "antibiotic, pesticide, and growth hormone free" products on the market. Are these organic formulas worth the hefty price tag? It's your call. The good news: stores like Wal-Mart now sell generic organic formula at lower prices.

◆   *Organic formula*–> Similac Organic, Enfamil Simply Organic, Gerber Natura, Earth's Best, Walmart (Parents' Choice

Dr. Young's tip: Ingredients matter. Remember, the protein source of the formula will make the biggest difference to your baby's comfort. I recommend finding the right protein source for your baby first and then trying to get it organic if that is important to you.

DR B'S OPINION: DON'T SNEAK TODDLER FORMULA!

ALL "toddler" formula bypasses the FDA process and the formulations are NOT appropriate for babies under 12 months of age. Be honest with your pediatrician if you are contemplating this product (that is, don't lie and use this behind your doctor's back).

Carrageenan additive.

Carrageenan, a seaweed derived food additive, is an ingredient used in some ready-to-feed and liquid-concentrate formula to keep it stable. The World Health Organization deems it safe in small amounts, but some experts do have concerns about an association with gut irritation. While we are not too worried about this ingredient, we do prefer powder formula anyway for the cost savings alone!

◆ *Carrageenan-free formula–>* powder formula

Decision tree for your wallet:

Generic or store brand baby formula in powder form is the least expensive way to provide optimal nutrition for your baby. Even if you opt for organic baby formula, organic store-brand in powder form is available from several retailers.

Helpful Hint

Do not switch formulas without asking your doctor. Most babies who are gassy and fussy will be gassy and fussy for the first three months of life no matter what they are eating.

Dr Young says, "If you do switch formulas, I recommend going slowly if possible. Start by mixing a little of the new formula in with old formula in each bottle. Then slowly increase the amount of new formula as you decrease the amount of old formula so that it takes a couple of days to get fully onto the new formula."

BOTTOM LINE

All marketed infant formulas are tested extensively and required by law (Infant Formula Act 1986) to contain minimum levels of 30 different nutrients.

Soy Formula

Considering soy formula? There are very few reasons why any baby would need this product. The American Academy of Pediatrics (AAP) recommends soy formula for the following limited reasons:

FORMULA FOR PREEMIES

There are higher-calorie formulas made especially for babies who are born before 34 weeks gestation or less than four pounds. These formulas have more calories, more protein, more calcium, and more phosphorous than standard formulas. Some babies will switch to standard formula, but the premature formulas can be used for a whole year if necessary for growth. (*AAP Committee on Nutrition*)

◆ Full term babies who are not breastfeeding and whose parents want a vegetarian alternative to cow's milk-based formula. Soy formula is considered a safe alternative.
◆ Full term babies with galactosemia or hereditary lactase deficiency.
◆ Full term babies with documented (diagnosed) transient lactase deficiency.
◆ Babies with documented (diagnosed) IgE-mediated allergy to cow's milk.

The AAP does NOT recommend soy formula for:

◆ Preterm infants with birth weights less than 1800g (4 lbs).
◆ Prevention of colic or allergy.
◆ Infants with Food Protein Induced Allergic Proctocolitis (FPIAP) or Food Protein Induced Enteropathy (FPIE) (*AAP Committee on Nutrition*)

Q. I am primarily breastfeeding, but will need to supplement with formula once I return to work. Any advantage to buying the formulas especially designed "for supplementation"?

In our opinion, no. Enfamil first came up with this idea and competitors Similac and Gerber soon followed with formula "designed for supplementation."

There are very few, if any, differences between the product specifically labeled for supplementation and the standard cow's milk infant formula made by the same manufacturer. As Dr. Young points out, "If you are providing formula as a supplement to breastfeeding, I still recommend starting off by finding the right protein source that keeps your baby comfortable. That should guide your choice." We would suggest using the regular infant formula and calling it a day.

Q. What are "comfort proteins" and "gentle formulas"? Should I believe claims that some formulas are easier to digest?

As discussed earlier, some infant formulas contain partially broken down or predigested cow milk protein. And yes, they probably are a little easier to digest. Look for the words "partially hydrolyzed" in the ingredients. Goat milk-based formulas naturally contain A2 beta casein, which, according to some studies, is easier to digest than standard cow milk protein.

Q. So which is better, cow,goat milk protein-based formula or soy formula?

The consensus according to the American Academy of Pediatrics: cow or goat milk protein-based infant formulas are perfectly acceptable as optimal infant nutrition for non-breastfed babies or those needing formula supplementation in the first year of life. Cow milk and goat milk are adapted for baby formula to support normal growth and development (*HealthyChildren.org Oct 2023*). Soy formula is acceptable infant nutrition for specific health circumstances or families seeking a non-animal product.

Q. I have seen other formulas on the shelf at the grocery store. What are they used for?

These would be classified as the "gourmet formulas." Most are made for babies with particular problems. A few are made as optional products, which are not based on a medical necessity. See the following section for more on gourmet formulas.

? ?

LIQUIDS

Insider Tip

Baby formula is really expensive. Gourmet baby formula is even more expensive. Choose your formula based on the big picture (macronutrients including protein, fat, carbohydrates) ingredients that your baby tolerates. The other stuff lacks enough evidence for the cost, but feel free to spend your money on it.

The Gourmet Formulas

1. Lactose Free Formula

Lactose intolerance occurs in older children and adults. Babies are rarely born with this problem. Lactose intolerance can occur temporarily after an infant has a stomach virus. Some stomach viruses break down the human enzyme "lactase" which digests the lactose sugar, creating a temporary intolerance. This can go on for one to six *weeks* after the virus.

When babies are allergic to formula, it is usually the milk *protein* that is the problem, as it is the most allergenic part of the food. It is rare for a baby to have a problem with the milk sugar (lactose). Human milk has lactose in it and it is perfect nutrition.

2. Similac for Diarrhea

This delicacy is made for babies who are experiencing a stomach virus. Not only has the lactose sugar and cow's milk protein been removed, but 6 grams of fiber are added per liter of formula. You're thinking, why give fiber to a child with the runs? Believe it or not, fiber actually bulks up watery stools. This formula can be used for the duration of a stomach bug to cut down on the water loss that occurs with intestinal infections. However, it should only be used when your baby's doctor recommends it.

3. Enfamil AR / Similac for Spit-Up

All babies spit up a little. But babies who suffer from heartburn (a.k.a. gastroesophageal reflux or GERD) spit up a lot or are very uncomfortable at meal time. Historically, pediatricians would recommend thickening a formula to keep it from coming back up. The science does not really support this treatment but it is worth a try. Add a teaspoon of rice cereal to each bottle to make the formula heavier. After trying this at home, however, I can tell you that the formula gets clumpy and it requires minor surgery on the rubber nipple to get it out of the bottle.

Enfamil AR or Similac for Spit-Up solves this problem by adding rice starch to their regular cow's milk formula. This is much easier to use, reducing your frustration. You will still need to use bottle nipples with a larger hole to get the formula to flow, however.

4. Formula with probiotics

Human milk has lots of good bacteria, so now some formulas have them, too. The potential benefits include fewer illnesses, less severity/frequency of diarrhea, and yes, maybe less colic. And there do not seem to be any significant risks with this type of formula. (*Weizman*)

Are the health benefits worth the added cost? Maybe, but only time and more research will tell. A cheaper option: Buy a L reuteri probiotic supplement and toss it into whatever your baby is eating once a day. (see Appendix B, Complementary Medications, for details)

FYI: If you use a probiotic-enhanced formula, be sure to mix it with water less than 100 degrees or you will kill all those little good germs!

LIQUIDS

? ?

5. Formula with prebiotics

Found naturally in human breast milk, prebiotics feed good germs in the gut. Hence, probiotics (see above) are good bacteria, while prebiotics are food for good bacteria. Prebiotics may aid in digestion, boost immunity to disease, and reduce allergies—but most of the research on these benefits is only in its infancy.

Most of the major brand infant formulas now contain prebiotics, including Similac, Enfamil, Gerber, and Kabrita. Cow milk-based formula add a biosynthetic product called human milk oligosaccharide (HMO). Oligosaccharides are naturally present in goat milk-based formula.

6. Formula with MFGM

MFGM stands for Milk Fat Globule Membrane which is basically a brain superfood. It is found in both human and other animal milks. It promotes brain development and supports the baby's microbiome. Older version baby formulas removed MFGM in the manufacturing process but Enfamil is touting inclusion of this bioactive nutrient based on a Swedish study showing better cognitive scores in babies who ate MFGM enriched infant formula. Note: this study made no adjustment for mom's IQ or educational level, did not have a breastfeeding baby control group, and had no long term follow up after the study. *(Hernell O, 2016)*. Our take: it's not worth the additional cost for this formula based on available data.

7. Formula with Lactoferrin

Lactoferrin is a protein found in breastmilk, particularly colostrum, that helps with iron absorption. It also has antimicrobial properties. This bioactive ingredient may be useful for a newborn who is formula fed from the start, but may be less useful for a baby who is primarily breastfed and formula is being used as a supplement or for a baby who starts formula after six months of age.

8. Older baby and toddler formulas

According to formula companies, toddler formulas are designed for older babies who are eating solid foods. This product contains more calcium than standard infant formula. The pitch: babies over nine months have a higher calcium requirement than younger infants.

The issue: companies are trying to hook parents with "next step" or follow-up formula for 9-24 month olds and "toddler formulas" designed for one to three year olds. The formulas, with added vitamins, are pitched to parents as an allegedly better substitute for cow's milk.

Is any of this necessary? We say no. Follow-up and toddler formulas are generally a waste of money. The calcium content of standard infant formulas is appropriate for birth to 12 months of age. After one year of age, a baby can drink whole or 2% milk—and milk is 85% cheaper than toddler formula! The American Academy of Pediatrics Committee on Nutrition concurs. They do not recommend using toddler or follow-up formulas for healthy children who have low risk of nutritional deficiency. (*Georgieff*)

Q. I've heard commercially prepared infant formula contains a ton of artificial ingredients. What do you think of making our own formula? I've seen recipes online.

No, we discourage DIY formula. We, too, have also seen these recipes circulating around the blogosphere, along with warnings not to tell your child's pediatrician that you are doing it.

Simply put, moms who came along before us tried to create a breast milk alternative in their kitchens—it worked out okay for some babies, and was an epic fail for others. Pediatricians want their little patients to get the exact combination of nutrients they need to thrive and grow. That is why we prefer products that are regulated to ensure that happens.

The most recent DIY formula disaster pulled from the headlines: three babies were treated for severe Vitamin D and calcium deficiency rickets (a bone disorder) due to consuming an alkaline diet-based DIY formula. *(Calello)*

If you are trying to save money, then buy generic infant formula. If you are seeking a GMO-free, organic, corn syrup-free product, then opt for buying an organic infant formula like Earth's Best, Happy Baby, Burt's Bees, Bobbie, or ByHeart.

Bougie Formulas

Q. Several friends told me to buy European formula online because it is healthier for my baby. Is it worth the cost and hassle?

So glad you asked—our opinion is no. This is the hot question of the moment. While there are stricter food standards in the European Union, there is no regulation when they are boot-legged and sold by third party vendors in the U.S. We want you to be aware that Kabrita is the ONLY European infant formula that is FDA-approved and sold in stores and online in the US.

You can find less expensive, organic, non-GMO offerings and even grass-fed cows on this side of the pond. Also note: European formulas contain less iron than the U.S. standard requirement.

The main concern about buying European formula through unregulated sources is that the shipping and storage are not guaranteed. Remember, infant formula is food for your little one—and its freshness depends on the temperature and length of time it is sitting in storage.

Q. What about Bobbie formula? It is European-style formula but made in the U.S.?

Sure, it checks all the boxes. This U.S.-made (Vermont) infant formula meets the FDA and U.S. infant formula standards, and you don't need to find a middleman to buy it under the cover of darkness from Berlin. Specifically, Bobbie uses lactose for the sugar component, a 60:40 whey:casein milk protein ratio, oleic and coconut oil for the fat component, and it is non-GMO. They were the first organic formula made in the U.S. and contain the ingredients that draw Americans to the European formula market.

Q. What about ByHeart formula? It's really expensive. Is it worth the cost?

We will give you the scoop on this unique American-made baby formula and then you can decide if it is worth it.

New to the market in spring 2022, ByHeart is made in their own manufacturing facility in

Reading, PA. This baby formula is innovative because it is the first U.S. company that uses organic whole milk (from grass-fed cows) for the fat component.

The milk cream in the fat blend means that it DOES NOT contain palm oil or soy oil and it DOES contain MFGM, omega-3 fatty acids, and fat-soluble vitamins naturally. The sugar source is 100% lactose. The protein source is a mix of many proteins including regular cow's milk whey and casein, partially hydrolyzed whey in a 70:30 whey:casein milk protein ratio, alpha-lactalbumin (the most common protein in human breastmilk, making it very digestible) and lactoferrin (another common protein in human breastmilk, which helps with iron absorption).

The return-on-investment decision is up to you. But, kudos to this company for creating a very competitive new product that may change the baby formula paradigm in the U.S.

Q. Are goat milk based infant formulas okay to use?

Yes. The milk of both cows and goats have been used for over 200 years to provide nutrition in non-breastfed babies. In fact, the proteins are similar enough that a baby with a true cow milk protein allergy should also avoid goat milk protein (goat milk formula is not an alternative for cow milk allergic babies).

Cow milk became the preferred base for commercially prepared infant formula primarily due to cost. Both cow and goat milk must be modified to fulfill the nutritional needs for human babies. So, commercially made goat milk based infant formula is perfectly appropriate to meet a baby's dietary needs. Some studies show that goat milk based formula is actually more tolerated or "gentler" than cow milk based formula (aka worth the higher price tag) but it is certainly equivalent nutritionally.

Goat milk based infant formula is popular and readily available in Europe and Asia. At the time we are going to print, Kabrita, a Dutch-based formula company, is the first FDA-approved goat milk based infant formula sold in the U.S. It has gone through the arduous process to achieve long-term FDA authorization, ensuring that it is legally and safely imported.

Q. Do you have a preference for powder, concentrate, or ready-to-feed?

As we mentioned above, we pointed out the cheapest option formula is powder. But is it best for baby? The answer: it's complicated. And cost isn't the only factor to consider.

The American Dental Association suggests using ready-to-feed formula to avoid excess fluoride intake (see discussion of this in the previous chapter). Or if you choose powder or liquid concentrate formula, the ADA recommends mixing it with purified, demineralized, deionized, distilled, or reverse osmosis filtered water.

Powdered formulas are heat-treated but cannot be commercially sterilized like ready-to-feed formula. Thus, powdered formulas contain low levels of microorganisms. One particular germ, Cronobacter sakazakii, can cause serious infections in babies who are low birth weight, born prematurely, or immune compromised. (*Centers for Disease Control*) That's why we recommend boiling bottled water before mixing with powdered formula.

Given those concerns, we STILL recommend powder formula as the best option for baby. But we do so with the following caveats:

1. Mix powder formula with purified, demineralized, deionized, distilled, or reverse osmosis

? ?

LIQUIDS

filtered tap water *that is boiled* (the water must be over 158 degrees to kill the germs).

2. Cool or chill the prepared formula slightly before giving it to your baby (test it on your inner wrist to check the temperature).

3. Refrigerate and use the prepared formula within 24 hours of preparation.

4. Toss any unused formula after a feeding.

5. Don't use a blender to prepare it—blenders can harbor bacteria.

6. Refrigerate any bottled water after opening it to prevent germs growing in the water.

7. Don't use powder formula if your baby was low birth weight, premature, or is immune compromised.

It's perfectly fine to use liquid concentrate or ready-to-feed formulas, but they are significantly more expensive.

FYI: the nutrients are the same for all types of formula!

Old Wives Tale
The ready to feed formula is easier to digest.

The Truth: The ready to feed is convenient, a little thicker, and a lot more expensive. All products are digested exactly the same way.

Q. Do I need to sterilize the bottles, boil water, or use bottled water to mix the formula?

No, maybe, and yes.

You don't need to sterilize bottles. Yes, we do suggest a run through the dishwasher when you first open the packages. Thereafter, you can clean bottles with warm, soapy water. That's clean enough.

You don't need to boil the water you use to mix *liquid-concentrate* formula because the American water supply is pretty clean. You DO need to boil the water you use to mix powder formula (see the previous question). Note: if you have well water, you need to get your water tested before your baby arrives to make sure it isn't contaminated.

Yes, we do recommend bottled water to mix *powdered* formula—see the above discussion in the previous question for more details. We also discussed this issue (fluoride and formula) in the previous chapter, Chapter 5, Nutrition.

Real Talk: Do NOT use alkaline water to prepare infant formula. Your baby's pH does not need to be altered.

Helpful Hint
Look at the mixing instructions on the formula can. Powder requires one scoop per two ounces of water. Liquid concentrate is one ounce of formula per one ounce of water. Ready-to-feed is ready to go (DON'T ADD WATER). This may seem obvious to you. But if you screw up, your baby gets either half of the calories he needs or rocket fuel.

My mother-in-law (who was a very bright woman) mistakenly bought ready-to-feed formula for her third baby (my future husband) and added water because she thought she had purchased concentrate. Her astute pediatrician identified the problem at the baby's two-week well check when he wasn't gaining weight. Sure, this baby ended up nearly six feet tall as an

LIQUIDS

? ?

adult, but we figure he could have topped Shaq's height if this mistake was caught earlier.

 Reality Check

Formula preparation is pretty quick and easy. We do not recommend using gadgets that mix formula like the Baby Brezza Formula Pro. Our opinion: the device is not precise enough to mix formula in correct concentrations and can be a potential health hazard.

Q. Which bottles/nipples do you recommend?

Walk into any baby store and you'll see the Wall of Bottles—a mind-numbing array of baby bottles and nipples, each claiming to be the best choice for your newborn. While we review baby bottles in depth in our other book, *Baby Bargains*, here is a quick primer.

Bottles come in several different types: glass, plastic and polycarbonate. Any type is fine.

Which nipples are best? Lactation consultants we've interviewed seem to like the Avent nipples best. They believe there is less nipple confusion when alternating between breast and bottle. Note: There are newborn nipples (low flow), older baby nipples (higher flow), and cross cut nipples (highest flow). You can switch to the older baby nipples at three months. The cross cut nipples are better for babies with reflux who drink thickened formula.

 Reality Check

Feeder bottles (solid food dispensers) are unnecessary. Your baby needs to learn how to eat, *not drink* their solid food. (See the next chapter for more).

Q. How much and how often do I feed my baby?

For the first few days of life, a newborn might take up to an ounce (30-60 ml) every few hours. After the first few days, offer him three ounces in a bottle and see what he does with it. From day three to two weeks old, babies usually eat about 2-3 ounces every 3-4 hours. They gradually want more to eat over the next several weeks. But as you might guess by the standard bottle size, babies eventually max out at eight ounces per feeding.

How will you know when your baby wants more to drink than what you have offered? Easy. He will finish off what you gave him and look for more! And the beauty of babies is that most of them just eat what they need to and then stop when they are full. So if you follow your baby's lead, he will probably eat just the right amount.

Using the "Big Picture" guidelines below, you will have a decent idea of how much and how often you can expect your baby to drink.

The Big Picture: Formula Feeding for the First Year

Birth to 2 weeks: (14-20 oz)

Newborns tend to eat two to three ounces every three to four hours. For the first two weeks, wake your baby if it has been more than four hours since the last feeding. Once baby has regained birth weight, they can sleep as much as they want (good luck)!

2 weeks to 2 months: (17-25 oz)

You will see a gradual increase in volumes at feedings. By two months, babies usually take around four ounces per feeding, about every three hours.

2 to 4 months: (21-30 oz)

Your baby will eat six to eight ounces per feeding, usually 21-30 oz. with a max *at about 40 oz per day at about four months of age.*

When the volumes go up, the number of daily feedings go down. So, a baby who chugs eight ounces at a feeding can eat five times a day and sleep through the night. Parents often ask if they can space out the frequency of daytime feedings. NO! Use common sense here—if your baby eats every two to three hours during the day, you will all be sleeping at night. (Get used to it. This frequency of meals continues into preschool, when kids still eat three meals and two snacks a day.)

Babies who take smaller volumes at each feeding will need to eat more often. These tend to be babies who suffer from heartburn (**GERD**). We'll have more on this in Chapter 8, The Other End.

4 to 6 months: (25-32 oz)

Babies continue to take a ballpark of 25-32 oz, up to a max of 40 oz per day of formula. Even if you begin offering your baby a nibble or two of solid food, *there should be no reduction in the volume of formula.* Initially, you should view complementary solid food as dessert.

6 to 9 months: (24-36 oz)

You'll be going full speed ahead on solid food. Your baby will start to wean—decreasing volumes of formula as their intake of calories from solid food increases. By seven to nine months, you will see this start to happen.

9 to 12 months: (20-30 oz)

Your baby will decrease drinking formula to a minimum of 20 oz per day. At one year of age, your baby will usually drink about three 8 oz bottles. This will then be replaced by whole or 2% milk that is Vitamin D fortified. *The goal is 16 oz a day (which is two cups a day) of milk.* The equivalent in dairy products is also fine.

It's time to kick the bottle habit at a year. Don't get stuck here. You don't have a baby anymore. You have a toddler. If you want a baby in your house, go have another one. Yes, your child will be quite capable of drinking via a cup or a cup with a straw. They will not go thirsty.

Other Liquids

Q. Does my baby need any water?

LIQUIDS

? ?

Not until six months of age.

The reason: your baby is already getting water. It's naturally in breast milk and added to prepared formula. Your baby gets plenty of water. After six months of age, your baby should start to drink some water every day. How much? Even though there is no official guideline, we think four to six ounces of water a day is adequate. It is fine to drink water from a baby bottle (see below). It does not take six months to learn how to drink from a cup!

No matter what other liquid babies are drinking or how it is prepared (breast milk, ready-to-feed formula, or powder/liquid concentrate formula), babies *over six months of age* should all drink some fluoride containing water (0.7ppm) on a daily basis. Again, four to six ounces a day is our best estimate on what is needed.

If your baby has no source of fluoride-containing water in their diet for whatever the reason (using fluoride-free bottled water, reverse osmosis filtered tap water, etc), then you should discuss getting a fluoride supplement with your doctor or dentist. For details on this whole fluoride issue, check out the section on Vitamin Supplements in Chapter 5, Nutrition.

Reality Check

Bottled water is not any safer than tap. A Dutch study compared bottled water from 16 countries. Of these samples, 37% were contaminated with bacteria and 4% were contaminated with fungus! Hence, for older children, tap water is preferred, since it usually contains fluoride. The only reason that we recommend using *distilled* bottled water to prepare formula is to ensure your infant doesn't get too much fluoride.

Q. When can I give my baby juice?

Pediatricians hate juice. The AAP actually came out with a policy statement saying that juice is "absolutely unnecessary for children under one." *(Heyman)* Sorry, juice producers of America. Here are the reasons:

1. **Juice provides little nutrition.** Vitamin C has to be added to many juices to give them any nutritive value. Otherwise, juice is just a form of liquid sugar.
2. **Juice is filling,** which decreases a child's appetite for more nutritious foods.
3. Drinking juice throughout the day (especially in a bottle) causes sugar buildup on the teeth. This, in turn, creates **high dental bills.**

DR B'S OPINION:
SIPPY CUPS

Yes, I know they are popular: the no-spill sippy cup. I have never been a fan of these because the sucking mechanism to get the fluid out is similar to a bottle. Dentists dislike sippy cups because the flow of liquid heads straight to the back of the top front teeth. In short, sippy cups can promote tooth decay.

I'd prefer to have your baby drinking from a straw if they haven't quite mastered the art of drinking from a cup. Another cool option: The Reflo drinking cup (reflo.net) which controls the flow of the liquid and reduces the mess while a child is learning how to hold and tilt a cup.

4. *A sugar-loaded diet causes diarrhea.*

 BOTTOM LINE: Children with poor weight gain, chronic diarrhea, or rotten teeth often are juice-a-holics. The American Academy of Pediatrics recommends no more than six oz of juice a day for 1-6 year olds.

Q. When can my baby drink from a cup?

You can try introducing a cup any time after six months of age, but there is certainly no rush. There is no reason to begin any type of trainer cup until your baby's first birthday.

It only takes a few days or weeks to learn to drink from a cup when child is developmentally ready—that is, around your baby's first birthday! Your long-term goal is to have your baby drinking from a cup around that time.

We repeat, it does not take six months to learn how to drink from a cup! Let your baby drink breastmilk, formula, or water from a baby bottle until they turn one.

DR B'S OPINION

"Don't offer juice. Give your baby or toddler some orange slices, strawberries, or papayas for some Vitamin C."

 ### Reality Check
Once your baby has teeth, you need to wipe them or brush them after the last feeding (before bedtime). Your baby shouldn't be falling asleep while they are eating by the time they have teeth anyway. (See Chapter 9, Sleep for details.)

Q. When and how do I switch to cow's milk?

At one year of age, cold turkey.

Your baby still needs a high fat diet because their brain development is on overdrive. The American Academy of Pediatrics recommends whole or 2% milk until *two years of age*. Previously, it was recommended that all children drink whole milk until age two. But the guidelines changed because many toddlers already eat a high-fat diet and obesity begins early in life. You and your child's doctor can decide whether whole or 2% is best for him, depending on your family history and your child's growth. (*American Heart Association*)

After the second birthday, your child should drink what the rest of the family is drinking. This should be *skim milk (nonfat or 1%)* for everyone. The fat will clog your baby's arteries just like it clogs ours.

 ### DR B'S OPINION: ALTERNATIVE MILKS

From 12 to 24 months of age, your child needs some dietary fat to build a healthy brain and calcium and Vitamin D to build healthy bones. I really don't care what your child eats or drinks to get those needs met. So if you or your child has some issue with cow's milk, choose an alternative milk . . . but compare labels to make sure it includes those nutrients.

? ?

LIQUIDS

Q. What do you think of alternative dairy products compared to cow's milk?

While some products have nearly the same calories as whole milk, less of those calories come from fat (and 12 to 24 month olds still need more fat than you do). Whole cow's milk is the preferred dairy beverage because it contains almost half of its calories from fat, 35% of your child's daily calcium requirement, and 20% of your child's Vitamin D needs per cup. Other products have trouble measuring up to that. If you select an alternative beverage, just be sure your child gets fat, calcium, and Vitamin D needs met elsewhere in their diet. Here is a comparison:

8 OZ SERVING	WHOLE MILK (3.5% FAT)	SKIM MILK (0.1% FAT)	SOY MILK	RICE MILK	ALMOND	RIPPLE
Calories	150 calories	80	150	130	30	100
Total fat	8 grams	0	4	2	2.5	4.5
Sodium	115 mg	125	140	105	125	130
Carbohydrate	11 grams	12	22	26	2	6
Cholesterol	35 mg	0	0	0	0	0
Protein	8 grams	9	7	1	1	8
Vitamin A	yes	yes	yes	yes	yes	yes
Vitamin C	yes	yes	no	no	yes	no
Vitamin D	yes	yes	yes	yes	yes	yes
Calcium	50%	50%	60%	<10%	45%	45%
Other nutrients				iron	B12	

2% or "reduced fat" cow's milk contains 2% fat and about 120 calories per 8 oz serving.

Q. What do you think of organic milk?

It's expensive.

Some families prefer to buy organic, pesticide free products. Others don't. There is no public health group that recommends the use of organic milk over store brand cow's milk. Some parents have concerns about bovine growth hormone in "regular" milk causing precocious puberty. Currently, medical evidence is lacking to support this claim. It's your call.

While organic milk is fine, we don't recommend raw or unpasteurized milk. We discuss the hazards of raw milk in Chapter 13, Infections.

Q. I've heard that goat's milk is healthier than cow's milk. Is this true?

No. When it comes to nutrients, cow's milk is about the same as goat's milk. Goat's milk contains less B12, folate, and iron. Goat's milk contains slightly more fat, and slightly less sugar (lactose) but that's about it.

It's totally fine if you prefer pasteurized goat's milk fortified with Vitamin D for your toddler. Just find other food sources for B12, Folate, and iron.

We do not recommend that you buy a goat to provide fresh milk for your family (check your local zoning ordinances first!).

Q. Is it okay to use formula after a year of age?

It is not the appropriate diet for a child over age one. For babies who are failing to thrive, your doctor might recommend a dietary supplement (such as Pediasure, Carnation Instant Breakfast). Using formula for convenience when you are out and about isn't harmful, but is unnecessary. Using formula for nutrition is a waste of money.

Now that you're an expert at liquids, let's move on to a topic that truly indicates your baby is growing up: eating solid food! Up next, your guide to solid foods, food allergies and more.

SOLIDS

Chapter 7

"Raising kids is part joy and part guerrilla warfare."
~ Ed Asner

WHAT'S IN THIS CHAPTER

◆ **HOW TO TELL IF YOUR BABY IS READY TO EAT SOLID FOOD**

◆ **GETTING STARTED: 4 TO 6 MONTHS**

◆ **MAKING YOUR OWN FOOD**

◆ **WHAT IS BABY-LED WEANING? FEARLESS FEEDING?**

◆ **6 MONTHS+**

◆ **FOOD ALLERGY SPECIAL SECTION**

◆ **THE BIG PICTURE— HOW MUCH TO OFFER AND WHEN**

This is the chapter you have been waiting for! After months of feeding your baby a liquid diet, you're looking forward to those photos with peas all over your baby's cute little face.

You are welcome to read this chapter at any time, but know that solid food doesn't enter the picture until your baby is four to six months old. Note: Although it's fine to try a limited amount of solid food between four and six months, breast milk or formula is the mainstay of nutrition.

When your baby is taking larger amounts of solid foods (six to nine months of age), solid food will start to replace some of the nutrients that liquid nutrition offers.

Before we get going, we need to tell you a little secret. There is nothing special about baby food. In fact, we are on a mission to banish "Baby Food" from the dictionary. We want your baby to eat Food . . . basically, the food you are eating. So when you see Food in this chapter with a capital F, that's what we mean.

Prepared commercial baby food is not in any way superior to the food you prepare in your home. It is just ready-made like a frozen pizza at the grocery store. Sure, it is convenient to pack up a jarred food or squeeze pouch when you are on the go or bringing meals to childcare, but we are hopeful that this chapter will help you make Food that is just as easy and portable.

We also want you to view your child's experience with solid food like any other developmental milestone. You give them the opportunity, and they master it when they are ready. Despite what all your family and friends will tell you, there are very few rules about introducing Food.

Here are five simple guidelines:

1. Let your baby try **any food** (except for raw, uncooked honey)*. In fact, we encourage introduction of food (including high allergy foods) at four to six months of age.

2. **Food diversity ASAP is the goal.** The age-old paradigm of offering one single ingredient food every few days to identify a food allergy has created generations of paranoid parents. While updated policy guidance from major medical organizations is forthcoming, it is MUCH easier to offer multiple new foods and then do some detective work if a food allergy concern arises. And eating higher allergy foods regularly reduces the risk of developing a food allergy. Fear not, let your baby eat your food.

3. **Use your seasonings and spices to flavor food.** Just keep salt to a minimum for everyone's health.

4. **Prioritize iron-containing foods.** Your baby needs an additional dietary source of iron in their diet, beyond breast milk or formula. We'll teach you which foods contain iron later in this chapter.

5. **Eating is a developmental milestone.** Your baby will start out eating very little solid food until they figure out how to move food around in their mouth, chew, and swallow. Most babies figure this out by eight to nine months of age. At that point, aim for three solid meals a day and your baby will cut back on liquid food intake on their own.

*Raw honey carries a risk of botulism for babies under one year of age.

Pretty easy, right? We will go into greater detail in this chapter, but really, this is not rocket science.

When to Start Solid Foods

Q. I hear that solid food helps a baby sleep through the night. Can I feed my two-month-old some cereal?

No. Starting solid foods will not make your baby sleep through the night. Most babies start sleeping through the night by four months of age. It is not because their tummies are full of rice cereal, but because they are developmentally able to by that age.

The right time to start solid food is somewhere between four and six months of age. There are some good reasons why you do not want to start before four months of age:

1 **INTRODUCING SOLID FOODS BEFORE FOUR MONTHS OF AGE CAN LEAD TO OBESITY.** Some research suggests that a parent who jumps headfirst into solid foods is more likely to misinterpret a baby's fussiness for being hungry—and overfeed them. (*Huh*) Babies who begin eating solid food before four months of age have a one in four chance of obesity later in life. Babies who start between four and six months of age have a one in 20 chance.

2 **INTRODUCING SOME SOLID FOODS BEFORE FOUR MONTHS OF AGE CAN LEAD TO DIABETES.** Recent studies suggest that babies who *first* eat wheat or barley (gluten-containing grains) before four months of age or after seven months of age can develop an inappropriate autoimmune response that leads to Type 1 Diabetes. (*Snell-Bergeon*)

PREEMIES & SOLID FOOD

Because eating solid food requires a certain level of oral motor skill, many premature babies are not ready to eat solid food until their adjusted age (based on due date) is at least four to six months old. Also, preemies tend to need lots of extra calories for catch up growth. Liquid nutrition is a much better source for calories than solid food.

---

3 SOLID FOOD DOES NOT PROVIDE ANY NECESSARY NUTRIENTS FOR AN INFANT UNDER FOUR MONTHS OF AGE. Breast milk and formula are the only items that should be on the menu for babies from birth to at least four months. These products contain 50% fat and thus, are loaded with calories (20 calories per oz). So unless you are serving lard for dinner, you will never get that many calories in solid food! Breast milk and formula also contain all the essential nutrients a young infant needs (with the exception of Vitamin D—see Chapter 5, Growth and Nutrition for the discussion on that issue).

Q. My baby is four months old now. Are they ready to eat solid foods?

It depends. The advice on this topic can be confusing, but experts at the AAP and the National Institute of Allergy and Infectious Diseases recommend starting solid food sometime between four and six months of age when a baby shows signs of readiness. *(NIAID)* Babies DO need to eat foods beyond breast milk or formula around six months of age for additional nutrients and for prevention of food allergies.

But you may hear contradictory advice for the four to six month old age group—even the AAP doesn't agree with itself on when to start solid foods. While the AAP Nutrition Committee says go for it, the AAP Breastfeeding Committee says wait to start solids until six months if your baby is breastfed (because it promotes continued breastfeeding).

So what defines "readiness" for solid food? Your baby is ready when they know what to do with food in their mouth (**ORAL MOTOR SKILLS**). Some babies are ready at four months; some aren't ready until six months. Your baby will tell you if they are ready. Let your baby sit at the dinner table with you and join the mealtime experience. If they watch every bite you are taking, let them have a bite, too.

If your baby swallows it, they are ready. If they spit it back out at you, try again another day. But being at the table at mealtime is a good social experience to start now—even if no food is eaten!

BOTTOM LINE: There is a great deal of variability amongst babies (and their doctors) about when they are ready to eat solid food. Anywhere between four to six months is fine. But remember, solid food is a developmental experience from four to six months and not really for nutrition.

Reality Check

One-third of parents do not listen to the pediatrician's advice and start feeding babies solid food *before* four months of age. The reasons are unclear. Whatever the case may be, please wait until your baby is at least four months of age. Trust us.

How to Start Solid Foods

Q. I have some friends who recommend baby-led weaning. What is it, exactly?

This is a great question because learning *how* to feed your child is just as important as learning *what* to feed your child.

Baby-led weaning advocates suggest that babies who are six months of age and older do not need pureed food and do not need to be spoon-fed. Their position: the whole point of eating solid food is learning how to gnaw, chew, and swallow. Babies can be given bite-sized pieces and stick shaped "finger food," such as broccoli, cucumber sticks, bananas, or a soft chicken leg. Advocates admit that most babies will do more exploration than eating initially and that gagging (not choking) does occur. The argument: bypassing baby food purees and parental control of feeding simplifies the process and reduces food battles later on.

We agree with many of these principles. We want your baby to eat Food. We want your baby to be an adventurous eater. And we'd like to minimize the high chair battlefield over eating a spoonful of pureed peas. However, there are two concerns with this feeding method:

Babies over six months of age need a dietary source of iron beyond breast milk or formula. If you rely on your baby to eat enough iron-containing foods on their own, they may become anemic by nine to twelve months of age. That's because babies will not master self-feeding for several months.

There will be gagging. Nothing ruins a perfectly good meal more than a baby who gags and vomits at the dinner table. If a solid-food novice eats a big chunk of food, it may come right back out. It's true that gagging is no big deal, but accidental choking is also possible— and calling 911 during dinner is a real buzzkill!

Bottom line: Spoon-feeding your baby some pureed foods at the beginning is fine. It is particularly important to offer iron-containing foods like soft meats, beans, eggs or fortified cereals. At the same time, you can let your baby try soft pieces of food and put them in charge. If you prefer the more traditional way to introduce solid food, advance from purees, to chunky texture, and then bite-sized pieces over 2-3 months. The take home message: find a feeding method that works for you and your little one.

Getting started: Four to Six Months

Before we get rolling, remember one key point: pretty much every "rule" about starting solid food has changed in the past few years.

Q. Is there a particular order to introduce new foods?

Nope.

Just one generation ago (ahem, when you were a baby), your parents dutifully fed you

? ?

SOLID FOODS

rice cereal, then single ingredient vegetables, then fruits, and so on. You didn't get to eat eggs until your first birthday and your first taste of peanut butter was at age three. These guidelines were supposed to prevent food allergies and make kids like vegetables. They failed at both! Lucky for you, introducing solid food to your baby is a whole lot easier than it used to be.

According to the American Academy of Pediatrics, "no comprehensive research has been conducted on which specific complementary foods [solids] to provide or in which order." *(AAP Committee on Nutrition)*.

Just be sure to offer iron-containing foods daily and high allergy foods regularly starting around six months of age. We will discuss in detail later in the chapter.

Reality Check

Commercially prepared baby food is nothing special, plus it is five times more expensive than cooking the same food at home.

Q. What is the first solid food I should offer?

It does not need to be rice cereal, and honestly it really doesn't matter. Just start and don't look back.

Yes, get ready to have your mind blown—let your baby eat whatever you are eating. In Austin, Texas, that very well may be a breakfast taco.

In all seriousness, a bite of mashed avocado, pureed beans, or queso is a great introduction to real food. Allergy experts want to de-medicalize the process of introducing solid food to babies and encourage parents to practice Fearless Feeding.

Allen Lieberman, MD, a pediatric allergist and medical advisor for our book, advises parents of low-risk infants (no severe eczema or egg allergy) to feed their babies "whatever they want, whenever they want" and not delay introducing any foods.

Q. Which foods contain iron?

Full-term babies are born with a full tank of iron, which gets depleted by four to six months of age. And breastfed babies get very little iron from breastmilk (formula is fortified with iron). The important point: at or around six months of age, your baby needs a daily source of iron in their diet.

Back in the day, rice cereal was the perennial "first food" to feed a baby. It's rare to be allergic to rice and it is fortified with iron and zinc, two key nutrients a baby needs. But there is nothing magical about it.

That's why some experts suggest making meat one of your baby's go-to foods instead. Why? Meat contains both nutrients in abundance . . . plus iron and zinc in meat are better absorbed by the body than in iron-fortified infant cereal. Steak is a choking hazard, but you can start with a meat puree (beef, lamb, pork, turkey, chicken), ground meat, meat sauce, or a chicken salad. *(AAP Committee on Nutrition)* Other iron-containing foods include eggs, beans, lentils, tofu, green leafy vegetables, and yes, iron-fortified cereals (rice, oatmeal, barley, wheat).

SOLID FOODS

? ?

411 FEARLESS FEEDING IDEAS!

Fruits and Vegetables, Single Ingredient

Applesauce
Apricots
Asparagus
Avocados
Bananas
Broccoli
Carrots—cooked, pureed
Green beans
Guava
Mashed potatoes
Mango
Melons
Nectarines
Papaya
Peaches
Peas
Pears
Plums
Prunes
Pumpkin
Squash
Sweet potatoes

Fruits and Vegetables, more interesting textures

Bell peppers
Blueberries
Grapefruit
Kale and other greens
Kiwi
Oranges
Pineapple
Rhubarb—cooked
Spinach—cooked
Strawberries
Tomatoes

Dairy, Single Ingredient

Whole milk yogurt
Soft cheeses (cream cheese, sour cream)

Dairy, More interesting textures

Cottage cheese
Shredded cheese

Dairy, Combination foods

Yogurt and fruit smoothies
Mac & cheese (made with real cheese!)

Grains, Single Ingredient

Iron-fortified infant cereal
Rice, Barley, Oatmeal, Wheat
Millet cereal
Quinoa cereal

Grains, More interesting textures

Cheerios/Oatios or generic
Corn tortillas
Oat bran cereal
Pasta such as wagon wheels
Puffed kashi
Rice cakes

Grains, Combination foods

Cornbread
Enchiladas
Grits
Lasagna
Oat bran muffins
Polenta
Quinoa salad
Whole grain pancakes (*Add sweet potato or pumpkin to pancake/waffle batter to add nutrients!)
Whole grain waffles

Meats, Beans, Legumes, Single Ingredient

Beans: *red, kidney, white, black-eyed, navy, etc*
Beef; Chicken; Lamb; Pork; Turkey
Lentils
Split peas
Tofu
Garbanzo beans

Meats, Beans, Legumes, More interesting textures

Edamame; Egg; Fish
Peanut sauce, cashew/almond butter*

Meats, Beans, Legumes, Combination foods

Chicken salad
Egg salad
Falafel
Hummus

*Whole nuts are a choking hazard for kids under age three.

SOLID FOODS

Reality Check

If your family maintains a vegan or vegetarian diet, you do not HAVE to offer meat to your baby at all. There are dietary alternatives to meet your baby's/growing child's nutritional needs. If you plan on feeding your baby a purely vegan diet, chat with the pediatrician about potential vitamin supplements for iron, zinc, calcium, Vitamin B 12, and Vitamin D.

Q. What is rice cereal, anyway?

Rice cereal for babies is packaged in a box as dry flakes and sold in the baby food aisle. The brand doesn't matter, as long as it is labeled iron-fortified infant cereal.

Mix it with either expressed breast milk or formula—otherwise it tastes like cardboard. (Truth be told, even when you doctor it up, it still tastes like cardboard!). You can make it watery or slightly thick. Make about two tablespoons worth. If that isn't enough, you can always make more.

Helpful Hint

If you do feed your baby iron-fortified cereal, you may want to experiment with tastier cereals beyond rice. Try oatmeal, barley, or wheat. These grain cereals also offer another advantage: FIBER. Rice cereal contains no fiber . . . therefore, if your baby eats a fair amount of it, they may become constipated.

Q. Does rice cereal contain arsenic?

Yes, arsenic has been found in baby rice cereal, as well as in brown and white rice and other rice-containing products like rice milk and rice cakes. For details, check out Chapter 15, Safety. In a nutshell, we think rice cereal for infants is safe. But it is important to offer a variety of grains to reduce the arsenic exposure.

Q. How should I give my baby his first solid meal?

Offer it as a snack *after* your baby has had breast milk or formula. If you try to feed them solid food when they are hungry, they will only become impatient and frustrated. By six months of age, your baby could probably win a chugging contest with the speed they guzzle down 160 calories (eight ounces of liquid).

High chairs are a convenient way to let your baby have a seat at the kitchen table. Let them join you at mealtime, and offer a few bites (or spoonfuls) at a time. FYI: If your baby cannot sit upright and hold their head and neck up, they are not ready to eat solid food! (Our sister publication, BabyBargains.com, has recommendations for high chairs).

If you are spoon-feeding, your baby will tell you when they are no longer interested in eating by turning away or blowing raspberries at you. Do not force your baby to eat. This is meant to be fun, not nutrition.

For babies who are six months of age and up: if you are aiming for self-feeding, offer a few soft sticks or pieces of food (think banana or avocado) on their tray and let them smell, touch, mash, play, and taste their food. Food is a multisensory experience.

With either method, prepare for a mess—on your baby, high chair, and kitchen floor.

Q. What other foods should I offer as we get started?

Remember, there are no rules on which "order" to progress through these foods.

It is absolutely fine to let your baby eat what you have in your fridge/on your dinner table— assuming you eat a healthy diet. We fully support Fearless Feeding. Try everything (really)! And offer different textures of foods so your baby gets to practice new skills. There will be a learning curve.

If your baby has been diagnosed with a cow's milk protein allergy, ask your baby's doc first before offering yogurt or cheese products. And, get your pediatrician's guidance first if your baby has severe eczema or a known egg allergy.

Q. Are there any other foods my baby shouldn't eat?

Yes. Here are three:

- *Honey*: Wait on honey until your child is one year old. Honey contains *clostridium botulinum* spores that can cause botulism in an infant. (Infants' digestive systems are relatively sterile compared to ours and can't kill the spores).
- *Choking Hazards:* Raw carrots, celery, popcorn, potato chips, nuts, hard candy, hard meat, fruits with seeds, raisins, hotdogs, and grapes (unless cut lengthwise). Wait on these foods until your child is really good at chewing (two to three years).
- *Artificial sweeteners:* There is no official party line on this one, but there is no reason to offer these products to babies.

Q. I've heard I need to introduce one new food/ingredient at a time. Is this true?

Eh. Probably not. The age-old paradigm is to offer one new ingredient every three to four days in addition to what food has already been introduced. The concept: introducing one food at a time makes it easy to identify a food allergy if a reaction occurs. And full disclosure, *the AAP currently recommends no more than three new foods per week*. This policy may be changing soon, so stay tuned.

However, some allergy experts feel this approach delays the introduction to a variety of foods, which ultimately increases the risk of developing a food allergy! They advise offering multi-ingredient foods from the start instead of the old stepwise one-food-at-a-time approach. And if an allergic reaction occurs, the problem food can be teased out with allergy testing. (We will explain allergic reactions in the food allergy section later in the chapter.)

DR B'S OPINION: FEARLESS FEEDING

The paradigm of slowly introducing solid food may change soon. Giving fear-based advice for decades likely led to delaying introduction of many high allergy foods and hence, the huge rise in food allergic kids!

DR B's OPINION: While this advice deviates from the current AAP policy, I encourage you to dive in to solids by offering multi-ingredient foods. It is much easier and may prevent food allergies (and picky eaters).

Q. How often do I feed my baby solid foods?

Three times a day. There is more to the meal experience than nutrition. Mealtime should be a social, joyous experience when families gather together. It is about sitting around the kitchen table with loved ones—literally and metaphorically breaking bread together. That said, let your baby participate at breakfast, lunch, and dinner every day—even if there is not much food consumed initially.

The definition of a "solid food meal" for a four to six month old is a few bites or spoonfuls of food.

Until about eight to nine months, always feed your baby his breast milk or formula first. Your baby's primary source of nutrition is still breast milk or formula until they eat a large amount of solid food (we are talking about at least 12 oz. of solid food daily). So when your baby is just getting started with solids, view solid food as a snack between those liquid meals.

Looking ahead, your nine-month-old baby will eat significantly more solid food. They will naturally drink less of their calories as they consume more calories from solid food. Solid food will no longer just be a snack between nursing or bottle feedings. You will be able to offer liquid and solid food together at mealtime and your baby will drop a nursing session/bottle or two.

Reality Check

To give you some perspective: rice cereal has 60 calories per 1/4 cup (5 calories per tsp) and a 4 oz pouch of carrots has 50 calories. Your baby would need to eat almost 3/4 cup of cereal or three whole pouches of carrots to replace one bottle or breastfeeding session. You'll be lucky if your baby eats two tablespoons of cereal or 1 oz of carrots in a feeding session in the first weeks of starting solids.

Old Wives Tale

Introducing fruits before vegetables will give your baby a sweet tooth.

The truth: Your baby will either like vegetables or not. The order of introduction has

DR B'S OPINION: RECIPES

You can easily go to Instagram and find millions of recipes and "baby friendly" meals. But, I intentionally chose not to include an exhaustive list of suggested meal plans for your baby in this chapter. Why? Because I don't want you to make a separate meal for your baby! In the grand scheme of things, no one has time to be a short order cook and prepare different meals for each family member. Some parents say they make healthy baby food because they rely on Uber Eats for their next meal. While I support your parenting goals, don't forget about yourself. Spend your time making one healthy family meal for everyone.

? ?

SOLID FOODS

nothing to do with it. When your baby is a toddler, they won't eat *anything*.

Q. My baby started solids and now their skin is turning yellow—HELP!

You are what you eat!

Babies are often first introduced to a series of yellow vegetables (carrots, squash, sweet potatoes). All of these vegetables are rich in Vitamin A (carotene). This vitamin has a pigment that can collect harmlessly on the skin producing a condition called **CAROTINEMIA**. The difference between this condition and jaundice (high bilirubin level) is that jaundiced babies have a yellowing in the whites of their eyes. Sweet potato lovers don't have that. See Baby411.com (click on "Bonus Material") for a great picture.

Q. Can I make my own baby food?

Absolutely. But there is that phrase we hate, "baby food." We want you to offer Food from your table! That way, your baby will get used to your cooking! Yes, you can use seasonings, herbs, and spices. Just limit the amount of salt, and use iodized salt if you must add it. It's not that hard.

Of course, this assumes that you and your partner are preparing home-cooked meals for your family. When we refer to Food, we are not talking about a Big Mac and a side of fries. If you were a take-out/eat-out couple before you had a baby, now is the time to rethink mealtime . . . and get cooking.

Trust me, I'd never make it on "Top Chef" but even I could make food for my kids. Here's the secret: take the food that you are eating and mash it up into a texture your baby can handle. That's it. And it doesn't take that much time . . . you just need a blender or food processor. If you are on the go, pick up a cheap handheld baby food grinder or mill for about $10.

Feeding your baby gets even easier as they expand their repertoire of foods and figure out how to manage different textures and pieces of food. When your baby begins to work on self-feeding (at six months of age or older), cut up soft food into thin sticks or small pieces that her tiny fingers and hands can grasp.

Reality Check: Table salt vs fancy salt

Our bodies need iodine, a mineral that makes thyroid hormone. Iodine is found naturally in fish, kelp, and dairy products. Prior to 1924, many people developed goiters from iodine deficiency. An easy solution: salt manufacturers added iodine to standard table salt (hence the term "iodized"). But thanks to our diets and love of fancy salt, there is a modern-day resurgence of iodine deficiency. Sea salt and kosher salt do not contain iodine. Opt for table salt if you are going to add a little to your home-cooking.

Q. Is baby food in squeezable packages (pouches) safer or more healthy?

Baby food is baby food—regardless of the packaging. But, pouches are extremely popular with parents and kids on-the-go. Because babies and older kids can suck the pureed solid food directly out of the package, they don't require parental assistance. A parent can hand a pouch to a hungry child sitting in the back seat of a car and keep on driving through rush hour traffic. And, some parents report that pureed veggies are the only kind their kids will eat.

BEHIND THE SCENES: WHAT IS "ORGANIC"?

The USDA regulates the labeling of all of these "natural" products so that people know how natural a product really is. Organic products are meats, poultry, eggs, and dairy products made from animals that did not receive antibiotics or growth hormones or fruits and vegetables grown without pesticides or petroleum based fertilizers. Organic farms are certified by a government inspector. Here are the rules:

♦ *100% Organic* must have a USDA seal on it.
♦ *Organic* is made of 95% to100% organic ingredients.
♦ *Made with Organic Ingredients* is made of at least 70% organic ingredients.

So where's the downside, right?

For babies, learning how to eat foods of different textures is important. So, while pouches are certainly a convenient option, they should not be the only way you introduce solid foods to your fledgling eater. They also cost significantly more than jarred baby food (which already rivals a three star Michelin restaurant's prices in cost per ounce).

Bottom line: baby food pouches are fine when used in moderation.

Q. Is it ever a good idea to pre-chew food for my baby?

Um, no. Celebrity Alicia Silverstone was captured on video doing that, but remember she starred in *Clueless*.

Seriously, yes, some cultures practice "premastication," but there is no need to take the health risk in the modern age of utensils and food blenders. Mixing baby food with an adult's saliva increases the chance of spreading germs that can lead to infection, as well as germs that can lead to cavities.

Q. What do you think of organic baby food?

It's a lifestyle choice.

DR B'S OPINION:
PICKY-EATER TODDLERS

After years of watching babies grow up to be picky-eater toddlers, I can tell you those who acquire a taste for their parents' cooking early on, eat a broader range of healthy food in the toddler and preschool years. If you were a couple who usually ate out or ordered take-out in your pre-baby years, now is the time to make a permanent change in your food lifestyle. It really does take a family to eat healthy.

? ?

SOLID FOODS

As we have discussed, some parents make this a priority. Others don't. What does the science show? We will save that discussion for Chapter 15, Safety.

If you do opt for going organic, we advise you to prepare your own food from organic fruits and vegetables rather than to buy commercially prepared organic baby food, which is very expensive.

We'll delve into what we know about food-borne environmental exposures in Chapter 15, Safety.

Six months and beyond

Q. My baby is six months old now. What can he eat?

Full speed ahead! Let your baby eat what you are eating. This includes a variety of ethnic foods. Don't worry about herbs and spices you use in seasoning—just limit adding salt or sugar. Your baby needs to get used to your methods of food preparation.

Let your baby try different food groups and textures, and eat a larger volume as they demand it. They rarely overeat. Traditionally, we advised going from pureed to chunky (think apple sauce or guacamole) to bite-sized pieces or "finger foods". But it is fine to let your baby experiment with soft pieces or thin slices of foods at the same time you are feeding them purees and see what they can do. They may or may not like certain textures initially, but keep offering them. No pressure.

Q. How much solid food will my six-month-old eat?

Not much, initially. Real talk: you do not need to measure serving sizes for your baby's meals! You have too many more important things to do with your day. But to give you a rough estimate, a six-month-old may start out with an ounce or two of solid food and gradually move up to four ounces per meal. Your baby will tell you they are done by turning their head, spitting out their food, and/or throwing it on the floor.

Solid foods should still be a supplement and not replacement of calories. View solid food meals as snacks right now.

You are merely adding three solid food "meals" to your baby's liquid nutrition meals. And typically, six-month-old babies nurse or bottle feed five to six times a day.

Q. Is my six-month-old ready to eat eggs or peanut butter?

Yes. Your baby should start eating cooked eggs, egg containing foods, and peanut products (like peanut sauce or peanut powder mixed with other food) three times a week, starting now. We will take a deep dive on food allergies later in this chapter. But, in short, early introduction and frequent consumption of foods on the top food allergy list seems to reduce the risk of developing a food allergy—particularly for eggs and peanuts.

Q. Is it okay for my baby to eat fish?

Yes! Fish is an excellent source of protein, omega-3 fatty acids, Vitamin D, as well as other important micronutrients. There are two issues related to fish, though.

First, seafood and shellfish are both on the top food allergy list. So, introducing these foods in your baby's diet around six months of life may help reduce their risk of a lifelong food allergy.

The other concern is mercury exposure. Some fish contain high levels of mercury so the Food and Drug Administration has recommended that shark, swordfish, king mackerel, and tilefish be avoided for young children. It is also recommended to contact your local health department about any warnings on fish caught in area lakes. Canned tuna is okay in small amounts (less than six ounces/week).

Q. My baby doesn't have teeth yet. Are they really ready to chew and eat bite-sized pieces without teeth?

Yep. Your child can be toothless and still chew up pieces of food. They can gum just about anything.

Q. How will I know if my baby is ready to eat bite-sized pieces? I am so afraid they will choke!

Your baby is probably ready to eat bite-sized pieces and do some self-feeding (pick up and put food into their mouth) when they use their index finger and thumb to grasp things, otherwise known as the *pincer grasp*. Finger foods include: Cheerios, pieces of banana, pieces of pears or peaches, avocados, mashed beans, shredded cheese, whole wheat toast, boneless fish, wagon wheel pasta, pancakes, graham or whole grain crackers, falafel, and ground or shredded meats.

Just be sure to avoid choking hazard foods which are firm in texture and the same size as a baby's airway. Those include spherical/cylindrical foods such as uncut grapes, hot dogs, and sausage, hard foods like raw carrots, celery, raisins, nuts and peanuts, popcorn, potato chips, fruits with seeds, and hard chunks of meat.

Helpful Hint

Now is a good time to take that CPR class you have been meaning to take. It's unlikely you will ever need to utilize your skills, but it's always good to be prepared.

Q. My eight-month-old loves eating solid food and is less interested in nursing now. Is that okay?

Yes, that is normal, as long as they don't go on a total nursing strike. As babies get more excited and proficient with eating, they will naturally titrate their daily liquid and solid food intake. Your baby may drop a nursing session or two entirely, or simply drink less at each nursing session. This gradual taper begins somewhere between six and nine months. This is usually when a solid food meal is at least a four to six ounce serving.

If you reach a complete nursing strike, you can try offering expressed breast milk in a bottle with solid food meals.

See the handy table at the end of this chapter for the big picture on liquid and solid food intake.

? ?

SOLID FOODS

Q. My baby is nine months old. What can they eat now?

Aim for all types and textures of food. Encourage self-feeding, but you can still assist with some foods. (It's frustrating to eat soup with your fingers!)

If you thought solids were messy before, just wait...do not make a big deal out of it—just clean it up. Kids sense frustration and will have mealtime anxiety if you make it an issue.

As far as amounts, your baby should be taking enough solid food at a sitting to cut back on the volume of liquid nutrition. Aim for three solid meals per day (six to 14 ounces of solid food). See the "Big Picture" table at the end of this chapter.

You can view breakfast, lunch, and dinner as real meals now and not just snacks between nursing or formula feedings. Your baby will start and end the day with a breast or bottle feeding, but the liquid nutrition (breast milk/formula) during the day can be given in conjunction with the solid food mealtime. In summary, your baby still eats about every three hours or five times a day.

Feedback from the Real World: Multiples

Cutting the finger foods ahead of time reduced my stress. Patience is not exactly a baby or toddler's strong suit! Less fussing and crying made mealtime a little more enjoyable for me.—*Agustina, mom of twins Gael and Malena*

Q. My nine month old refuses any food that has a texture to it. Help!

This is called **TEXTURE AVERSION.**

Some babies prefer smooth, pureed foods well into their second year of life. If they are otherwise developing normally, I'd consider your baby a little eccentric, but normal.

Babies with texture aversions, adverse reactions to sensory stimulation, and developmental delays may be worth talking to your doctor about (see **PERVASIVE DEVELOPMENTAL DISORDER, SENSORY PROCESSING DISORDER**).

Q. My one year old refuses to let me feed her, but can't use utensils yet. Any ideas?

Try letting her dip foods. Yogurt, applesauce, guacamole, hummus, and beans will stick easily to a cracker that your baby can lick off.

Remember, getting your toddler to eat anything is a real challenge.

Q. What are the food expectations for a one-year-old?

To join the family at the dinner table, and eat what the family is eating.

They should eat three meals and two snacks per day. In reality, it's probably more like five small meals, spaced about three hours apart. Snacks should be nutritionally dense (such as egg salad, avocado or hummus dip) and not just a filler (such as crackers, Goldfish) until the next meal is served. Those snacks may be your toddler's best meal of the day! And some days, toddlers will decide not to eat anything. The 5-small-meals feeding routine continues through kindergarten, by the way.

They no longer need baby formula. And, despite the marketing hype, they do not need toddler formula, either. You may continue nursing as long as you and your child desire.

However, solid food is the mainstay of a one-year-old's nutrition. Liquids are not a meal now, they are a beverage. A one-year-old should drink whole or 2% milk (16 oz. or dairy serving equivalent), juice (less than six oz. per day), and water out of a cup. Say goodbye to bottles.

Reality Check

Your one-year-old, who is now officially a toddler, is a little person who should eat their meals just like you. I don't know why, but kicking the bottle habit is often very unsettling to parents (possibly more so than for the child). Maybe parents enjoy having a baby, and somehow leaving the bottles behind is an emotional step forward in acknowledging they have a toddler. Or, maybe they fear their child will not get enough milk if they don't chug 8 oz. in a sitting.

Don't worry. Kids only need 16 oz. of milk (or even less if they eat cheese and yogurt) in an entire day and that intake can be spaced throughout the day. It's usually pretty easy to reach that goal.

The reason why it's important to move on from the baby bottle is that chugging formula or milk in it is in essence, a meal replacement. Your toddler should be eating real meals now, not drinking them.

Special Section: Food Allergies

Q. What are the signs of an allergic reaction to food?

Warning: detailed medical content ahead. But let's take a moment to nerd out together because understanding allergic reactions will make you more confident about introducing solid food and knowing if there is a problem.

There are adverse reactions to food and then there are true allergic reactions. Adverse reactions are unpleasant to be sure, but they typically do not involve the immune system so the symptoms are less serious. For example, lactose intolerance (trouble digesting the sugar in milk) leads to gas, cramping, and watery diarrhea. It's not fun, but it is also not life-threatening. And adverse reactions, fortunately, are more common than true allergic reactions.

True allergic reactions are due to an abnormal immune response to a particular food, and that category breaks down further into Immunoglobulin E "IgE-mediated" and "non-IgE medi-ated". (To make things more confusing for you, some true allergic reactions can have manifestations of both IgE-mediated and non IgE-mediated responses.)

IgE-mediated allergic reactions are the red alert ones. Most IgE allergic responses occur within minutes or at most four hours after an exposure. (Although it's quite rare, some serious reactions can occur up to three days after an exposure.) *(Sampson)*

A chemical in the body called **HISTAMINE** is released in massive quantities. Histamine can cause a tingling or itchy mouth, mouth or lip swelling, shortness of breath, profuse vomiting, abdominal pain and dramatic diarrhea. You may also see skin flushing, sweating, and hives (raised borders of red plaques that look like mosquito bites with circles around them). See our web site at Baby411.com (click on "Bonus Material") for a picture.

The extreme scenario is called an **ANAPHYLACTIC REACTION**. This is when loss of consciousness and airway swelling occurs—obviously, this is life threatening and you need to call 911.

solid food

? ?

SOLID FOODS

Milder forms of IgE-mediated responses include something called oral allergy syndrome where someone just gets lip/tongue/throat itching and swelling with eating certain fresh, uncooked produce. When we refer to food allergies and the top high allergy foods in this book, these are the foods (in general) that cause IgE-mediated allergic reactions.

Non IgE-mediated allergic reactions can also be pretty significant. Celiac disease, for example, is a non IgE immune-mediated inflammatory disease due to gluten sensitivity. We discuss this disease and symptoms in-depth later in this special section.

COW MILK PROTEIN ENTEROPATHY (also known as cow milk protein intolerance/sensitivity or infant proctocolitis) causes streaks of blood in the poop that has a consistency of mucous (the poop looks stringy, like snot from the nose).

And then there is FPIES (Food Protein-Induced Enterocolitis Syndrome), which can cause severe vomiting, diarrhea, lethargy, and paleness of the skin one to four hours after eating a certain food that can mimic a really bad case of food poisoning or a severe bloodstream infection.

We point this out because FPIES often gets misdiagnosed at first—until the same reaction happens repeatedly after ingesting certain foods (cow milk, soy, rice, barley, and oats are the top offenders). Our allergy expert for this book, Dr. Allen Lieberman, points out that FPIES to peanuts, bananas, avocados, and sweet potatoes are on the rise. The good news is that FPIES is relatively rare and most people outgrow it.

Bottom line: True allergic reactions are not subtle. If your baby has a few dots of a rash or a diaper rash, it's not because of the food you just introduced.

Reality Check

True allergic IgE-mediated reactions produce boatloads of the chemical, histamine. This is why taking an anti-histamine (Benadryl, Zyrtec, Claritin) can help reduce the allergic response temporarily. For more serious allergic reactions, like anaphylaxis, antihistamines alone may not be enough to help. Antihistamines will not help for adverse reactions. Make sense?

Q. I have a food allergy, is my baby at greater risk of having a food allergy?

Yes, genetics play a role in allergic disorders. For better or worse, your baby inherited some of your genes. Infants who are more at risk for food allergies are those with parents who are very allergic. These babies' risk of having a food allergy may be as high as 20%. A baby whose sibling has a peanut allergy has a seven-times greater risk of having a food allergy. Compare that to the general population, which has about a 2% risk of food allergies. Children who have asthma have a higher risk of having a more serious allergic reaction if they have a food allergy.

Reality Check

Acidic foods such as berries, lemons, grapefruit, oranges, and tomatoes can cause redness or even hives when it touches the skin. This is NOT an allergic reaction. Just wipe the food residue off your baby's cheeks and chin if this response occurs.

If this happens with regularity, apply petroleum jelly or another barrier ointment to the chin and cheeks prior to mealtime.

FOOD ALLERGIES AND ECZEMA: CHICKEN OR EGG?

Food allergies and eczema can go together, but not always in the way you might think. Yes, 37% of kids with severe eczema have a food allergy and the food ingestion flares up the eczema. The severe eczema improves when the food offender is eliminated from the diet. The vast majority of food offenders are the top high allergy foods. (*Eigenmann*) For those of you keeping track, eczema is a non IgE-mediated allergic response to a food protein.

However, the hot topic in allergy literature right now is the "epithelial barrier hypothesis."

In a nutshell (no pun intended), when babies are exposed to food proteins through the gut, the gut's immune system acknowledges and welcomes them in a good way.

But babies with an impaired skin barrier (that is, eczema), are exposed to food proteins such as peanut dust through the skin. The skin's immune system is not so welcoming—in fact, it may sensitize the body and lead to a food allergy. Bottom line: keeping eczema under good control with thick emollients reduces itchy skin may also reduce the risk of developing a food allergy. (*Bird 2019*)

solid food

Q. What is food intolerance?

As a recap, this term refers to an adverse reaction to a food or food product, not an allergic response.

Allergic reactions produce histamine. Food intolerances do not. If a baby has intolerance to a food, they might have stomach cramps or bloating. You'll probably avoid that food in the future, but they'll never have a life-threatening (anaphylactic) reaction if they are exposed to it.

(Example: An adult with lactose intolerance has gas or diarrhea when they drink milk, but don't get hives).

Q. What foods are more likely to cause food allergies?

1. *PEANUTS/Peanut Butter.* We'll discuss this in detail next.
2. Egg whites. (the *white* part—egg protein is the problem)
3. Shellfish (crab, lobster, shrimp, scallops, oysters).
4. Fish.
5. Tree nuts (walnuts, cashews, etc).
6. Wheat.
7. Cow's milk protein.
8. Soy protein.
9. Citrus fruits, berries.
10. Cocoa.
11. Sesame seeds.

HIDDEN SOURCES FOR DANGEROUS FOODS

If you have a food allergic child, the world can be a scary place. Are you aware of how peanuts and other potential food allergy dangers are hidden in other products? Candy and cookies, as well as fresh baked goods, are a flash point—undeclared soy, wheat, nuts, and eggs are common in baked goods. Today most processed foods are required to list allergy facts, but some products still are not covered by these laws.

And let's talk about restaurants. Unfortunately, there is no law requiring restaurants to disclose the use of allergenic foods as ingredients. As a parent, you have to take charge: inform the waiter of your preference to avoid peanuts (or a child's allergy) and ask what dishes are a problem. If you get a blank stare in return, ask to see the manager. Ditto for quick-serve restaurants.

Watch out for stealth uses of allergenic foods like peanuts—for example, some Chinese restaurants seal their egg roll wrappers with peanut butter!

Now, we're not trying to make you overly paranoid here. But as a parent, you have to be vigilant—especially when your child goes over to friends' or relatives' homes. For more information, check out the Food Allergy Network (FoodAllergy.org), which provides an FAQ, alerts and school resources.

Food Allergies Stats

- 2.5% of newborns have a cow's milk protein allergy. 80% outgrow it by age five.
- 1.5% of children are allergic to eggs protein. 80% outgrow it by age ten.
- 0.8% of children are allergic to peanuts, but of those with the allergy, only 20% will outgrow it.
- 1/3 of people who are allergic to peanuts are also allergic to tree nuts. FYI: Peanuts are actually legumes (like soybeans), not nuts!
- Most food allergies occur in the first three years of life (8% of all children).
- Fun fact: Children who live in urban areas of the U.S. are more likely to have a food allergy than those who grow up in rural areas. (*National Food Allergy Survey 2009-10*)
- Only 2% of adults have a food allergy, and of those, 50% are allergic to either peanuts or tree nuts. (*Sampson, AAP*)

Q. Can my baby have a cow's milk protein allergy if I am breastfeeding?

Yes. Food proteins are passed into mom's breast milk, and cow's milk protein is no exception. Babies with a milk protein allergy may have blood streaked or slimy snot-like poops and poor growth. If your baby is fed a cow's milk-based formula, this allergy may pop up in the first few weeks of life. In breastfed babies, it may not be a problem at all. Or, it may take a few months to become apparent because there is less exposure to the cow's milk protein.

If you are nursing and your baby is diagnosed with a cow's milk protein allergy, you will need to eliminate ALL cow milk products from your diet. That means no milk or dairy products—no cream in your coffee, no parmesan cheese sprinkled on your spaghetti, etc. We discussed this in Chapter 6, Liquids.

And yes, your baby may not get their doctor's blessing to eat dairy solid food products like yogurt or cheese until they outgrow the allergy.

Q. My baby was diagnosed with a cow's milk protein allergy. I am nursing and I've removed all milk and dairy products from my diet. But they are still having blood in his poop. Am I doing something wrong?

No, you are probably doing everything right. It takes at least six to eight weeks for the irritated, inflamed gut/rectum to heal. So, even if your baby is not ingesting any more milk protein, it can take time to see the results in their poop. The poop often returns to seedy and watery, but it's okay if it continues to be somewhat slimy. As pediatric gastroenterologist Dr. Bryan Vartabedian says, "the goal is good poo, not perfect poo." The good news: most parents report that the baby seems happier and less uncomfortable after the dietary changes occur. Babies with persistent bleeding should see a pediatric gastroenterologist (a specialist in childhood intestinal disorders).

Food allergy testing is usually not helpful in situations where the baby is only having bloody or mucousy poop (because allergy testing identifies IgE-mediated reactions and infant proctocolitis is a non IgE-mediated reaction). Most babies with a cow milk protein allergy will have negative allergy tests. But their symptoms gradually improve when their diet changes. (Ruffner MA)

Reality Check

Many babies with a cow's milk protein allergy also are allergic to soy protein. Studies report that up to 40% of babies are allergic to both proteins. Milk from other mammals (like goat's milk) can also be problematic for these babies. Nursing moms often opt for rice milk or coconut milk in their diets.

Q. So when can I feed my child a peanut butter and jelly sandwich?

Okay, let's talk peanuts and peanut butter.

Here's the scary fact about peanut allergy: it can be life threatening. That's right, some kids with a peanut allergy can die from ingesting less than one peanut. Another scary fact: only 20% of kids who have peanut allergy will outgrow it!

So here are more details about the latest guidelines. The American Academy of Pediatrics and the National Institute on Allergy and Infectious Diseases both recommend you offer solid food (including high-allergy ones) at four months of age and beyond. This includes children who are born to families who have a history of food allergies.

Yes, you read that correctly. Experts believe eating the top high-allergy foods early in life may be protective! This reverses the advice of years past, when doctors urged parents to hold off introducing high-allergy foods until later.

For example, a major study on peanut allergies found that Israeli children who typically got their first taste of peanuts between eight and 14 months of age (thanks to a popular Israeli snack food called Bamba) were LESS likely to have a peanut allergy than their British peers who didn't start eating peanut products until after 14 months. In fact, the British kids were TEN times more likely to have peanut allergies! (Du Toit) And the landmark "LEAP Study" (Learning Early About Peanut) led to the current advice: introduce peanut products to allergy prone babies by around

CELIAC DISEASE: ON THE RISE

Celiac Disease, a disorder caused by an abnormal immune response to a protein found in certain grains called gluten, used to be rare. Today 1% of the U.S. population has Celiac Disease.

Here is what you need to know. People with celiac disease have an unfortunate combination of genetics (predisposition that is passed down from family) and exposure to gluten. The exposure leads to injury of the intestinal lining and then, difficulty with digestion (malabsorption). The result: chronic diarrhea, failure to thrive, vomiting, and bloating to name a few symptoms. But some people have no or subtle symptoms while their guts are being irritated.

Wheat, barley, and rye grains all contain gluten protein. And, there are a variety of other gluten-containing foods that might surprise you—who knew Communion wafers could be a problem? See the list below for more problematic foods.

As babies start to eat cereal grains (wheat, barley, and rye), Celiac Disease can become apparent. More subtle symptoms include trouble gaining weight or anemia.

If you have a family member with this disorder, or notice a change in your baby after introducing these foods, check in with your baby's doctor. Children with Down syndrome, diabetes, and other genetic syndromes are also at risk and should be tested if they have worrisome symptoms. The first thing to do is a couple of blood tests (IgA endomysial antibody and IgA antitissue transglutamate) after a child is on a gluten-containing diet for at least two to four weeks. If the blood tests are abnormal, a biopsy of the small intestine (done via an outpatient procedure) confirms the diagnosis.

Recent research shows the ideal time to introduce gluten-containing foods is between four and seven months of age. Introducing gluten-containing food *before or after* this time frame actually increases the risk of developing celiac disease!

Fun fact: children with celiac disease who receive the Hepatitis B vaccine prior to diagnosis may not form an adequate response to the vaccine. A simple blood test will confirm if your child mounted a response. If they are not immune, they can be revaccinated. *(Celiac.org)*

Gluten-containing foods:
Always contains gluten
Wheat (einkorn, durum, faro, graham, kamut, semolina, spelt), rye, barley, malt, malt flavoring, malt extract derived from barley, malt vinegar, triticale

May contain gluten
Breading, brewer's yeast, broth, bouillon, brown rice syrup, cake frosting, candy, coating mixes, Communion wafers, certain condiments, croutons, dates rolled in oat flour, drink mixes, flavored teas and coffees, flour/cereal products, gravies, imitation bacon, imitation seafood, licorice, marinades, matzah/matzah meal, some medications, some oats, panko, pasta, processed lunch meats, rice pilaf, roux, some salad dressings, some sauces and spreads, some seasonings, seasoned chips/nuts/seeds, self-basting poultry, smoke flavoring, soup stock, soy sauce (often made with soy and wheat), stuffing for poultry, some nutritional supplements. *(Hill)*

six months of age. *(Du Toit)*

A quick caveat here: eating whole peanuts are a no-no until after age three because they are a choking hazard. *(AAP Committee on Nutrition, NIAID.)*

Here are the specific guidelines for peanuts:

Guideline 1: Baby with SEVERE ECZEMA and/or egg allergy: peanut skin prick testing by allergist and if negative, introduce peanuts at 4-6 months.
Guideline 2: Baby with mild/moderate eczema—> introduce peanuts around 6 months of age
Guideline 3: Healthy baby without eczema—> introduce peanuts with other solid foods around six months of age

Q. If introducing peanuts earlier protects against a peanut allergy, does this strategy work for other high allergy foods?

Currently, egg is the only other food that may follow this principle. Both the Australian/New Zealand (ASCIA) and British (BSACI) allergy societies encourage introducing cooked egg around six months of age based on the research. *(Bird 2019)*. But as our pediatric food allergy expert, Dr Allen Lieberman points out, "this benefit has not been demonstrated for other foods such as milk, wheat, or fish. It demonstrates the complexity of food allergies and food allergy prevention is not a one size fits all."

 BOTTOM LINE
Peanut butter is pretty tough to swallow for a young child, so a nice peanut sauce is a safer bet. Mix 2 tsp. of peanut butter with 2-3 tsp. of hot water, cool, and voila! Peanut sauce.

Since peanut butter and peanuts are both choking hazards, there are some clever products that might make your life easier.

Bamba puffs are popular Cheeto-looking snacks from Israel that are dusted with peanut powder. They are sold online and in many U.S. grocery stores.

Inspired Start (inspired-start.com) and Spoonful One (spoonfulone.com) make pouches, powders, and dusted puffs, some containing multiple food proteins (the highest allergy offenders) in one serving.

The data that led to development of Spoonful One indicates that introducing multiple allergens at once may protect against developing food allergies—and while more research is needed to confirm those findings, we feel it is safe to offer multi-ingredient foods.

While the amounts of each food protein is unlikely to cause an allergic reaction (no reactions in 10,000 babies studied), if there is a reaction it will just be harder to decipher which food is the problem. They are definitely a great option for snacks once all these foods have been introduced.

Key point: the goal is to offer these foods regularly in the diet, not just as a science fair project.

 Reality Check
Do people with food allergies have other allergy problems? Sometimes. We've already discussed the eczema and food allergy pairing. The most serious combination

? ?

SOLID FOODS

is asthma plus a food allergy. Those children are more likely to have a scary respiratory emergency (wheezing/anaphylaxis) with an allergic reaction to a food, because that is the way their body responds to an allergen. That doesn't happen to everyone, mind you. However, kids with these combo allergies need to be particularly careful to avoid allergenic food(s).

Feedback from the Real World: Ben's Story

Want to hear something really scary? How about the story of Ben, (Denise's son), and how we discovered his life threatening peanut allergy. When Ben was one year of age, we decided we could add peanut butter into his life. Being a confessed peanut nut (I've searched the Southern U.S. for the best peanut butter pie–haven't found it yet but I'm still looking), we thought this would be a tasty addition to his diet. Besides we had no history of severe food allergies in our families.

Shazam! He immediately swelled up like a tomato. This was our first experience with an allergic reaction. Hives hit him like a ton of bricks. We practically threw him in the car and raced down the mountain (yes, we did live in the mountains at the time) to the doctor's office. There we were informed that he was allergic to peanuts. After treating the hives, the doctor mentioned that this would probably be allergic for life and the next time could be life-threatening anaphylaxis (after eating one peanut he could stop breathing and die). We next visited with an allergist who confirmed the diagnosis with a "peanut challenge" test.

So what now? Well, we see the allergist once a year. And we have to carry an epinephrine injectable pen with us everywhere we go. In fact, there is an Epi-Pen at school, at Nanna's, at our house and in my purse. We had to teach Ben to read labels on food, never share at school and never, ever take food samples without first checking with us (Sam's Club is a nightmare sometimes!). It's no wonder a recent study showed that kids with a peanut allergy suffer from more stress than kids with diabetes.

The good news: oral immunotherapy (OIT) is a new option for some food-allergic kids. Patients take a tiny amount of the food substance they are allergic to on a daily basis–forever. While it is not curative, it may lower the odds of having a life-threatening allergic reaction.

Helpful Hints

1. If your baby does have a food allergy, get educated about hidden sources of the problem food.

2. Know how to read an ingredient label. Products containing milk include: casein, sodium caseinate, whey, or lactoglobulin.

3. Be a detective. Deli slicers are often contaminated with milk because both cheese and lunchmeat are sliced on the same machine. Many candies without peanuts are processed in the same location as those with peanuts.

Q. What is the best way to prevent food allergies?

Breastfeed for at least four months. Since human milk is made for human babies, it is the least likely to be problematic.

Is there any benefit to a breastfeeding mom avoiding high allergy foods in their diet? No. A fair amount of research has been done on nursing mothers eliminating highly allergenic foods from their diets to prevent "sensitizing" their infants. It is true that the breakdown products of foods mom eats end up in their breast milk. However, this exposure does not put a baby at any greater risk of developing a food allergy. A nursing mom only needs to make dietary changes if a problem is identified.

Q. Okay, so when can I try these high allergy foods with my baby?

Again, your baby can try any solid food, even the high allergy ones (eggs, fish, peanut containing products) after four months of age as long as you have a low-risk baby (ask your doc if you have questions). Offer a small amount in the comfort of your own home (not at childcare or at a restaurant!). Then, let your baby eat larger quantities of that food regularly *(Fleisher DM)*

New Parent 411

I had one mom bring in a jar of peanut butter in at their baby's well check so baby could try it in front of me. You do not have to be that anxious about it! If you want to be uber-cautious, offer these foods during daylight hours and have an antihistamine (Benadryl, Zyrtec, etc) nearby.

Reality Check

The recommendations for starting highly allergenic foods represent a MAJOR change from past years' advice on this topic. So have a discussion with your child's doctor if you have questions or concerns. It is particularly important to talk to your doc if your baby already has eczema, wheezing, or a milk protein allergy.

Q. What is a good reference if my baby does develop a food allergy?

Check out the Food Allergy Network, foodallergy.org. (800) 929-4040.

Q. How are people tested for a food allergy?

There are four basic ways to test for a food allergy, but be aware that there is no perfect science:

1 **ELIMINATION DIET.** Eliminate the food from the diet for three to six weeks; see if there is an improvement in symptoms (i.e. eczema, diarrhea, etc).

2 **SKIN TESTING.** Skin prick tests detect a true allergic response (see IgE below) to a food. If skin testing shows an allergic response, RAST testing can be done for confirmation.

3 **CAP-RAST TEST.** Blood test detects an elevation of the body's IgE antibodies (an allergic response chemical). RAST testing is useful because it can identify some food allergies. However, not all food allergies cause an elevation of IgE levels. In English: a positive test is useful. A negative test does not rule out a food allergy. The newer CAP-RAST tests have been shown to be 95% predictive in food allergies for milk, eggs, peanuts, and fish.

4 **FOOD CHALLENGE.** When a person is known to be allergic to a certain food, periodic (annual) RAST testing may show a decrease in allergy response levels. A person can try a certain food again in a controlled medical setting to see if he is still allergic to a particular food. (This does not mean at your kitchen table). (*Sampson*)

Q. Can you outgrow a food allergy?

Most kids outgrow food allergies to milk, eggs, soy, and wheat by the time they are five years old. Over 50% of kids will outgrow their food allergies by the age of one. The foods that tend to be lifelong problems are peanuts, tree nuts, fish, and shellfish. (*Wood*)

The Big Picture For Liquid And Solid Nutrition

AGE	LIQUID NUTRITION	SOLID NUTRITION	SOLID SERVING SIZE
4-5 months	25-32 oz. **5-6 meals**	Food, prioritize iron-containing foods, introduce high allergy foods **0-3 feeding/day**	2-4 Tbsp (1-2 oz.) 1-2 items at each meal. *Mostly pureed foods.* **0-4 oz./day**
6-9 months	24-36 oz. **4-5 meals**	Food, prioritize iron-containing foods, egg and peanut products 3x weekly and all other top allergy foods regulary **3 feedings/day**	3-4 oz. per meal *More textures, bite-sized pieces.* **6-14 oz./day**
9-12 months	20-30 oz. **3-4 meals**	Food, prioritize iron-containing foods, egg and peanut products 3x weekly and all other top allergy foods regulary **3 meals/day**	4-6 oz. per meal *Bite size pieces.* **10-18 oz./day**

For more information, check out our online community for more fun food tips and videos!

THE OTHER END

Chapter 8

"Gil, why are you standing there?"
"I'm waiting for her head to spin around."
~ Parenthood

WHAT'S IN THIS CHAPTER

◆ **NORMAL NEWBORN POOP**
◆ **THE TOP 5 WORRISOME POOPS**
◆ **TRADE SECRETS FOR CONSTIPATION RELIEF**
◆ **FUN FIBER FOODS**
◆ **SPIT UP, REGURGITATION, AND VOMIT**
◆ **WHAT IS GER GASTROESOPHAGEAL REFLUX?**
◆ **TOP 5 WORRIES ABOUT VOMIT**
◆ **URINE AND BLADDER INFECTIONS**
◆ **BURPING, HICCUPS, AND GAS**

This chapter addresses a subject taboo at most dinner tables. We are going to have a candid discussion about poop (as well as gas, burps, pee and spit up, too). Why spend a whole chapter on poop? Let's be honest—you'll have LOTS of questions about this subject. And you'll be looking at lots of it too! The average baby goes through 2300 diaper changes in the first year alone.

Parents have concerns because baby poop does not look like theirs. If it does, your baby has a problem. And as you might imagine, changing at least eight diapers a day also results in a pre-occupation with diaper contents.

Before we go too far, it's a good idea to go over the terminology we'll be using in this chapter:

◆ **Stool.** Digested food garbage that is eliminated through the anus. Stool also has bacteria germs in it (these germs help us digest our food). Just so we're on the same page—it's also known as poo, poop, feces, caca, Number 2, bowel movement . . . for this book, we will use the term **POOP.**

◆ **Urine.** The garbage that the kidneys clean out of the bloodstream that is eliminated through the urethra (the hole in the penis or the hole above the vagina). Urine is sterile (germ free). Otherwise known as pee, pee-pee, wee-wee, wet diapers, urinating . . . for this book, we will use the term **PEE.**

◆ **Gas.** The air inside the intestines that is a by-product of the food transit through it. When babies

? ?

THE OTHER END

eat 24 hours a day, their intestines move 24 hours a day, *and* make a whole lot of gas. The gas slows down when the intestinal transit slows down, around six weeks.

◆ **Burps.** The air that gets swallowed comes back out of the esophagus. Because babies exclusively suck and swallow their nutrition for the first four months of life, burping feels good after a big meal. Some babies suck very aggressively and ingest a large air bubble. When this air bubble comes up, often so does the whole meal.

◆ **Hiccups.** This is caused by a muscle spasm of the diaphragm (the muscle that divides the chest and abdomen). All babies have some hiccups. This sometimes is a sign of sensory overload (i.e. over stimulation). There is nothing wrong with your baby. You may just want to soothe them.

Newborn Poop

Q. What should my newborn's poop look like?

Black tar.

In the first 24 hours of life, your baby should pass a poop called **MECONIUM**. This has the color and texture of black tar. It looks like this because the baby has swallowed some blood while inside the womb. The black tar contains some digested blood. (Good to remember if you ever see poop that looks like this again from your baby or a family member).

As your baby starts to eat breast milk or formula, the poop will change color and texture. This happens on about the fourth day of life. (Remember, they don't eat much the first few days.)

Q. My newborn is breastfed. What should their poop look like?

Grey Poupon (or crab mustard, as my Baltimore friends would say).

Breast milk poop is very watery. In fact, many parents worry that their baby is having diarrhea if they have never changed a breastfed baby's diaper before. It's watery because the breast milk is so easily digested, it goes right through the intestines and leaves very little solid garbage to be pooped out.

Parents often wonder how they will know when their baby is having diarrhea. The answer is the *frequency* of poop increases. Breastfed babies often poop with every feeding for the first six weeks of life. Some babies will poop less frequently than that, sometimes only once every few days. Do not worry unless the consistency of the poop looks like yours.

The color is often yellow. But, *any shade of yellow, green or brown is okay.* Florescent green is okay too.

Q. My newborn is formula fed. What should their poop look like?

Strained peas. Or wasabi if you are a sushi fan.

Formula poops tend to be greener than breast milk poop. But, as we mentioned, any shade of yellow, green or brown is okay.

Formula poops are also thicker and pastier than breast milk poop. It takes longer to digest

DR B'S OPINION:
GREEN POOP AND FOREMILK?

Some mothers hear that green poop is a sign that their baby is only getting the foremilk and not the richer hindmilk. (For a discussion of foremilk and hindmilk, see Chapter 6, Liquids). While this may be true, a better way to tell if a baby is getting hindmilk is to look at the feeding patterns and growth charts, not the poop color. Babies who get foremilk only tend to be snackers who eat frequently (they don't fill up as well). They also gain less weight if they miss out on the fatty hindmilk.

formula in the intestines, so more water is absorbed before the "final product" comes out.

Q. How often do formula fed babies poop?

Formula fed babies poop less often because the "transit time" through the intestines is longer. These babies may poop three or four times per day or once every couple of days. The frequency slows down even more at six weeks of life.

RED FLAGS: Worrisome Poop

If you see/note any of these, call your doctor immediately:

1. Your baby doesn't poop in the first 24 hours of life (see **MECONIUM PLUG OR ILEUS**).
2. Your baby's poops look bloody, tarry, or mixed with mucous (see **BLOOD IN STOOL**)
3. Your baby's poop looks like yours. (see **CONSTIPATION**)
4. Your baby has a stomachache and poop that looks like grape jelly (see **INTUSSUSCEPTION**)
5. Your baby's frequency of poop increases two or three fold (see **DIARRHEA/GASTROENTERITIS**)

Q. My baby grunts and their face turns red while pooping. Is this normal?

Yes.

Try lying down and pooping some time. See what your face looks like. This does NOT mean your child is constipated. There is actually a term for this phenomenon—The Grunting Baby Syndrome.

Q. My three-week-old usually poops with every feeding. Now, they haven't gone in 24 hours. Are they constipated?

No. The Poopapalooza has ended.

Please read this carefully. Constipation is diagnosed by the FIRMNESS of the poop, NOT THE FREQUENCY (or infrequency) of pooping. *Concerned parents often think their baby is constipated when they are not.* Newborns to six week olds usually poop several times a day. Occasionally, though, they may take a day off. That's when you call the doctor in a state of panic.

? ?

THE OTHER END

The answer is, "Be prepared for the Mother Load." Some babies may poop once or twice a week. That's fine, as long as it is soft when it comes out.

Your baby is constipated when the poop looks like logs, rock balls, marbles, or deer pellets. See below for tricks of the trade for relieving constipation.

Trade Secrets For Relieving Constipation

1 **RECTAL THERMOMETER TRICK.** If your baby is straining and not having any success, insert a rectal thermometer in their anus for about a minute. Trust me—this is the most dispensed advice by any pediatrician's office. You can read the exact details on how to insert a rectal thermometer in Chapter 15, First Aid. This usually provides the inspiration your baby needs to get moving. (And no, they don't mind it!)

2 **PRUNE JUICE COCKTAIL.** If your baby is regularly irregular, they may need some extra fiber to move things along. Try one teaspoon of prune juice per feeding (mixed in formula or given separately to breastfed babies) until you get the desired consistency of poop. You can adjust the volume to what your baby needs (that is, anywhere from one to five teaspoons a day). Prune juice has both fiber and sorbitol (sugar) that pull water into the poop to make it softer. Hint: Buy store brand prune juice—not the stuff in the baby food section. "Baby" prune juice is mixed with apple juice and is very expensive by comparison.

3 **GLYCERIN BULLET.** For immediate relief, use a glycerin suppository to get dramatic results. These suppositories can be purchased without a prescription at the grocery store or pharmacy. Frequently, the label will read "infant" suppository. The suppository looks like a bullet made of soap. Insert it directly into the anus. It dissolves as you push it in. Be prepared for the fireworks.

If these tricks don't work, call your doctor. Pediatricians always have a few more tricks like this up their sleeves!

Q. My six-week old breastfed baby used to poop at every feeding. Now they only go once a day. Should I be worried?

No. This is normal and you should be thankful.

Babies are born with intestines that work 24/7. They work that way to keep the nutritional juices flowing. By six weeks of age, things start to slow down. This is called slower intestinal transit time. Mature breast milk is also mostly digested, so there is very little garbage to eliminate.

As long as the poop is soft, your baby is fine. So be grateful you have fewer diaper changes!

New Parent 411
We said it before and let's say it again: babies poop less often after six weeks of life!

Solid Food Equals Solid Poop: Older Babies

Q. My five month old started rice cereal and now they are constipated. Help!

Rice cereal has this effect on some babies. And in general, solid food leads to solid poop. Although it has been the traditional first food for babies, there is nothing magical about rice cereal. There is also a concern for arsenic in rice cereal. Opt for cereals that actually contain fiber such as oatmeal, whole wheat, or multigrain varieties. Add pureed prunes or berries for an extra fiber punch.That should help move things along! See below for more fun fiber foods.

Reality Check

There are no rules stating that babies must eat cereal. Through trial and error, you will soon figure out the appropriate amount of fiber foods your baby needs to eat every day to pass soft, formed stools regularly.

Q. How much fiber does my child need to eat?

Truthfully, daily needs vary from baby to baby and there are no established guidelines. Breast milk contains no dietary fiber, but it is so easily digestible that constipation rarely is an issue. From six to twelve months, fiber is introduced in the diet via solid foods. Fiber turns out to be pretty important since it pulls water into the poop, making it bulkier and softer to pass. Studies have shown that children who are constipated eat significantly less fiber than their "regular" peers. (*McClung*) So, while there are no official guidelines, it makes sense to aim for your baby's diet to include about five grams of fiber daily.

Reality Check

You, Mom and Dad, need 25 to 30 grams of fiber per day no matter how old you are. Most Americans do not eat enough fiber. The way to get your child to eat fiber is for you to have it in the house and eat it yourself. If you don't realize this yet, your baby is watching every move you make!

Q. Which foods are high in fiber and more importantly, which ones will my child eat?

This is my favorite fiber food list. Some foods will be off limits under a year of age and are designated with an asterisk (*)—these are choking hazards. Kids usually find the bread/grain category the most appealing. Take careful note of serving sizes. The sizes listed below are sometimes more than even a one-year-old will eat. In general, a serving of fruit, vegetable, or oat/barley/multigrain cereal will contain about one gram of fiber. (See the next two pages).

PRODUCT	SERVING SIZE	FIBER GRAMS/SERVING
Bread/Grains		
Whole wheat Bread	1 slice	2 grams
Pepperidge Farm HeartyWheat Crackers	3 crackers	1 gram
El Galindo Wheat Tortillas	1 tortilla	9 grams
Hodgson Mill Whole-wheat pasta	2 oz	6 grams
Brown Rice	1/4 cup	0.9 grams
Farro	1/4 cup	3 grams
Cereal		
Baby Oatmeal	1/4 cup	1 gram
Cheerios	1/2 cup	1.5 grams
Mamma Chia Squeezes	3.5 oz	4 grams
Quaker Oat Bran	1/2 cup	2.4 grams
Quaker Oatmeal Squares	1/2 cup	2.5 grams
Kellogg's Nutragrain bars	1 bar	1 gram
Wheat germ	1 Tbsp	1 gram

(I like wheat germ because you can sneak it into food and your child might not even notice)

Fruit (raw)
Note: The peel is often the part of the fruit that contains the fiber. Since most kids hate the peels, the fiber ends up in the compost pile and not in your child.

PRODUCT	SERVING SIZE	FIBER GRAMS/SERVING
Apple (with peel)	1/2 medium	1.8 grams
Apricots	1/4 cup	0.8 grams
Banana	1 whole	2.7 grams
Blackberries	1/4 cup	1.8 grams
Grapefruit	1/4	1 gram
Grapes	1/2 cup	0.5 grams
Orange	1/2	1.5 grams
Pear (with peel)	1/2	2.1 grams
Prunes	1/4 cup	3.5 grams
Raspberries	1/4 cup	2 grams
Strawberries	1/4 cup	0.8 grams
Watermelon	1/2 slice	0.5 gram

PRODUCT	SERVING SIZE	FIBER GRAMS/SERVING
Vegetables/Legumes		
Avocado	1/4 cup	2.5 grams
Broccoli	1/4 cup	1.4 grams
Corn	1/4 cup	1 grams
Green beans	1/4 cup	0.7 grams
Green peas	1/4 cup	2.2 grams
Lentils	¼ cup	2.5 grams
Lima beans	1/4 cup	3 grams
Pinto beans	1/4 cup	3.7 grams
Refried Beans	1/4 cup	3 grams
Squash (baked)	1/4 cup	2 grams

Q. Now that my nine month old eats a large amount of solid food, what should their poop look like?

Soft and solid.

The more your baby eats like you do, the more their poop will look like yours. It should always be easy for your baby to pass. It has a cow patty appearance when your baby sits on it after they poop.

By the way, some foods don't get completely digested as they pass through the intestines. It's normal to recognize last night's corn, carrots, etc. in your child's poop.

RED FLAGS:
Worrisome Poops For Older Babies

1. **Streaks of blood.** If the streak is on a hard, firm poop, it's probably due to a tear in the anus as the poop was passed. It's worth checking out, though.
2. **Streaks of blood/mucous.** This is more concerning for infection, particularly if poop is loose/diarrhea. Be prepared for a homework assignment (providing your doctor with a fresh poop specimen). This can also be a sign of a food allergy, especially if the poop looks slimy and stringy like snot from the nose. Sorry to gross you out.
3. **Clay (white) colored poop.** The official name is **ACHOLIC STOOL.** This can occur in conjunction with a stomach virus. But inform your baby's doctor. This is more of a medical concern if the skin is yellow (jaundice) AND the poop is white.
4. **Looks like meconium again.** Black, tarry poop can be a sign of bleeding in the upper part of the intestinal tract (because the blood has had time to get digested). This may indicate irritation and inflammation in the intestines. Your doctor will do a test to check for blood in the poop.
5. **Grape Jelly poop.** The doctor term for this is actually "currant jelly stool." This is a medical emergency. It is a worrisome sign of **INTUSSUSCEPTION** where the intestines have kinked.
6. **Bulky, REALLY stinky, greasy, floating poops.** This may indicate difficulty with absorption (see **MALABSORPTION**).

Helpful Hint

Pepto Bismol makes poop look black like meconium. Pepto Bismol is *not* currently recommended for infants. Just thought you'd be interested for your own sake.

Q. My baby just had a BLUE poop. Help!

Your baby is not an alien. It's either natural or artificial food coloring.

To the best of my knowledge, blue poop is never a sign of illness. Blue colored kid juices (Hi-C) and kid yogurts are often the culprits.

Beets cause a dramatic red hue in both poop and pee.

Q. I am interested in toilet training my baby. Is it too early to think about this now?

Yes, in our opinion. Your baby will be in diapers for a long time.

Being toilet trained is a developmental milestone, just like learning to talk and walk. Milestones can be encouraged, but the child has to achieve it on their own. Your child needs to be able to sense the urge to pee and poop (not just after they have gone). Their only incentive to be toilet trained is the desire to be clean (regardless of how many toys you buy them). If they run around in a poopy diaper and could care less, they are miles away from this milestone.

Girls usually train around 2 1/2 years of age. Boys train around 3 or 3 1/2 years. There is no need to purchase a potty seat any time soon. All it will do is collect dust in your bathroom. Good news: we cover this topic in depth in the sequel to this book, *Toddler 411* (see back of this book for details).

We should note there is another school of thought on this topic: Elimination Communication (EC). Proponents say babies give subtle clues that they need to poop or pee and it is up to the parent to respond to those cues. These babies go diaper-less, and parents put them on the pot every time they think their kid needs to go. If you want to learn more about this method, check out DiaperFreeBaby.org. We admit our skepticism about EC—it seems that the parent is potty-trained, not the child.

Spit Up, Regurgitation, And Vomit

Q. My newborn spits up all the time. Should I be worried?

No. Most babies spit up after meals. They are born with a loose muscle between the esophagus (swallowing tube) and the stomach. This muscle, called the *lower esophageal sphincter* (see picture at right), will tighten up by about six months of age. Until then, liquids travel down into the stomach. Then some will return into the esophagus and mouth. By definition, most babies have **GASTROESOPHAGEAL REFLUX (ACID REFLUX OR GER)**. They spit up effortlessly and with small volumes.

GER is not a problem (other than forcing you to spot treat all the shoulders on your shirts). According to Dr. R. Jeff Zwiener, Medical

? ?

THE OTHER END

Director of Pediatric Gastroenterology at Dell Children's Medical Center of Central Texas, GER only becomes a problem called **GASTROESOPHAGEAL REFLUX DISEASE (GERD)** if it leads to these unpleasant consequences:

◆ irritation of the esophagus (esophagitis), making babies irritable, fussy, or refuse to eat.
◆ respiratory/airway problems that make babies wheeze, gag, choke, or have trouble breathing.

RED FLAGS: When to worry about acid reflux

1. If your baby spits up large volumes consistently, they won't gain weight (see **GERD TREATMENT**).
2. If your baby cries or arches after feeding, with or without spitting up. The stomach acid is irritating their esophagus (See **GERD TREATMENT**).
3. If your baby has Exorcist-style, projectile vomiting after every meal, call your doctor immediately (see **PYLORIC STENOSIS**).

Q. My baby is four-months old now and is spitting up more than they did when they were younger. Should I be worried?

No.
It takes about six months for the sphincter muscle to tighten up. As your baby takes larger volumes of breast milk/formula, larger volumes will come up. Hence, it gives the appearance that your baby's reflux is getting worse instead of better. The spit up is usually at an all-time high around four months of age.

Q. Okay, my baby is nine-months old and still spitting up. Should I be worried?

No. You're just at the end of the bell curve. Many babies graduate from spitting up by six months, but there are a few stragglers. Almost all babies stop spitting up by one year of age.

Reality Check
No, it's not just your baby who is an Olympic-caliber spitter. Consider this:
Of all babies 0-3 months of age, 50% spit up.
Of all babies 4-5 months of age, 67% spit up.
Of all babies 6-7 months of age, 21% still spit up.
By 12 months of age, less than 5% of babies are still spitting up. (*Nelson*)

Q. How can I tell if my baby is suffering from acid/gastroesophageal reflux?

Everyone is usually miserable from this. Your doctor can help you make the diagnosis on this one.

This is usually the problem behind fussy, "colicky" infants. Most parents are convinced that their infant either has horrible gas pains, a milk allergy, or colic. They also think that they are inadequate as parents because their baby is always fussy and they haven't figured out how to make them feel better. Some adventurous parents will unsuccessfully try Mylicon drops (an over-the-counter medicine which makes big gas bubbles into little gas bubbles), switching formulas, or eliminating dairy from breastfeeding Mom's diet before scheduling an appointment with their doctor.

How do we make the diagnosis? We look at the time the fussiness occurs, and what seems to make it worse. *The first rule: babies with reflux don't always spit up—(spitters are really easy to diagnose).* Some babies experience heartburn when the stomach acid comes up into the esophagus with the milk. If it doesn't make it all the way up to the mouth, you won't see it. Babies with heartburn often cry during and shortly after feedings. They can also cry when lying down (for example, on the changing table) because this allows the acid to come up. They may try to arch their backs or thrust their heads back to alleviate the pain. This happens around the clock, making a very unhappy baby.

Babies are born with immature guts that can cause symptoms of colic. Colic is ruled out

TRICKS OF THE TRADE TO TREAT ACID REFLUX

If your baby is uncomfortable from the heartburn associated with acid reflux, or is not gaining weight, there are many options to reduce the severity of the symptoms. Start by using the following tricks at home. If that doesn't work, consider a medication (which will require a prescription). Medication is obviously a last resort, but it is an option for miserable babies with severe reflux symptoms.

1. Keep your baby upright for 20 minutes after feedings. This lets the food travel out of the stomach into the small intestine before moving baby around.

2. Let your baby plan mealtimes. Babies often figure this out themselves. They have more discomfort with large meals, so they learn to become snackers. It's not great for parents' schedules, but is more comfortable for baby.

3. Dream Feeds. Reflux babies associate eating with pain. They want to eat, but avoid eating to avoid the pain. Try feeding your baby when they are too tired to fight or think about it—and they may have a better meal. While it is ideal to eliminate night feedings as soon as possible, it may not be possible for reflux babies.

4. Get a therapist. Feeding therapists (usually occupational therapists or speech therapists) can train reflux babies and their parents to enjoy mealtime. Ask your baby's pediatrician or pediatric gastroenterologist for a referral. You may want a therapist, too, but one of the talking kind. Just kidding, not kidding. This parenting stuff can be very stressful.

5. Medications. Babies use the same antacids as adults. Many products are over the counter for adults, but are by prescription-only for kids. Some products are not approved by the FDA for use in children, but are routinely used by both pediatric gastroenterologists and pediatricians.

by the frequency of the behaviors. Babies with colic are also unhappy. However, they are only unhappy for three hours a day (say, around 5 pm to 8 pm). Colic starts at three weeks of age and lasts until three months of age. We'd recommend a daily probiotic to help relieve those symptoms. If your baby has been fussy since two weeks of age and is always fussy, it's probably not colic and most likely acid reflux. (See Chapter 11, Discipline and Temperament for more about colic).

Cow milk protein allergy or intolerance is ruled out by exploring some details about baby's poop. A true milk allergy causes mucous and/or blood in loose poop, really horrible eczema, or worse—hives or immediate vomiting. If you have a fussy baby with normal poop, the food is unlikely to be the problem. A therapeutic trial of using a hypoallergenic formula or Mom's dairy elimination will not improve a reflux baby's symptoms.

Q. Can't we just do a test to look for acid reflux?

Yes, tests are available. Here's an overview:

Doctors typically try Pepcid first and move on to proton pump inhibitors (or "PPI's") if symptoms are not improving. The options are listed below. (For details, see Appendix A on medications.):

Histamine 2 Receptor Antagonists: Axid (Nizatidine), Pepcid (Famotidine)
Proton Pump Inhibitors (PPI's): Prilosec, (Omeprazole), Prevacid (Lansoprazole)

If you reach the point that your baby needs medication, they likely have a pretty irritated esophagus lining from constant stomach acid burns. The medication prevents further insults, but it takes at least a week for the irritation to heal. So, don't expect a miraculous change in your baby's behavior after just one dose of medicine. Give the medicine for a week to see if it is working.

Helpful hints: The medication is dosed based on your baby's weight. In some cases, if your baby gains a pound or two, they may no longer be getting a therapeutic dose of their meds. Remind your doctor to recalculate the dose every month or so. And medications like Prilosec that have to be specially mixed (compounded) need a monthly refill.

Parents are often leery of giving medication on a daily basis (sometimes for a few months) to their babies. Understandable. There are a few rare, but potentially significant adverse side effects. But if your baby is miserable and refuses to eat due to pain, medication is definitely the right choice. Once a baby starts to feel better, doctors will try to reduce the dosage and wean off the medication over a couple of weeks.

FYI: we used to recommend thickened feedings (using rice cereal or formula with added rice starch) and a wedge for babies to sleep on an incline. Unfortunately, studies show that neither of these home remedies give babies much relief from GERD.

An Upper GI or "barium swallow imaging study" (see Appendix C, Lab Work and Tests) can be done to rule out other problems that cause regurgitation. If the baby happens to reflux while the test is being done, you have an answer. But having a "normal" barium swallow can simply mean your refluxing baby didn't do it during the test.

An esophageal pH probe can be inserted through the baby's nose to their esophagus and acid levels can be monitored for 24 hours. While the test is about 70% accurate, performing the test on all babies is impractical for obvious reasons—keeping this lovely tube in a baby's nose for a day is no fun, nor is the time baby isn't allowed to eat (several hours).

Then, there's always the option of doing an endoscopy. That involves anesthesia—a tube with a camera at the end of it that is inserted through the baby's mouth and throat to look at the esophagus. Biopsies (tissue samples) can also be taken at the same time to make the diagnosis. This test is 100% accurate, but very expensive.

Given the unpleasant and imperfect nature of these tests, most doctors rely on a simple examination of baby (and parent reports) to make an acid reflux diagnosis.

What's your baby's I-GERQ score?

Here's a free and painless way to assess for possible reflux disease (GERD) in your baby. It's called the I-GERQ-R score. If your baby experiences many of these symptoms, they may be suffering from at least mild heartburn.

This quiz is pretty good at screening for babies who have troublesome heartburn. But it's not 100% accurate and some normal, healthy babies who "fail" the test do not need treatment.

Take the quiz and get your baby doctor's opinion on the problems they are experiencing. Your doc may suggest monitoring for worsening symptoms, additional testing, or treatment. (*Orenstein*)

The test is on the following page.

(I-GERQ-R; Author I-GERQ, Susan Orenstein, MD, © 2004, University of Pittsburgh) To be filled out by primary caregiver of baby. Please read each of the questions carefully, answer to the best of your ability, and do not skip questions. There are no right or wrong answers.

DR B'S OPINION:
GERD . . . AND PATIENCE

Having a baby with GERD can be miserable for everyone. Feeling helpless and sleep deprived (thanks to the symptoms worsening when reclined) makes any parent rethink the number of kids they want to have. These are normal feelings. I promise it gets better with time. Patience is key. And call on friends and family for help.

If your baby is not improving while taking medication, contact your baby's doctor.

Infant Gastroesophageal Reflux Questionnaire

1. **During the past week, how often did the baby usually spit-up (anything coming out of the mouth) during a 24-hour period?**
Less than once / 1 to 3 times /4 to 6 times /More than 6 times

2. **During the past week, how much did the baby usually spit-up (anything coming out of the mouth) during a typical episode?**
Did not spit up
Less than 1 tablespoonful
1 tablespoonful to 2 ounces
More than 2 ounces to half the feeding
More than half the feeding

3. **During the past week, how often did spitting up (anything coming out of the mouth) seem to be uncomfortable for the baby, for example, crying, fussing, irritability, etc.?**
Never / Rarely/ Sometimes
Often /Always

4. **During the past week, how often did the baby refuse a feeding even when hungry?**
Never / Rarely/ Sometimes
Often /Always

5. **During the past week, how often did the baby stop eating soon after starting even when hungry?**
Never / Rarely/ Sometimes
Often /Always

6. **During the past week, did the baby cry a lot during or within 1 hour after feedings?**
Never / Rarely/ Sometimes
Often /Always

7. **During the past week, did the baby cry or fuss more than usual?**
Never / Rarely/ Sometimes
Often /Always

8. **During the past week, on average how long did the baby cry or fuss during a 24 hour period?**
Less than 10 minutes
10 minutes to 1 hour
More than 1 hour but less than 3 hours
3 or more hours

9. **During the past week, how often did the baby have hiccups?**
Never / Rarely/ Sometimes
Often /Always

10. **During the past week, how often did the baby have episodes of arching back?**
Never / Rarely/ Sometimes
Often /Always

11. **During the past week, has the baby stopped breathing while awake or struggled to breathe?**
No / Yes

12. **During the past week, has the baby turned blue or purple?**
No / Yes

13. **Overall, how would you rate the severity of your baby's Gastroesophageal Reflux Disease (GERD) symptoms during the past week?**
No symptoms
Very mild
Mild
Moderate
Severe
Very severe

the other end

? ?

THE OTHER END

Again, if you have concerns, fill out the quiz and ask your baby's doctor to evaluate your child for possible heartburn or GERD.

BOTTOM LINE

Most babies outgrow their symptoms of acid reflux when the esophagus muscle tightens up (around six months of age). A few babies will continue to have problems up to their first birthdays. Babies who suffer with daily reflux symptoms from 6-12 months of age are more likely to have feeding problems in their second year of life (even if the reflux is gone). (*Nelson*)

Reality Check

Your baby does not have acid reflux because your Great Uncle Harry has acid reflux. Nor will your baby develop a hiatal hernia because of acid reflux. However, there are a few babies with GERD who grow up to be adults with GERD.

Insider Tip: Acid Reflux . . . a reason for wheezin'

Some babies with acid reflux have respiratory symptoms such as chronic cough and wheezing. This happens because the milk is coming up and irritating the baby's airway. Again, even babies with severe reflux may not be spitting up large volumes of milk. If a baby is having this much trouble with reflux, doctors are pretty aggressive about a treatment plan (for good reason!).

The flip side: if your baby wheezes and a diagnosis of asthma is being considered, get them evaluated for acid reflux (GERD)—that may be the reason for the wheezing.

Q. Occasionally, my baby will throw up their whole feeding. Should I worry?

No.

When babies eat aggressively, they suck in a lot of air. When that big air bubble comes back up with burping, often the whole feeding does too. Unlike adults, babies often throw up and then want to eat again.

The only time to worry is when the whole feeding gets thrown up at *every* feeding. This is a red flag for **PYLORIC STENOSIS** (see picture at right). This is a medical emergency caused by a narrowing of the muscle between the stomach and small intestine (called the *pyloric sphincter*). It usually occurs at six to eight weeks of age because the muscle seems to narrow over time.

RED FLAGS: Vomiting

1. Vomiting bile. Bile is a fluorescent green/yellow color that can indicate a blockage in the intestines. It is especially worrisome if associated with stomachache or a bloated looking tummy, or fever. Call your doctor ASAP.

2. Vomiting blood or "coffee grounds." In newborns, blood in baby's spit up is

? ?

THE OTHER END

often from Mommy's cracked and bleeding nipples. Beyond that time, blood in vomit warrants a call to the doctor. Blood that has been partially digested by the stomach looks like coffee grounds when it is thrown up. Both of these symptoms can be caused by bleeding in the esophagus or stomach.

3. **Vomiting repeatedly over six hours**. Excessive vomiting can be caused by stomach viruses (see **GASTROENTERITIS**), food poisoning (see **BACTERIAL ENTERITIS**), or an intestinal blockage (see **ACUTE ABDOMEN**). Most of the time, it's a stomach virus. It's time to check in with your doctor after six hours because your baby can get dehydrated.

4. **Vomiting associated with fever and irritability.** This is how meningitis presents in a baby. Babies have a unique "window" to the brain with their soft spot (fontanelle) on their heads. A full, bulging soft spot occurs with meningitis. Call your doctor immediately.

5. **Morning vomiting.** Babies don't get morning sickness. It's incredibly rare, but vomiting exclusively in the morning is a symptom of increased pressure in the skull. This can be caused by abnormal fluid collections or a mass (i.e. **HYDROCEPHALUS, BRAIN TUMOR**). Both of these abnormalities cause a full, bulging soft spot (fontanelle). This definitely needs to be checked out.

Q. What should I feed/let my baby drink while they are vomiting?

Nothing.

When your baby is actively vomiting, give them nothing to eat or drink unless you want to see it come right back out.

Wait until it has been at least an hour since the last vomit to test the waters. Start with Pedialyte or a generic brand oral rehydration solution sold at most grocery stores and pharmacies (or see the recipe to make your own in Appendix B).

This is basically Gatorade made specifically for babies. Give one teaspoon every five minutes. Don't let your baby chug as much as they want. They will be very thirsty. If they take a full bottle worth on an unsettled stomach, it's destined to be thrown up. They'll get about two ounces an hour for the first couple of hours. If the Pedialyte test fails (more vomiting occurs), call your doctor.

Once the Pedialyte stays down, resume formula or breast milk.

Q. What are the signs of dehydration?

Lethargy, dry skin and lips, sunken soft spot (fontanelle), and peeing less often (less than three wet diapers in 24 hours—or no wet diaper in eight hours).

Another measure is weight loss, which is checked in the doctor's office. If your child is vomiting and/or having diarrhea, *start tallying how many wet diapers your baby is having*. Your doctor will ask you that question when you call or come in for an appointment. For more info, check out Chapter 15, "First Aid."

Pee/Urine

Q. My newborn urinated only once in their first day of life. Is this normal?

Yes.

All you can expect is one wet diaper on baby's first day. We just want to know that the pipes are working. Your baby might pee twice on the second day of life. The wet diapers will start to accumulate once your baby is drinking more. By day four of life, you should get at least four wet diapers. This should reassure you that your baby is getting something to drink when you are breastfeeding.

Q. These diapers are so absorbent, how can I tell if my baby has urinated?

Many diapers now have a urine sensor line. If you don't have those fancy diapers or you are using cloth diapers, put a tissue in the diaper and you can see the pee.

In the first week of life, keep track of wet diapers. This information is also useful if your baby is vomiting and has diarrhea.

Another hint: diapers with pee in them feel heavier than dry ones.

Q. My newborn looks like there is blood in his pee. What is it?

Take a closer look. Does it look like brick dust? Is it powdery and on the *surface* of the diaper?

If the answer is yes to these questions, it's not blood. These are **URIC ACID CRYSTALS**. When newborns are a little dehydrated (in the initial 10% weight loss mode), the pee is more concentrated and less watery. This causes one of the ingredients of pee, uric acid, to separate out. That's what you are seeing. Uric acid crystals are nothing to worry about if it is just one newborn diaper. Call your doctor if this is persistent or you see it in an older baby. For a picture of this, see Baby411.com/bonus (click on Visual Library).

Q. There looks like blood in my baby's diaper. What is it?

This is the equivalent of a menstrual period. It's not in the pee.

Baby girls' bodies respond to their mother's hormones. There is frequently some bleeding and vaginal discharge in the first few weeks of life. This is normal.

Q. I've heard that baby girls are prone to bladder infections. How can I prevent them?

Good hygiene.

A brief anatomy lesson here. Girls have a very short tube (urethra) that attaches the bladder to the outside. The urethral opening sits just above the vagina. Just below the vagina is the anus. Remember that poop has bacteria in it and urine is sterile. If the poop ends up in the nooks and crannies surrounding the urethra, the bacteria (usually E.coli) can climb into the urethra and grow in the bladder causing a bladder infection. Girls in diapers are particularly prone to infections.

The best ways to prevent infection are:

♦ *Change a baby girl's poop diaper ASAP.*
♦ *Wipe "front to back."* This means start cleaning your daughter at the urethra and wipe downwards to the anus. Never go the other direction! Gently separate the labia and be sure to clean well in there.

Boys rarely get bladder infections because the urethral tube is much longer from the bladder to the opening (the urethra tube is inside the penis and the opening is at the tip). It's much harder for those bugs to travel that far.

Q. How do you diagnose a bladder infection in a baby?

Foul smelling urine, cloudy urine, and particularly, *fever in a baby with no obvious symptoms* (i.e. no runny nose, cough, or diarrhea).

This is one of the top reasons why we want to hear from you if your baby under three months of age has a fever. *Untreated* bladder infections can quickly lead to kidney infections (and even meningitis) in infants under six months of age.

If your baby is in diapers, and has a fever with no obvious symptoms, your doctor will need a urine sample to look for infection.

Q. Are some babies more prone to bladder infections than others?

Yes. Although most bladder infections occur due to poor hygiene (poopie diapers) and bad luck, about 30-45% of all children who have a bladder infection have a rare abnormality of the urinary system that causes urine to flow backwards into the kidneys. This is called **VESICOURETERAL REFLUX (VUR)**. See pictures at right.

There are five grades of VUR, with Grades 4 and 5 being the most severe. Kids with the most severe VUR are at the greatest risk of kidney infection and permanent damage. The good news: most children with VUR outgrow this disorder by age seven—even 70% of kids with Grade 3 VUR will outgrow it.

However, those with Grade 4 or 5 are the least likely to outgrow VUR and may need surgery to correct the problem.

Because of the potential for permanent kidney damage, pediatricians have always been cautious about little ones who have bladder infections.

Normal urine flow.

Vesicoureteral reflux.

Historically, *any* child with their first bladder infection **before reaching puberty** would have been tested for VUR. That testing involved an ultrasound of the kidneys (easy and relatively cheap) and either a Voiding Cystourethrogram "VCUG" or a radionuclide DMSA scan (more involved and expensive). See Appendix C, Labs and Tests for details on these studies. If the child was diagnosed with VUR, girls were prescribed a low-dose antibiotic to take at bedtime to prevent future infections. This antibiotic was taken every night until they outgrew the VUR (monitored by repeating these fun imaging studies annually.)

This evaluation and preventative antibiotic treatment for kids with VUR has been evolving and there is no official consensus here. Evidence shows that kids with severe VUR will likely be sicker, and have their first urinary tract infection before being potty trained. So, is it worth the time, money, and discomfort of the procedure to test every child with their first bladder infection? And should all babies who have VUR be on a nightly dose of antibiotics until they outgrow the condition? Even children who have mild to moderate (Grade 1-3) VUR may never have another infection and may not end up with kidney damage anyway.

The American Academy of Pediatrics and American Urological Association have slightly different advice, but here is what all experts can agree on:

Any infant under two months of age with a bladder infection needs to be tested for this abnormality. Other children at high-risk for having VUR should be tested. That includes those with: more than one bladder infection, a bladder infection with bloodstream infection, poor urine stream, a bladder infection with unusual bacteria, abnormal urinary tract on prenatal ultrasound, or continued symptoms after being on antibiotics over three days.

Here is the summary of recommendations for who should get tested for VUR:

- ◆ All children under two months of age who have a fever with a bladder infection.
- ◆ Kids ages two to 24 months old with more than one bladder infection with a fever.
- ◆ Children whose infections do not clear up quickly. *(Finnell)*

And, newborns who have abnormalities detected on a prenatal ultrasound (Grade 3-4 hydronephrosis, hydroureter, abnormal bladder) should have a VCUG screening test for reflux shortly after birth. *(AUA 2010)*

Reality Check

There is a 60% chance of a child having vesicoureteral reflux if a parent has the disorder. There is a 30% chance of having VUR if a brother or sister has the disorder. *(AUA 1996)*

Siblings (or offspring) of affected children may be screened as well. The American Urological Association says that healthcare providers may opt to screen healthy siblings of children with reflux via a kidney (renal) ultrasound. Then a VCUG test should be performed if an abnormality is detected on the kidney ultrasound. It's also an option to just observe siblings and then promptly evaluate these kids if they have a bladder infection. The same logic applies to offspring of adults who had reflux in childhood.

BOTTOM LINE

Your doctor may want to screen your child for VUR, even if they doesn't fall into the high-risk category. There is no harm in following the precautionary principle. *(AUA 2017)*

Burping

Q. Do you have any tips on burping my baby? I spend 20 minutes trying to burp them and nothing happens.

It's either going to happen or it won't. It's not your technique or patience that does the trick.

Burps are the result of swallowed air during feedings. Once your baby is an efficient eater (by four months old), they're also likely to be an efficient burper.

For the first few months of life, stop in mid-feed to burp your baby. There are basically three techniques.

1. Baby is upright on your shoulder, and you rub upwards on thier back.
2. Baby is sitting in your lap, upright, and you rub upwards on their back.
3. Baby is lying face down on your lap, and you rub upwards on their back.

If it has been more than ten minutes, the burp ain't happening on your watch. Unfortunately, your baby may sleep for 20 minutes, then wake himself up when he burps. Welcome to parenthood. Just do what you can.

> **DR B'S OPINION**
>
> *"Note that the burping technique involves rubbing. I watched my brother burp his twins once and considered reporting him to child protective services. Patting and hitting aren't really necessary!"*

Hiccups

Parents ask a lot of questions about hiccups. Here is what you need to know:

1. Hiccups don't hurt.
2. Don't worry about hiccups—doctors don't.
3. Only *excessive* hiccupping is associated with acid reflux (GERD).

Gas

A nice way to exit this chapter.

Q. My baby has more gas than me. Should I be worried?

No.

Your baby has more gas because they suck in a lot of air and because their intestines are on high alert 24 hours a day.

Most of the time, babies don't really care that they have gas. And don't be embarrassed, it's the only time in your child's life when people will think it's cute.

Q. What can I do about my baby's gas? Are Mylicon drops okay to use?

Not much, and sure, it won't hurt.

Gas is one of the biggest obsessions of newborn parents. Some parents believe it is the root of all evil . . . the reason that the baby is unhappy . . . the reason why nobody is sleeping.

NEW PARENT 411: HELPING YOUR BABY PASS GAS

Here are some tips from seasoned parents:

1. Infant massage. This is a comforting way to help your baby relax. Pressing gently on baby's belly sometimes gets the gas out.

2. Warm bath. This also works by relaxing your baby.

3. Mylicon (simethicone) drops. This over the counter medication is safe for babies, including newborns. It makes big gas bubbles into little gas bubbles. Some parents swear by it, others see absolutely no difference in their baby's demeanor. Gripe water, a combo of ginger and fennel, is also a popular remedy. Using daily probiotics such as Lactobacillus reuteri, is another option for babies who were born full-term.

4. Support and lean your baby forward and facing away from you. It may help reduce the tummy pressure and get rid of the uncomfy feeling.

The truth is—IT'S PROBABLY NOT THE GAS. But, if you feel compelled to do *something* (which is a common feeling of all parents), it's okay to try those Mylicon (simethicone) drops. See above for gas tips. If you have a baby who was born full-term, it is also okay to try some daily probiotics as a digestive aid. See Appendix A, Medications for more information on probiotics such as Lactobacillus reuteri and Bifidobacteria infantis.

The good news; the gassy phase will pass by age two or three months.

Q. I'm breastfeeding. Will eliminating high fiber foods from my diet fix my baby's gas problem?

No, but it will give you, Mom, a constipation problem.

This is rarely the cause of baby's gas. You can try an elimination diet, but it's usually not the problem.

Q. My baby is colicky. Is it because of gas?

No. Gas gets a bad rap.

See Chapter 11, Discipline and Temperament, for information on colic. Eliminating gas won't solve your colic problem.

Section 3

*Sleep,
Developmental Milestones,
Temperament & Soothing*

Sleeping Like A Baby

Chapter 9

"Whoever coined the phrase, 'sleeps like a baby' never slept with one!"
~ Anonymous

What's in this Chapter

- ◆ The science of sleep
- ◆ Newborn sleep issues
- ◆ Sleep safety tips
- ◆ Deciding on your family's sleep routine (family bed vs. solo)
- ◆ Setting up good habits
- ◆ Undoing bad habits
- ◆ Top 10 Mistakes parents make
- ◆ Gradual, rapid and gentle training.
- ◆ Naps and "wake windows"
- ◆ Special situations— Multiples and Preemies

Who needs sleep?
well you're never gonna get it

Who needs sleep?
tell me what's that for

Who needs sleep?
be happy with what you're getting
There's a guy who's been awake since
the Second World War
    —Barenaked Ladies

New (and veteran) parents struggle with their baby's sleep habits—it's a fact of life. Everyone warned you about it, but you weren't buying it. At first, the excitement of being a parent gives you the momentum to make it through the first few weeks of sleep deprivation. Then, the novelty begins to wear off. You are exhausted and desperate for a good night's sleep. Don't worry, we are here for you! And if this 45-page chapter isn't enough, pop over to our online community and watch our sleep videos.

If you are reading this chapter before your baby is born, good for you. You will be prepared for what lies ahead. If you are already in the desperate category—don't worry—we can help you, too.

Before we give you all of our sage advice on this subject, it is *essential* that you understand the science of sleep. Knowing the basics will help you appreciate the advice and avoid the common mistakes parents make.

The Science Of Sleep

Q. Do newborns have the same sleep patterns that adults do?

NO. That's why you cannot expect them to sleep like we do. Here are four important concepts you need to understand:

1 TYPES OF SLEEP. There are two basic types of sleep: REM and Non-REM. REM stands for **R**apid **E**ye **M**ovement. Here are the differences between the two.

	NON-REM SLEEP	REM SLEEP
Muscle movements	relaxed	active (stretches, sucks, vocalizes)
Brain activity	relaxed	active (dreams)
Occurrence	1st part of night, PM nap	2nd part of night, AM nap

Newborns spend 50-80% of their sleep in REM sleep while adults spend only 25% of their sleep in REM. The result: babies are very active when they are asleep. Your baby will be noisy and moving around, but they are not awake.

BOTTOM LINE: Your baby's sleep activity and noises do not mean you need to feed/help them.

2 SLEEP CYCLES. Humans go through a series of sleep cycles throughout an evening's rest. Adults tend to bunch all the Non-REM cycles first, and then go through REM cycles. Babies do more flip-flopping of Non-REM and REM cycles. Each sleep cycle has a beginning and an end, where a person goes from light sleep to deep to light again, before entering the next cycle. Humans recheck their environments and body comfort at that time. At the end of each sleep cycle, a partial wakening occurs. Babies may whimper or briefly cry out during this time.

BOTTOM LINE: Leave your baby alone when they have a partial wakening. If left alone, they will enter into the next sleep cycle. If you intervene, you will wake them up. As the say- ing goes, let sleeping babies lie.

3 LENGTH OF CYCLES. The average adult sleep cycle lasts 90 minutes. The average newborn sleep cycle lasts 60 minutes.

BOTTOM LINE: Your baby has shorter sleep cycles than you. It can take several months until they have mature sleep patterns like an older child.

4 CIRCADIAN RHYTHM. The human body has a biological clock that registers 24.5 to 25 hours in a day. This is called a circadian rhythm. It is affected by both light exposure and a body chemical called melatonin. Babies follow their mother's circadian rhythm in the womb probably because of melatonin levels. Once outside the womb, they have exposure to light and must form their own circadian rhythm.

BOTTOM LINE: It takes several weeks for a baby to get their circadian rhythm sorted out. If you lived in the dark for nine months, you'd probably be a little confused too.

Newborn Sleep Issues

Q. Okay, now I understand why my newborn has erratic sleep patterns. But, how can I get my baby to sleep at night instead of during the day?

This is called Day-Night Reversal. It usually takes three or four weeks to resolve.

The best way to help your baby through this is to stimulate them during the day and keep things low key at night. Talk to your baby during daylight hours and encourage any wakeful periods he has. At night, do your feeding routine with little interaction. Only turn the lights on if you have a poopy diaper to clean. If your baby decides they want to have a slumber party, they can party (coo, grunt, etc.) on their own. You don't have to be by your baby's side to entertain them.

These nocturnal habits usually resolve by three to four weeks of age. See "Sleep Tips" below in this chapter for more advice on the first couple weeks of life.

Q. How much should a newborn sleep?

About 14 to 18 hours total a day.

But here's the cruel part: most newborns will not sleep more than four hours at a stretch. They need to eat frequently and their little bodies know it.

Check out the table in the Setting Up Good Habits section later in this chapter to get an idea of how sleep changes through the first year of life.

BOTTOM LINE: Most newborns have six or seven stretches of sleep every 24 hours. Feedings occur in between these stretches.

Helpful Hints
Three Sleep Tips for the First Two Weeks of life

◆ *Wake your newborn up if they have slept longer than three hours during the day.* When your baby has day-night reversals, they may have their one and only long stretch of sleep in the middle of the day. Encourage your baby to wake up and eat, if possible. Otherwise, you will be in for a long night of cluster feedings.

◆ *Do not let your newborn sleep more than four hours straight during the night.* They need nutrition to grow. They also need to stimulate your milk supply to come in if you are breastfeeding. Once they have regained their birth weight and your doc gives you the green light, you can let the baby sleep at night (they won't, but it's fine if they do).

◆ *Your job is to sleep when baby sleeps.* Become nocturnal. Don't even think about doing laundry when your baby crashes in the afternoon. Go to bed!

Q. When can I expect to sleep through the night?

Now that you are an expert in "sleep-ology," you can appreciate the following fact: it takes (on average) *17 weeks of life* for an infant to develop mature sleep patterns. Yep, that's about four months. Think about that for a moment.

The definition of "sleeping through the night" is six hours of uninterrupted sleep. That will feel like a great night's sleep by the time you get there! (*Kleitman*)

FYI: Even parents with school-aged kids will be awakened by middle-of-the-night announcements ("I just had a nightmare, Mom" . . . you get the picture). The concept of "sleeping through the night" is only a fuzzy and abstract concept that exists for childless couples.

BOTTOM LINE

There is a popular baby sleep book entitled *Twelve Hours' Sleep by Twelve Weeks Old*. If the author were honest, it would be really entitled Six Hours by Seventeen Weeks. Of course, then no one would buy it! Bottom line: Don't fall for the marketing hype of sleep "experts" that promise the Holy Grail for sleep-deprived parents.

Old Wives Tale

Giving your baby rice cereal helps them sleep through the night earlier.
The truth: Food has nothing to do with it.

Q. My friend says that their baby slept through the night at four weeks of age! That's not fair! How can this be?

Odds are, your friends are exaggerating—or will soon be proved wrong when their baby reverts back to a normal sleep pattern (that is, waking up during the night). Sure, lightning sometimes strikes and a one month old will sleep through the night . . . for one night. Or even a month. But then, as we'll discuss later, they may relapse into waking up during the nighttime.

By the way, some babies *will* sleep up to 12 hours a night as early as two months of age, but it's not the norm. If your baby is a terrific sleeper, don't brag about it—you'll jinx yourself for the next baby!

DR B'S OPINION

"If your full term, healthy baby is still not sleeping six hours straight by six months of age, you need help. Read the section 'Undoing Bad Habits' later in this chapter."

Q. How do I get my newborn to fall asleep? They seem to have trouble relaxing.

It would be nice to have the baby who awakens to feed and then goes right back to sleep. More likely, you have the baby who eats and then fusses until you help them return to the Land of Nod.

After you and your baby get to know each other better, you will figure out what helps them settle down.

Newborns are born with immature nervous systems. That means, they don't have the ability to pull it together, relax, and fall asleep. The most reliable way babies know how to settle down is to suck. See the box nearby for our Newborn Sleep Tips.

NEW PARENT 411: TOP 5 TIPS FOR GETTING A NEWBORN TO SLEEP

1. **Suck to soothe**. If you are so inclined, your breast may become the human pacifier. If this approach is not for you, use your finger or a pacifier in your baby's mouth to encourage sucking. This is fine for the first few months of life (more on pacifiers later in this chapter).
2. **Move around.** Rocking, swaying, and bouncing (you will have the veteran-parent-bop down quickly) are effective.
3. **Sing**, in or out of tune.
4. **Snug as a bug.** Swaddling, sleeping in a bassinet, or even sleeping in a wearable baby carrier may do the trick.
5. **Go for a car ride.**

Q. How long should my newborn sleep in a bassinet or use the Snoo with the swaddler feature?

Two or three months max.

You are not setting up any permanent habits the first two months of life. Babies become aware of their surroundings as their brain and nervous system matures around three to four months of age. That's when you can and should establish a healthy sleep routine.

For now, newborns prefer to be snug. They like to sleep in bassinets or cradles until they decide they want and need to stretch out and move. We'll explain the expiration date for swaddling (which is also two or three months of age) a bit later in this chapter. But spoiler alert: your baby may love the Snoo bassinet but they need to be able to move around in it by three months of age. They will graduate from the swaddler feature (which will deactivate all the bells and whistles that go along with it).

Another tip: do not use inclined sleep products—where the head of the bassinet is elevated or so called "infant lounger" or sleeper devices. The extremely popular Fisher Price Newborn Rock 'n Play (an inclined sleeper) was recalled a few years ago due to over 30 infant deaths while using this product. Please do not use a hand-me-down or buy one from a resale shop. FYI: It's okay if your baby falls asleep in their car seat while you are driving. Just don't use the car seat as a sleep space at other times. We know it is tempting, but it is designed like an inclined sleeper and carries the same risks. Later in this chapter, we'll discuss sleep products in more detail.

I recommend transitioning over to where you want your baby ultimately to sleep around two to three months of age. Another factor: some playpens with a bassinet insert have weight limits that are usually exceeded by two or three months of age.

Old Wives Tale
Too much holding and rocking will spoil your baby.
The truth: You cannot spoil a newborn. Remember, babies don't have the ability

to settle on their own. Do what it takes to get your baby to sleep. *However,* you *need to grow as your baby does. Your six-month-old will be quite capable of settling down on their own.*

Reality Check

Many babies will sweat while they are asleep. Don't be alarmed if your baby awakens in a pool of water (well, you might want to check the diaper, too).

Q. My baby will only sleep on me. If I put them down anywhere (bassinet, etc.) they wake right up. What do I do?

Remember, babies are not born with self-soothing skills. They are used to being snug, warm, and next to your heartbeat. While you can simulate that environment (you can even buy a device that makes heartbeat noises), your baby may still sleep better when they are skin to skin with you.

During the day, it's fairly easy to do this. Wear your baby in a front carrier (example: the ERGObaby 360°). Just continue your daily activities with your baby in tow.

During the night, it's a bit more of a challenge. You'll need to come up with a safe way for both of you to get some sleep. One solution: the Halo Bassinest Swivel Sleeper. That way, each of you will sleep in your own space, but you can swivel the Bassinest for easy access to baby.

We also like the pricey but awesome Snoo, especially since there is a rental option for it. See more information about this product later in this chapter.

You are not setting up any bad habits. By two or three months, your baby will want to stretch out and won't need to be carried continuously. You're welcome to continue using a carrier as long as you'd like for transportation, but we'd suggest discontinuing its use as a sleep aid at three months.

Q. How do sleep patterns and needs change as baby grows?

Check out this information as well as the handy sleep requirements chart nearby for details. Remember, these are general guidelines. No need to freak out if your baby doesn't follow

DR B'S OPINION: CONTACT NAPS

Advocates in the gentle parenting camp believe in the concept of "contact naps" where older babies (over three months of age) and toddlers continue to take daytime snoozes on/with their parents. If you have the desire (and time) to rest with your baby, you are welcome to do so. I wish I could take a nap every day! The downside is many parents also complain about being "nap-trapped" and perpetually "stuck under a baby." And speaking as someone with over 25 years of infant sleep expertise, it is my opinion that contact naps lead to the same expectation for night-time sleep and co-sleeping in a family bed. So, if you love this concept, go for it. I just want you to be fully aware of the habits and expectations you are setting up.

SLEEP

Sleep requirements, birth to 2 years (in hours)

	Nighttime sleep	Daytime sleep	
1 week	8	8	4-5 naps
1 month	8	6	3-4 naps
3 months	8.5	4.5	3-4 naps
6 months	9.25	3.25	2-3 naps
9 months	9.5	2.75	2 naps
12 months	10	1.75	1-2 naps
18 months	9.6	2	1 nap
2 years	9.6	1.9	1 nap

these numbers to a tee!

◆ **Birth to two months.** Newborns sleep 14-18 hours a day. They have day-night reversals, and rarely sleep for more than a four-hour stretch at a time. Yes, you have our blessing to do whatever it takes to get your baby to fall asleep and stay asleep, as long as it is safe. Swaddling, rocking, nursing to sleep, wearing your baby in a front carrier, going for a car ride, using a pacifier, etc. You are not spoiling your baby or setting up any permanent bad habits. Remember: your baby does not have the neurologic maturity to pull it together, relax, and fall asleep on their own yet.

(Continued on page 234)

DR B'S OPINION:
IT CAN BE ROUGH AT THE START

WE GET IT. Newborns do not sleep very well or very long. This makes for some extremely exhausted parents looking for solutions that will help their baby sleep. And yes, the best way to reduce a baby's risk of SIDS—sleeping alone, on their back, in a naked crib—seems to make it even harder for everyone to get a few precious moments of shut eye. This is even more painful when parents have to get up in the morning for work.

Just remember this is all temporary and your agony will be a distant memory (that you can remind your child of throughout their life). Your baby will mature over the first 8-12 weeks of life and will become more capable of settling down at night. The goal is to have your baby sleep safely.

BABY 411'S SAMPLE SLEEP SCHEDULE FOR YOUR BABY'S FIRST YEAR

AGE	BEDTIME	AWAKE TIME BETWEEN NAPS	# NAPS

*Morning naps are usually shorter catnaps (30-45 minutes), the afternoon nap is usually longer (1-3 hours).

1 WEEK — Good luck — 30-60 mins — 5+ catnaps

—Newborns eat often and take short snoozes between meals. Expect variability and lots of night wakings for feedings.

1 MONTH — Good luck — 60-90 mins — 4 catnaps

—The feeding frenzy continues for another month or two. Expect short naps between feedings and lots of night wakings for feedings.

—Begin a short, relaxing wind-down-to-bed routine beyond feeding. Start reading, singing, and snuggling for 15-20 minutes if your baby is still awake to enjoy it.

3 MONTHS — 9-10 PM — 1-2 hours — 3-4 naps*

—Make a schedule for your baby's day, and put your baby down for naps at regular intervals.

—Your baby will have more wakeful time to play between naps and feedings. Watch your baby's cues, but in general, they can/should be awake for 1-2 hours between naps.

—Consistently use your relaxing wind-down-to-bed routine for naps and night time. Make it short and sweet (15-20 minutes of wind down, not hours).

—Start trying to put your baby down relaxed, but not asleep. No swaddling.

—Aim for a reasonable bedtime, but know that there will probably still be some night feedings. You are not done with those quite yet.

4 MONTHS — 7-8:30 PM — 2-3 hours — 3-4 naps*

—You have a schedule! Put your baby down for naps at regular intervals. They are usually awake for 2-3 hours for playtime between naps and need to eat about every 3 hours during the day.

—Consistently use your short and sweet wind-down-to-bed routine for naps and night time.

—Put your baby down relaxed, but NOT asleep. Give them at least 10-15 minutes to try to self-regulate. Be consistent and let them try to figure it out without you jumping in to the rescue.

—Morning naps are restorative catnaps, lasting 30-45 minutes. The afternoon nap is the big Kahuna, usually 1-3 hours in duration.

—Aim for a 7-8:30 PM bedtime. Your baby may still need one night feeding after the first six hour stretch of the night (yes, six hours is the goal for an appropriately growing full-term baby).

—Make sure the last nap of the day ends two hours before bedtime (by 5-6 PM) to ensure your baby is ready to go to bed for the night.

SLEEP

Baby 411's Sample Sleep Schedule for Your Baby's First Year

AGE	BEDTIME	AWAKE TIME BETWEEN NAPS	# NAPS

6 MONTHS   7-8:30 PM   2-3 hours   2-3 naps*

—Follow your schedule. Put your baby down for naps at regular intervals. They are awake for about 3 hours for playtime between naps and need to eat about every 3 hours during the day.

—Consistently use your short and sweet wind-down-to-bed routine for naps and night time.

—Put your baby down relaxed, but NOT asleep. They've got this self-regulation thing down now, let them fly! Yes, they are all capable little beings if you allow them to be.

—The morning nap lasts 30-45 minutes. The afternoon nap is usually 1-3 hours in duration.

—Aim for a 7-8:30 PM bedtime. Your baby is done with night feedings. Really. They can sleep 10-12 hours without needing to eat (or needing your help to fall back asleep)—the key is setting up the right self-regulation routine at the beginning of the night.

—Make sure the afternoon nap ends 2-3 hours before bedtime (by 4-5 PM) to ensure your baby is ready to go to bed for the night.

9 MONTHS   7-8:30 PM   3 hours   2 naps*

—Follow your schedule. They have 3 hour playtime sessions, 2 naps a day, and eat every 3 hours (usually 5 meals a day and none at night).

—Consistently use your short and sweet wind-down-to-bed routine for naps and night time.

—Your baby falls asleep without you. Yes. If you aren't there yet, read the rest of this chapter!

—The morning nap lasts 30-45 minutes. The afternoon nap is usually 1-3 hours in duration.

—Aim for a 7-8:30 PM bedtime. They can sleep 10-12 hours a night, without food or you.

—Make sure the afternoon ends 2-3 hours before bedtime (by 4-5 PM).

12 MONTHS   7-8:30 PM   3 hours   1-2 naps*

—Toddlers have morning and afternoon playtime sessions, usually 2 naps a day, and 3 meals and 2 snacks a day.

—Some toddlers instinctively drop the morning catnap, others will be forced to stop at daycare. The afternoon nap is usually 1-3 hours in duration.

—Aim for a 7-8:30 PM bedtime. They can sleep 10-12 hours a night, without food or you.

—Make sure the afternoon ends 2-3 hours before bedtime (by 4-5 PM).

◆ *Two to four months.* On average, babies sleep 12-14 hours a day. They are usually taking three or four naps per day. Babies who prefer catnapping may take four shorter naps. If you are lucky, your baby may sleep for a six-hour stretch at night. It is still too early to train your baby to sleep. Your goal: set up *healthy sleep routines*. We'll have more on this subject later in the chapter.

◆ *Four to six months.* The average four to six month old sleeps a total of 11.5-13.5 hours a day, with two or three naps included. Your baby should be sleeping AT LEAST six hours at night. Some babies will sleep up to 12 hours at night. Yes, everyone in the house should be getting sleep by now. . .but if this is not happening, you need help. Do not be convinced that your baby NEEDS to be up at night. In fact, everyone will be happier if your child is sleeping at night. Sometimes parents aid and abet their baby's bad sleep behaviors. We'll discuss the reasons why babies this age continue to wake at night later in this chapter.

◆ *Six to 12 months.* On average, these babies sleep 11–13.5 hours per day, with two naps included. Many babies sleep ten to 12 hours straight at night. Yes, your prayers were answered! If your baby is still waking up for night feedings or comfort, you need help. See "Undoing Bad Habits" later in this chapter.

Feedback from the Real World: Multiples

Keeping your sanity with one newborn's erratic sleep habits is difficult enough. Imagine the juggling act when you have two (or more) newborns! You can't control or force them to sleep, but you can encourage them to eat (sometimes!) and that helps synchronize their sleep. Here's what worked for us: wake the sleeping baby for a feeding within 30 minutes of the first baby waking up. Feeding twins at the same time gives you more time to rest between feedings especially in the beginning when feedings are so close together.
—*Agustina, mom of Gael and Malena, 18 months*

Sleep Safety Tips

Q. I've heard about sudden infant death syndrome (SIDS). What is the official recommendation about infant sleep position?

For the past thirty years the American Academy of Pediatrics and various other health organizations have recommended that babies sleep on their backs from birth to at least six months of age to reduce the risk of SIDS (90% of SIDS cases occur in babies under six months old). This recommendation has reduced the number of SIDS deaths by 50%. Just take a look at the graph on the next page that shows the SIDS rate plummeted as parents stopped putting baby to sleep on their stomach.

SIDS seems to be caused by a suffocation-like event—a pocket of carbon dioxide forms around the baby's face when they are face down on a mattress or soft bedding. Babies don't have the neck muscles to move their heads and, sadly, that's how some SIDS deaths occur.

BOTTOM LINE: When it comes to SIDS prevention, follow the ABC's.

US SIDS rate versus the % of babies sleeping on their stomach

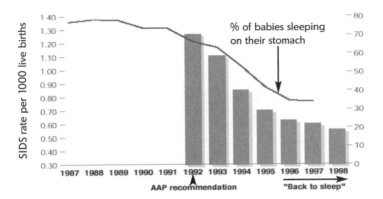

Source: Contemporary Pediatrics, Vol 17, No. 9

A stands for the baby sleeping Alone in their own sleep space.
B stands for the baby sleeping on their Back.
C stands for the baby sleeping in a naked Crib. Just add a fitted sheet and your baby.

Q. Are there any other known risk factors for SIDS?

Yes. Here are the top six:

1 ROOM TEMPERATURE. Stuffy rooms with poor ventilation are a SIDS risk. The cooler the room, the better. SIDS occurs more frequently in the winter months when babies are bundled and the heat is on. Believe it or not, the recommended "safe" room temperature to reduce SIDS risk is 68 degrees. And a fan in the baby's room can also reduce the SIDS risk. (*Coleman-Phox*)

2 SOFT BEDDING. All those beautiful bedding sets need to stay out of the crib. Heavy quilts, pillows, bumper pads, and blankets cause the ambient temperature of the crib to go up. Babies can also smother themselves in soft bedding. All your baby's crib needs is a sheet and mattress.

MEMO TO GRANDPARENTS: BACK TO SLEEP

Here's a scary fact: babies who are used to sleeping on their backs and are placed on their sides (and roll over) or stomachs to sleep have a significantly greater risk of SIDS than those babies who are used to sleeping on their tummies.

The message: make sure that your childcare provider or occasional grandparent-as-babysitter puts your baby on their back to sleep. Childcare providers should be well versed in this sleep safety recommendation, but it never hurts to ask about their policies.

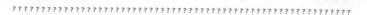
3 **SMOKING.** Babies whose parents smoke have a higher risk of SIDS. So, if you can't do it for yourself, stop smoking for the most important thing in your world.

4 **ETHNICITY.** Native Americans and African Americans have a much higher risk of SIDS than other babies. New research suggests a genetic defect may be passed on in certain ethnic groups.

5 **FAMILY HISTORY.** There may be a higher incidence of SIDS when a previous family member has had it.

6 **BIOCHEMICAL ABNORMALITY.** Recent studies point to a deficiency in serotonin (a neurotransmitter necessary for a baby's arousal system) as a reason why some babies do not wake up during life-threatening situations (like when they're sleeping face down and not getting enough oxygen.) This is a major medical breakthrough, but there's no practical way of testing babies for this disorder right now. (*Paterson, Duncan*)

Obviously, there are risk factors on this list that you cannot control. But try to avoid the ones you can—like bedding, sleep position, and smoking.

Q. I've heard conflicting information about SIDS prevention and when a baby can sleep in their own room. What is the right answer?

Great question and yes, it is very confusing! The AAP SIDS Task Force encourages "room sharing", not "bed sharing." And, they advise that babies sleep in the parents' bedroom (known as "room sharing") for at least six months but "ideally" the entire first year of life. Why? Room sharing promotes breastfeeding and breastfeeding protects against SIDS.

But once a baby is sleeping through the night and no longer night nursing, there is no data to show that room sharing prevents SIDS. Authors of a 2017 study raised that key point. In their research, they found that room sharing families of 4-10 month olds often end up *bed sharing* in order to get a better night's sleep. And that actually **increases the risk of SIDS**. It seems like a safer choice to move the baby to the nursery! (*Paul*)

More research is obviously needed. If your baby is sleeping 10-12 hours at night, though, you can certainly consider moving them to their own room.

New Parent 411:
Sleeping on the sofa is risky business.
Over the past decade, sofa sleeping led to over 10% of sleep-related infant deaths in the U.S. Soft sofa cushions can enable a baby to roll to the back of the couch and get stuck. And babies who nap with a snoozing parent can roll off the parent's chest (and couch), leading to injury, entrapment, and suffocation. (*Rechtman LR*)

Reality Check: Pacifiers Reduce SIDS Risk
Believe it or not, there is substantial evidence to show that pacifiers actually reduce the risk of SIDS. It is unclear why, though. It may be that the pacifier keeps a baby's airway open. Or, sucking on a pacifier prevents a baby from forgetting to breathe. FYI: 90% of SIDS cases occur between one and six months of life. (*AAP SIDS Task*

? ?

SLEEP

Force) For a quick look at the latest recommendations to avoid SIDS, see the Top Ten Take-Home Messages on Sleep Safety later in this chapter.

Helpful Hints

◆ *What should you do with that baby quilt you got as a gift?* Use it as a wall hanging. Or buy a special quilt rack for your baby's nursery. You can always use it on the floor as baby gets older. Put a few toys out and encourage some supervised tummy time.

◆ *Don't borrow a crib or use a hand-me-down.* Over two million cribs have been recalled in recent years for safety hazards. As a result, the federal government rolled out tough, new crib safety standards a few years ago. The take home-message: we strongly recommend buying a new crib for your baby instead of using a hand-me-down or that Facebook marketplace find.

Q. What bedding items are acceptable to place in the crib?

A fitted sheet over a mattress is all you need. We like to call it the Naked Crib. See nearby picture for an example.

What about blankets? While it is acceptable to swaddle a newborn to eight-week old baby in a receiving blanket, we discourage any other loose blankets for babies under a year of age.

A baby can just sleep in sleeper pajamas or be swaddled. Or consider a "wearable blanket" (an example is the SleepSack from HALO Innovations, halosleep.com). These provide warmth but cut the SIDS risk, as babies can't crawl under them or become entrapped. Again, the key goal here is to not over-heat your baby—putting your child in a wearable blanket and cranking up the thermostat is a no-no.

What about crib bumpers? Safety experts, including the American Academy of Pediatrics, discourage using them. The risk of SIDS with crib bumpers is greater than the protection bumpers offer from minor injury. (*Thach*) And, no, you don't need a mesh crib bumper to

---

HOW TO SWADDLE A BABY—AKA BABY BURRITO WRAP

And now, the seven steps to swaddling your baby:

1. Take a square receiving blanket and turn it diamond shaped on a flat surface.
2. Take the top corner and fold it towards the center of the blanket. You now have a horizontal line at the top.
3. Place your baby on the blanket with his neck at the level on the horizontal line.
4. Bring the bottom corner up to the baby's belly button.
5. Bring one side corner over the baby and fold over the other side of the belly.
6. Bring the other side corner over the baby and fold over on the other side. *Voila!*
7. Remember to keep the legs loosely wrapped to allow the hips to develop normally.

keep a baby's arm or leg from getting stuck between the crib rails. The risk of a trapped limb in the crib slats is minor compared to SIDS.

Save your money, skip the bumper.

Reality Check

Another item you DON'T need: a sleep positioner—a device pitched to parents as a way to keep their baby sleeping on their back. Sleep positioners have been responsible for 12 U.S. infant deaths over the past 15 years, due to suffocation or the baby rolling onto his belly. Both the American Academy of Pediatrics and the Consumer Products Safety Commission advise against their use.

Q. I've heard that standard crib mattresses are a risk for SIDS and organic mattresses are safer. Is this true?

Short answer: no. Evidence-based medicine says conventional crib mattresses are not a significant risk factor for SIDS. And buying an organic mattress is not going to prevent SIDS. We'll delve into this debate a bit more in Chapter 16, Safety.

Q. Is it okay to swaddle a baby in a crib?

Yes, with a few caveats. You need to know *how* to swaddle and know *when* to stop.

Your friendly nurses from the hospital probably taught you the "burrito wrap" technique of swaddling your baby. If not, see the box nearby. It's fine to wrap your baby's arms snugly but leave the legs loose enough to be able to move them around. Experts advise this technique to possibly prevent hip dislocation from spending hours positioned like a mummy. A good tip if Baby Houdini lives with you: The Miracle Blanket ($30; miracleblanket.com). This is one blanket your baby will not be able to squirm out of.

Newborns like to be snug for the first six to eight weeks of life. Think about it. They are used to being in a confined space. Swaddling works well; until baby wants and needs to stretch out. But, after eight weeks, ditch the swaddling trick. It is important for a baby to move and turn during sleep—otherwise you will end up with a flat-headed baby.

Q. My 2 month old sleeps really well when we swaddle. Why does our pediatrician want us to stop doing it?

Because your baby is growing up.

For the first two to three months of life, newborns have very immature nervous systems which includes a dramatic startle reflex when placed on their back. You've been there—just when your baby has peacefully fallen into a blissful sleep, you put them down, their arms flail out in the breeze and, yep, it's back to square one again.

Parents quickly find that swaddling keeps those little arms contained and their little baby remains asleep. So, it's no surprise that most parents have a look of terror on their faces when the baby's doctor says it is time to stop swaddling.

But here's the thing—a baby's nervous system matures and that startle reflex goes away by three months of age. And, babies, like all other humans, like to move around a bit in their sleep.

If a baby remains wrapped like a mummy beyond three months of age, it adversely impacts his head shape, leading to a flat head and possibly a $3000 helmet. Snoo users take note: The same rules apply to the Snoo swaddler feature, even though the product literature says it is intended for use up to six months of age. The flat head risk is real.

The swaddle blanket also becomes a strangulation or SIDS risk because babies figure out how to squirm out of it. So, the short answer is: there is a time to swaddle and a time to stop. Don't worry, your older baby will sleep well without it.

Q. Do I need to transition my baby out of a swaddle?

No, go cold turkey.

Sure, we see lots of products on the market that promise to transition baby out of a swaddle. These are unnecessary and, in our opinion, concerning since they all restrict baby's movement to one degree or another.

Q. Okay, I put my baby on their back to sleep. What do I do if they roll over?

Let them sleep!

Your baby probably won't figure out how to roll over until they are at least four months old. Once they start, you can't stop them. The next morning, you will find them in a completely different position than the way you left them!

If it makes you feel any better, once babies are good at clearing their nose and mouth by turning their heads, the risk of SIDS is lower.

Q. I'm concerned my baby might choke if they sleep on their back. Should I be?

No.

Babies have a gag reflex that protects their airway when they vomit (all humans do). There is no increased choking risk. Even babies with gastroesophageal reflux who puke all the time do fine in this position.

Q. Can I cheat, and let my baby sleep on their side?

We can't recommend it. Babies who sleep on their sides may accidentally roll onto their tummies. And babies who are not used to being tummy sleepers have an 18 fold increased risk of SIDS if they end up sleeping that way.

Q. Can I buy one of those breathing motion detectors and let my baby sleep on their stomach?

These products are not worth the expense—a gadget can't prevent SIDS. It leads to more parent anxiety and disrupted sleep when the alarm goes off accidentally. The motion detectors you buy at the store are not the same as "apnea monitors" that some premature infants use after they are sent home from the hospital.

Wearable baby health monitors will probably improve over the coming years. But right now, they are still a work in progress and largely unnecessary.

Q. My baby has a flat head and a bald spot on the back of their head from this sleep position. Is this permanent?

No. This is called **POSITIONAL PLAGIOCEPHALY** and most kids do not need helmets to fix the problem. As your baby starts to roll over, the head shape will round out. All babies lose their hair around four months, and then grow new hair in.

You can help with the head shape issue by scheduling daily tummy time. This also promotes neck and back muscle strength. And, it helps them learn how to roll over. (It's easier to roll from stomach to back than the reverse). For details on tummy time and positional plagiocephaly, see the section on Flat Heads and Tummy Time in Chapter 5, Nutrition & Growth.

Our Warning on Sleep Devices: Loungers, Inclined Sleepers & Nests

We get it. You are sleep-deprived, desperate parents, but safety comes first when it comes to infant sleep aids.

Sadly, babies have died from using products that have bypassed regulations for bassinets, cribs, and play yards by calling themselves "loungers," "inclined sleepers," or "in-bed sleepers." It has taken way too long for the Consumer Product Safety Commission (CPSC) to create a uniform federal safety standard for all infant sleep products, but it is finally happening. Here is our hot take, based on hands-on reviews:

1. DockATot: *Not recommended*
Parents like Kourtney Kardashian may love it but we don't. The pitch: the soft-padded sides make it a snug place to "chill out." But that's not how folks are using it on social media, where the DockATot shows up in cribs, adult beds and, yes, even airline seats. We believe the DockATot used for sleep in ways like this could be a SIDS risk. Health Canada went so far as to ban its use in their country.

2. Crescent Womb Hammock: *Not recommended*
This product, which is basically a hammock that's installed over a crib, is structurally similar to a recalled product called the Crib Cuddle that led to at least one infant death in the 1980's. Because hammocks are not technically cribs, there are no safety regulations for them. We are concerned because babies sleeping in this chin-to-chest position can obstruct the airway and lead to asphyxiation.

3. Baby Merlin Sleep Suit: *Not recommended*
We have serious concerns about the potential for a baby to overheat in what essentially is a padded snowsuit. This product also restricts a baby's movements. The company states that the point of this product's use is to help with the transition out of swaddling and inhibit the baby's startle reflex. It is "not intended for use" once the baby rolls over. Problem is, these milestones all occur around the same time. And keeping a baby in one position for several hours a night is a risk for developing a flat head (positional plagiocephaly).

Good news: there are two products we do like and recommend:

4. Halo Bassinest: *Recommended*

It is a small sleep space, which newborns tend to prefer, with mesh sides for good airflow. It is portable and easy to take your baby out for late night feeding sessions. And for the price point, we think it is one of the better products on the market.

5. Snoo Smart Sleeper: *Rental Recommended*

This infant sleeper was created by my pediatrician colleague and friend (full disclosure), Dr Harvey Karp, also of *Happiest Baby on the Block* fame. It has all the bells and whistles from both a safety and soothing standpoint and may help lull your newborn to sleep with white noise and gentle rocking. It also has a swaddler that can be removed when the baby ages out of it. The nearly $1600 price tag seemed ridiculous when the product first launched but the rental option for $5.30/day* makes it more reasonable if you are desperate for your baby to have better, but also safe, sleep (*one month rental minimum—check Snoo's web site for details and rules).

Q. Is there any risk to having a family bed?

When it comes to infants, the answer is yes. Babies who sleep in a family bed are at greater risk of SIDS and Sudden Unexplained Infant Death (SUID) The family bed increases the risk of smothering and entrapment, both of which can be fatal. Waterbeds, comforters, pillows, and exhausted or intoxicated parents in the family bed are suffocation hazards. That is why the American Academy of Pediatrics supports *room* sharing, but NOT *bed* sharing for infants.

However, toddlers (older than one year) can safely sleep in a shared family bed if this is your preference.

For room sharing and safe infant sleeping, try these two tricks:

◆ Use a bassinet.
◆ Move the crib next to your bed.

BOTTOM LINE

Here are the latest American Academy of Pediatrics recommendations to prevent SIDS:

1 **NO TO SIDE SLEEPING.** Babies who sleep on their sides are more likely to roll onto their tummies and increase their risk of SIDS. And infants who are back sleepers that sleep on their tummies increase their SIDS risk by 18 times.

2 **NO TO BED SHARING.** The risk of smothering or entrapping an infant is greater when parents and baby share a bed.

3 **YES TO ROOM SHARING.** The AAP encourages room sharing to support breastfeeding and reduce SIDS risk. See earlier discussion for advice on duration of room sharing.

4 **YES TO PACIFIERS.** For unknown reasons, the binky is protective. Just know when to start (after breastfeeding is well established) and when to stop (when the risk of SIDS is over) using it.

SLEEP

? ?

Top Ten Take-Home Messages on Sleep Safety

1. Put your baby to bed on their back.
2. Keep soft bedding out of the crib.
3. Keep the room temperature cool (68 degrees).
4. Keep the room well ventilated. Consider using a fan.
5. Don't over bundle your baby with too many clothes. Swaddling in one light blanket is okay. No need for a hat or cap.
6. No smoking.
7. Avoid hand-me-down cribs (new safety rules took effect in 2012).
8. Buy a new, firm crib mattress.
9. Make sure the mattress fits into the crib snugly, without gaps.
10. Lower the mattress height to the lowest level *before* your baby starts to pull on the railings to stand up.

Deciding On The Family's Sleep Routine: a.k.a. The Family Bed vs. Sleeping Solo Debate

This debate is worthy of an introduction before we get to the details. Where your baby sleeps is completely your decision. This is a judgment-free zone. We just want your baby to be safe.

Here are two things you need to know:

1. The American Academy of Pediatrics endorses room sharing—but not bed sharing— as a way to promote safe sleep and successful breastfeeding.
2. Attachment Parenting International states that paying attention to a baby's needs at night is the priority, not the sleep location.

We'll give you the information to make an educated decision about what is best for you, with your baby's health and wellness in mind.

Your options:

◆ **The Family Bed (Co-sleeping):** Parents and children sleep together in the same bed.
◆ **Sleeping Solo:** Each child sleeps separately in their own sleep space (crib, bassinet, or cradle).
◆ **The Desperation Move:** Parents prefer that their baby sleep in a crib, but end up having baby in a family bed out of sheer exhaustion and frustration with their inability to get their baby to sleep in a crib. (See undoing bad habits section later in this chapter.)

Q. What are the advantages of a family bed?

Convenience is a big advantage. And many parents who practice attachment parenting view the family bed as a way to maintain secure parent-child bonds and work the nighttime parenting shift.

For a breastfed newborn, it's very easy to eat at night. As soon as they stir, a nursing mom

DR B'S OPINION

"Having a well-adjusted and happy child has nothing to do with where they sleep!"

is there for them. This is also convenient for Mom, who might fall asleep shortly after (or during!) those middle-of-the-night feeds. Recent data suggest that co-sleeping babies nurse more frequently and take larger volumes of breast milk at night than their solitary sleeping peers.

Many parents choose this option simply because it feels good to snuggle up with their baby.

Just a bit of trivia: in the U.S., 12.8% of infants regularly sleep in a family bed. And it's hard to know how accurate that figure is, as some folks may not admit to sleeping in a family bed when surveyed.

Q. What are the disadvantages of the family bed?

Potential for SIDS and SUID (Sudden Unexplained Infant Death).

The American Academy of Pediatrics policy position warns against family bed sharing with infants due to the increased risk of death. They strongly encourage infants to have their own sleep space.

Solitary sleep advocates argue that co-sleeping families get poor sleep and prolong the time before a baby starts sleeping through the night. They also feel that co-sleeping interferes with a baby's ability to become an independent being.

BOTTOM LINE
An eighteen-year study on parent-child bed sharing

A landmark study evaluated children who slept in a family bed as infants and young children and compared them to their solitary sleeping peers. These children were studied from birth through age 18 years. *The data showed that co-sleeping had no statistically significant problems or benefits.* (Okami)

Q. What are the advantages of sleeping solo?

Safer sleep for babies. And, better quality sleep for parents and children.

Bed sharing for infants, in short, is risky business. And as stated above, breastfed babies who co-sleep are up more often at night to feed.

Q. What are the disadvantages of sleeping solo?

Consistency is required.

A baby who is used to sleeping alone in their own bed may have more sleep disruptions when families travel or sleep away from their home. It also requires taking a portable crib on trips or making arrangements to borrow one at your destination.

Babies who sleep alone need a consistent sleep ritual to wind down.

Q. With all of these night feedings, my baby ends up falling asleep on me. Will this be a problem in the future?

? ?

SLEEP

For the first two months, do anything that is safe for your baby and buys you some sleep.

Babies are very malleable for the first two to three months of life. You are not setting yourself up for having long-term sleep problems. If your baby nurses and falls asleep on you, just try to peel them off of you and put them into the bassinet afterwards.

However, your goal should be to have a consistent sleep routine by four months of age.

Setting Up Good Habits (Two to Four Months)

Note: as we discuss the steps to establishing good sleep routines, these are general age ranges for healthy, thriving babies. Babies who are born prematurely or those with medical problems (such as failure to thrive or acid reflux) may go through these sleep milestones a little later.

For the first two months of life, when it comes to you and your baby's sleep, you gotta do what you gotta do—nursing, rocking, a car ride, etc. You know the drill.

INSIDER SECRETS: TOP 10 COMMANDMENTS FOR ESTABLISHING A

1 **TEACH YOUR BABY TO FALL ASLEEP ON THEIR OWN.** Remember those sleep cycles? The cycle consists of light to heavy to light arousal before entering the next cycle. At the end of each cycle, humans re-check their environment and change body position (move a pillow or blanket, roll over). By three to four months of age, your infant will be aware of their world. If they fall asleep on a parent's shoulder and get moved to a crib, or fall asleep when they are drinking or sucking a pacifier, that is what they will be expecting when they arouse at the end of their sleep cycle. Translation: be careful of sleep "crutches" like the pacifier. Put your child in a crib or bassinet when they are relaxed. . . but before they fall asleep. If the child always falls asleep on your shoulder, they will expect to see that shoulder at the end of every sleep cycle.

2 **BE CONSISTENT. KIDS DO BEST WITH ROUTINES.** Predictable is comfortable. You will learn that rapid transitions and unexpected activities promote anxiety and outbursts in your child (see Chapter 11 Temperament & Soothing for details). Have a routine for both nap and bedtime and stick with it by the age of four months.

3 **YOUR CHILD SHOULD SLEEP IN THE SAME PLACE FOR NAPS AND NIGHTTIME.** Reality check: yes, every now and again your child may fall asleep in a car seat, especially after a long trip on the weekend for example. That's OK on an occasional basis. But when you are at home, keep the sleep place the same.

4 **NAP TIME AND BEDTIME SHOULD BE APPROXIMATELY THE SAME TIME EVERY DAY.** That goes for vacations, visits to relatives, etc.

Guess what? Your baby is now nearly four months old. It's time to stop those old habits.

Why? Your baby is becoming more aware of their environment. They will respond better when things are *predictable*, anticipating what is next. They will also start to form sleep *associations*. That means your baby will rely on certain routines to fall asleep. Those routines are the good sleep habits you want to keep. And now is the time to punt the bad habits. Think about it—you really don't want to be rocking your five-year-old to sleep every night, do you?

For the nitty gritty on forming good sleep habits, check out our Ten Commandments for establishing a healthy sleep routine in the box nearby.

Q. When can I start to schedule my baby's naps and bedtime?

Between two and four months of age, your baby will start to have some regular sleep and feeding patterns (finally). Keep a sleep/feeding diary for a week and you'll know your baby's preferences.

Then you can put your baby down for naps and bedtime *before* they show you that they are tired (cranky, rubbing eyes—you've seen it all before). The key word in that previous sen-

---

SLEEP ROUTINE (2 TO 4 MONTH OLDS)

5 **ALWAYS FOLLOW YOUR SLEEP RITUAL.** Bath, feeding, (teeth brushing), story-time, songs, prayers...you might do the abbreviated version of a book or song if it has been a long day, but still do it.

6 **START YOUR SLEEP RITUAL BEFORE YOUR CHILD IS TIRED.** Don't wait for the yawns and eye-rubbing to begin the routine.

7 **EARLY TO BED, LATE TO RISE.** Sounds like it wouldn't work this way, but it does. Babies actually sleep better when they go to sleep early. An "overtired" baby does not sleep longer —so, you are not buying time to sleep in by putting your baby down later in the evening. Trust me on this one.

8 **GET RID OF THE PACIFIER BY FOUR TO SIX MONTHS OF AGE.** Your baby is very aware of their world. If they fall asleep with a pacifier in their mouth, they will cry when it falls out. At 3am. And 5am.

9 **BABIES NEED REFRESHER COURSES ON SLEEP ETIQUETTE AFTER TRAVEL, ILLNESS, OR TEETHING.** When consistency is broken, it takes a few days to get back on track. If you don't remind your baby of what to do, they will remain on a disrupted sleep schedule.

10 **DON'T TREAT YOUR FOUR MONTH OLD LIKE A NEWBORN.** Your baby will take advantage of your naiveté. Many four month olds are capable of falling asleep on their own if given the opportunity to do so.

SLEEP

? ?

tence is BEFORE. Once you see those sleepy signs, they are actually overtired.

Start your wind down routine before that happens by aiming for nap/bedtime about 20 minutes earlier than what your sleep diary shows. Not only will you have some idea how to schedule your day, but you'll give your baby the best shot at falling asleep on their own.

You're in the driver's seat now and can put your baby on a schedule they already like—yes, YOU have the power!

Q. My three month old only falls asleep while feeding. How do we change that habit?

You will be walking a fine line between two and four months of age. We like the mantra, "Eat, Play, Sleep" or at least separate the feeding from the falling asleep part. Your goal is to *separate* the eating experience from the sleeping experience. Your baby may not need to eat to fall asleep, but you won't know until you try! And if you fail the first time, try again the next week. Your baby is maturing at the speed of light. At this stage, a week older is a week smarter.

In the middle of the night when you hear your baby cry . . . walk, don't run, to your baby's bedside. They might just go back to sleep without your intervention.

You can also try soothing your baby without offering food if you have frequent night wakenings. Your baby may not need to eat every time and is just relying on you to help them get back to sleep. If you are breastfeeding, let your non-nursing partner try to be the soother. There will be less expectation of food. But if it has been more than four hours or so since the last feeding, you will probably have a hungry baby on your hands who needs to eat.

The Big Transition: (Four to Five months)

Q. My four month old still needs help falling asleep. What do I do?

You can gradually cut the virtual umbilical cord. Your goal is for your baby to fall asleep on their own—without feeding or rocking them to sleep.

Now that they are four months old, set up a consistent sleep ritual. If your baby falls asleep during the feeding, wake them up before putting them in bed so your baby is aware of where they are going. You are creating a healthy bedtime ritual—and one that lets your baby be in charge of falling asleep.

DR B'S OPINION:
FOUR MONTH OLDS AND SLEEP

Your four-month old baby is aware of their surroundings. If they fall asleep in your arms and you sneak them into bed, they will awaken at the end of their sleep cycle (every 90 minutes) looking for comfort. If your child is awake when you leave the room, they will fall asleep alone and content. You'll hear them on your baby monitor discussing the day with inanimate objects. Your baby is growing up. Our advice: relax and trust your baby.

DR B'S OPINION:
CRYING IT OUT, LET'S DISCUSS

I encourage you to give your baby a chance to fall asleep on their own. Obviously, you have to do what you feel comfortable with . . . but it is not cruel or inappropriate (from a child development perspective) to give a healthy baby the freedom to self-soothe from four to six months of age. Otherwise, I'd never advise it!

Yes, there are parenting circles that vehemently oppose this sleep training approach. They like to cite research that it causes permanent emotional damage to the child. I'm here to say that is absolutely untrue. In fact, a recent study looked at five-year-old children who went through sleep training as babies and guess what? They were completely normal, well-adjusted kiddos. *(Price)*

There is no middle of the road when it comes to sleep training. Every parent wants their baby to sleep through the night without any crying to get that happy place. While I wish there was a noise-free solution, your baby is probably not a unicorn.

Give your baby at least ten minutes to try to fall asleep on their own. Yes, they may protest (code word for cry) and that is okay. They are learning they have a superpower to self-regulate and calm down. If they cannot fall asleep, go back in and do as little as possible to help your baby relax. Try patting, singing, and cuddling for a few MINUTES (not hours). Rocking your baby until they are dead weight on your shoulder or nursing them to sleep is the last resort.

The exact method of transitioning to a better sleep pattern varies for each baby. Basically, you do as little as possible and give your baby more time to work things out on their own. Thirty minutes is a reasonable amount of time by five months of age.

If your healthy, thriving baby still does not fall asleep on their own by five months, you can use the gradual or rip-the-band-aid-off rapid training methods so they can figure out how to self-regulate (more info later in this chapter). The same rules apply for frequent night wakenings.

Consistency is key. Do the same ritual for both nap and bedtime.

Q. I've heard babies are more likely to sleep through the night if their tummies are full. What do you think of "dream feeds"?

For newborns, feeding and sleep patterns are intimately related. Babies under two months of age need to eat frequently, usually every two to three hours day or night. That means they can't sleep very long because they get hungry. Babies start to stretch out feedings at night (and give parents a small break) at two to four months.

However, as babies get older, their ability to sleep through the night has more to do with their brains than their guts. Your healthy, growing four month old is capable of sleeping at least six hours without needing to eat. Don't let them fool you. The key to Mr. Sandman's house resides in your ability to teach your baby self-soothing skills . . . not stuffing them full of milk.

For a full-term, healthy thriving baby (who doesn't have acid reflux), here are some helpful feeding parameters:

◆ Four month olds: Can sleep SIX hours without needing to eat.
◆ Five month olds: Can sleep NINE hours without needing to eat.
◆ Six month olds: Can sleep TWELVE hours without needing to eat.

Some parents will try to feed a sleeping baby (a.k.a. Dream Feed) before they go to bed, hoping to catch that six-hour stretch during the hours they want to actually sleep. For example, instead of your baby fasting from 8 pm–2 am, they fast from 11 pm–5 am. While this sounds great in theory, I am not a big fan of this strategy. I think it sets up a habit of feeding a child when they aren't hungry, and it in no way guarantees you'll sleep until 5 am. Second problem: cavities. Many parents continue night feedings long after their baby has teeth (around six months of age). Unless you plan on brushing your child's teeth after that dream feed, you will be paying for your dentist's kids to go to college.

If your baby learns how to self-regulate, you'll have better odds of sleeping through the night.

Undoing Bad Habits (Five to 12 months and beyond): Solving the Sleep Problems

If you have a healthy baby who is still not sleeping at least six hours a night, or you are bringing your child to bed with you out of desperation (and not choice), this section is for you. Admitting you have a problem is the first step! Don't say we didn't warn you: if you set up healthy sleep routines up front, you won't have to endure the (often) highly emotional experience of sleep training.

The International Pediatric Sleep Education Task Force found that 25% of ALL parents report problems with their baby's sleep patterns . . . no matter what country they live in. You are not alone. (*Touchette*)

Behind the Scenes
Is there a correlation between parents' behavior and infant's sleep?
A recent Canadian study showed that many infant sleep disorders were based on parents' excessive intervention in comforting them to sleep. These parent behaviors with their five month olds included these sleep crutches: (Continues on page 250)

DR B'S OPINION:
SLEEP STATS TO KNOW

These stats are based upon my 25 years of experience working with babies of all shapes and sizes:

◆ At least 50% of healthy four month olds can fall asleep on their own.
◆ At least 75% of healthy five month olds can fall asleep on their own.
◆ 100% of healthy six month olds can fall asleep on their own.

THE TOP TEN MISTAKES PARENTS MAKE WITH INFANT SLEEP ROUTINES

1. Sneaking baby into bed. Your baby falls asleep in your arms, and then you sneak them into their crib. Compare this to the following scenario, courtesy of acclaimed sleep expert Dr Ferber. You fall asleep on the couch in front of the TV. Your spouse picks you up and carries you into your bed. When you wake up in your own bed, you are disoriented and alarmed. Your baby feels the same way—and hence, wakes up and wants your arms back!

2. Falling asleep while eating. Your baby falls asleep when they are drinking (breast or bottle). When they stir, they are in a different place and not eating anymore.

3. Falling asleep with a pacifier. Here is the comparison, again credit to Dr Ferber: You fall asleep with your head on your pillow. In the middle of the night, your spouse steals your pillow. When you wake up, you are confused and probably annoyed. (Ferber)

4. The Trained Night Feeder. Your baby gets used to eating a snack or a meal in the middle of the night, so they continue to be hungry at that time. Equate this to working the night shift and having your lunch break at 3 am. Yes, your body will work up an appetite if you are used to it. Stop eating at 3 am., and your body will no longer be hungry. Parents frequently continue these feedings well beyond six months of life because they don't know any better and their babies continue to demand it.

5. Inconsistent schedules. Babies are creatures of habit. Adjust your schedule as much as possible around your baby's. Don't change your baby's bedtime because you got home late from work and missed spending time with him. Your baby loves spending time with you, but tomorrow is another day. You'll both be happier if your little one gets better sleep.

6. Missed naps. The better your baby sleeps during the day, the better they will sleep at night. Being overtired actually creates sleep disturbances. So, don't run errands when it is your baby's naptime.

7. Late to bed equals EARLY to rise. This is really true, even though you would think the opposite. As we've said, overtired babies sleep poorly.

8. Interventions at partial wakenings. Just because your baby stirs at night, does not mean they need your help. We all stir at the end of each sleep cycle (every 90 minutes). If you go in "to help," you will wake your baby up. If these partial wakenings are waking you up, turn off the baby monitor. If your baby really needs you, you will hear them (or see what's up on the video monitor).

9. Bringing baby into bed when you don't want them there. Babies get used to routines. If you consistently bring your baby into your own bed when they cry, this is what they will expect. They will continue to cry until they get what they want. If the expectation is not there, the behavior won't exist. Make a plan between BOTH parents and STICK WITH IT.

10. Not letting your baby learn how to self-regulate. The ability to soothe one's self is a learned skill. This skill can be mastered by six months of age, if your baby is given the opportunity. Yes, both thumb sucking and comfort objects (see below) are acceptable. It's true that newborns need help to relax, because they are born very immature neurologically. Older babies are more mature neurologically, and thus, more capable of pulling it together.

SLEEP

? ?

1. Putting a baby in bed *after* they were asleep.
2. Remaining in the room *until* the baby was asleep.
3. Taking the baby out of their bed to comfort them.
4. Parent feelings of inadequacy.

A significant percentage of these babies continued to have sleep problems well into their third year of life.

BOTTOM LINE: Don't just wait for your baby to outgrow sleep issues—it may be a long time waiting. And the issues may belong to the parent and not the baby. (*Willinger*)

New Parent 411

I've had parents resort to some pretty crazy strategies in the name of sleep. One mom admitted to sleeping with her baby *in the crib*. Another mom turned her blow dryer on for an hour every night as a form of white noise. Both agreed to share their stories to protect our readers from making the same mistakes!

Q. My friends have all warned me about the "four month sleep regression." What is it and how can I avoid it?

Honestly, I hate the phrase "four month sleep regression." The four-month milestone is a sleep *progression*—not regression.

Newborns have young, developing brains for the first three months of life. As a result, parents are not setting up any bad habits by doing whatever it takes to help a baby fall asleep.

By four months of life, it is a different story. Those little brains are aware of routines and become capable of self-regulation and self-control. That is why it is time to create a healthy wind-down routine before bed and let a four-month old figure out how to use self-regulation skills.

When parents talk about having a sleep regression, it is because they were lucky enough to have a baby who started sleeping through the night without a sleep ritual before this four-month mark. They just fell asleep eating and were placed into bed. Now they have a baby who thinks they need to be rocked or fed to fall asleep (and fall back asleep) at the end of every 90 minute sleep cycle. That's when they know their baby's current sleep routine has backfired.

If you set up the right routine at the beginning of the night, this will not happen to you. Start using a sleep ritual that lets your baby fall asleep on their own.

DR B'S OPINION:
BEEN THERE, DONE THAT

I am a parent. I have walked in your shoes. I know that irrational thoughts seem rational at 3 am. It SEEMS EASIER to just bring your baby in bed with you or nurse them to sleep. But it is not the right answer anymore.

Once you are on the other side (sleeping through the night), you'll say, "What was I thinking?" I am happier and so are my children when we have all slept at night.

SLEEP

DR B'S OPINION:
DON'T BE THE UBER

Here is a good analogy. Your baby knows how to drive their own car to the Land of Nod. But, when the Uber arrives for them, why would they bother driving? You are the Uber here.

Q. My baby uses a pacifier to fall asleep. When should we stop offering it?

We'll discuss the Great Binky Debate in the section on Soothing a New Baby in Chapter 11, Temperament and Soothing. But when it comes to healthy sleep routines, we suggest saying goodbye to the binky by six months of age.

In the first two or three months of life, babies have very few ways to soothe themselves. Parents usually figure out within the first few days of bringing their baby home that a pacifier buys everyone some sleep. This approach is fine for the first few months.

BUT, do not use a pacifier beyond six months of life. Trust me. This is the time when you need to set up the routines you plan to keep. What if someone stole your pillow while your were sleeping? If the pacifier falls out in the middle of the night, your baby will be looking for it.

You don't want to have a baby who is capable of sleeping through the night waking *because* the pacifier is out. If the pacifier isn't there to begin with, they won't be looking for it.

Helpful Hints
◆ Don't place dozens of pacifiers in your baby's crib so they can find one on their own.
◆ Don't go in every 90 minutes to put a pacifier back into your baby's mouth.
◆ Don't buy a glow-in-the-dark pacifier so your baby can find it at night. I promise that your six-month-old can fall asleep without the pacifier.
◆ Don't get stuck treating your older baby like a newborn!

Q. My eight month old can only fall asleep nursing/taking a bottle. When will my baby outgrow this?

Your baby has been capable of it since four or five months of age. But they will continue to do it much longer if you continue this routine. Feeding has become their crutch to fall asleep.

Again, for the first two months of life, anything goes. The optimal time to change this behavior for a full-term, healthy baby is around four months. But if you missed the window of opportunity, it's not too late. Babies are resilient and adaptable. If your baby falls asleep while feeding, wake them up just enough so they know they are getting into bed and you are leaving the room. Be prepared for some protesting the next few nights, but they will quickly adjust to the new routine soon.

It's much easier to change these behaviors now. Your child isn't going to wake up one morning and move on from this routine—you need to actively change it. (I once consulted with a family whose five YEAR old still drank milk to fall asleep every night. Don't let this be your kid!)

Q. Are comfort objects okay to put in the crib?

Yes, at one year of age.

You can offer a comfort object during the day at any point, but it's safest to use—a little blanket or **small** stuffed animal that can go to bed with your baby, starting at one year of age. Remember, SIDS occurs in babies under age one. Just make sure the comfort item you select is small/light enough that it is not a smothering or suffocation hazard.

Q. My nine month old still has a middle of the night feeding. Is this normal?

Well, it has become "normal" for your baby because they are a trained night feeder. There is nothing wrong with them. You've just allowed your baby to get part of their nutritional needs met during the night beyond when they need them. Healthy, full term babies are all capable of fasting for up to 12 hours at night by six months of age. As long as your baby is growing well, read on.*

Stop the night feeding and your baby will stop being hungry. That's easy to say, right? Offer water at 3 am and see what happens. It's likely to be rejected the first night. And yes, your child will protest. The second night, offer water again. The protesting will be less lengthy. By the third night, your baby won't bother to wake up.

*Some babies nurse all night long because mom's milk supply has diminished and they are truly hungry. If this is a possibility, it is best to visit the doc and do a weight check before making any interventions.

Reality Check

It's likely that your nine-month old has at least one tooth. Therefore, offering milk at night without brushing their teeth afterwards may be a set up for cavities (milk has sugar in it). Be honest—you aren't getting out the toothbrush at 3 am after your child has crashed on your shoulder. The answer: STOP THE NIGHT FEEDING.

Q. What sets off disrupted sleep patterns?

Travel, teething, and illness. Any change in routine will disrupt a child's perfect sleep pattern.

Q. How do I get my baby back on track after a disrupted sleep schedule starts?

A quick refresher course in the preferable, normal sleep routine is helpful. It's quick, I promise! It may take just one or two nights, but be consistent with the routine you want to re-establish. Let them fall asleep on their own. Do not offer an additional night feeding. Do not bring them into your bed if your baby usually sleeps in a crib.

If you continue to intervene (a.k.a resorting to whatever it takes to get everyone back to sleep), your baby will demand the new "normal" routine. And trust me, these disrupted and sleepless nights are not what you or your child wants in the long run. As a doc, I am very comfortable recommending either gradual or rapid training methods depending on how you feel about it. Key point: it is okay to take charge of the situation. More on this below.

Q. My nine month old sleeps through the night, but they like to start the day at 5 am. Can we change that?

You can adjust it somewhat, but some kids are early risers. Some tips:

First, pick a reasonable time to start the day–like 6am (sorry about that!). When you hear your little one making noise at 5am, wait until 5:15 or 5:20 before going them. The next morning, wait until 5:45. By the third morning, you can begin the day at 6am.

Next, try to put them down a little earlier at night.   Early to bed often means late to rise–the opposite of what you might think.

Finally, try putting a few board books in the crib. Your baby can look at them for a while until the sun comes up. Some babies will decide to play, others will go back to sleep. But it's fine to leave them alone for a little while. Your presence signals the beginning of the day.

Helpful Hint

A baby's bedtime usually falls between 7pm and 8:30pm. Just because your baby or toddler is bouncing around the living room doesn't mean they aren't tired. Don't fall for this trick! They are probably actually *overtired*. Wired = tired.

Q. There are so many infant sleep training techniques. What do you think about them?

If you really want to go down this rabbit hole, there are plenty of books, videos, and online/in-person sleep coaches to help you and your baby get a good night's sleep! Better yet, pop on over to our online community (see back of book) and watch our handy sleep videos!

To keep it simple, there are three basic categories of sleep training: gradual methods, rapid methods, and gentle methods. Do not be fooled by the names. All of them involve crying...because babies don't like change and will cry. Parents may cry a little bit, too. In general, we support any mindful, intentional way that leads to a healthier sleep routine. You have to decide what feels the most comfortable for you and commit to making a change in your own behavior.

If you are looking for more information, we also recommend the Pediatric Sleep Council's free website, babysleep.com, for evidence-based sleep advice.

Here are our opinions of the leading sleep advice. And, if you are a co-sleeping, attachment parent family, you can just skip right past this section of the chapter.

GRADUAL TRAINING. *Based on Dr. Richard Ferber Method. Theory*: "What parents view as abnormal wakenings in the night are actually normal. What they do to treat the 'abnormal' wakenings—namely going in to help their child go back to sleep—is actually causing the disturbance."

For the first four months of life, parents need to create positive sleep associations, routines, and rituals. If your baby is not sleeping through the night (six hours of uninterrupted sleep) by five or six months of age, it is time to train or un-train (break bad habits) your baby to stop the night wakenings.

Note: Babies under four months of age are not neurologically mature enough to settle and console themselves. This method is not intended for that age group.

SLEEP

? ?

Ferber Method, in a nutshell:

1. Provide a consistent sleep ritual (books, songs, cuddling) at nap and bedtime.
2. Have your baby sleep in the same place for naps and bedtime.
3. Avoid sleep crutches and sleep associations that require your participation. Examples: pacifiers, white noise machines, falling asleep feeding, being rocked, being stroked.
4. Put your baby down relaxed, but not asleep.
5. Gradual, progressive waiting. If your baby protests, you make a brief appearance at increasing intervals (add five minutes each time) to reassure your baby that you have not abandoned them. This is NOT intended to console your baby. In fact, they will yell louder. Eventually your baby falls asleep on their own.

Pros: This method works! And it works quickly—usually in three or four nights. Dr. Ferber is truly one of the world's experts on sleep disorders in children. His book, Solve Your Child's Sleep Problems, thoroughly explains the science of sleep at a level that parents can understand. He explains his method clearly with good detail and examples.

This book also addresses the gamut of all childhood sleep disorders, not just infant sleep problems. It is an excellent reference for night terrors, bedwetting, sleep walking, etc.

Cons: Yes, your child will cry. Yes, the first night will be ugly. The second night is less ugly. The third night is manageable. The fourth night, your baby has a smile on their face and so do you. Your baby will be fine. More on this later.

Table: Sleep Techniques Compared

METHOD/AUTHOR	BACKGROUND	THEORY	GRADE
GRADUAL			
Ferber Solve Your Child's Sleep Problems	M.D.-Director of Sleep Lab, Boston Children's Hospital, Harvard	Ferber method. Intervals of intervention extinguish night wakenings. Progressive waiting.	A
RAPID			
Weissbluth Healthy Sleep Habits, Happy Child	M.D.-Founder of Sleep Disorders Program Children's Memorial Hospital, Chicago	Sleep deprivation creates a vicious cycle. Break cycle cold turkey. Rapid extinction.	A
GENTLE			
Sears The Baby Book	Pediatrician	Attachment parenting. Babies belong in contact with parents—asleep and awake.	B-

As in every method, there are occasional setbacks. Illness, teething, and travel create sleep disturbances. Kids need an occasional refresher course (shorter than the initial training) to return to the normal routine!

Note: the popular Taking Cara Babies video series, and many other sleep guides, have a similar philosophy on gradual sleep training. The secret sauce to all of them is how the information is presented, but the methods are not unique.

Reality Check

There is no one-size-fits-all approach to infant sleep training. But babies thrive on consistency and routines. And, setting up good sleep habits up front prevents sleep problems down the road.

RAPID TRAINING. *Based on Dr. Marc Weissbluth's healthy Sleep Habits, Happy Child, Weissbluth.* Establishing healthy sleep is critical to good behavior and functioning. Overtired children have a lower frustration tolerance (short fuses), more behavior problems, and more difficulty falling asleep. Parents, with good intentions, perpetuate their child's poor sleep habits unintentionally with their actions.

Weissbluth Method, in a nutshell:
1. Set an earlier bedtime to get baby down BEFORE they are overtired. This may limit the evening playtime after a working parent comes home, but makes for a happier child.
2. Naptime should be preserved at all costs.
3. Let your baby learn the process of falling asleep by letting them do it on their own.
4. *Rapid extinction*. If your baby is already in a vicious cycle of being overtired, end this cycle abruptly by letting them cry until they fall asleep on their own (after four months of age). This strategy is called the "Let Cry" Plan, and it takes one night to accomplish.
5. Weissbluth offers the "Maybe Cry" and the "No Cry" Plans which are more gradual approaches for parents who can't handle crying.

Pros: This method works quickly—in one or two nights. Dr. Weissbluth provides an understandable, in-depth discussion of sleep physiology in his book, Healthy Sleep Habits, Happy Child.. He teaches you how to set up healthy sleep habits so you won't have to resort to breaking bad habits down the line.

Cons: Breaking the vicious cycle can be one very long night of crying (both on the part of the baby and the parent). Many parents don't have the stamina to let their child cry for more than 15 minutes, even if it is in their child's best interest.

Reality Check

Sleep expert Jodi Mindell, PhD gives a bit more wiggle room for parents who are squeamish about the whole crying thing. However, her take home message is essentially the same. As she says, "Setting limits for your child is part of being a good parent . . . it's a tough job, so don't feel guilty when your child doesn't like what you just told him to do." Her writing style is warm and engaging. It's the easiest to read, and thus, probably my favorite of the sleep books.

GENTLE TRAINING *Based on attachment and gentle parenting methods.* The granddaddy of attachment parenting, Dr. William Sears feels that babies need positive sleep associations. To Dr. Sears, this means your baby should be skin to skin with you during sleep. Dr. Sears once said in a Child magazine interview (1998), "Why would a parent want to put her child in a box with bars in a dark room all by herself?"

Method: The family bed fosters attachment parenting. There is no reason to force your baby to sleep through the night or discontinue night feedings.

Pros: Many cultures use the family bed. Attachment parenting, for those who desire it, is rewarding for both parents and baby.

Cons: Our opinion: we know that there is no one-size-fits-all approach to infant sleep training. We don't have a problem with attachment parenting advice, but the way the Sears' present their method as the *preferred* way to have happy well-adjusted child. We think parenting should be guilt-free.

Some parents in the gentle parenting camp eventually want their own beds back or at the very least, want a baby who sleeps through the night. And, the longer the co-sleeping routine continues, the more challenging it can be to change your child's mind about it.

The Batelle Sleep School is a newer online offering for families seeking a gentle sleep training program. It takes longer to accomplish, but has more hands-on parental involvement. And yes, even with this approach, your child is going to cry. The current price tag for this program is $1500.

Reality Check

Some of these gentle training methods may take up to *eight weeks* to be successful. Perhaps a prescription for Prozac could be included for the parents when they buy these books or videos. Most sleep-deprived parents are at the end of their rope at week ONE!

Q. I tried letting my child "cry it out" and it didn't work. Help!

There are a couple of reasons why attempts at sleep training fail:

1. A determined child.
2. A tired parent.

Let's tackle the child issue first. Yes, some babies protest more than others. It is completely normal for a child to push back when they are asked to change and try something new.

Most babies will cry for 45 minutes and then fall asleep. A few, really vocal ones, may go on for an hour or two. Most babies will adapt to self-soothing and be capable of self-regulation after a few nights. A few, really determined ones, may protest for a week or more.

We understand that if you are living with the vocal, determined baby that you will only have so much will power to follow through with this self-soothing, baby-in-charge-of-falling-asleep

GRADUAL VS. RAPID TRAINING

Let's break this down so you understand how to implement these techniques in the real world. Both gradual and rapid methods work. It just depends on your tolerance level. Do you prefer to suffer in small doses over a period of nights (gradual training). . . or suffer one long sleepless night (rapid training). Remember: Your child is going to be fine.

Gradual Training (a.k.a. Ferberizing)
1. Do a relaxing wind down routine (read a book or two, sing, cuddle) with your baby, put your baby in their crib, and say goodnight.
2. Your child will start complaining.
3. On night one: Wait three minutes before returning to the nursery.
4. When you enter the nursery, make your response short and sweet (no more than 60 seconds). Tell your child you love them and say goodnight. Do NOT pick them up, rock or feed them. Leave the room. The purpose is for you to see that your baby is just fine and for your baby to know you have not gone to Brazil.
5. Your baby cries louder. (No surprise here.)
6. Wait *five minutes* before returning.
7. Repeat step 4.
8. Your baby sounds possessed. (They usually get louder once you leave).
9. Wait *ten minutes* before returning.
10. Repeat step 4.
11. Wait ten minutes before returning (this continues for the rest of the night).

This process requires *your baby* to do the work to fall asleep (yes, they are quite capable). The first night will be very difficult to tolerate. **Don't back down once you have committed to this plan.** When your baby wakes up the next morning, they will be happy to see you.

The second night is much easier. The night's events will last half as long as the first night.

The third night may last only ten minutes. By the fourth night, your baby will have adjusted to the new sleep schedule.

Rapid Training
Do a relaxing wind down routine (read a book or two, sing, cuddle) with your baby, put your baby in their crib, and say goodnight.

If you are looking for steps #2 or #3, you won't find them. Yes, this is one long night. But guess what? Your baby will figure it out and move on to a new, healthier sleep routine of falling asleep and staying asleep.

Some final thoughts:
1. These techniques only work when your baby is neurologically mature enough to settle on their own—five or six months old. If you set up healthy sleep routines in the first place, you won't have to break the bad ones.
2. I always recommend doing this over a weekend. Otherwise, you will be cursing me the next day at work.
3. You can't give in or give up once you start.

FIVE REASONS PARENTS CAN'T LISTEN TO THEIR BABY CRY

1. You feel like you are helpless and not "doing anything" for your baby (not true).
2. You are a working parent and feel guilty (don't).
3. You think you will cause your baby to have long-term emotional scars (you won't).
4. You think you are an inadequate parent if you can't get your baby to settle down (you aren't).
5. You think something must be wrong with your baby (probably not).

game plan. If this is your situation, it's okay to go in for a brief intervention. Do some snuggling or singing but don't completely rock your baby to sleep...because then you just taught your baby that a long tirade achieves the objective: a parent's shoulder to fall asleep on.

Note: although most babies adapt very quickly, there are a handful of kids who may not be ready for this approach quite yet. For those babies, take a complete break from sleep training and try again in a few weeks.

Now, let's talk about you. Most parents are unsuccessful because they are either too exhausted or don't feel right about letting their baby cry. We know it can be nerve-wracking.

Admitting there is a problem is the first step. You probably need a change in your current routine if:

1. Your older (six months and up) baby's wind-down-to-sleep routine takes HOURS.
2. Once you finally get your older baby to sleep, you're not done. The process occurs over and over again with frequent night wakings during the night.
3. Your older baby will only take catnaps on you.
4. You are exhausting and reconsidering if you will have any other children.
5. You are co-sleeping by default, and your spouse is sleeping in the guest room.
6. You can't remember the last time you were intimate with your partner.
7. You feel hopeless.

Here is my pep talk to give you the incentive to persevere.

1. What you are doing currently is not working.
2. Nothing is medically wrong with your child.
3. Nothing will happen to your child if they cry.
4. Your child will not hate you or feel you have abandoned them. Your baby will be HAPPY to see you the next morning and you'll be happier to see them.

Feedback from the Real World: Multiples

One parent wrote of her nine-month-old twins:

"You'll be interested to know that they slept through after the second night. I guess they were as ready as I was."

? ?

SLEEP

DR B'S OPINION:
WHICH SLEEP METHOD IS BEST?

By far, my patients' families have had the most success with gradual or rapid training methods. Which works better for the individual child depends on the parents' ability to cope. Some parents prefer to go into the nursery to check on their baby. Others prefer to avoid seeing the drama unfold. Either way, the baby learns to self-soothe. If you have a video baby monitor, you may be more willing to wait it out outside the nursery.

Yes, your baby will probably (okay, almost definitely) cry. If you avoid our "top ten mistakes" and follow through with your plan, the crying is a one night to one week (at most) experience. Your baby is resilient and has the wings to fly. Give them the chance to use them!

For parents who "just can't let their baby cry," I offer these words from Dr. Weissbluth: "Have the courage to do what is best for the child."

As Dr. Mindell points out in her sleep book, sleep training will NOT a) cause your child harm, b) affect your child's attachment to you or c) make your child emotionally scarred for life. In fact, studies have shown that kids who sleep well are well adjusted and have fewer behavior problems than kids who are up several times a night. Studies have also found that "young children are **more securely** attached to their parents following sleep training." (*Mindell*)

Anti-CIO (Cry It Out) activists claim that infant crying causes elevated stress hormone (cortisol) levels and permanent damage. However, the studies that critics refer to were NOT done on the impact of sleep training techniques. Those studies looked at babies who cry all the time (not just at bedtime) beyond three months of life to detect early signs of neurological or developmental delays. (*Rao, Stifter*)

According to Dr. Mindell, "The positive results of weeks and months of a good night's sleep clearly outweigh a few nights of sleep training. Not only are babies happier and more alert during the day after a good night's sleep, but moms and dads are also better parents when they get the sleep they need."

I'd argue that a few nights of crying is insignificant compared to MONTHS (or, gulp, years!!) of disrupted sleep. That, I believe, takes a huge toll on growth, development, and parent-child relationships.

Here's another reader comment from a mom of twins:

"'Crying it Out' is a frightening term to most parents. But truth be told, fear is often times worse than the actual event itself. It was such an intimidating undertaking for us, but once we started, it only took two nights before they learned how to self-soothe. And contrary to what you might think, the crying twin rarely awakens the other twin. They have been sleeping through the night since six months for 12+ hours a night!"
—*Agustina, mom to twins Gael and Malena*

Q. I know I am being a wimp, but I don't think I can listen to my baby cry.

Be strong. You can do it.

As a baby sleep consultation expert, here is my perspective. Yes, your baby is mad that they are not getting their way. You will see a lot of this behavior in the years to come (a preview of the toddler and teenage years)! Remember when you were 16 and your parents didn't let you borrow the car? Did you still love them? Your child will still love you, even when you set limits on their behaviors (including sleep).

I know, easy for us to say. But as moms, we've been there and know what you are going through. Follow the advice in this chapter and you can do it.

Real talk: Babies don't like change so they will cry. So, yes, there will be crying.

So now that we've picked apart all of the other sleep gurus, it's our turn to summarize our approach to sleep. Yes, it's the BABY 411 SLEEP PLAN. Drum roll please . . . we've cleverly used the acronym S.L.E.E.P. (Heck, you all are so exhausted, it would be hard to remember otherwise!)

S Set up a sleep routine. Babies and kids thrive on consistency. Follow the SAME routine at naps and bedtime. Make it short and sweet. Example: one book, one song, a few minutes of rocking, bed.

L Less is more. The less you intervene, the more everyone sleeps. Babies who learn to self-soothe won't need you to help them fall asleep or go back to sleep after every sleep cycle.

E Empower the child. Babies (by four to six months) are capable of going to sleep, and falling back asleep on their own . . . if you let them!

E Earlier bedtime. Babies who are overtired have more trouble falling asleep. The earlier they go to bed, the better and longer they sleep.

P Plan together and stick to it. Make a plan *with* your partner that you BOTH agree to follow. And then don't cave at 3am. If you need to do a sleep "intervention," start it over a weekend so no one has any excuses.

Feedback from the Real World

"Consistency is key. Keep your bedtime wind-down routine simple, and one that works for both you and your partner. Don't lock yourself into an elaborate ritual that you will later regret!"

—*Agustina, mom to twins Gael and Malena*

Nap Schedules

Q. How much should my baby be napping?

Here's the timeline:

◆ *Birth to one month:* Four to five naps per day (mostly waking up to eat and going back to sleep)
◆ *One to three months:* Three to four naps per day (still not much wakeful playtime in between feedings and naps)
◆ *Four to six months:* Two or three naps per day
◆ *Six to 12 months:* Two naps per day
◆ *12 months:* One to two naps per day

Babies usually cut back to one afternoon nap a day shortly after their one-year birthdays. Some will keep that nap until kindergarten. Most (like my own kids) give it up by three years old.

Q. When will my baby be on a nap schedule?

By four months, maybe earlier. Follow your baby's lead.

At two months of age, you will have more predictability in your lives. Your goal, at this point is to start having a schedule by four months of age. You follow your baby's plan and work around it. In general, babies are awake for a couple of hours and then it's time for a nap. More on this to come.

Naptime can begin within 30-45 minutes of your daily goal. But try as much as you can to be consistent. Overtired babies are not exactly the life of the party. Things happen and delays sometimes are unavoidable. Just be prepared. . . you will pay for it!

Remember, from birth to two months, anything goes. If your baby falls asleep in the car, that's fine. This is a popular parent trick. But by four months, avoid it.

Yes, by four months of age, it's time to put your baby down awake and follow your same sleep routine as at bedtime. View naptime as your baby's downtime. If they choose to talk for 30 minutes instead of sleep, so be it.

By six months, you should have the nap thing down. If you don't, it's time for an intervention. The only difference with naps versus night sleep is that if your intervention goes on for more than an hour, that is the end of naptime. As a result, you may have a baby who is not actually sleeping during naptime for a few days.

Q. How long should my baby be awake between naps? I've heard the term, 'wake windows."

Some sleep consultants use the phrase "Wake Windows" to describe the times your baby is alert, awake, and interested in engaging and playing. In other words, it's your kid's day. So, we will refer to it as wakefulness!

Your newborn is using most of their energy to grow, so they are not awake and playful initially. Their wakeful periods will increase over the first year of life. We will give you some ballpark numbers here, but every baby is different and it's best to watch for tiredness cues (less engaged and less interested, eye rubbing, yawning) in the 0-3 month age group and follow their lead. Once your baby is a little older, you will see a routine emerge. You can plan their day and put them down for naptime before they show signs of being tired.

0-1month: 30-60 minutes of wakefulness
1-3 months: 60-90 minutes of wakefulness
3-4 months: 1-2 hours of wakefulness
4-6 months: 2-3 hours of wakefulness
6-12 months: 3-4 hours of wakefulness

Q. How long are naps supposed to be?

Thirty minutes to three hours.

It depends on the child. By four months of age, your baby should have two to four naps per day. The more naps, the shorter they all are in duration. Once baby is down to a couple of naps a day, one is likely to be a morning catnap and the afternoon nap (30-45 minutes) may be a three-hour marathon.

By a year of age (12-21 months), the morning nap is lost, and your baby will probably take a 90-minute to three-hour afternoon siesta.

Q. My baby never naps at daycare and comes home cranky. Help!

Some babies just don't do well with group naptime. They prefer solitude.

See if your daycare center is willing to put your baby in a private area to take naps. If this is not a possibility, you may need to rethink your childcare options or aim for a very early bedtime.

Insider Tip

Avoid letting your daycare baby come home and take a catnap at the end of the day while you make dinner. It seems like a good idea, in theory, but ends up delaying bedtime when the quality of sleep is deeper and better. Just get them fed, cleaned up, and ready for bed. And then you can enjoy your own dinner.

Q. My nine-month-old talks and plays during the second nap of the day and rarely falls asleep. Is it time to cut that nap out?

It's reasonable for naptime to last one hour. What your baby chooses to do with it is up to them. They are having downtime (and likely, so are you). They may look at books, talk to teddy bears, or complain. But they still need that opportunity to rest or sleep. The second nap is usually dropped around 12-21 months.

Q. I have an older child that is in school. My baby's naptime falls right at the time I pick them up from school. We either miss that nap or they fall asleep in the car, only to be awakened when we get home.

Naps are an important part of your baby's schedule. Enough that it is worth looking into carpool options. Perhaps you could drive in the morning and a friend could pick your child up from school. Don't sacrifice that nap if you can help it. However, flexibility is sometimes required, especially when you have multiple kids.

Q. My baby takes a late afternoon nap and then wants to stay up all night. I don't. What should I do?

It's wise to *end* that afternoon nap by 4 pm or 5 pm at the latest. Otherwise, your baby won't be tired enough to go to sleep at a reasonable hour. Try putting your baby down for the last nap of the day by 1pm or 2 pm. If your baby plays in their crib for an hour and then finally falls asleep, you will probably need to wake them up to stick to the game plan.

Insider Tip

Once your baby is four months of age, bedtime should be around 7-8:30PM. Make sure the last nap of the day ends at least two hours before bedtime.

Beyond The First Year

Q. How long will my baby sleep in their crib before graduating to a big bed?

As long as they still like it.

That can be as old as three years of age. We don't recommend toddler beds or convertible beds because they are a waste of money. When your child starts trying to climb out of their crib, take the mattress out and put it on the floor. Put up a safety gate in front of the doorway. That way, your toddler will have free reign of their room, but not the whole house.

Q. We have a one year old and are expecting again. Should I take the older baby out of the crib when the new one arrives?

No.

A bassinet will buy you a couple of months with the newborn. Then, see if the older child still likes their crib. If the answer is yes, borrow or buy a crib for the younger baby until the older one graduates. We do suggest a new mattress for each baby.

Otherwise, you are asking to have a toddler roaming free around your house at night.

Q. Can we use a small travel pillow in the crib?

After a year of age, it's okay.

Special Situations

Q. I have twins. Is it okay to let them share a crib?

Yes. Until they start waking each other up.

For the first two months, both babies will sleep snugly and not get in each other's way. After two months, it's probably wise to give them the space they need to move around—that means two cribs. It's fine to have them share a room.

SLEEP

Q. Do you have any recommendations for how to get both babies to sleep through the night?

The answer is the same as for single babies. Set up the right routines and rituals.

The only difference is with feeding times. See Chapter 6, Liquids for how to coordinate night feedings with multiples.

Q. I have a baby who was born prematurely. Will it take longer for them to sleep through the night?

Yes. It may be as long as 17 weeks beyond your baby's *due date*, not their birth date.

Premature babies are neurologically immature. They also need more calories for "catch up growth." Night feedings will be necessary for a longer period of time than full term babies need.

Q. My baby has acid reflux (GERD). Will this make any difference in their ability to sleep through the night?

Yep. Babies with reflux take longer to sleep through the night for a few reasons. For starters, their heartburn symptoms are worse at night when they are lying down. You can't really blame them for having trouble falling asleep. If your baby is taking medication to control the symptoms, be sure they haven't outgrown their dose of medication (get the dose re-calculated by your doctor every month). You don't want your child lying there in misery.

And crying can make the acid reflux worse. So it's probably not the best idea to let your baby cry it out for an hour. It's okay for five or ten minutes, but not for the duration an otherwise healthy baby would cry. The good news: most kids outgrow reflux by six months of age. Get the green light from your doc or gastroenterologist, and then proceed with your sleep plan.

BOTTOM LINE

Some final thoughts: the National Sleep Foundation found that infants and young children are not getting enough sleep (and neither are their parents—but you already knew that). Tired kids are not only cranky, but they are less interested in learning new information. Make sure both you and your baby get enough sleep!

DEVELOPMENTAL MILESTONES
Chapter 10

"I have found the best way to give advice to your children is to find out what they want and then advise them to do it."

~ Harry S Truman

WHAT'S IN THIS CHAPTER

◆ **HOW DO I KNOW MY BABY IS DEVELOPING NORMALLY?**
◆ **WHAT IS THE DEVELOPMENTAL CHECKLIST?**
◆ **FAILING MILESTONES AND EARLY CHILDHOOD INTERVENTION**
◆ **AUTISM**
◆ **INTELLECTUAL (COGNITIVE) DEVELOPMENT**
◆ **SOCIAL & EMOTIONAL DEVELOPMENT**
◆ **KEEPING KIDS SAFE WHILE THEY EXPLORE**
◆ **DEVELOPMENTALLY APPROPRIATE TOYS AND BOOKS**

"There should be a warning label in bold at the beginning of this chapter: 'Caution: all overachievers and/or first-time parents. Your baby may not develop at the same rate as we have listed in this chapter as normal. You should neither jump off a bridge nor sign your child up for Sylvan Learning Center. These are just averages.'"

—Adventures in the Life of NGL, blogger and fan of *Baby 411*

Okay, you've heard the conversations on the playground: "Janey was walking at only ten months." "Well, my little Henry was saying his first words at four months." You know—competition starts early. Now if you're pregnant as you read this you're probably wondering when they should start walking and talking. If you have a child already, you may be one of those quiet moms who doesn't join in the above boasting conversation. But, you may still be wondering if your baby is behind. That's what this chapter is here to tell you.

When can your child roll over, when should he, and when is a baby developmentally delayed? And what is important to worry about and bring up to your doctor during well check visits? This chapter provides the key to understanding how your child's brain works. Knowing what to expect will help you know how to respond to your child's needs as they are growing.

Your first lesson: DO NOT COMPARE YOUR BABY TO OTHER CHILDREN. We know, you just can't help it. You watch other kids in playgroups, at the park, and in your own family and then look at your baby. Don't do it. Every child reaches developmental milestones at their own pace. Yes, there is a certain timeline to reach these milestones, but there is a broad range of "normal."

Q. What do development and developmental milestones mean?

The way a child evolves in muscle skills (large and small muscles), language skills, social and personality skills, and intelligence. This is different from the term "growth" which refers to physical body changes. We'll define some key terms on this topic next.

Developmental milestones are individual skills that your baby progressively masters as they mature.

The series of questions your pediatrician asks are based on expected milestones at specific ages. Some babies will show off and demonstrate their new tricks in the office. In most cases, however, doctors rely on your descriptions for the rest. Remember, there is a range of time for when milestones are achieved.

1. Gross Motor Development. This refers to using large muscle groups to function (i.e. arms, legs, torso). *Milestones*: rolling, sitting, crawling, climbing, walking, running, throwing, and kicking a ball. *FYI: Gross motor development is mastered in a "Head, shoulders, knees, and toes" direction. Remember these milestones by the numbers 3-6-9-12:*

- ◆ Three-month-olds have achieved *head* control. (no more head bobs)
- ◆ Six-month-olds have *shoulder* and *trunk* support. (rolling over, sitting up)
- ◆ Nine-month-olds have *knee* control and can stand up holding on, and walk with support.
- ◆ 12-month-olds have control of their feet and toes, standing alone and taking steps.

2. Fine Motor Development. This skill involves using small muscle groups to function (i.e. fingers). *Milestones*: batting with hands, grabbing, picking up objects, feeding oneself, holding food utensils, holding writing utensils, coloring, and writing.

3. Oral Motor Development. The ability to use mouth and tongue muscles. *Milestones*: swallowing, chewing, and talking. Newborns only have the ability to suck, swallow, and cry.

4. Language Development. This refers to the ability to communicate with others. The prerequisites for language development are oral motor development and the ability to hear and process language (see receptive language skills below). *Milestones*: cooing, babbling, stringing sounds together, imitating noises, and using words purposefully. There are two different areas of language development:

- ◆ *Receptive* language skills. The "input" that babies get in the form of words is understood long before they start talking. Babies can follow directions (if they are in the mood) before they say any words.
- ◆ *Expressive* language skills. This is language "output." When people refer to a child having language delays, it is usually an expressive language delay (i.e. they aren't talking yet). If there is a concern for an expressive language delay, your doctor

? ?

DEVELOPMENT

should always check to be sure there is not a receptive language delay, too (a hearing problem, or an **AUDITORY PROCESSING DISORDER**).

5. Social-Emotional Development. This is how a child adapts to their world. *Milestones*: smiles responsively, knows parents, asks to be held, laughs, imitates, plays peek-a-boo, anxiety towards strangers, anxiety from being separated from loved ones, seeks independence.

Social skills are a learned process. And, parents are the most important role models for a child. Children interact in social situations quite differently at different ages.

6. Cognitive (Intellectual Development). This refers to how a child figures out their world. Babies are like big sponges. They absorb vast quantities of information on a daily basis and learn how to decipher it all. And you thought your learning curve was steep with this new parent experience. Imagine what your baby's brain is going through!

Milestones: follows people and objects in field of vision, expresses needs, explores toys, prefers routines, knows how to get people's attention, understands cause-and-effect (that is, banging this toy makes noise), object permanence (things still exist even if not in view), remembers frequent visitors, limited problem solving skills.

Q. How do I know that my baby is developing normally?

You visit your pediatrician or family doctor for well baby checks. Or schedule a special appointment to address any developmental concerns you might have.

Many parents think that well baby checks are "just for shots." They're not. At every well baby check, your doctor will ask a series of questions to be sure your baby is developing all five types of skills at an appropriate pace. Docs don't usually ask developmental questions at sick visits because those are "problem-focused" appointments.

If a delay in any of the developmental areas is detected, it may be followed for a period of time to see if your baby "catches up" or a referral may be made to a specialist in that particular field.

This is an extremely important part of both the parent and doctor's job description. If you have concerns about your child's development, don't be shy about it. There is never a downside to getting your concerns checked out.

Early intervention makes the greatest impact in lifelong outcomes. For more on this, see the section "Learn the Signs. Act Early."

Q. Can I have a milestone checklist so I can follow along?

Yes. We have included the test items in a box below.

Remember, no obsessing over this list. Do not tape it to your baby's crib and check off their accomplishments. This is by no means a perfect test, but it is a helpful guide for doctors to screen for developmental delays.

There is a very low criterion to "pass" a test so that children with normal skills are not falsely considered delayed. In light of this, if a child does "fail" a test on a developmental checklist, it is quite likely they have a developmental delay in a certain area. In such a case, the doctor will investigate this further either in their office or via referral to a developmental specialist.

BOOKMARK THIS PAGE! THE BABY 411 ALL-IN-ONE

Developmental checklists are designed to identify developmental delays in infants and young children. In general, the areas are divided into the following categories:

◆ Gross motor skills (large muscle groups)
◆ Fine motor skills (small muscle groups)
◆ Social/emotional development
◆ Language including all forms of communication (indicating wants, facial expressions, understanding language, and vocalization)
◆ Cognitive intellectual development

Because children accomplish these milestones at a range of ages, mastery of a particular milestone will vary over a period of time (i.e. walking may be mastered between 9-15 months of age). The Centers for Disease Control and American Academy of Pediatrics advise the cutoff for 'normal' (and when to refer for further evaluation) is at the level where over 75% of children have achieved a milestone at a particular age. In other words, if a child has not reached an expected milestone when 75% of their peers already have, they should get further testing and possible treatment. *(Zubler)*

For babies born prematurely (if your child was born before 36 weeks gestation and your child is under 2 years old): Subtract the number of months missed in pregnancy from the baby's current age and check at the adjusted age.

Gross Motor:	Age achieved:
Holds head up and steady when on tummy	2 months
Moves both arms and both legs	2 months
Holds head steady without support when you are holding them	4 months
Uses arm to swing at toys	4 months
Pushes up onto elbows/forearms when on tummy	4 months
Rolls over from tummy to back	6 months
Pushes up with straight arms when on tummy	6 months
Leans on hands to support self when sitting	6 months
Gets to a sitting position by themselves	9 months
Sits without support	9 months
Pulls up to stand	12 months
Walks, holding onto furniture ("cruising")	12 months
Takes a few steps on own	15 months
Walks without holding onto anyone/thing	18 months

Note: Crawling is not listed on the developmental checklist because many children skip crawling and are developmentally normal.

? ?

DEVELOPMENT

DEVELOPMENTAL MILESTONE CHECKLIST

Fine Motor:	Age achieved:
Opens hands briefly	2 months
Holds a toy when you put it in their hand	4 months
Brings hands to mouth	4 months
Uses fingers to "rake" food towards themselves	9 months
Moves things from one hand to other hand	9 months
Bangs two things together	9 months
Drinks from a cup without a lid, as you hold it	12 months
Picks things up between thumb and pointer finger	12 months
Puts something in a container, like a block in a cup	12 months

Social/Emotional:	Age achieved:
Calms down when talked to or picked up	2 months
Looks at your face	2 months
Seems happy when you walk up to them	2 months
Smiles when you talk to or smile at them (social smile)	2 months
Smiles on their own to get your attention	4 months
Chuckles when you try to make them laugh	4 months
Looks at you, moves, or makes sounds to get or keep your attention	4 months
Knows familiar people	6 months
Likes to look at self in the mirror	6 months
Laughs	6 months
Is shy, clingy, or fearful around strangers (stranger anxiety)	9 months
Shows several facial expressions, like happy, sad, angry, surprised	9 months
Looks at you when you call their name	9 months
Smiles or laughs when you play peek-a-boo	9 months
Reacts when you leave (looks or reaches for you, cries)	9 months
Lifts arms to be picked up	9 months
Plays games with you like pat-a-cake	12 months

Language/Communication:	Age achieved:
Makes sounds other than crying	2 months
Reacts to loud noises	2 months
Makes sounds like "ooo" and "ahh" (cooing)	4 months
Makes sounds back when you talk to them	4 months
Turns head toward sound of your voice	4 months
Takes turns making sounds with you	6 months
Blows 'raspberries' (sticks tongue out and blows)	6 months
Makes squealing noises	6 months

(Continued on next page)

DEVELOPMENT

DEVELOPMENTAL MILESTONE CHECKLIST

Language/Communication:	Age achieved:
Makes different sounds like 'mama' and 'baba'	9 months
Waves bye-bye	12 months
Calls a parent 'mama' or 'dada' or special name	12 months
Understands "no"	12 months
Tries to say 1-2 words besides mama/dada, like "ba" for ball or "da" for dog	15 months

Cognitive/Intellectual development:	Age achieved:
Watches you as you move	2 months
Looks at a toy for several seconds	2 months
If hungry, opens mouth when they see breast/bottle	4 months
Looks at hands with interest	4 months
Puts things in mouth to explore them	6 months
Closes lips to show they do not want more food	6 months
Looks for objects when dropped out of sight	9 months
Looks for things they see you hide, like a toy under a blanket	12 months
Tries to use things the right way, like a phone, cup, or book	15 months

---

Putting it all together

Here are the questions your baby's doctor will ask you at each well check during the first year. Complete these checklists ahead of time if you want to make sure your baby is tracking where they should be (or if you want to look really smart!).

Two months

Large Muscle

Can your baby hold their head up when on tummy?	Yes	No
Does your baby move both arms and both legs?	Yes	No
Can your baby open their hands briefly?	Yes	No

Language/communication

Does your baby make sounds other than crying?	Yes	No
Does your baby react to loud noises?	Yes	No

Social/emotional

Does your baby calm down when spoken to or picked up?	Yes	No
Does your baby look at your face?	Yes	No
Does your baby seem happy to see you when you walk up to them?	Yes	No
Does your baby smile when you talk to or smile at them?	Yes	No

? ?

DEVELOPMENT

Cognitive/Intellectual

Does your baby watch you as you move?	Yes	No
Does your baby look at a toy for several seconds?	Yes	No

Four months

Large Muscle

Does your baby hold their head steady without support when you are holding them?	Yes	No
Does your baby push up onto elbows/forearms when they are on their tummy?	Yes	No

Small Muscle

Does your baby use their arm to swing at toys?	Yes	No
Does your baby bring hands to their mouth?	Yes	No
Does your baby hold a toy when you put it in their hand?	Yes	No

Language/communication

Does your baby make sounds like 'ooo' and 'ahh' (cooing)?	Yes	No
Does your baby make sounds back when you talk to them?	Yes	No
Does your baby turn their head toward the sound of your voice?	Yes	No

Social/Emotional

Does your baby smile on their own to get your attention?	Yes	No
Does your baby chuckle when you try to make them laugh?	Yes	No
Does your baby look at you, move, or make sounds to get your attention?	Yes	No

Cognitive/Intellectual

If your baby is hungry, will they open their mouth when they see the breast or bottle?	Yes	No
Does your baby look at their hands with interest?	Yes	No

Six months

Large Muscle

Does your baby roll from tummy to back?	Yes	No
Does your baby push up with straight arms when on tummy?	Yes	No
Does your baby lean on their hands to support themselves when sitting?	Yes	No

Small Muscle

Does your baby put things in their mouth to explore them?	Yes	No
Does your baby reach to grab a toy they want?	Yes	No

Language/Communication

Does your baby take turns making sounds with you?	Yes	No
Does your baby blow raspberries?	Yes	No
Does your baby make squealing noises?	Yes	No

Social/Emotional

Does your baby know familiar people?	Yes	No
Does your baby like to look at the mirror at themselves?	Yes	No
Does your baby laugh?	Yes	No

Cognitive/Intellectual

Does your baby close their lips to show they do not want more food?	Yes	No

Nine months

Large Muscle

Does your baby get to a sitting position by themselves?	Yes	No
Does your baby sit without support?	Yes	No

Small Muscle

Does your baby use fingers to rake food towards themselves?	Yes	No
Does your baby move things from one hand to another?	Yes	No

Language/communication

Does your baby make different sounds like "mama" and "baba"?	Yes	No
Does your baby lift their arms to be picked up?	Yes	No

Social/intellectual

Is your baby shy, clingy, or fearful around strangers?	Yes	No
Does your baby show several facial expressions, like happy, sad, angry and surprised?	Yes	No
Does your baby look when you call his name?	Yes	No
Does your baby react when you leave (looks, reaches for you, or cries?)	Yes	No
Does your baby smile or laugh when you play peek-a-boo?	Yes	No

Cognitive/Intellectual

Does your baby look for objects when dropped out of sight?	Yes	No
Does your baby bang two things together?	Yes	No

One Year Old

Large Muscle

Does your baby pull up to stand?	Yes	No
Does your baby walk holding onto furniture?	Yes	No

Small Muscle

Does your baby drink from a cup without a lid as you hold it?	Yes	No
Does your baby pick things up between thumb and pointer finger?	Yes	No

Language/communication

Does your baby wave bye-bye?	Yes	No
Does your baby call parents "mama", "dada" or a special name?	Yes	No
Does your baby understand "no"?	Yes	No

Social/Emotional

Does your baby play games with you, like pat-a-cake?	Yes	No

Cognitive/Intellectual

Does your baby put something in a container, like a block in a cup?	Yes	No
Does your baby look for things they see you hide?	Yes	No

Autism Screening Questions:

Does your child have constant repetitive behaviors, like flapping of the hands?	Yes	No
Does your child have an unusual preference for a hard object, like preferring to carry a phone around instead of a doll or blanket?	Yes	No
Does your child avoid eye contact?	Yes	No
Does your child act like they are in their own world?	Yes	No
Is your child bothered by cuddling?	Yes	No

If you answer YES to more than one of these autism screening questions, please be sure to inform your doctor.

Q. What is the significance if my child fails in their milestones?

Maybe something, maybe nothing.

This is a non-committal answer, but it is the truth. Some children will have an isolated delay in one particular developmental area (that is, just motor skills, just expressive language skills, etc.). With a little help and encouragement, these kids catch up to their peers and you might never notice a problem later on. For others, it may always be an issue. For instance, a child with gross motor delays may grow up to be a non-athletic kid. A child with expressive language delays may turn out to have a learning disability. Both of these children might also be a varsity football player or the valedictorian. It just might take a little more work for that kid to succeed in those areas.

The children we are most concerned about are those with delays across the board, termed "global developmental delays." These children are more at risk to never catch up to their peers. There is a range from mild to severely affected children. Doctors evaluate these children for genetic and metabolic (the way the body breaks down certain chemicals) defects when they are diagnosed.

Autism Spectrum Disorders

Q. I've heard a lot about autism. But what is it, and when do I worry?

AUTISM SPECTRUM DISORDER (ASD) is a neurodevelopmental disorder defined by atypical/abnormal social and communication skills, and repetitive/restrictive behaviors. This is relatively common, occurring in one in 44 American children. One reason for the rise in number of cases is that a variety of disorders now fall under the autism umbrella. True to the name, there is a continuum or "spectrum" of symptoms and very broad range of severity.

Previously, specialists used the terms **PERVASIVE DEVELOPMENTAL DISORDERS (PDD), PERVASIVE DEVELOPMENTAL DISORDER, NOT OTHERWISE SPECIFIED (PDD-NOS)**, and **ASPERGER'S**

? ?

DEVELOPMENT

SYNDROME separately to describe people who fell on the autism spectrum. A child may be extremely intelligent, but socially awkward and anxious about deviating from routines. Or a child may be incapable of engaging with other people, and spend time rocking and hand flapping for stimulation instead of pretending and playing appropriately with toys. Both children have autism. And that is why the psychiatric diagnostic bible (DSM-5) eliminated these other diagnostic terms and gave everyone on the spectrum the same diagnosis—autism.

As you might suspect, children with severe problems are diagnosed much earlier than kids who can communicate but have trouble with social skills.

Children are usually diagnosed by 18-24 months of age when language delays are obvious. Many mildly affected children may not be diagnosed until preschool (or sometimes even later!)

However, clues to the diagnosis appear long before that time. Some early clues include: not smiling back at people, poor eye contact, not imitating, not gesturing (waving bye-bye), not responding to being called by name, and not trying to communicate/connect/engage with other people by one year of age. The social and communication deficit makes a person with ASD struggle to understand or interpret the intent of other people.

There are also some unusual behaviors. Cuddling may not be soothing. In fact, a child with autism may get very upset by being touched. Bright lights and noises often bother them. They have an atypical or adverse response to sensory input (smells, tastes, noises, touch, visual stimuli). Because they are bugged by the outside world, they may be anxious and distressed in certain situations. Children who are more severely impacted turn inwards and find comfort in repetitive behaviors (rocking, head banging, spinning). Children who are more severely impacted with autism may have little interest in playing with toys. Or they may play in an odd way—such as using a phone as a comfort object.

Children with ASD can have additional medical and behavioral diagnoses that seem to occur more often. These include Attention Deficit Disorder (ADD), anxiety, sleep and feeding issues, gastrointestinal problems, obesity, and seizures. *(Hyman)*

BOTTOM LINE: Children with autism have autism long before their first birthdays, even though their "official" diagnosis usually occurs in their second year of life. Remember this fact when we discuss the now debunked measles (MMR) vaccine controversy. (see Chapter 12, "Vaccines" for details).

Q. My baby bangs their head frequently. Is this a sign of autism?

No, not as the only sign. Many babies have behaviors that they perform repeatedly. The repetition is soothing for them. It becomes a red flag (see below) when the behavior goes on

---

LEARN THE SIGNS, ACT EARLY.

Check out the Centers for Disease Control campaign called "Learn the Signs. Act Early." It empowers parents with information on what is normal child development and what isn't. The key point: early diagnosis and intensive therapy leads to the best developmental outcome for the child. Kids who get help before age three (and earlier is even better) have the best chance of overcoming developmental challenges. You can access their info at www.cdc.gov/ncbddd/actearly

? ?

DEVELOPMENT

all day long and replaces meaningful play. And with autism, there are other also other atypical behaviors (lack of social skills, poor language, etc.). By the way, babies have the same self-preservation instincts that we do, so they really won't hurt themselves by head banging.

RED FLAGS for Autism

Although autism is usually diagnosed by age two or so, clues are apparent much earlier. Here are some things to be watching for by a child's first birthday.

- ◆ Lack of eye contact. Babies should make eye contact (and smile back at you) by two months of age.
- ◆ Failure to respond to name by first birthday.
- ◆ Constant repetitive behaviors (hand flapping, etc).
- ◆ Preference for unusual comfort objects (that is, not a doll or blanket).
- ◆ No babbling by first birthday.
- ◆ No gesturing by first birthday.
- ◆ Lack of social skills. Babies should try to engage and get someone's attention.

Insider Tip: Testing

All children who are being evaluated for autism should have chromosome testing done, called a chromosomal microarray (CMA). Testing can be helpful to determine prognosis and inheritance risk for future siblings.

Q. Is there a test for autism?

There's currently no blood test or imaging study that detects autism, although there is ongoing research to identify biomarkers in the blood. An autism diagnosis is based on the symptoms that a child displays (and lack of findings/results that would suggest a different diagnosis). Testing for metabolic disorders is only useful if there are other family members who have autism or the child's physical examination is concerning. Doing a blood lead test is helpful if a child has had a significant environmental exposure. (Kids with lead poisoning don't really have autism, but their bizarre behavior may be misdiagnosed as autism.)

What is NOT useful? Tests that look for heavy metal exposure in the hair/urine/poop, food allergy tests that look at "IgG" levels, or any "alternative lab" where you get your child's test results back on a pretty, four-color grid.

Your pediatrician can do an assessment in the office. If autism is suspected, your child's doctor can make a referral to a developmental pediatrician or multidisciplinary assessment program.

The American Academy of Pediatrics has an extensive Autism Toolkit to help educate families. Go to healthychildren.org for more information.

Q. I have a friend whose child has autism. She said he was "perfectly normal" until he was about 18 months old. Does this happen?

About 25% of children with autism appear to have normal language and social milestones and then regress. Although the cause is not entirely clear, the current theory it may be due to the brain "over-pruning" the nerve synapses in children with ASD as a part of the disorder.

Without getting too technical here, the brain naturally turns off neurochemical pathways that are not needed anymore (hence the name, pruning, like a gardener would do to promote new plant growth).

We also know this fact about brain anatomy: primitive brain parts control early language development from birth to 18 months. At 18 to 24 months, the mature brain parts turn on and language takes off. With children who have autism, mature language does not take off. But from a parent's perspective, it may look like a loss of skills.

For most kids with autism, parents and doctors just miss (or dismiss) the early signs in the first year of life and the child's atypical development only becomes apparent at 18 months.

Doctors rely heavily on parents to point out concerns. And parents (especially first timers) don't know what is normal and what isn't.

One of my patient's mothers told me that she only realized how unusual her son's development was after she watched her second child, without autism, breeze through her milestones. Even the most vocal autism activist mom of all, Jenny McCarthy agrees. Her son was five months old when he first smiled at her (that's abnormal), when all of her friend's babies smiled at two months of age (that's normal).

Some parents report that their child with autism spoke a few words and then "lost" the ability to say them. If you delve a bit deeper, the child may have randomly said a few things, but was not consistently using words like "juice" or "no" to communicate his needs.

And again, children with subtle atypical behaviors may be harder to diagnose early on. Reviewing home movies of a child once the diagnosis is made often shows that early signs are overlooked. (*Maestro*)

Q. Okay, so what causes autism?

The million-dollar question.

In the 1980's, one in 10,000 kids were diagnosed with autism. Today, about one in 44 American eight-year-olds have some form of autism. Boys outnumber girls four to one. But since girls are more difficult to diagnose, that ratio may be inaccurate. The U.S. is not the only country seeing this trend. It is increasingly diagnosed worldwide.

For starters, is it really an epidemic? Or are more people being diagnosed? Many children who were diagnosed with mental retardation (yes, this is an outdated term) thirty years ago are children who are diagnosed with classic autism today. And mildly disabled kids with autism today are children who never would have had a diagnosis thirty years ago. Those verbal, but socially awkward, children account for the majority of new autism cases.

So what are the hotbeds of research into the causes of autism?

GENETICS. There's no question that genetics play a role. Autism runs in families. I have a family in my practice and all four children have a diagnosis on the autism spectrum.

Studying twins is an obvious way to detect genetic disorders. If one identical twin has autism, up to 90% of the time, so will the other twin. To date, studies suggest there is more than just one "autism gene"—there appear to be several.

Children with autism have several different abnormalities with their DNA. However the X chromosome is one of interest because of the high prevalence of boys with autism. (*Jamain*)

Fragile X Syndrome, which is a known genetic cause of autism, also points to a defective

X chromosome in autism spectrum disorders. And Rett Syndrome, which is a disorder causing developmental regression and autistic behaviors in girls, is caused by a defective MECP2 gene located on the X chromosome. (*Chahrour*)

2 ABNORMAL BRAIN GROWTH. Children with autism spectrum disorders have problems with brain growth. Babies are born with immature brains that grow rapidly and make nerve connections called synapses . . . like an information superhighway. In the normally growing brain, some branches of this superhighway get "pruned." In the autistic brain, this pruning process seems to be defective. This may explain why babies who are autistic have abnormally rapid head growth under one year of age. No one has yet figured out what causes that defective nerve growth. There is limited data looking at people with ASD who had brain autopsies after death, the "vast majority of brain abnormalities seen originate during prenatal development" according to the most recent clinical report by the American Academy of Pediatrics. (*Hyman*)

3 ENVIRONMENTAL TRIGGERS. Is there some environmental exposure that sets off abnormal brain development in a genetically predisposed baby? Maybe. And that exposure may happen at or shortly after conception, before a mother even knows she is pregnant. The embryo has a critical period of brain development at 20-24 days after conception. That is when the developing brain is most sensitive to injury. Studies done by the Environmental Working Group have detected over 280 environmental toxins in umbilical cord blood, so clearly pregnant moms are exposed to a variety of toxins—could one of these be the autism trigger? We don't know.

Viral infections during pregnancy may also be a key environmental trigger that causes abnormal genes in the fetus. Those infections include rubella, CMV, and influenza (yes, "the flu"). (*Fatemi*.) Having prolonged fevers during pregnancy also seems to be a risk factor. (*Atladottir*)

What about vaccines as an environmental trigger? Researchers and scientists have taken a long, hard look at vaccines—and there is conclusive evidence that vaccine exposure is NOT the turn-on switch for autism. (*AAP*) Flip over to Chapter 12, Vaccines for an extended discussion.

The bottom line: there's evidence that newborns who are later diagnosed with autism already have abnormal levels of certain proteins in their brains. So, whatever the trigger is (if there is one), it has been fired before the baby even enters the world.

4 PREMATURITY. A developing brain is quite vulnerable. Premature, very low birth-weight babies (under three pounds) have a 25% chance of developing an autism spectrum disorder. (*Limperopoulos*)

5 OLDER PARENTS. Another possible reason for the increase of autism: the trend of parents having babies at a later age. Moms who conceive after the age of 40 have a 30% increased risk of having a child with autism. Dads who conceive after the age of 40 have a 50% increased risk of having an autistic child. (*Croen*) Scientists speculate that an older dad's sperm may have defective genetic material, possibly altered by environmental toxins. Dads who are 20 years old at conception pass on 25 different gene mutations. Dads who are 40 at conception pass on 65 genetic mutations.

6 CLOSELY SPACED PREGNANCIES. One intriguing study compared children who were conceived at least three years after their sibling was born, to closer spaced pregnancies and found that babies conceived less than 12 months after the birth of the first-born child were THREE times more likely to be diagnosed with autism spectrum disorder. Babies conceived from 12 to 23 months after the birth of the first-born child had almost two times the risk of autism. And, even babies conceived 23-35 months after the first-born child had a slightly greater risk of autism.

Unfortunately, researchers have no idea why the odds are greater when the spacing between pregnancies is shorter.

Thus study alone should not necessarily influence your decision on how long to wait between pregnancies. However, the current recommendation from the Centers for Disease Control is to wait at least 18-23 months between pregnancies for a mother and baby's optimal health. (*Cheslack-Postava*)

7 OBESITY. Researchers at UC Davis and Vanderbilt medical school found women who were obese (Body Mass Index of 30 or greater) at the beginning of their pregnancies were more likely to have a child diagnosed with autism. Perhaps the altered metabolism affects the intrauterine environment, and thus affects the intricate process of fetal brain development. More research is definitely needed in this area. (*Krakowiak*)

8 FOLIC ACID DEFICIENCY. A Norwegian study showed that women who took folic acid (or prenatal vitamins) at least four to eight weeks before becoming pregnant lowered the risk of having a child with an autism spectrum disorder by 40%. We've known for a long time that folic acid is clearly necessary for proper brain and nervous system development (deficiencies in pregnancy cause spina bifida). So, it isn't a crazy stretch to think this nutritional deficiency in pregnancy could also lead to autism. (*Suren*)

Follow our online community for new information on this topic.

Q. My child has autism. What therapy do you recommend?

The first place to start with is your child's medical provider. They can help with both diagnosis and referrals locally in your community. National resources to help you get started include:

The Centers for Disease Control: cdc.gov/ActEarly
American Academy of Pediatrics: healthychildren.org

Early, intensive therapy with developmental specialists is key. Please beware of unproven (and possibly dangerous) therapies that promise a cure for autism. We realize that parents will do anything to help their kids. But we also know that leaves them prey for unscrupulous folks selling snake oil.

Other developmental differences

Q. My baby has Down syndrome. What steps do I take to get help?

Down syndrome is the most common of all the known chromosome abnormalities that cause intellectual disability. So it's important to get your baby hooked up with developmental specialists from the start. The AAP recommends that kids with Down syndrome receive early intervention services from 0–3 years of age. That's good news because it means most insurance companies will foot the bill for it!

Down syndrome also causes other potential health problems that need to be assessed. Most large pediatric hospitals and academic centers offer a Down syndrome clinic where an affected child can see all their specialists on the same day (convenient, one-stop shopping!)

Here is a checklist for the health issues associated with Down syndrome:

- *Growth*: Assess at regular well child visit intervals.
- *Sleep*: Evaluate for sleep apnea (snoring, restless sleep) beginning at 1 year of age.
- *Thyroid screening*: Assess as part of newborn metabolic screening, recheck at 6 months of age, 1 year of age, and then annually.
- *Hearing screen:* Formally assess in newborn period, recheck at five years of age, 13 years of age, and then annually. Referral to specialist between 1–2 years of age. Assess for frequent ear infections.
- *Vision screen:* Referral to specialist by six months of age. Formally assess as needed until 13 years of age, and then annually.
- *Heart defect screening:* Heart ultrasound (echocardiogram) performed at prenatal visit. Referral to specialist for periodic assessment in teenage years and adulthood.
- *Blood count:* Newborns need a complete blood count, recheck annually between 13–21 years of age.
- *Celiac disease screening:* Perform at two years of age. Repeat assessment if symptoms of gluten intolerance develop.
- *Periodontal disease screening:* Referral to dentist for regular dental visits every six months.
- *Neck/spine stability screen:* Assessment by neurologic exam, and possibly a screening x-ray. (*AAP*)

For more information and parent resources on Down syndrome, check out the Association for Children with Down syndrome at acds.org.

Q. If my child has a developmental delay, where can I get help?

Want to use a service that makes house calls?

Most states offer an early childhood intervention (ECI) program—Google your state name and "early child intervention" to find a local agency. Your child's development will be screened over the phone. If your child qualifies as having a delay, a specially trained physical therapist (large muscles), occupational therapist (small muscles), or speech therapist (language, mouth skills) will show up at your doorstep and do a formal assessment. If help is needed, regular therapy will be scheduled.

Like most government programs, needs often exceed resources of early intervention agencies. Our advice: be a strong advocate for your child. ECI is a great program in theory, but your child may need more intensive services than what the program can offer. If your child qualifies for speech therapy once a month but really needs it once a week, speak up or seek alternative programs.

Besides ECI, another option is to get a referral from your pediatrician to a private specialist in your area. Easter Seals also has a national program that provides services based on ability to pay. Contact them at easter-seals.org or at (800)-221-6827.

Denise's opinion: We've all been at the park and noticed a child who seems to be "hyper" or "slow" or "aggressive" or non-communicative. But no matter how tempting it is, keep your opinions to yourself. Besides, behavior problems on the playground probably have more to do with kids who are tired or hungry than with some kind of serious brain dysfunction.

As the parent of a learning-disabled child, I can tell you that no outsider would have known he was anything but normal until he got closer to school age. And kids who *seem* to have delays and problems often sort them out and have no issues by the time they reach kindergarten.

But if you notice your child doesn't seem to be keeping up with other kids his age physically or socially, be sure to bring it up to your doctor at the next well visit. If you don't say anything, your doctor may not notice subtle signs in a ten or 15-minute visit.

Feedback from the Real World
Special babies, Extraordinary Parents: Meredith's Story

"When we first learned of Meredith's diagnosis (developmental delays) our first worry was that there would be nobody to take care of her in the future when we were gone. We now realize that dwelling on that is giving up any hope for the present. When Meredith was finally able to throw a ball, we celebrated all the years in therapy that got her to that moment. When she was able to catch the ball, we marveled that it happened the very next day."—Sarah B. and Jim H., parents of Meredith (diagnosis: agenesis of the corpus callosum).

Q. My baby was born prematurely. Does the same developmental checklist apply to preemies?

Yes, but not at first.

Your baby's chronological age will be adjusted by subtracting the number of weeks born prematurely. So, the expectations will be lower initially. Your baby's "age" won't need to be corrected once they are is 2 1/2 or 3 years old.

FYI: Because very low birth weight babies (under three pounds) are at greatest risk of developmental delays, they should have a formal developmental screening (in a developmental assessment program or Early Childhood Intervention) at nine to 15 months corrected age, and again at 21-30 months corrected age.

Babies who are born between 32 to under 37 weeks are at higher risk for having learning issues (particularly reading skills) than babies born full term. So, even if your kiddo was a "late preterm infant," they should still be followed closely for developmental delays. (*Chyi*)

Now that we've talked about general developmental milestones and delays, we want to explain a bit about intellectual development and social/emotional development. We'll explore theories from two prominent doctors with their thoughts on the stages your child will go through throughout his life.

How Your Baby Learns

Ever wonder how your baby learns all the amazing things they do? How do they go from being a little lump at birth to a smiling, talking independent being by their first birthday? Dr. Jean Piaget, the father of the major accepted theory for cognitive (intellectual) development, believes that a child's brain processes and understands information in different ways at different ages. As a parent, it's helpful to know what "stage" of brain development your child is at, *because your child's reasoning will be different than yours*. And if you are educated about those differences, hopefully, you'll be less perplexed and frustrated by them.

So here is the big picture, stage by stage:

Sensorimotor: Age birth to two years

Babies learn by hearing, feeling, tasting, smelling, moving, and manipulating (that is, using their Five Senses). Babies are **EGOCENTRIC**. In their minds, the world revolves around them. They continue to think this way until about age six or seven years old (although you might think that some adults haven't outgrown this stage yet!).

◆ *Birth to one month:* A newborn comes equipped with immature reflexes (sucking, rooting, grasping). They will learn how to use and coordinate them. Newborns have no concept of "self."

◆ *One to four months:* Babies realize that they have body parts, and can control them. If you see your baby staring at their hand, it's because they have discovered it.

◆ *Four to eight months:* Babies are more interested in the world. They realize their actions can make other people do things. They start to manipulate objects and explore with their mouths. But, people and things don't exist unless they are within a baby's visual field. They do well with routines and predictable events with their limited memory banks.

◆ *Eight to 12 months:* Babies grasp the concept of *object permanence*. A baby realizes that a person still exists even when they leave a room. The same goes for toys, food, etc. A baby this age has a limited repertoire of techniques to explore a new situation. They use their *memory* of what worked in the past to approach something unfamiliar.

◆ *12 to 18 months:* Toddlers have more sophisticated approaches to problem solving (although it won't feel that way to their parents). They experiment systematically. Toddlers go through a trial and error method of attack. Things are explored more with hands than with mouths. They CAN follow directions. (It's a matter of whether or not they CHOOSE to).

◆ *18 to 24 months:* As these kids approach two years of age, they can do "trial and error" in their minds, and figure out the solution to a problem (i.e. simple puzzles). They will figure out language, and start to pretend.

Pre-Operational: Age two to seven years

Kids have the concept of symbols representing things (i.e. language, pretend play). Their level of reasoning is based on *their* viewpoint. They are not capable of taking someone else's perspective. They have primitive logical thinking. For example, a full juice cup will look like it has more in it than a half-full water glass.

Concrete Operational: Age seven to eleven years

Kids this age can think logically, order and classify items, compare, and sequence information. But, everything is black and white—there is no *gray* zone.

Formal Operational: Age 12 to Adulthood

This is the age of abstract reasoning— when a child can "think outside of the box." A teenager can take a hypothetical situation and reason it out. (*Brainerd*)

Your Baby's Social and Emotional Growth

Prominent psychologist, Erik Erikson is the OG of social and emotional development . His theory suggests that personality development rests on how a person deals with a series of stages in their life. A person's sense of identity depends on the outcome of eight crises or conflicts. If a person does not successfully resolve a particular conflict, the unresolved issue persists in later life.

People can also regress to prior stages during times of stress (that is, a four-year-old returns to the Terrible Two's when a baby sister is born).

Again, the big picture....

Trust vs. Mistrust: Birth to 18 months

Infants learn to trust their parents. They learn that their needs are met. Babies who do not get appropriate care have a sense of distrust and apprehension around others.

Autonomy vs. Doubt: 18 months to three years

Children are seeking independence and are trying to gain confidence in their abilities. This happens while parents are trying to set limits on inappropriate behaviors. (This meeting of the minds is also known as the Terrible Two's). Children need some autonomy to rely on their own skill, or else they will begin to doubt themselves.

Initiative vs. Guilt: Three to six years

Children thrive on decision-making and accomplishments. If parents do not support these experiences, the child feels guilty for trying to be independent.

Industry vs. Inferiority: Six to 12 years

Children gain confidence in their skills and want to learn. With failure or lack of support, children feel inferior to others.

Identity vs. Role Confusion: 12 to 18 years

Simply put, teens either figure out who they are and what they want (sense of self) or they are confused and reliant on their peers. (*Harder*)

DEVELOPMENT

Now you know the theories behind how babies develop. So you're probably wondering how to put them to work. This is the section for you. Here we're going to discuss how to foster appropriate development for each age and stage. Keep in mind the idea is not to "train" your child to be the next Beethoven, Mary Cassatt or Bill Gates.

Birth to Two Months of Age

Q. So what is a general idea of how my baby will develop in the first two months?

Here is a thumbnail sketch.

You may think that your newborn spends their whole life eating and sleeping, but they are actually learning a great deal. Babies are born with an immature nervous system (brain, spinal cord, nerves). So, most of what you see develop is not dramatic in the first two months of life. Instead, development is happening with a baby's neurological system. *Milestones*:

◆ *Newborn reflexes.* Babies suck and turn their head instinctively when you rub their cheeks. They will also grasp anything placed in the hands. If you gently drop their heads back, they will flail their arms out and open their eyes. These reflexes should go away by six months of age.

◆ *Motor skills.* Babies are born with poor head and neck stability. Over the first two months of life, they gain better head control. They should move both arms and legs equally well. A dominant side or hand preference is NOT normal.

◆ *Vision.* Newborns have 20/200 vision. They are not blind. But, they can only see clearly about eight to ten inches in front of them. Putting your face right up to theirs is very entertaining for them. Babies like contrasts (hence, all of the black and white toys at trendy baby stores). By the time your baby is two months old, they will be able to see one to two feet in front of them. They should also be able to fix their eyes on an object and follow it side to side.

◆ *Hearing.* Newborns are born with normal hearing. They startle to loud noises. Babies recognize their parents' voices. They have heard you inside the womb.

◆ *Social.* Newborns are interested in your face. By two months of age, if you smile at or talk to your baby, they will smile back (called a social smile). Under six weeks of age, any smiling is a mere coincidence, or gas. By two months, they should be happy to see you!

◆ *Language.* Initially, babies cry to express all of their needs. By two months, they should start to make sounds other than crying.

Q. What kind of developmental stimulation should I provide my birth to two month old?

Give them lots of time with you. Here is a breakdown:

DEVELOPMENT

1. Sensorimotor:

◆ Give your baby interesting things to follow with her eyes (your face, colorful toy).

◆ Listen to music; play with rattles, music boxes.

◆ Let your baby touch different objects (your face, your hair, the dog).

◆ Give your baby short bursts (five minutes) of time on their tummy (a.k.a. Tummy Time) to work on shoulder and stomach muscles. Not only does it strengthen neck and shoulder muscles, it also prevents the flat head issues we discussed earlier in the book (**POSITIONAL PLAGIOCEPHALY**). Many babies hate tummy time at first because it's a lot of work for them! The earlier and more often you do it, the more comfortable they get with tummy time. Get down on the floor and give them some encouragement (and entertainment).

2. Language:

◆ Start a *reading ritual*. Set aside reading time EVERY day until your child packs up and goes to college. There is a great deal of research that proves infants who are read to at early ages have stronger language and cognitive skills than their peers.

◆ Infants respond best to rhymes and good illustrations. See the end of this chapter for a list of good books for kids age birth to one.

3. Social:

◆ Spend time talking and smiling at your baby.

Q. **My newborn does not have good head control yet. Is it okay to use an infant baby carrier?**

Yes. Holding your baby in your arms 24/7 gets old quickly. Carriers provide enough head support and allow you to use two hands to get something done. See our sister site, Carriers.BabyBargains.com, for suggestions.

Q. **My two month old's eyes cross frequently. Should I worry?**

No. A baby's eye muscles are weak initially and frequently are not in sync with each other.

Doctors start testing for lazy eye muscles (see **AMBLYOPIA**) from six to nine months of age. If you notice that one eye turns in, turns out, or only one eye has a "red eye" effect in photographs, let your doctor know. Note: a two month old can follow your face as you move it in front of him. A three month old can follow it for a full 180 degrees.

Old Wives Tale
Letting an infant bear weight on their legs will make them bowlegged.
The truth: Babies like to bear weight on their feet with your support. It's fun—and it won't make them bowlegged.

Two to Four Months of Age

Q. **What milestones should I expect my two to four month old to achieve?**

- *Gross Motor.* Your baby should have good head control by three months of age. If you lift your baby from a lying position, their head should come up at the same time and not lag behind. Babies may or may not roll over. By four months old, they should bear weight on their legs if you stand them up. Most babies can lift their heads up and push up onto their elbows and forearms when they are lying on their tummy.

- *Fine Motor.* Your baby will start to realize that their hands are useful. At first they will bat at objects, then try to grab around four months. (This is when moms usually stop wearing hoop earrings and pull their hair back). They should also be able to bring their hands to their mouths.

- *Language.* Babies are really experimenting with their voices at this age. They will move on from cooing ("ooo" and "ahh") to laughing and squealing. They also experiment with the volume of their voice.

- *Vision.* Your baby's vision improves to about 20/40 by four months of age. So they will be able to see you across the room.

- *Social/Personality.* Your baby will try to imitate social contact with you. Smiling, tickling, and laughing are very entertaining for your baby.

Q. What developmental stimulation can I provide for my two to four month old?

- *Motor.* Give your baby more tummy time (five to ten minutes) several times a day. They will let you know when it's time to turn over. Activity gyms are fun because they can start to bat and grab at the objects.

- *Language/Social.* Keep that reading ritual going. When you are out and about, talk to your baby. They are your companion, so treat them like one. Tell your baby where you are going and what you are doing. You may feel silly telling them what you are putting in your grocery cart, but all those vocabulary words will be recorded in your baby's growing brain.

Reality Check: The Value of Talk Time

A recent study looked at three-month-old babies' brain activity in response to hearing simple phrases. Guess what? Their little brains lit up when they heard phrases they had heard before! While you may not hear your baby talk back to you for a while, there is a lot going on in there. This study validates the importance of talking to your baby early in life. (*Dehaene-Lambertz*) While it may seem awkward conversing with your baby during a Costco outing, keep it up. These seemingly insignificant moments are actually pretty significant.

Four to Six Months of Age

Q. What developmental milestones will I see with my four to six month old?

- *Gross Motor.* Your baby will sit up with your assistance, then "tripod sit" with their hands supporting them between their legs. Eventually, they will sit up without support. They should also be able to roll from tummy to back now and push up with straight arms when they are on their tummy.

◆ *Fine Motor.* Your baby has mastered grabbing. They will start to use their fingers more than just their hands. They will "rake" objects to get them into the palm of their hand by six months. And they will put everything into their mouths to explore them.

◆ *Oral Motor.* Your baby will figure out how to maneuver their tongue to swallow solid food by six months of age (see Chapter 7, Solids). This is one of several reasons why it is not recommended to offer solid food before four to six months of age.

◆ *Language.* Your baby will start making the first recognizable sounds of language. Consonant sounds usually progress from B's to D's to M's. This means, you'll first hear "ba-ba" then "da-da" then "ma-ma". You may start to hear "Ba-Ba" around six months of age. Your baby should also turn to you when you are talking to them by six months. They may start to "blow raspberries" (spray saliva). This is particularly fun at mealtime.

◆ *Social/Cognitive.* Your baby is very aware of their surroundings. They know their family and friends. They know their room and their crib. Four month olds already thrive on the routine and the expected. But even at six months of age, your baby will not have the concept of "object permanence." So, if a toy leaves their sight, it no longer exists.

Q. My six-month-old is sitting up but never rolled over. Should I be worried?

No. Welcome to the SIDS-prevention generation.

It is easier to roll from tummy to back, than from back to tummy. Babies spend significantly less time on their tummies because of the "Back to Sleep" recommendations to prevent Sudden Infant Death Syndrome. As a result, babies these days often master rolling over about the same time as sitting up (or skip rolling over entirely). Rolling over used to be a four- month milestone. Sitting up is a six-month milestone.

NEW PARENT 411: READING PROGRAMS

Reach Out and Read (reachoutandread.org) is a national program that encourages 15-20 minutes a day of reading to young children. In participating doctors' offices, books are given free of charge at well child visits from infancy to five years of age. This allows parents to build a developmentally-appropriate reading library in their homes.

You can also seek out local libraries and national bookstore chains that offer free story times for both infants and toddlers.

The benefits of reading to children at an early age are clear. Set aside special time everyday for reading with your little one!

DEVELOPMENT

Q. What can I do to promote my four to six month old's development?

◆ *Gross Motor.* Because babies of this age group aren't quite sitting alone yet, the stationary Exersaucer toys are great. They give babies a sense of independence, and free up their hands to play. However, we don't recommend using them for more than ten or 15 minutes at a time. Also, be sure to give babies lots of floor time to work on rolling and balancing.

◆ *Fine Motor.* Give your baby large plastic or plush toys to grab, manipulate, and mouth. Yes, mouth is used as a verb here. Everything your baby examines will go into their mouth to test out. Toys that make noise are fun. The plush caterpillars that have different sounding objects in each segment are popular.

◆ *Language.* You know the drill by now. Read to your child on a daily basis. Use board books and those designed for tub time (that is, they're waterproof)—these give your child a tactile experience as well. But, for safety reasons, no chewing on vinyl books.

◆ *Social/Personality.* Babies are keenly aware of facial expressions. Get a cheap plastic mirror for hours of fun—your baby will sit there and stare at themselves.

Six to Nine Months of Age

Q. What are your expectations for a six to nine month old?

◆ *Gross Motor.* The milestone over these three months is locomotion. Your baby will try to figure out how to get where they want to go. That may be achieved by rolling, crawling, or "cruising" (walking while holding onto furniture). Some babies skip crawling. Because of this, if you look at the Developmental Checklist, you'll notice that crawling isn't listed. Meanwhile, your baby should also be able to get from lying down to sitting, and be able to sit up independently.

RED FLAG: AVOID WALKERS

The American Academy of Pediatrics strongly discourages the use of walkers. Canada banned walkers over a decade ago. Why? Babies drive these things without taking a driver's ed course. Walkers allow babies to get places that their knees or feet would never take them. This sometimes means falling down a flight of stairs.

New walkers now have some safety devices built in meant to keep them from falling down stairs. Because of the newer safety requirements, there has been a marked decline in the number of injuries caused by walkers.

Even with the new safety standards, pediatricians see numerous head injuries every year as a result of walkers. Even if a child doesn't fall down the stairs, they can still run into low tables and chairs and knock items off tables (like hot drinks and glass vases, for example). And older, used walkers without the new safety devices are definitely death traps.

◆ *Fine Motor.* Your baby will have mastered their reaching and grabbing skills. They will work on refining their crude "raking" to a "pincer grasp" (picking things up between index finger and thumb). Things like lint and dirt on the floor will suddenly become very interesting. This correlates with the ability to self-feed (see finger foods in Chapter 7, "Solids").

◆ *Oral Motor.* Your baby should be able to maneuver their tongue and chew food with teeth (or gums).

◆ *Language.* Your baby should be progressing from "Baba" into the D's and M's. We expect a nine month old to say "Baba" and maybe "Dada" and "Mama", but don't expect them to know the meaning of those words until about 12 months. Everything you are saying is recorded in your little one's big brain. Their receptive language is quite good (that is, they understand what you are saying). *Your nine month old understands the word, "No." Whether they choose to respond to it is another story.*

◆ *Cognitive/Social.* Ah, the light has turned on. Somewhere between six and nine months, your baby will have achieved "object permanence." This is a MAJOR concept. They realize that people and things still exist, even if he can't see them anymore. So, if you leave the room, they will look for you. This, understandably, creates some anxiety (see "separation anxiety" in the next chapter).

◆ *More social issues.* Another concept that arises is stranger anxiety. Not only will your baby want to know your every move, but they won't want to hang out with anyone but you. Don't get too frustrated. When your baby is so independent that they want nothing to do with you, you will look back fondly at these days. Your baby also is picking up social cues. They will smile to engage others. They are also starting to figure out how to express their needs non-verbally. Finally, your baby will start testing the limits of their world. At nine months old, your real parenting job begins. You need to set limits on your baby's behaviors STARTING NOW (see Chapter 11, Discipline).

◆ *Vision.* Your baby's vision is 20/20 by six months of age.

Old Wives Tale

A baby who skips crawling and walks first won't be able to do higher math.
The truth: Where did this one come from? I crawled before I walked and still couldn't figure out calculus—so there. It has no bearing on intelligence.

Q. What developmental stimulation can I provide for my six to nine month old?

◆ *Gross Motor.* Provide a SAFE environment for your baby to move around in (see safety tips in Chapter 15, Safety). Your house is now their playground.

◆ *Fine Motor.* Provide SAFE toys for your baby to feel, touch, maneuver, and taste. Babies explore with their hands first, then their mouths. If you are buying toys, pick ones that make sounds or lights when manipulated. Before you order a bunch to toys online, look around your kitchen. Old measuring cups, Tupperware, seasoning bottles (sealed shut), pots, pans, and wooden spatulas are often a hit with this age group. If you actually venture to a restaurant, those individually wrapped crackers are a real crowd pleaser until your meal arrives.

♦ *Language.* Now would be a good time to take the book plunge–reading books to your baby is key to language development. Use your local library as your baby gets older, but for now buy some cardboard books (called board books) of your own. Your baby's library will double as their teething toys.

♦ *Even More Language.* When you speak to your baby, use single words and short phrases. Otherwise, you will sound like the teacher in the Peanuts cartoon to them. Your baby will start to show you what they want. Instead of saying, "Oh, do you want the rubber ducky?" say, "Duck?" That will teach them the vocabulary word they are looking for. The same language rules apply for discipline. Instead of saying, "Oh, no, Honey, don't bite Mommy's shoulder!" say, "No biting." (Yes, there is more coming on this in the next chapter).

♦ *Social/Personality.* Your baby is a social being and is very responsive to family members. Your baby will imitate the way you respond to situations. They follow your lead. Be a good role model. Since your baby now has object permanence, playing peek-a-boo is fun. It's also fun to hide toys under a blanket and let your baby look for them. How easy it is to amuse a child this age!

Nine to Twelve Months of Age

Q. What are the developmental milestones for a nine to 12 month old?

♦ *Gross Motor.* Your baby should definitely have their sea legs. As they approach 12 months, they should be able to stand holding on to someone's hand or a piece of furniture. By their first birthday, they will be able to pull up to stand and get back

DR B'S OPINION:
BABY SIGN LANGUAGE

We know that children are capable of understanding language and communicating nonverbally long before they are able to speak. So, teaching an older baby or toddler hand gestures to communicate makes sense. And there is scientific proof that signing is beneficial. One study found that infants and toddlers that were "sign talkers" spoke earlier and performed slightly higher on IQ tests at age eight that their non-signing friends. (*Brenner*)

While your baby may only learn a few signs, sitting down with your child to learn any new skill has its merits. You don't need to buy a book to learn sign language. You can create the hand gestures on your own (check out *Meet the Fockers* on Netflix sometime). If you choose not to teach your child sign language, do not fear...your child will master the universal "point and grunt" skill to tell you what they want.

down to a sitting position. One day, you'll go into the nursery and be shocked to find your baby standing up in their crib grinning at you. Your baby may or may not be taking his first steps at his birthday party. It's still within developmental limits to be walking by 15 months old.

◆ *Fine Motor.* Your baby should be good at picking up small items. They will also start banging objects together. Babies this age get really good at pointing.

◆ *Oral Motor.* Your baby should learn how to drink liquids from a cup. Ideally, by 12 months old, they will be able to drink from a real cup as you hold it, but most parents seem to prefer the no-spill sippy variety. Drinking from a straw is also something that works well for a child this age. By one year of age, your baby should graduate from a bottle to a cup (see Chapter 6, Liquids for details).

◆ *Social/Personality.* As your baby approaches their birthday, they will be very good at expressing their needs non-verbally. There is a universal "point and grunt" that babies around the world know how to do.

◆ *Anxiety.* Separation anxiety peaks at nine to 12 months, then again at 15 to 18 months. Remember that anxiety stems from the fear that you are leaving permanently. Ease these fears by kissing your baby goodbye and telling them when you will be back. Keep it short and sweet, and make your exit.

◆ *Language.* From nine to 12 months, your baby may start to say "Mama" and "Dada" and mean it. Your baby will speak with great confidence in some foreign language. If you listen to them (via monitor) in the crib at night, you should hear a whole monologue going on. This singsong intonation of speech is called "jabbering." Even though there aren't any vocabulary words, you know your baby has been listening to you.

Babies start to imitate their parents' activities. You may catch them pretending to dust and sweep. You may have a cleaning buddy!

Your baby will make it clear that they want to be in charge and independent (in simple terms, it's their way or the highway). It is important to begin discipline and setting limits.

Your child will have conflicting moods. They may happily leave you behind, but then call for your help. Your availability as a consultant teaches your child to turn to adults for problem solving. Your child's sense of self (ego) is developing. Praising your child for small accomplishments gives them confidence.

Q. We speak two languages in our house. Will our child learn both?

Yes. They will have excellent receptive language skills in both languages (that is, they'll understand both) long before they speak either language.

Q. What can I do to promote my baby's development from nine to 12 months?

◆ *Gross Motor.* Offer a wide-open space for your child to roam. Start playing with a ball. Toys that can be pushed are fun for babies who are walking (lawn mower, grocery cart, baby buggy).

- ◆ *Fine Motor.* Play pat-a-cake. Offer toys that your baby can bang together. It's also fun to get "cause and effect" toys (your baby pushes a button that causes a toy to move or make a noise; Jack-in-the-Box). Now is the time to buy "the classics." These toys are called stacking cups (plastic cups of various sizes) and shape sorters (cylinder with plastic shapes and matching holes in the top). Toys that can be filled and dumped are also entertaining.

- ◆ *Social.* Let your child participate in activities of daily living. While you are cooking dinner, let your baby "cook" their own meal on the floor with old pots and pans. While you are cleaning up, give them a towel, too. Start reviewing body parts with your child as a part of their vocabulary. You can also begin giving jobs to your baby. They should be able to follow one-step directions (such as "Bring me the ball.")

- ◆ *Language.* Books, books, and more books. Picture books with a single picture and word on each page encourage vocabulary words. Remember to converse with your child as your companion. Continue to identify items in single words and short phrases. Singing songs helps with language skills, and helps pass the time in traffic. Your baby doesn't mind if you can't carry a tune.

Don't forget friends' toys. When you take your child to another kid's house for a play date, they get exposed to a whole other set of toys. Some parents even get together and toy swap so their kids get different toys but don't have to spend oodles of money on them.

Feedback from the Real World: Multiples
"Don't buy two of everything! Twins learn to share early on. Instead, have a few different options and swap them around to keep them entertained."–*Agustina, mom of Gael and Malena.*

Q. When should I buy shoes for my baby?

When they are a good walker.

There is no medical reason to wear shoes. Most babies use their toes to grasp the floor when they are trying to walk. For this reason, we encourage your baby to travel the house in bare feet. If you are out in public, by all means, put shoes on your child. You don't need to buy expensive shoes. (Yes, we are looking at *you*, Golden Goose baby sneakers). But, it is a good idea to get your child's foot measured when you buy that first pair of shoes to ensure proper fit.

Q. When can my baby start using media (TV, smartphones, touchscreens)?

I'm so glad you asked! As the lead author of an American Academy of Pediatrics policy statement on media use in kids under age two, I can answer this question and explain the rationale behind it. Note: because technology (and research about how it impacts kids) is evolving, the AAP updates their policy statements and continues to examine this issue.

Here is the current statement from the AAP: "For children younger than 18 months, [the

AAP discourages] use of screen media other than video-chatting. For parents of children 18 to 24 months of age who want to introduce digital media, [parents should] choose high quality programs/apps and use them together with children, because this is how toddlers learn best. Letting children use media by themselves should be avoided." *(AAP)*

Despite that recommendation, 90% of kids under age two watch TV/videos every day and 26% even have a TV/screen in their bedrooms. *(Kaiser Family Foundation)*

For children 2 to 5 years of age, the AAP says to limit screen use to one hour a day of high-quality programming and have the parent participate with the child if possible. *(AAP)*

Why are the experts so down on technology? What's the harm, you say?

Sure, we know that a 30-minute kiddie video might buy you time to take a much-needed shower. And don't "educational" shows help kids learn?

Here's why screen time (other than FaceTime with Grandma) is bad for babies under age 18 months of age:

1 **WATCHING A SHOW ON A SCREEN IS A LOW ENERGY ACTIVITY.** If a screen is turned on, your child is sitting down (unless you are doing an exercise video). The average school age child has three to eight hours of daily screen time. Yep, that's a third of a day sitting on their butts. Do you want to start this couch-potato habit in infancy? In fact, preschoolers who are heavy media users are also physically heavier. That may be a path to obesity later in life.

2 **IT'S ONLY EDUCATIONAL WHEN YOU CAN UNDERSTAND IT.** Studies have shown that educational programming is beneficial for kids ... BUT only for children who understand the content. The magic age to understand traditional digital media is 15 months to 2 years of age. For younger babies, it gets lost in translation. Toddlers from 18-24 months of age can learn from digital content when a caregiver watches with the child, participates, and reteaches the information. The reality: those baby videos that *claim* developmental stimulation have no data to back up those claims (heck, why spend money doing a study when the product sells like hotcakes). Bottom line: even Sesame Street, which is an educational show, is not appropriate for your baby to watch. *(Anderson)*

3 **SCREEN TIME DISPLACES OTHER ACTIVITIES.** The time kids are using media is time they are not spending with their family, engaging in conversation, playing with someone, or playing independently. These are important activities for kids of all ages. *(Vandewater) That* is the harm of screen time for babies. We know you can't sit down and play with your child 24/7. But realize that independent or solo play is a valuable use of your child's time. That is how kids fine-tune skills that they need in this world (like problem-solving or using their imagination).

4 **SCREEN TIME INTERFERES WITH TALK TIME.** If a parent and child are in the same room (even if both are working on individual tasks) and screens are off, a parent is more likely to chat with a child. That "Talk Time" is a necessary part of learning language and social skills. When screens are on, parents talk time goes down by 85%.

5 **MANY PROGRAMS ARE INAPPROPRIATE FOR CHILDREN.** For instance, cable news can be very graphic and disturbing (and don't think your baby/child isn't watching because it's "your" show). Even children's programs can be problematic. Have you watched a cartoon lately? The average cartoon has 20 violent scenes per hour. The violence that occurs does have an impact.

Studies have shown a direct influence on children's behaviors after watching cartoons. (*AAP*)

So, here are some suggestions:

◆ *After your child turns two or older, limit your child's screen time (a daily limit is good).* Have house rules and stick to them.

◆ *Content matters.* Any PBS show is usually a good bet. Cartoon Network shows require a parent preview. Yes, that means sitting down and watching without your child to see if that show is appropriate. Go to commonsensemedia.org to get expert and parent reviews of programs.

◆ *Co-viewing matters.* Participate WITH your child. Watch shows or play apps/games together. Talk about it.

◆ *Keep screens out of your child's bedroom.* Let's get real here—your kids will learn how to master just about any screen you put in front of them…probably better than you. So, any screen that lives in a child's room gives your little one free access without supervision. Bad idea.

◆ *No screens at meal times*—no exception for kids' shows or checking your Instagram. This not only interferes with important time together as a family, but it also encourages people to continue eating after they are full.

BOTTOM LINE

Many baby videos and apps have clever marketing pitches—watch THIS and your child will be smarter! Stronger! Wealthier!

The truth: your baby will be smarter if *you sit down for 15 minutes and play with him*—no screen time required. Children learn much better when they are actively participating in a learning activity. No kiddie program will make your child an Einstein or a Mozart.

Reality Check: Distracted Parenting

Have a media management plan for everyone in your family—that includes YOU. Screen time is distracting for parents. That all-important "talk time" gets reduced when a parent is immersed in their devices or even has the TV on in the background while preparing dinner. And even if the TV show is intended for grown-ups, a child playing in the same room will look up at the screen about every 20 seconds and be less attentive to his their play. Just turn it off and watch your shows later.

And don't get us started on parents who check Instagram or get lost watching TikTok videos while their little ones play on the playground, or worse, in the pool. Turn it off!

Q. But I just need 15 minutes to take a shower or prepare dinner. Is a little screen time okay to entertain my child?

We hear you—as parents of four children ourselves, we know there are times you just want to take a shower. Or cook dinner. Yes, this means taking your attention away from your child. But what is your child to do during this brief period of time? We know the simple answer is to use a kiddie video as a digital babysitter. While there are no studies that suggest this will leave a permanent scar on your child, here is an alternative:

It's called *independent play.* Crazy, eh?

Yes, you have our blessing to let your child find something to do with their time! And yes, it stimulates your child's creativity and problem solving skills. They can be sitting in the bathroom while you take a shower. Or on the floor in the kitchen with some age-appropriate toys (plastic bowls and wooden spoons do nicely).

We'd argue this is time well spent. Our kids have become the Entertained Generation—if they aren't plugged in, they're bored. The take home message: you do NOT have to entertain or find entertainment for your child 24/7. Let them play on their own.

Q. What about educational apps on touchscreens? Are these ok?

Great question. "Babies need laps, more than apps," according to Dr. Dimitri Christakis, Director of Child Health, Behavior, and Development at Seattle Children's Hospital. He also happens to be one of the nation's leading researchers on how media affects young children's minds.

It is true that young children are hands-on learners and some toddlers get pretty good at pointing and swiping on a touchscreen. But that does not always mean they are actually learning something. The AAP suggests that parents who opt to introduce their 18-24 month olds to technology should explore it together. And wait until your child is two or older to hand them your smartphone!

Our advice: the answer depends on how much you trust your baby with an expensive piece of equipment (does AppleCare cover drool damage?) and how you decide to manage your family's media time. Trust us, once the cat is out of the bag, your child will be as addicted to it as you are.

There are some great interactive apps that let kids test cause and effect, learn vocabulary words, and practice problem-solving skills. Just know that an app can never replace some toys. There is real value in figuring out how to take two blocks in your hands and stack them up on top of each other so they don't fall over. You can't do that on an iPad. Remember that young children are tactile learners and need to experience real people and real things—not just virtual ones.

Q. What do you think of "Parent and Me" and other community programs for babies?

For babies, these are a mixed bag. For the most part, the parent gets more out of these programs than babies less than one year of age. But that parental peer support network may be worthwhile for your own sanity! Look for programs that focus on singing, story time, and finger plays. The more motor oriented programs (Gymboree, Little Gym) are more appropriate for toddlers (over one year in age). One tip: watch a class or two before you sign up so you aren't wasting your time.

Q. Should my baby take an infant swim class?

Sure. It can be a fun way to bond with your baby and get out of the house. And it may actually help prevent a drowning.

Swim classes are an important part of drowning prevention—which is why the American Academy of Pediatrics recommends beginning swim lessons when a child shows signs of interest and developmental readiness. Children ages 1-4 who have had some formal swimming instruction are less likely to drown.

The other keys to prevention include pool fencing, adult supervision (and we really mean supervision—without distraction), and a CPR-trained parent or caregiver sitting poolside. (*Brenner*) For more water safety information, check out colinshope.org, an advocacy group founded by a family who lost their son, Colin, in a drowning accident at a community pool. Not only is it chock full of useful information, it's near and dear to my heart because Colin was my patient.

Many community pools offer "parent and me" classes. Check with a local office of the Red Cross or your city's parks and rec department for more info.

Reality Check

By swimming instruction, we are NOT endorsing the Infant Swimming Resource (ISR) programs where babies are repeatedly immersed in water until they learn to roll to their backs and float. Look for Red Cross approved lessons.

Q. What books do you recommend if I want to learn more about child development?

Touchpoints by Dr. T. Berry Brazelton. He has a beautiful style to approaching development, developmental stimulation, and the challenges within these topics. Brazelton has a "cup is half full" way of viewing your child's struggles with growth and independence.

BOTTOM LINE

The most critical developmental stimulation for your baby is the time you spend with them. You don't need to buy expensive toys or park them in front of "developmentally appropriate" videos or apps. Nor do you need to enroll your baby in a special preschool program. We'll discuss preschool at length in our Toddler 411 book (see the back of this book for details). For now, just concentrate on spending time with your baby.

Q. Can you give me some ideas for age appropriate toys for babies?

Here are some guidelines:

Infants birth to six months:
Look for: bright primary color, clear lines, features, human faces
Fine Motor (manipulatives): soft blocks, rattles, squeeze toys, keys on a ring, activity gyms.
Other sensory activities: Audio recordings of you singing or reading a story, music boxes, mobiles, mirrors, hand held puppets

Infants six to 12 months:
Look for: things safe to go in the mouth, things to stack, pour, dump, things to push, turn, or press, things to open and shut
Gross Motor Play (large muscles): Push toys, Low climbing platform   *Fine Motor:* soft

DEVELOPMENT

? ?

blocks, easy puzzles, squeeze-squeaky toys, pop-up boxes
containers to empty and fill, nesting cups, water toys
Other sensory: music boxes

This list is derived from The Consumer Products Safety Commission guide called *Which Toys for Which Child: A Consumer's Guide for Selecting Suitable Toys, Ages Birth Through Five.* Check out their website at cpsc.gov for your own copy.

Recommended books for birth to age one

We suggest buying the board book versions if you can find them. Not only will your baby enjoy listening to the stories, but they'll want to help turn the pages. Babies are also likely to use them as a teething toy at some point (as we discussed earlier). If you want the books to have a decent lifespan, go cardboard.

Here are some favorite titles:

Margaret Wise Brown: *Good Night Moon, Runaway Bunny*
Eric Carle: *The Very Busy Spider, The Very Hungry Caterpillar*
Eric Hill: *Where's Spot?*
Bill Martin, Jr.: *Brown Bear, Brown Bear, What Do You See?*
Golden Books: *Pat The Bunny, The Pokey Little Puppy*
Nancy White Carlstrom: *Jesse Bears' Yum Yum Crumble*
Dr. Seuss: *Mr. Brown Can Moo! Can You?*
Sandra Boynton: *Barnyard Dance!*
Tedd Arnold: *Five Ugly Monsters*
Jan Pienkowski: *Little Monsters, Oh My a fly!*
Paul Strickland: *Dinosaur Roar!*
Stephen Losordo: *Cow Moo Me*
Adam Rubin: *Dragons Love Tacos*

NEW PARENT 411: FINDING THE BEST TOYS

The best place to find great toys are to look in your own home. Old bowls, wooden spoons, measuring cups, and Tupperware can entertain a child more than you think.
But, if you are in the market for toys, it is worth doing a little research. The Oppenheim Toy Portfolio is a great resource. Visit their website at toyportfolio.com.

TEMPERAMENT & SOOTHING

Chapter 11

"Any child can tell you that the sole purpose of a middle name is so he can tell when he's in trouble."
~ Dennis Fakes

WHAT'S IN THIS CHAPTER

- ◆ FIGURING OUT YOUR BABY'S TEMPERAMENT
- ◆ THE HIGH MAINTENANCE BABY
- ◆ TIPS FOR SOOTHING THE SAVAGE BEAST
- ◆ PACIFIERS
- ◆ COLIC
- ◆ INFANT MASSAGE
- ◆ TIPS ON PLANTING THE SEEDS OF DISCIPLINE
- ◆ SEPARATION ANXIETY
- ◆ MASTURBATION
- ◆ THUMBSUCKING
- ◆ BITING AND BEING BITTEN

Now that you know all about child development, you can take all that knowledge and apply it to guiding your child's behaviors today and into the future.

If you just rolled out of the maternity ward, you will probably feel like this is way too soon to even think about how you will teach your child to be a good citizen. Guess what? How you respond to your baby's emotions and behaviors (the good, bad, and downright ugly) now is setting up the foundation for what seems like a lifetime of discipline.

But before we get to discipline, we'll need to discuss temperament. Call it the "getting to know the real you" section of the book. Once you figure out your little angel's temperament, you can tailor your discipline issues to fit them like a glove. Or at least that's the theory.

Believe it or not, your baby's doctor may be a good resource to help you sort through these issues. If they don't have all of the answers, they can point you in the right direction to get the answers.

Temperament, soothing and discipline issues are the toughest part of your job description. Here is a general list of what you will be facing this first year:

SOOTHING

? ?

AGE	FUN CHALLENGE
0-3 months	Learning your baby's temperament
	Soothing issues
3-4 months	Night feeding/sleep issues
9 months	Separation anxiety
	Stranger anxiety
	Night awakenings
	Limit setting
12 months	Aggressive behaviors (biting, hitting)

(*Harriett Lane Handbook*)

Temperament: Getting to know YOUR baby

Every baby is different. We know that's not news to you. No matter how much advice you get, or how many books you read, no one can tell you what YOUR child's emotional needs will be. You will realize when you have a crying baby on your hands that you'd better figure out your child ASAP . . .

Q. What are the typical temperaments of babies?

Landmark research done in the 1970's described the three main types of temperaments. Every child doesn't fit into only one category all the time, but here are the groups:

1 **EASY CHILD.** Surprisingly, 40% of kids fit in this category. These babies have regular eating, sleeping, and elimination habits. They are usually happy and easy going. They are interested in exploring new things and don't mind change.

2 **DIFFICULT CHILD.** Only 10% of kids fit in this category. These babies have more irregular eating, sleeping, and elimination schedules. They have trouble with change, transitions, and new experiences. These babies are intense.

3 **SLOW TO WARM UP CHILD.** About 15% of kids fit here. These kids are also difficult because it takes them a while to adjust to change in environment or care provider. They hide in their shells when they encounter a new situation.

4 **THE REST.** Thirty-five percent of kids don't fit into any of the above categories and have "mixed" temperaments. (*Thomas*)

BOTTOM LINE
Figuring out what type of baby you have will help you to *anticipate* how your child will react to certain situations. Plus, you'll have a better idea how to make their world (and yours) a better place. For example, a difficult baby needs extra time getting into a car seat without a fight. Plan extra time in your schedule for coaxing if you have some place

you need to be.

Real world parent story: It always amazes us to watch our child-less friends decide to go somewhere (like a restaurant). They just pick up their keys, lock the door and poof! They're gone. For parents of children, it is a 20 (or 30 or 40) minute odyssey that first involves finding shoes/socks, coats, toys, books, etc. Then someone has to have a diaper change. It then takes more time to buckle in the car seat, only to discover a child has forgotten their toy and then the process repeats. As a parent, outings require the pre-planning that usually goes into staging a small-scale military invasion—remembering to bring that diaper bag (honey, do we have any wipes?), wallet, purse, keys . . . as well as your sanity. Then add in a "difficult" baby and you may as well just stay home.

> **DR B'S OPINION**
>
> *"View your baby's temperament . . . as a cake mold. While you can't break the mold, you can control how the cake is baked. How you interact with your baby can positively impact the future!"*

Q. When will I be able to figure out my child's temperament?

By the time a baby turns one, most parents have their baby's number—you know what kind of child you have on your hands.

Of course, some temperaments are more difficult to live with than others. But all have their strengths. When you are feeling frustrated with your baby, think about how successful they will be in the future with those traits!

Here are seven questions to help you understand your child's temperament:

1. *Adaptability*: How does your baby respond to change or new situations?
2. *Regularity*: Does your baby follow a schedule with sleep and mealtimes?
3. *Mood*: Is your baby's attitude positive or negative about life?
4. *Persistence*: Does your baby persist at activities or give up easily?
5. *Sensitivity*: Is your baby sensitive or oblivious to environmental changes (like noises, smells, tastes, lights)?
6. *Intensity*: Is your baby laid back or intense?
7. *Energy*: Is your baby energetic or quiet? (*Kurcinka*)

Q. As a doc, what is your view of infant temperament?

There are high-maintenance babies and low-maintenance babies. If you are blessed with a high maintenance baby, recruit family and friends to help out.

High-maintenance babies require more physical and emotional strength from their parents. These babies get walked around, rocked, and soothed more than their low maintenance friends. Parents of these babies are exhausted and frequently at wits end. They have irrational thoughts about giving their baby up for adoption. Don't worry—you are not alone.

Low-maintenance babies need little intervention, and therefore need little discussion here.

Q. Can you predict a child's future personality based on their temperament as an infant?

Yes.

soothing

SOOTHING

? ?

Elements of a child's temperament will persist through a lifetime. However, all humans adapt to succeed in the face of life's challenges. The way you respond to your child has a *tremendous* impact on your child's personality. It's that heredity vs. environment thing—both have an influence on behavior.

Q. I have an extremely active baby. Can you tell if they have Attention Deficit Disorder (ADD)?

No.

Attention Deficit Disorder is a diagnosis based on the shortened attention span of a child compared to peers their age. All babies under one year of age have fleeting abilities to pay attention to anything for very long. It's virtually impossible to make a diagnosis of ADD in a child less than three years of age.

Will your very active baby ultimately have ADD? Only time will tell. As we discussed in the previous chapter, armchair quarterbacks (namely, other parents at your local park) may be quick to offer a diagnosis for your child on this subject. Don't listen to them!

Q. Why is my baby crying?

Because they can't talk. The average baby cries one to four hours a day.

If you had no other way of communicating you'd be crying, too. Babies are trying to tell you something when they cry. It's your job to play detective and figure out what it is. Yes, there are certain types of cries (I'm hungry, tired, in pain), and that will give you some clues. The truth is, when you spend 24 hours a day with your crying baby, you will get each other figured out—we have no doubt about it. Welcome to Hell Week—you are about to be initiated as a parent.

Read the next box for a reasonable cry management approach.

Reality Check
A study done at a clinic for babies with colic showed that two-thirds of the babies referred actually had gastroesophageal reflux (that is, heartburn). (*High*)

BOTTOM LINE
The mistake most parents make is that they give their newborn more credit than they deserve. Newborns have simple needs. They don't cry because you are a bad parent, because they are lonely, or because you have gone back to work and they are mad at you.

Most of the time, your baby just can't pull it together to fall asleep and needs some soothing. Depending on your baby's temperament, that may mean a little—or a lot—of soothing.

Old Wives Tale
Picking your newborn up every time they cry will spoil them.
The truth: Your newborn does not have a neurological maturity to relax and settle down on their own. You need to do the work to comfort them—*given their age*. From birth to two months, you do whatever it takes. There is no such thing as spoiling a newborn. As babies reach four to six months of age, they become more capable of self-soothing. Wait

a minute to see if your baby can settle on her own before intervening immediately.

Top Ten Tricks for Soothing a New Baby (under three months of age)

1 **LET YOUR BABY SUCK ON YOUR FINGER.** Sucking is incredibly soothing for newborns. Pacifiers are okay, too. (More on this below).

2 **DO THE BABY BURRITO WRAP.** Swaddle your baby in a receiving blanket. They are used to being snug in the womb, without limbs flailing around. See the How to Swaddle a Baby box in Chapter 9, Sleep for a how-to lesson.

3 **ROCKING.** Either sitting in that expensive rocking chair you bought, or walking around and gently swaying baby back and forth in your arms. (Much as YOU would like to be sitting in that chair, babies often prefer you to walk around.) Singing or humming is also helpful.

4 **GO FOR A WALK IN THE STROLLER.** A change of scenery often helps baby and parent.

5 **GO FOR A CAR RIDE.** When parents call me about prolonged (over two hours straight) crying, I tell them to go for a car ride. If a few trips around the block don't make the crying

NEW PARENT 411: THE 3 RULES OF CRY MANAGEMENT

Rule #1: DON'T PANIC—the most important advice!

Rule #2: Go through your baby's To Do List. Is your baby crying because they:

- ◆ Need to eat?
- ◆ Need a diaper change?
- ◆ Is overtired and having trouble falling asleep?
- ◆ Is a high-maintenance baby and doesn't know what they want?

Rule #3: Rule out medical causes if crying persists over two hours straight. A good rule of thumb is that medical reasons for crying are generally not fixed by holding and rocking your baby. For example, your baby may be saying:

- ◆ I'm having heartburn. (This is probably the most common medical reason—see **GASTROESOPHAGEAL REFLUX DISEASE**).
- ◆ I have colic/PURPLE crying. I do this every night. (See later in the chapter for more discussion on colic.)
- ◆ I have a fever. (If your baby is under *three* months old, call your doctor ASAP.)
- ◆ I have gas, constipation, or cow milk intolerance (Memo to new parents: usually this is NOT the cause, but every parent is convinced that this is the problem).
- ◆ I have a really serious medical problem (also rare, but that's why you should call your doctor).

? ?

SOOTHING

stop, I'll tell them to keep on driving to the nearest emergency room.

6 **USE A VIBRATING INFANT SEAT OR INFANT SWING.**

7 **TAKE A TRIP TO THE LAUNDRY ROOM.** Put your baby in their car seat and place on top of the dryer. Turn on the dryer. Vibration is particularly helpful for colicky babies. Don't leave your child unattended, however.

8 **GIVE YOUR BABY A BATH.**

9 **TRY SOME INFANT MASSAGE** (see later in this chapter for more info).

10 **PUT YOUR BABY IN BED AND LEAVE THEM ALONE.** If you have tried everything and now you are crying, too, it's time to let your baby cry it out. They are truly exhausted at this point and will fall asleep on their own.

Feedback from the Real World: Multiples

"My twin stroller turned out to be my best friend, both indoors and outdoors. I used it whenever my two hands weren't enough. If necessary, I could simultaneously bottlefeed them in the stroller. During bath time it was the best way I found to focus all my attention on the one in the water and know that the other one was safe and secure in the stroller next to me. It was also my crutch anytime they were crying in unison. I would strap them in and do laps around my kitchen and living room which calmed them every time!"—*Agustina, mom to twins Gael and Malena*

The Great Binky Debate

Q. Is it okay to use a pacifier?

Sucking is soothing. And it is one of the few skills a newborn possesses. That's why pacifiers and thumb sucking are such popular pastimes for the diaper-clad set.

Yes, by four to six months of age, babies have other ways to calm themselves. And by the time babies reach their first birthdays, they are more than developmentally ready to lose the binky and move on. But do they *need* to? And, is there any harm in clinging to the pacifier after a birthday or two (or more)?

We've all seen binky-addicted preschoolers. Case in point: years ago, then five-year old Suri Cruise graced the tabloids with a binky in her mouth (which sadly clashed with her Dolce&Gabbana handbag).

So let's tackle the Great Binky Debate! Where do the experts weigh in? Pediatricians, lactation consultants, speech pathologists, and orthodontists all have their own opinions.

The American Academy of Pediatrics states that pacifiers offer some protection against

Sudden Infant Death Syndrome, which occurs exclusively in babies under one year of age (90% of cases occur in babies less than six months of age). That's all the AAP says on the matter.

However, pacifiers can potentially increase the risk for ear infections. They are also a sleep crutch, requiring a parent to repeatedly return to the crib-side for re-insertion when the child pops it out of their mouth. For those reasons, many pediatricians advise kicking the pacifier habit sooner rather than later.

The International Lactation Consultant Association (ILCA) has no official position. Although many lactation experts feel that pacifiers sabotage breastfeeding success, research shows that pacifiers don't have an impact—that is, when a family is motivated to breastfeed. (*Jaafar*)

Do pacifiers cause speech impediments? The research is inconclusive, according to Shelley Solka, MS, CCC-SLP, an Austin-based speech language pathologist. "Pacifier-using children plug themselves up and don't have a chance to use their words," she said. "Instead they point and grunt to communicate. Speech starts developing earlier than parents think and if a child is using the pacifier, they may not experiment with sounds and putting sounds together to make words." Her perspective: with respect to speech development, it's best to get rid of the binky in infancy.

Perhaps the greatest concern about pacifiers is their potential impact on a child's teeth and mouth structure. You'd think the major orthodontic organization in the country would have something to say on the matter, but they don't. So, we asked Randy Kunik, DDS, an orthodontist in Austin, TX, for his advice on binkies as well as thumb sucking. Here are his answers:

Q. Is there any harm in letting my child use a pacifier beyond a year of age?

Dr. K: As long as parents use a "Nuk" style pacifier after a year of age and the baby is not turning it upside down, there is no significant dental issue in using them until 24 months of age. It's rare to see any long term consequences if discontinued before then.

Q. How old is "too old" for a binky?

Dr. K: From a purely dental standpoint, any child over 24 months is too old for a pacifier. Kids who use pacifiers between two and three years of age risk having additional nasty habits such as tongue thrusting or lip sucking. These habits can adversely alter the growth of the mouth and teeth, which makes future orthodontic treatment more complex. It may take longer to correct the problems and may be difficult to maintain permanent results.

Q. Are there any other dental risks?

Dr. K: Yes. Pacifiers are germ-laden. The bacteria S mutans can be present on a pacifier and increase the risk of caries (dental decay)…especially if a parent licks the binky after it drops on the floor. (Yuck, right? It's gross but many parents use this "cleaning" tactic.)

DR B'S OPINION

"I cringe when I see a three-year-old walking around the mall with a pacifier in their mouth. In fact, my daughter enjoys pointing these kids out to me to see my reaction."

Q. What do you say to parents who say, "My child might need braces even if they don't use a pacifier"?

Dr. K: Well, it's true that your child may need braces anyway. But long-term binky users or thumb suckers (and the associated habits of tongue thrusting and lip sucking) can create some really challenging orthodontic problems, particularly in people who have longer, less round facial structures. Those cases require oral surgery for optimal results. Bottom line: prolonged binky use or thumb sucking may be the tipping point that results in oral surgery and not just braces if a child is already genetically predisposed to having tooth misalignment.

Q. Which is worse? Pacifiers or thumb sucking?

Dr. K: Pacifiers (beyond three years of age) cause more orthodontic damage, but truthfully, it is much easier to break a pacifier habit than a thumb sucking habit. Thumb sucking pushes the erupting permanent teeth outwards, increasing the risk of injury. And, if the finger or thumb isn't clean, thumb or finger sucking increases the risk of bacterial and fungal infections.

Q. How old is "too old" for thumb sucking?"

Dr. K: From an orthodontist's perspective, a child needs to stop by kindergarten. By age six, there is a much greater risk of significant and complex orthodontic problems.

BOTTOM LINE: The longer the pacifier remains in your baby's world, the harder it will be to kick the habit. Babies adjust very quickly to life without a pacifier and forget about it within a day or two.

Linda's tip

If you are breastfeeding, it's probably wise to wait until things are going well (at least four to seven days) to introduce a pacifier. That way your baby learns good sucking etiquette at your breast first.

Another concern: WHICH pacifier to use. A newborn who uses an "orthodontic" pacifier (such as "Nuk" brand) may suckle (or bite!) at mom's breast the same way, leaving a nursing mom with some very sore and cracked nipples. I recommend Phillips Avent brand's "Soothie" pacifiers for newborns since they're shaped like the human nipple—lowering the odds of gnarly nipples! Orthodontic pacifiers are fine for a seasoned breastfeeding team.

DR B'S OPINION: PACIFIERS

Pacifiers are okay to use for babies *under six months of age*, at most, a year. After one year of age, there are absolutely no medical or developmental benefits—only risks. While it's not a dental issue before age two, binkies can lead to ear infections and inter-fere with a good night's sleep for everyone in the house.

Colic and PURPLE Crying

Q. What is colic and PURPLE crying, anyway?

Both of these terms refer to a very unpleasant ten weeks or so of prolonged crying every night. Yes, the newborn is the one doing the crying but everyone in the household suffers.

The traditional term, colic, follows the Rule of Three's. It starts around three weeks of age. The baby cries for about three hours straight from about 5–8 PM every night (otherwise known as the "UN-happy hour"). And it lasts until the baby is three months old.

PURPLE crying is a newer term for colic. It's an acronym to help describe the symptoms, not the color of your kid's body when it is happening. The developmental pediatrician who coined this term (The Period of PURPLE Crying is a registered trademark) likes to say it is a "period" because it is a crying phase that has a beginning, and thankfully, an end. All babies experience this period of life, so it is normal, but some are more vocal about it than others. Here's the acronym:

P is Peak of Crying: Crying gradually gets worse every week of a newborn's life until about two months of age and then improves around three months of age.
U is Unexpected: There is really no good reason for the crying. So give up worrying about the why.
R is Resists Soothing: The baby struggles to calm down even when a parent pulls out all their tricks.
P is Pain-Like Face: The baby looks really unhappy, but they are not in pain.
L is Long Lasting: The crying can last for up to five hours a day.
E is Evening: Crying occurs at a time when you would prefer to have a baby who is going to bed and not one who is crying nonstop.

Q. What causes colic/PURPLE crying?

Although scientists have been studying colic for years, no one knows exactly what causes it. Many experts think the problem is due to immaturity of the gastrointestinal or digestive system. It may be because newborns enter the world without the gut microbes that help humans digest food. Once the good germs move in, the fussy phase goes away. Coincidental? We don't really know. Previously, doctors treated colic with medications to reduce gas, relax the intestinal muscles, or cause sedation. None of these medications really help. The best treatment for colic is time….all babies eventually outgrow colic. And for healthy full term babies, daily probiotics may help.

Some babies who seem "colicky" actually have a medical diagnosis. So it is important to check in with your baby's doctor if you've got a chronically fussy baby on your hands. Some babies have heartburn (gastroesophageal reflux disease or GERD). Those babies are usually miserable all day and night or around feedings—not just for a three-hour period everyday. Other babies may have a cow's milk protein allergy and don't start to show signs of discomfort until several weeks of being exposed to the milk protein going through mom's breast milk or in standard cow's milk-based formula.

Insider Tip

The difference between a baby with colic and one with heartburn (gastroe-sophageal reflux, GERD) is that colicky babies act this way for specific periods during the day. Babies with heartburn do it all day long.

Q. My baby has colic/PURPLE crying. Help!

We know you want to do something. As parents, we are compelled to help our babies feel better even when the doc tells us there is no treatment but time. After browsing the net, you'll no doubt find many colic treatments that make miraculous (and unregulated) claims.

My advice before starting any treatment is to ask yourself this question: Am I treating my child to make myself feel better (because I feel I am doing something), or does the therapy really work?

Q. Do any complementary therapies for colic really work?

Eh, doubtful.

While there are over 1700 studies in the medical literature looking at colic, fewer than ten studies were well designed. And, only two treatments had more than one single study showing beneficial results to treat colic. *(Perry)*

Therapies included spinal manipulation, massage therapy, reflexology, herbal remedies (chamomile, fennel, licorice, vervain, mint tea or fennel seed extract), sugar solutions, and probiotics. Of those, the most effective therapies were fennel-containing remedies, sugar solutions, and probiotics.

Fennel may relax the gut and increase the gut's motility. Sugar solutions may have a pain-relieving effect. And probiotics may kick-start a colicky baby's (presumably) immature gut.

We know you just want your baby to be happy and stop crying but the best remedy truly is time.

Q. Is it worth it to try probiotics for my colicky baby?

Sure, why not? It may actually help. Sold in capsules, powder, or concentrated drops, probiotics are the good germs in your body that help improve intestinal function. Babies are born germ-free and then acquire good germs in the gut to help digest food (you have millions in your adult gut as you read this).

One of the first studies published on colic & probiotics compared 90 exclusively breastfed babies with colic. Half received over-the-counter gas drops (simethicone) and the other half got one capsule a day of a probiotic containing the germ Lactobacillus reuteri (commonly known as L. reuteri). (*Savino*)

The results? Pretty darn impressive . . . the gas drops group saw a 7% reduction in crying. *The probiotics group had a 95% reduction in crying.* No, that isn't a typo. *Babies who cried two to three hours a day were crying less than an hour after one month of treatment.*

Several studies have shown similar results, including research on Bifidobacteria infantis that also show positive results. While we won't promise that it will cure your baby's colic, probiotics are certainly less expensive than hiring a babysitter every night for two months!

The most popular products are Gerber Soothe, BioGaia Protectis, and Evivo. Just follow the directions on the package. Mix into a bottle of formula or expressed breast milk or place on the baby's tongue.

Q. Do you have any other tips to help us survive the next 10 weeks of colic?

We know it is a nerve-wracking experience. So, here are a few tips to help you keep your sanity:

1. Recruit loving friends and family to come over from 5 to 8 pm a night or two a week. You leave.
2. If #1 isn't an option, put your baby in their crib and step outside for a few moments.
3. Put your baby in a sling or carrier and run the vacuum cleaner. You probably haven't had a chance to clean the house in a while anyway. We're not being cruel, just realistic here.
4. Seek professional help for yourself if you can't take it anymore—this is not a sign of weakness or poor parenting skills.

Tips and tricks for dealing with colic could fill an entire book—and, in fact, one doctor has already written an excellent book on this. Dr. Harvey Karp, a retired pediatrician in Santa Monica, CA, has developed a terrific method for soothing colicky babies. His *Happiest Baby on the Block* book (Bantam, $13.95) focuses on five steps to mimic the baby's experience in the uterus: swaddling, side/stomach position, shhh sounds, swinging and sucking. We highly recommend Karp's book.

Reality Checks

◆ *A common parent thought is, "I can't listen to my baby cry."* That is exactly the way nature intended it to be. All animals have a certain noise that is disturbing to their elders and that prompts them to take action. As a doctor, I listen to children cry all day long in my office and completely tune it out. When I get home and my own children cry, it drives me nuts. Parents (including me!) need to learn to take their own emotions out of the picture. View crying as a form of self-expression and it won't raise your blood pressure. Remember this rule: Most of the time, YOUR CHILD IS FINE.

◆ *Parents at the end of their rope need to walk away from their baby. NEVER SHAKE a baby.* Babies who are colicky or high maintenance have a significantly higher risk of being abused. A baby's brain is very fragile. If they are shaken, the motion can lead to blindness, brain damage, or death.

Q. When should I encourage my baby to have a favorite toy?

The official term is *transitional object*. You can introduce it starting at six months of age, but it is safest to keep it out of the crib until a year of age.

Remember that *object permanence* concept from Chapter 10, Developmental Milestones? Babies start to realize that parents still exist when they leave their viewing field between six and

12 months of age. The transitional object or toy is the friend that travels with your child when you aren't there. They are making an emotional "transition" to seeking an alternative source of comfort. The object may be a doll, blanket, or even a piece of parent's clothing.

Your child will likely have their comfort object for a while. They will give it up before going to his first slumber party (age seven to eight years is normal).

 ### Helpful Hint

Try to pick a transitional object you don't mind carrying around everywhere. One of my patients clung to his mother's satin nightie. Another important point: buy EXTRA objects. Once your child has a favorite "lovie" (such as a stuffed animal or blanket), be sure to buy extra identical ones. Odds are, the lovie will get lost or destroyed—and that isn't a pretty scene. Having back-ups is important for everyone's sanity. Also: be careful when you attempt to wash a lovie—a much-loved stuffed animal can easily fall apart in a washing machine. Hand washing or using the delicate cycle (and not drying) is important.

Q. What do you think about infant massage?

Everyone benefits from a massage.

The power of touch has known therapeutic value. Not only are babies soothed, but parents are too. Learning infant massage teaches parents how to feel more comfortable holding and handling their babies.

Infant massage classes are very popular. Check online for information in your area.

DR B'S OPINION

"Spouse massages are also very important. Often our energies get focused on the baby and our spouses get treated like chopped liver."

Self-Regulation and Planting The Seeds Of Discipline

As parents, we all want to raise good kids. In general, that means raising a child with a good moral compass, empathy and compassion for others, and emotional self-regulation. It starts by being a good role model and demonstrating the behaviors you want to see in your child.

But how exactly do you teach your child right from wrong? (The word discipline literally means, "to teach".) How do you get them to listen to you and follow your advice? How do you help them navigate big feelings? And when is the time to start working on this little project?

Spoiler alert: we definitely don't have all the answers to these burning questions. But knowing how your baby's brain works is the first step. And establishing a good foundation for discipline with your baby will prepare you for the tougher times to come, like the toddler years and the teenage years. We can help with that!

Q. At what age should I start to discipline my baby?

By nine months of age.

Planting the seeds of discipline is CRITICAL. From birth to eight months, your parenting job is easy. It is physically exhausting but doesn't require too many mental strategies to succeed.

SOOTHING

At about nine months old, you will start playing chess with your child and will continue to play for a lifetime. Here are the rules of the game:

Discipline is the process of teaching your child to be an independent being. Your job is to give your child a **SUPER-EGO**. This is a Freudian term that refers to self-control and self-regulation—a person's internal control that limits inappropriate behavior from occurring. In other words, your discipline implants a device in your child's hard drive that they will carry with them wherever they go. That way, your child will do the right thing even when you aren't around.

Let's review your child's development. A nine to 12 month old is exploring, not purposefully destroying, their environment (your house). They use their memory of what has worked before to approach the unfamiliar, so everything ultimately ends up in their mouth (and hence, a safety hazard). They have figured out how to get other people to repeat behaviors (if you scream when they bite you, they will bite you again). They are egocentric—the world revolves around them (how could a phone call be more important than them?) They want independence, but don't quite have the motor skills to accomplish their goals (refusing to let you feed them). They have developed a sense of trust with their parents and caretakers. They don't want anyone to leave them, even to go to the bathroom (separation anxiety). Are we having fun yet?

BOTTOM LINE

Consistency is the key to making a discipline plan work. If there is an adult who ignores a behavior that other adults reprimand, the behavior will continue to occur.

Q. What should be included in our House Rules?

Anything dangerous or potentially painful to the child or others.

These are behaviors that are *never* acceptable. These include pulling on cords, touching the stove, putting fingers in electrical outlets, turning on bathtub water, biting, hitting the dog and so on. Look around your house and add to your list.

NEW PARENT 411: PLANTING THE SEEDS OF DISCIPLINE

1. Make your house kid safe, so you don't have to say "No" to everything your child touches.
2. Make up a set of "House Rules" that all caretakers enforce.
3. Make up a discipline management plan with consequences—again, that all caretakers enforce.
4. Know that your nine-month old understands the word "no", but wants to be sure you really mean it. Yep, this is "testing limits."

Remember, you are planting the seeds of discipline. Don't expect a tree to grow overnight. You won't see your child's behavior change immediately. It takes months (and sometimes years!) to see the fruits of your labor. Be calm and consistent.

Q. What is a discipline management plan?

How adult caretakers will respond to inappropriate behaviors.

Everyone has their own style. Most parents will think back to their own parents' approach and remember what worked. You and your partner need to come up with a uniform strategy that both of you feel comfortable enforcing.

Q. Do you think it's okay to spank my child?

No.

We never recommend using physical force to punish a child. Your child learns from you. If you are violent when you are angry, your child will be that way, too. We know that your first reaction when your child hits you is to hit back—DON'T. You're older than your child remember?

BOTTOM LINE: The goal of discipline is to *teach*. If you want a well-behaved child, you need to be well behaved as their role model.

Q. At what age does the Terrible Two's start? My one year old is already acting terrible.

The Terrible Two's is a misnomer. It actually starts when your child declares independence from you. This behavior starts around 12 to 18 months and lasts until age three or four.

My advice is to have a glass of wine at dinner for the next two years. Just kidding—sort of. My other advice is to give your child the opportunity to feel like they are in control of their world. You are really in charge, but they don't need to be reminded of that 24 hours a day. When there is an opportunity for *your child* to choose something, let them (picking out a snack, a toy to play with, etc.). Also, don't bother to discipline for minor infractions. It's not worth it and limits the amount of conflicts that arise.

Q. What is a temper tantrum and how should I respond to it?

A physical release of anger. Your child needs to let it out. You need to let it happen.

Tantrums are frequently seen in toddlers, but some kids like to start early. When your child is at the end of their rope, they may have an emotional breakdown. This involves kicking, screaming, crying, and flailing around on the floor.

The top priority is to give them a safe place to have it out. The next part is the soufflé of parenthood (it's tricky!) *Validate your child's emotions without validating the behavior/event that led to the tantrum*. In simpler terms: tell your child it's okay to be upset. You can stay there with them and even hold them during the tantrum (if that helps to soothe them). But wait until they are calmed down to have the conversation about why grabbing the dog's tail is not okay.

Just for fun, as parents, we also like to rank our children's temper tantrums much in the way scientists score hurricanes. There are Category 1 and 2 fits, which like minor hurricanes involve a minimal amount of damage. Then there are the serious tantrums—up to and including the big ones we like to call Category 5.

11 Steps to Raising a Self-Regulated Child

1 **Avoid as many conflicts as possible**. Make your house kid safe. Don't push your child past their threshold. For example: running too many errands, missing naptime, waiting forever at a restaurant. For eating out, we have a ten-minute rule—if the wait is over ten minutes, it's time to go elsewhere. Obviously, eating early is a good way to avoid lengthy waits for a table.

2 **Anticipate conflicts**. If you see your child heading towards the dog food, move it elsewhere or offer a toy. Obviously, parents develop a sixth sense for this—soon, you'll be able to scan a room and predict the future (that is, zeroing in on your baby's next conflict).

3 **Anticipate attention-seeking behavior**. Be prepared for trouble when your attention is turned elsewhere. If your child gets into trouble when you are cooking dinner, let them "cook" on the kitchen floor.

4 **Pick your battles**. Saying "No" twenty times a day loses its effectiveness. Believe it or not, I had a parent tell me her child thought his name was "No." Categorize behaviors into major errors, minor ones, and those too insignificant to bother with. Minor infractions are negotiable with an older child.

5 **Act Immediately**. Discipline when the behavior occurs, not after the fact. Otherwise, your child won't remember what they are getting in trouble for. Never say: "Just wait till your father/mother gets home!"

6 **Make your comments short and sweet**. Speak in short sentences such as "No hitting." This is much more effective than, "Johnny, you know it's not nice to hit the dog." Believe us, you lost Johnny right after "you know."

7 **Focus on the behavior, not the child**. Be sure to state that a particular behavior is bad. NEVER tell your child that THEY are bad.

8 **Remind your child that you love them**. Always end your intervention with a positive comment. It reinforces the reason that you are teaching them how to behave.

9 **Use age-appropriate and temperament-appropriate discipline techniques**. You need to adapt to your baby and find a discipline style that works well with your individual child. What works at nine months might not work when your child is two. They've had time to figure out your strategy!

10 **Don't yell**. It's not the volume of your voice, but the tone that gets your point across. Remember *The Godfather*? He never needed to yell. Some of the most effective discipline we've ever seen has been whispered.

11 **Catch your child "being good."** Praise for good behavior is so important and helps encourage more of it. Think of it as fertilizer for their conscience.

Once we took our two-year-old to a train show, something he absolutely loved. Until it was time to go. They were closing it down and turning out the lights (we had been there for an hour or more). Suddenly, our son launched into the most amazing Category 5 tantrum—a one-hour scream-fest. You just had to marvel at the intensity of it all. Of course, at the time, we wanted to give back our parent license and go into the Federal Parent Witness Protection Program.

Reality Check

A word of caution: If you give in to a situation when your child has a tantrum, you have just taught him that a tantrum is an effective way to get what he wants. Be strong!

Q. What sets off a temper tantrum?

Anything and nothing.

Look at your child's world through your child's eyes. They have poor language skills and can't tell their parents everything they need and want. They haven't mastered many motor skills to accomplish certain tasks. They aren't sure where their activity boundaries are and are told "no" numerous times a day. Add in an egocentric perspective that Mom and Dad can read their mind (if they think it, everyone must know what they are thinking). Finish with the unattainable goal of complete independence.

Being tired, bored, and hungry are also contributors to ugly behavior.

So, when you pick out the wrong pajamas at bedtime and your child explodes, don't think it's just the P.J.'s.

Special Situations: Tips & Tricks

Q. How do I deal with separation anxiety? Can I just sneak out of sight?

Before, you could leave the room and your baby might not have cared. Now, if you leave the room, they want to know where you're going. This is about the time you will keep your bathroom door open so your baby does not panic every time you answer nature's call. (That bathroom door often remains open for the next several years. I have to remind myself when we have company to close mine. But I digress). It is CRITICAL that you tell your baby where you are going. You will think it is better to "sneak out" of the house when you leave, so your baby doesn't cry. But, you are NOT helping your baby with their anxiety—you only make it worse. They don't know if you are leaving for a minute or for a lifetime. If your baby is prepared for your departure, they will protest for a few minutes and then move on.

Q. My child freaks out with strangers. How do I make them comfortable?

Be patient. All babies, but especially the slow-to-warm-up ones, are afraid of strangers. They need some time to check out these people and make sure they are okay. And "strangers" to a baby might include a grandparent who lives out of town.

To help the situation, let your baby watch this person before handing them over. Then, stay in your child's view for a while after the hand off.

It's probably a good idea to have consistent caregivers while your child is in their stranger anxiety mode (nine to 15 months).

Q. My baby is playing with their genitals. How do I make them stop?

Your child is normal and you don't need to stop them.

The official term is **MASTURBATION**. It is amazing how quickly babies find these body parts, and yes, it does feel good to touch them. P.S. Erections are also normal.

For now, there is little you can do to limit this behavior. As your child gets older (18 months) you can start explaining to them that it's okay to touch down there, but only when they are at home/in their room. This is a good segue into a discussion that no one else touches or looks down there except for Mom, Dad, and Doctor.

Masturbation is in the same category of self-soothing behaviors as thumb sucking. You won't be able to eliminate these behaviors, but you can limit where and when they are occurring.

Reality Check

Boys aren't the only ones exploring their pleasure zones. I had a female patient who would ride the high chairs at restaurants. Needless to say, her parents didn't take her out to eat much.

Q. My nine-month old enjoys having food fights in our kitchen. Help!

A budding John Belushi. Children start to play with their food when they are no longer eating it. When the food starts to fly, mealtime is over. Your child will quickly learn that they are excused from the dinner table when more food ends up on the floor than in their mouth.

Q. My one year old sucks their thumb. How can I stop it?

You can't. The thumb goes everywhere your child does. This is another self-soothing activity. As your child gets to be around 18 months, you can reason with them about where it is appropriate to thumb suck (in their bedroom) and where it is not (out in public). This will limit the behavior to certain times when your child needs to have some down time. Check out our other book, Toddler 411, for ways to end a preschooler's thumb sucking habit.

Q. My child holds their breath when they get angry. What do I do?

Nothing. At worst, they will faint. It is human nature not to inflict harm on oneself. If your child holds their breath long enough, they will lose consciousness and start breathing spontaneously. We know this is going to sound really cruel, but don't cave because you are afraid of the breath-holding spell. It's okay for your child to be angry, and for you to allow those big feelings to happen. Yep, your kid might faint.

Note: If your child has numerous breath-holding spells, check in with your doctor. Occasionally, this can be related to iron deficiency anemia.

Q. My child is biting me. What do I do?

Don't bite back. And whatever you do, don't scream.

When babies are teething, they often start to gnaw on whatever is available. This may be a parent's shoulder or Mom's nipple (OUCH!). It's not malicious. But, if you respond dramatically, it will encourage your baby to bite again.

Your response: Take your baby off your body and place them on the floor. Calmly and sternly say, "No biting." Do not pay any attention to your baby for one minute. Your baby learns that biting loses your attention. Lick your wounds later, out of sight from your baby.

It may take 20-30 times before your baby gets the message, but they will.

Q. My child is biting/being bitten at daycare. What do I do?

Talk to the daycare director and do an observation in the classroom.

There is a biter or hitter in every room. A good childcare program will be constantly watching the children and be able to prevent Dracula, Jr. from successfully drawing blood from another child.

Reality Check

My son's kindergarten teacher had a wonderful motto. "If I'm doing my job, I don't have to discipline these kids." The point is, children who have the opportunity to bite or hit are those that aren't being watched closely enough by an adult caregiver. If your child is biting, do an observation in the classroom.

Q. We are traveling with our baby. Do you have any tips?

For starters, lower your expectations. Then you can be pleasantly surprised when things go smoothly. How your baby does with a travel adventure depends on their temperament.

Regardless of the mode of travel, bring a "goodie" bag packed with old favorites and new toys/books to explore. Remember the New Toy Rule: whipping out a special new toy your child has never seen before can provide a valuable distraction. If your baby likes music, load up your music app of choice with some fun songs.

And try to travel at off-peak times—traffic delays and delayed flights make the experience that much more challenging. Here are our tips:

◆ *Get a seat for your baby, if possible.* The National Transportation Safety Board recommends that kids under age two be restrained in their own seats, but the FAA does not require it. Check to see if your airline will discount that seat—it's rare but worth a try.

◆ *Feed baby on takeoff and landing.* Babies don't know that yawning will equalize pressure in their ears as cabin pressure changes. Drinking works the same way as yawning.

◆ *What about drugs?* Parents often ask about giving Benadryl (diphenhydramine) to make their babies sleep through the flight. If your baby is under six months old or your flight is less than six hours long, I don't suggest it. If you are taking an international flight, it is a consideration but check with your doctor first.

◆ *Can my baby fly with a cold or ear infection?* Yes. For either issue, using decongestant nose spray (see Appendix A, "Medications") before takeoff reduces nasal secretions and makes cabin pressure changes less unpleasant (see Chapter 13, "Infections" for more info).

Finally, here's when you know you're getting through to your kids: My four-year-old was watching a football game on TV with my husband. One of the teams called time out. My daughter astutely asked, "Daddy, why is the team in Time Out?"

Section 4

Sickness &
How to Avoid It!

VACCINATIONS

Chapter 12

"It's a small world after all."
~Walt Disney

WHAT'S IN THIS CHAPTER

◆ **INFECTIONS AND VACCINES: HISTORY & PRESENT DAY**

◆ **THE TOP 15 VACCINE QUESTIONS**

◆ **THE VACCINATION SCHEDULE**

◆ **VACCINE PREVENTABLE DISEASES**

◆ **COVID-19 VACCINE**

◆ **CONTROVERSIES AND MISCONCEPTIONS**
  -MMR AND AUTISM
  -DELAYED OR SPACED OUT VACCINES
  -ALUMINUM

It's time to jump right into a hot topic that has reached a boiling point as we go to print with our 10th edition of this book. To be fair, the subject of childhood vaccines has pitted the quiet majority of believers against the vocal minority of disbelievers at family Thanksgiving dinners and playgroups for over twenty years now. But as the pandemic wears on, the silent majority of parents who believe in vaccinations are far from silent. And sadly, skepticism surrounding the COVID-19 vaccine has spilled over to all vaccinations, in general.

A head's up: since there is so much misinformation and disinformation out there on vaccines, you need to be armed with detailed, accurate information. And like the rest of this book, that is what you will get in this chapter. The information we provide is based on scientific evidence and solid peer-reviewed research. Remember our mantra: show us the science! Your child is too precious to make such important decisions on anything less. This chapter is *not* based on personal anecdotes, conspiracy theories, "research" study participants recruited at a children's birthday party (we are not kidding), or provocative podcasters.

However, before we get to our take on this debate, let's go back in time a bit. Well, more than a bit. How did the human race survive when other early humans didn't? Yes, making tools and efficiently finding food played a big role.

But here's another key element: we built civilizations. And we developed a sense of responsibility . . . to ourselves and to our society.

The pandemic should remind us how we are not just individuals living in our own little worlds. It's part of our civic duty to lend a hand and take care of our neighbors. It is our responsi-

? ?

VACCINES

bility to work together as a community to prevent the spread of infections, and that means getting vaccinated.

Consider a bit of history: in the 1890's, people would have seven or eight children in their families and only half of them would survive childhood. Just go to an old graveyard some time and look at the ages listed on the headstones. Many of the diseases that killed those children are now prevented by vaccination. It's a fact: vaccinations have increased the life expectancy of our nation's children. That's why our grandparents and parents embraced vaccines.

I think we all respect infectious diseases a whole lot more these days. Enduring a complete overhaul of life as we knew it due to a tiny little virus should have made all of us vaccine super-fans. Yet we know some folks still have concerns about vaccines and we hear you.

We would like to point out the next paragraph below was originally written in 2002 and unedited for this 10th edition of Baby 411, because it is still absolutely true.

Here's a crucial point: the key to a vaccine's success is that *everyone* in the community gets vaccinated. Vaccines won't work if a large number of folks just choose to opt out of the system and their responsibility. Germs are rather simple creatures . . . they just look for a new person to infect. They don't play politics.

Please keep this in mind as you read about vaccinations. Your decision (and every other parent's decision) affects your child. And society as a whole.

Reality Check

The concept of "public health" has been around since antiquity. Obviously, rulers had a vested interest in keeping their subjects healthy so they had a society to rule. Through the years, governments have been responsible for managing numerous programs. The most important advances in public health have been vaccination programs, water purification, and waste disposal/sanitation systems. The only way for public health to work, though, is for all members of the community to follow the same rules.

Q. Who came up with the idea of vaccinations in the first place?

It took centuries of observation as well as trial and error. (And sometimes, error meant death.) The first real step was describing the disease, in this case, smallpox. Smallpox was a deadly disease that, historically, wiped out entire civilizations. The earliest descriptions can be found as far

---

OUTBREAK: HISTORY REPEATS ITSELF

Full disclosure: the first nine editions of *Baby 411* included this content box, previously titled, "Outbreak: It Could Happen Today." It's not funny or even ironic, just predictable.

Fast forward to the present day. Well, hello COVID-19. Here's a new virus that in a matter of weeks spread around the world and killed over six million people worldwide thus far. Thanks to today's modern air travel system, a bug can go from a regional problem to a worldwide epidemic in a blink of an eye. COVID-19, like many of the diseases we vaccinate for, is a VIRUS. Besides a vaccine, there is little we can do to stop the spread of infection—despite our scientifically advanced world.

back as the ninth and tenth centuries among Turks. In fact, "inoculation" or the infecting of a person with the disease in hopes of introducing a mild form and then creating immunity was practiced first in Asia. In the 1700's an English aristocrat, Lady Mary Wortly Montagu, was living in Constantinople and learned of the practice of inoculation (known then as variolation). She had her son inoculated and subsequently, brought the practice back to England.

At about the same time, an English country doctor, Edward Jenner, made an interesting connection: milkmaids who had been exposed to cowpox (a common disease in cattle at the time) never seemed to get smallpox infections during epidemics. He began to study the idea that vaccinating humans with cowpox virus would make them immune to smallpox. In 1798 he published a paper on his idea and called it "Vaccination." Not to say, by the way, that Dr. Jenner's idea was accepted with completely open arms. In the nineteenth century there did emerge a group opposed to vaccination led by Mary C. Hume. See, even the anti-vaccination lobby has been around a long time! Of course, in those days, you could be prosecuted for refusing to vaccinate. (*UCLA*)

People were inoculated with a small amount of cowpox virus on their arm. It caused a localized infection at that site (hence, the scar that people over age 50 bear). And true to Dr. Jenner's hypothesis, it provided protection against smallpox disease. In 1972, the United States stopped vaccinating against smallpox because it was no longer a threat to the population. In 1977, the last case of smallpox occurred in Somalia. In 1980, the World Health Organization declared the world free of smallpox, thanks to a global effort to immunize all children.

The success of the smallpox vaccine and other scientific discoveries led to the evolution of many newer, safer vaccines that have made diseases like polio and diphtheria unheard of by most parents today.

DR B'S OPINION: TODAY'S PARADOX—ARE VACCINES TOO SUCCESSFUL?

Vaccinations are one of the greatest achievements in medical history. Long before COVID-19 (and the vaccine) ever showed up, vaccines significantly decreased infant and childhood mortality. Yet, amazingly, doctors have to convince some parents that immunizing their child is extremely important, not "optional."

Most parents have not spent a night in a pediatric intensive care unit with a child who has HIB meningitis, watched a child gasping for breath with whooping cough, or seen a child die from medical complications of chickenpox. I have. Sadly, every pediatrician has had one of these experiences and has known that the child's illness or death could have been prevented by vaccination. I don't want your child to be that child. And I refuse to let a child become a statistic because of online myths or fear mongering.

That's the bitter irony of today's vaccine "debate." As a vaccinated society, we've made diseases like measles so rare that parents have no idea today how devastating it was and still can be. I hope we have all gained more respect for infectious diseases and vaccines after living through COVID-19.

VACCINES

? ?

Q. Why do you care whether I vaccinate my child or not?

For starters, I want your baby to be protected.

But I also want you to realize that the decision to vaccinate your child impacts the health of other children in the community. Choosing NOT to vaccinate your child is choosing to put your child AND your community's children at risk. As a parent, you want to make the right choices for your child to protect them. I want you to ask questions. I want you to be informed. And I want you to get your child vaccinated. YOUR decision impacts ALL children. Why?

There are two critical points for vaccination to work:

1. You need to be vaccinated.
2. Your neighbor needs to be vaccinated.

If you followed pandemic news at all, you probably have a decent idea of what herd immunity means. Here is an another analogy. Think of germs as rain. Vaccination is a raincoat. Even with a raincoat on, you can still get wet. You need an umbrella, too. The umbrella is "herd immunity." Those who don't vaccinate expect someone to share their umbrella when it rains. But society can only buy umbrellas TOGETHER. And raincoats aren't made for newborns—they need umbrellas!

Or as comedian Jon Stewart once put it, herd immunity is like a zombie movie. You are in an isolated farmhouse and the occupants rely on each other to board up their windows to keep the zombies (germs) out. The zombies get in when some lady from Marin County decides not to board up her windows because she read an article on a wellness blog about the potential health risks of boarding up windows. I think you know what happens next!

Some decisions you make as a parent have little or no impact on the community at large. Deciding whether or not your child eats organic baby food, goes to preschool, or sleeps in a family bed is entirely up to you—your decision only affects your child.

However, your decision whether or not to vaccinate your child affects *all* our kids. If you

---

SEVEN BIGGEST MISCONCEPTIONS ABOUT VACCINES

Pop online to any of the anti-vaccine web sites out there today and you'll find a plethora of misconceptions, untruths and worse about vaccines. Here are the top seven we hear most often:

1. Diseases disappeared before vaccines were introduced. *No!*
2. Vaccines cause illness and death. *Reactions are very rare.*
3. Vaccine preventable diseases are rare. *No!*
4. Too many vaccines, given too soon overload the immune system. *No!*
5. Vaccines cause infertility. *No!*
6. Vaccines cause autism. *No!*
7. There is a government and Big Pharma conspiracy to inject microchips into the population to control them. *Dr. Strangelove, check your messages!*

SOURCE: CDC AND DR. BROWN'S PATIENTS.

---

are a parent who is considering delaying or skipping vaccinations altogether, please realize the impact of your decision.

If more than 10% of American parents choose to "opt out" of vaccines, these horrible infectious diseases of bygone days will return. Fortunately, very few parents decide to do this (see the stats below).

What is most concerning today is that there are pockets of under-vaccinated children. Birds of a feather flock together. Like-minded parents who don't vaccinate their kids tend to live in the same community and send their kids to the same schools. With lower immunization rates, there is no herd immunity. We have these "Ground Zero" areas to thank for recent measles and whooping cough outbreaks. (*Omer*)

Reality Check: The good news

While parents are asking more questions, they are still choosing to vaccinate their kids. The most recent CDC survey (2021) showed 99.0% of U.S. children aged 19 to 35 months are being vaccinated. Yes, 99.0%. Despite all the media stories on vaccine "controversy," only a tiny fraction of parents—less than1%—are choosing to forgo vaccinations. (*CDC*)

The Top 15 Vaccine Questions

1 **WHAT ARE VACCINES?** Vaccines are materials that are given to a person to protect them from disease (that is, provide immunity). The word vaccine is derived from "vaccinia" (cowpox virus), which was used to create the first vaccine in history (smallpox).

Modern medicine has created many vaccines. Vaccines PREVENT viral and bacteria infections that used to cause serious illness and death.

vaccinations

SEVEN TRUTHS ABOUT VACCINES

Let's contrast those misconceptions about vaccines with these truths:

1. Vaccines save lives. They have single-handedly reduced infant mortality rates.
2. Lower immunization rates mean higher disease & mortality rates.
3. Misinformation is everywhere—online, media, and playgroups.
4. The decision NOT to vaccinate is a decision to accept the consequences of the disease.
5. The decision NOT to vaccinate is a decision to put your community at risk for epidemics and pandemics.
6. Like any medication, vaccines are not 100% risk-free.
7. You know what a pandemic looks like now. Respect infectious diseases and the power of vaccines to protect us.

2 **HOW DO VACCINES WORK?** Here is your microbiology lesson for today. Your immune system is your body's defense against foreign invaders (viruses, bacteria, parasites). Vaccines prepare your body to recognize foreigners without getting infected. A vaccine revs up your immune system to make anti-bodies (smart bombs with memory) for the signature of a partic-ular germ. So, if your body sees the real germ, voila! You already know how to fight it off.

There are three types of vaccinations: inactivated, live atten-uated, and inactivated bacterial toxins.

> **DR B'S OPINION**
>
> *"I vaccinated my own kids to protect them. I wouldn't do anything differently for your kids. And, that includes the COVID-19 vaccine. I consider my patients to be my own children. I would not sleep at night if I knew they were not protected against preventable disease."*

♦ *Inactivated vaccines* do not contain any living germs. An immune response forms against either a dead germ, part of the germ (recombinant DNA, mRNA), or a protein or sugar marker that sits on the outer layer of the germ (its signature). Very cool. These vaccines are safe to give to immune-compromised people. The only down side is that several doses of the vaccine are needed to provide full, lifelong protection against disease. Some of these types of vaccines include: *Flu, Hepatitis A & B, HIB, Pertussis (whooping cough), Inactivated Polio, Prevnar.*

♦ *Live attenuated vaccines* are weak forms of the germs that cause infection. An immune response occurs just as if your body had the infection. So one or two doses of vaccine gives you lifelong protection. These vaccines are not given to immune compromised people because they can make them sick. Examples include: *MMR, Oral Polio, Smallpox, Tuberculosis, Varicella (chickenpox), Rotavirus.*

♦ *Toxoids* (inactivated bacterial toxins) are vaccines that create a defense against the toxin (poison) that a bacteria germ makes. Examples of toxoid vaccines include: *Diphtheria, Tetanus.*

3 **WHAT ARE THE DISEASES WE ARE PROTECTED AGAINST WITH VACCINATION?** Good question. You are probably unfamiliar with most of these diseases since we don't see them much anymore in the U.S. After you read about these diseases later in this chapter, thank your parents for immunizing you.

As you read through the vaccination schedule, note that some diseases are viruses. Antibiotics kill bacteria only. Doctors have no medications to cure the viral infections. See sec-tion on "vaccine specifics" for details on all of these diseases and the vaccines.

Doubt the effectiveness of vaccines? Just take a look at the sharp decline of illness and death rates from these diseases over the past 100 years. Here is the link if you want to check it out: http://j.mp/declineindeaths

Rather amazing, no? Diseases that used to kill *thousands* (if not hundreds of thousands) now only harm a handful of people—thanks to vaccines.

4 **HOW ARE VACCINES TESTED TO MAKE SURE THEY'RE SAFE?** Vaccines are researched extensively for an average of 15 years* before being approved for use. The reason why the FDA approved the COVID-19 vaccine so quickly was because the government eliminated many of the financial hurdles and expedited regulatory paperwork hurdles to make it happen. The scientific technology existed pre-pandemic era and the rigorous nature of the vaccine research and study format was the same as for other vaccines.

A pharmaceutical company conducts medical research trials in a series of stages. Once safety is proven, the vaccine is tested in several thousand volunteers to make sure the vaccine actually works. These volunteers are followed for at least one year to be sure that no serious side effects occur. The vast majority of adverse reactions to vaccines occur within 30-60 days of being vaccinated, not a year (or years) later.

Nothing in this world is 100% foolproof, including vaccine science. But the research trials that occur before licensing are very rigid. If you think there are a lot of vaccines on the market, imagine how many didn't make it through the research phase of development.

The Food and Drug Administration (FDA) governs this whole process. The FDA is the watchdog for any medication that is sold over-the-counter or by prescription. There are extremely high standards that must be met before any product is allowed for human use.

I know, I know, we have all now witnessed how sausage is made over at the FDA. But the transparency of the COVID-19 vaccine emergency use authorization and approval process should reassure you that these experts are extremely cautious, mindful, and data-driven. Making decisions in real-time during an evolving pandemic with more moving parts (scientific variables) is extremely challenging.

After a vaccine is approved for use, long-term follow-up studies are done to assess for side effects, adverse reactions, and potency over a lifetime.

5 **WHY IS MY CHILD GETTING MORE SHOTS THAN I DID?** Simple answer: we've been successful inventing vaccines to fight more diseases. It's one of the important advances in modern medicine—vaccines prevent disease, injury and death. More vaccines are a good thing!

An important point: many of the vaccine preventable diseases are viruses. These viral infections cannot be treated with medicine once an infection occurs (for example, Hepatitis B).

Vaccines that protect against bacterial diseases are often serious ones, and resistant to many antibiotics (for example, Prevnar).

And even though the number of shots has gone up, the total load on the immune system has gone down. Today's vaccines are smarter and better engineered than the shots from a few decades ago.

In fact, the total number of immunologic agents in *the entire* childhood vaccination series today is less than what was in just two vaccines in 1980!

Our children are getting smarter, safer vaccines today and better protection than we ever got as kids.

6 **ARE WE GIVING TOO MANY SHOTS, TOO SOON?** This is a false mantra of the anti-vaccine crowd: they say babies are receiving too many shots (compared to say, 1980) and too soon (infants can't handle all these shots, they say).

So, let's look at this scientifically. On any given day, your baby is exposed to literally thousands of germs (it doesn't matter how spotless your house is). Exposing your child to five to eight different germs in the form of vaccines is a spit in the bucket.

VACCINES

? ?

Young children have better immune responses to vaccines than adults and older children. So they will form adequate immune responses to various vaccines *simultaneously*. (This is studied extensively before a vaccine is licensed). Even if your baby got 11 shots at the same time, they would only need to use about 0.1% of their immune system to respond to them. (*Offit*)

Giving several vaccines at once does not damage, weaken, or overload the immune system. Vaccines boost the immune system.

Also, the diseases that the vaccines protect against are the most severe in infants and young children. Your doctor wants to get those vaccinations in as safely and effectively as possible. That's why the timing is so important (and why a staggered or delayed vaccination schedule is a bad idea—more on that in the controversies section of this chapter.)

Q. Can't you just give one big shot that has all the vaccines in it?

Medical science is working on it!

There have been a few combination vaccines licensed for use. The largest combination vaccines are Pediarix (DTaP, IPV, Hepatitis B) and Pentacel (DTaP, IPV, HIB). The reason there isn't just one big shot is that some vaccines are ineffective when they are sitting together in a solution. Your baby may still need more than one shot, but if your doctor uses a combo vaccine at least it will be fewer shots than if they are all administered separately.

More combination vaccines are on the horizon.

REASONS NOT TO VACCINATE

There are very specific medical reasons to discontinue or hold off on certain vaccinations:

1.   *An immune-compromised patient or family member.*
2.   *Had disease (for example, if you've had chicken pox, you don't need the vaccine).*
3.   *Encephalitis or degenerative brain disorder.*
4.   *Allergy to vaccine or an additive in vaccine.*

If your baby has a food allergy to eggs or gelatin, or an allergy to antibiotics (such as Neomycin, Streptomycin, Polymyxin B), notify your doctor before any vaccinations are given. Several vaccines are grown in chick embryo cells and therefore contain a small amount of egg protein: flu vaccine (Flushield, Fluzone, Fluvirin), MMR, rabies (RabAvert), and yellow fever vaccine (YF-VAX). The good news: people with egg allergy can safely receive both the MMR and Flu vaccine. The MMR vaccine also includes gelatin.

Several vaccines may contain trace amounts of antibiotics from the manufacturing process to prevent contamination of the vaccine itself. The antibiotics are NOT in the penicillin, cephalosporin, or sulfa categories. The most commonly used antibiotic is Neomycin. You can see a complete list antibiotics in vaccines here: chop.edu/centers-programs/vaccine-education-center/vaccine-ingredients/antibiotics. (*Schuval*)

Helpful Hints
Top Five Tips to Make Shots Less Painful
◆ **Distraction.** Blow in your child's face, or pull out a new toy.

◆ **A spoonful of sugar.** Put a little sugar water on a nipple or pacifier. It is a known pain reliever (analgesic).

◆ **Acetaminophen** (Tylenol). It's a great pain medicine. Be sure to check with your doctor for the correct dose for your baby's weight. *Remember, for your baby's immune system to respond optimally to his shots, wait at least four hours after the shots to give a dose of acetaminophen.*

◆ **Numb it.** There is an over-the-counter lidocaine anesthetic cream that can be applied one hour before shots are administered. The downsides: a) Pain is not just from the needle going through the skin but also from the fluid injected into muscle. b) You may not know where to place the cream.

◆ **Freeze it.** There is a cold "vapocoolant" spray that can be placed on the skin just before the injections. A few doctors use it. It works slightly better than the distraction technique. (*Reis*)

7 **WHAT GROUP MAKES DECISIONS ABOUT VACCINATIONS FOR CHILDREN?** There are four governing panels of experts in infectious diseases that make recommendations for vaccinations. These smart folks include: American Academy of Pediatrics (AAP), American Academy of Family Physicians (AAFP), Advisory Committee on Immunization Practices (ACIP), and the Centers for Disease Control (CDC). Because there are several groups involved in this effort, there is some variability in vaccination schedule recommendations. If you are really geeky like me, you could have watched several hours of ACIP meetings on YouTube as the group deliberated on the COVID-19 vaccine. It was impressive to see how these experts painstakingly reviewed and reflected on the data. It wasn't exactly riveting, but it was reassuring!

8 **MY BABY HAS A COLD. SHOULD I HOLD OFF ON VACCINATIONS?** No! This is a common misconception of parents. Even if your baby has a minor illness, they can still get their shots. We cannot stress how important it is to get your child vaccinated in a timely manner. So don't let a sniffle or two make you reschedule an office visit for shots. Your child can also get their shots even if they are on antibiotics.

9 **CAN I CHOOSE NOT TO VACCINATE MY CHILD?** Yes, but we wouldn't advise it. Choosing not to vaccinate is not a risk-free choice. It's choosing to expose your child to potentially serious infection. It's also choosing to expose other children in your community to serious, preventable diseases. And if you think your child will be safe because everyone else vaccinates their kids, you'd be wrong (and very selfish, we might add). You can also choose not to stop at a stop sign, but we wouldn't advise it!

Reality Check
Vaccine requirements for school entry vary by state. There is no one consistent policy. All 50 states allow vaccine exemptions for medical reasons, 44 states allow exemptions for religious reasons and 15 states allow exemptions for philosophical

reasons. After a significant measles outbreak in 2015, California revoked its philosophical vaccine exemption law. Limiting the exemptions improves vaccination rates and thus, protects more children.

10 **I'VE HEARD THAT GETTING A DISEASE PROVIDES IMMUNITY FOREVER AND VACCINATIONS MIGHT NOT PROVIDE LIFELONG PROTECTION. WOULDN'T IT BE BETTER TO GET THE DISEASE? ISN'T THAT A MORE "NATURAL" WAY OF CREATING IMMUNITY?**

No.

The diseases we prevent by vaccination are not minor illnesses (this includes chickenpox). For instance, would you rather have your child get meningitis and die or get the vaccine? Getting chickenpox or any other disease the "natural way" is a much greater health risk without any significant benefit. And just think of the discomfort, pain and perhaps serious injury that come with getting any of these diseases.

It is true that some vaccinations require a booster dose to keep antibody levels high. That is why we need a tetanus booster every ten years. (And we are learning about boosters as we go with the COVID-19 vaccine.)

11 **WHAT WOULD HAPPEN IF WE STOPPED USING VACCINATIONS?** That's an easy one. The diseases would come back.

Vaccinations keep us from getting sick from these infections. But, all of the infections we protect against are alive and well in our world. As of today, the only disease we have completely eliminated is smallpox. And when it was eliminated, we stopped vaccinating for it.

Anyway, it's a simple fact: when immunization rates drop, epidemics occur. Just look at states with lower immunization rates—their rates of pertussis (whooping cough) are twice the number seen in states with higher percentages of immunization rates. Children whose parents opt out of vaccines face a 23 times greater risk of getting whooping cough. (*O'Brien*) In the 2019 measles outbreak (the largest and preventable outbreak in 25 years), 88% of the cases occurred in close knit, under-vaccinated communities. (*CDC*)

12 **WHAT ARE THE TYPICAL SIDE EFFECTS OF VACCINATION?** Fever, fussiness, redness or lump at the site of the injection.

Inactivated vaccines cause an immediate immune response. The body mounts a response to the foreign invader as if it were being infected. The result, typically, is a fever within 24 hours of vaccination. Babies sometimes feel like they are coming down with a cold or flu (body aches, pains). Some babies prefer to sleep through the experience; some choose to tell you how they feel (fussiness, crying). All of these symptoms resolve within 24 to 48 hours of vaccination.

Live attenuated vaccines (MMR, Varicella) cause a delayed immune response. This occurs one to four *weeks* after the vaccination is given. Long after the doctor's visit, your child may wake up one morning and have a fever. This may be accompanied by a rash that looks like measles (pimples) or chickenpox (clear, fluid filled pimples). The rash can sometimes be dramatic. Both the fever and the rash tell you that your baby is forming an immune response to the vaccination. Babies are not contagious and aren't too bothered by the rash. You don't need to call your doctor. This reaction is expected.

Redness at the injection site is common. In particular, the fifth booster dose of the DTaP (at ages four or five years) can cause a pretty dramatic area of redness. No worries. We do get quite a few phone calls about it, though! A firm lump may develop at the injection site if some of the fat in the arm/leg gets nicked as the needle goes into the muscle. This is called **FAT NECROSIS**. It usually goes away within six to eight weeks. It doesn't hurt.

RED FLAG

If your baby has a fever *more* than 72 hours after being vaccinated, it's not from the vaccination. You need to call your doctor. The only exceptions are the MMR and chickenpox vaccines, which typically cause a fever one to four weeks afterwards.

Reality Check

To help reduce fever and discomfort from shots, it's okay to give your baby acetaminophen (Tylenol) as long as you wait at least four hours after vaccinations are given. The dose is not listed on the package. It says to "consult a doctor." That's because doctors don't want you giving this medicine to a baby *three months or younger* with a fever without checking in first. Other than with shots, you need to call your doctor about fevers in this age group—see the section on fevers in Chapter 16, First Aid chapter.

13 **WHAT ARE THE WORST REACTIONS TO VACCINATION?** These are called adverse reactions. This is the equivalent of an allergic reaction to a medication—and fortunately, they are all quite rare. With each generation of newer vaccinations, the risk of serious reactions is almost eliminated. Adverse reactions include:

1. Death.
2. Anaphylactic reaction.
3. Encephalitis.
4. Fever related seizure (convulsions).

Both the CDC and FDA keep close tabs on adverse reactions to vaccines via a Vaccine Adverse Event Reporting System (VAERS). Both doctors and patient families may submit a VAERS form if any adverse reaction occurs.

Keep in mind that medical illness reports do not prove an association of a particular illness with a specific vaccination. The job of both the CDC and FDA is to review each report that occurs and see if there is a pattern of subsequent illness after vaccination. VAERS data is publicly available at vaers.hhs.gov. To report a possible reaction, you can download a form at the same site. There is also a Clinical Immunization Safety Assessment Network comprised of six U.S. academic medical centers that evaluate adverse reactions to vaccines (vaccinesafety.net).

While we would be remiss if we didn't tell you that vaccinations have some risks associated with them, we want you to remember that the risk of adverse reaction is *significantly* lower than leaving your baby unprotected.

In 1988, recognizing that there are rare, serious reactions that occur as a result of vaccinating children, the U.S. Department of Health and Human Services created the Vaccine Injury Compensation Program. This program attempts to determine whether adverse reactions from vaccines are responsible for injuries or death and then to provide the victim with compensation.

Over the past 30 years, there have been 8767 claimants whose cases were reviewed and

VACCINES

? ?

received compensation. Several billion doses of vaccinations covered by VICP have been given during that same period of time. So the odds are literally about 1 in 1 million to have a vaccine injury. (Compare that statistic to one in 50 adults who have a food allergy!)

We agree that an adverse reaction only has to happen to one child for it to be heartbreaking. But if we look at the big picture, we can point to the millions of children who might have experienced illness, chronic disability, and death if diseases like smallpox or polio were not controlled by vaccinations.

RED FLAGS

Call the doctor if your baby does the following after a vaccination:
1. Inconsolable crying over three hours.
2. Fever over 105 degrees.
3. Seizure activity.
4. Extreme lethargy.

14 **WHO KEEPS A RECORD OF MY CHILD'S VACCINATIONS?** You and your doctor. Your doctor keeps a record of vaccinations in your child's records.

Some states have an immunization registry that also keeps records of vaccinations. The pandemic has brought more attention to this issue.

But ultimately, YOU need to have a copy of these in your personal medical record file. You will need proof of vaccinations for many things. Any childcare or school program requires this information. Summer camps and athletic programs want the records too. And with the pandemic, proof of vaccination is required for some travel destinations as well.

Helpful Hint

It's a good idea to have a personal medical file for your child. This summary should include an immunization record, growth chart, list of medical problems, list of surgeries, drug allergies, and name and dosage of any medications that are used regularly (such as asthma medicine).

Q. How do I know when my child needs booster shots?

Your doctor will remind you at each well child visit.

You can also bookmark the vaccination schedule on the page nearby or go to the Centers for Disease Control website at CDC.gov/vaccines/

15 **WHAT VACCINES ARE REQUIRED AND WHICH ONES ARE OPTIONAL?** The answer varies state to state. It also varies depending on the frequency of disease in particular counties within a state. Check out your state health department's website for details.

Q. Can I take my baby out before they get their first set of shots?

The short answer: yes. The pandemic, however, makes this answer a bit more complicated. You have to consider all infectious disease exposures when you are out in public.

Pediatricians usually recommend limiting human contact with babies under four weeks of life. Why? Because if your newborn gets any fever (of 100.4 or greater), that is an automatic ticket to the hospital for two days (see Chapter 15, First Aid for details). Even if your baby has the cold that the rest of the household has, we still need to rule out a serious infection. That said, you don't have to live in a complete bubble, but use discretion when planning your outings. In cold and flu season (October through April) or during a COVID-19 surge, avoid crowded places for the first three months of life.

With respect to an unvaccinated baby, the biggest threat these days is whooping cough. Whooping cough is spread by cough and sneeze droplets of an infected person. Babies get a series of four shots over the first two years of life to protect them from whooping cough. To keep everyone inside that long is crazy! But being cautious until your baby gets their first shot at two months isn't a bad idea.

As for measles, many babies from 0-6 months of age are protected by mom's antibodies passed on to them during pregnancy. The measles vaccine is usually not given to children until 12-15 months of age when they will mount a good immune response to it. So,the most vulnerable group is babies from 6-11 months of age.

Reality Check

Although newborns are too young to be vaccinated, a pregnant mom can pass their immunity to diseases like pertussis, flu, and COVID-19 if they receive these vaccines during pregnancy. Nursing moms also pass their immunity to their babies via breast milk. These forms of passive immunity offer a layer of protection to a baby who is too young to be vaccinated against these infections.

Q. I have a friend who does not vaccinate their child. Is it okay for our babies to play together?

Awkward, right? As we go to press, there is a quite a difference of opinion surrounding the COVID-19 vaccine. And unfortunately it has led to divisiveness among families and friends. But this uncomfy situation about childhood vaccines pre-dated the pandemic.

The most politically correct thing to do would be cancel a playdate when either child is ill. This is not a foolproof solution, however. As we now know all too well, a person with COVID-19 may be symptom-free, very contagious, and may readily spread the infection to others. And a person with measles is contagious for three to four days before the rash erupts.

If you want to make a statement (and potentially lose the friendship), be honest and explain to your adult friend that you feel uncomfortable with your kids being together—then it is their responsibility to consider their choices.

Vaccination Schedule

The schedule for vaccinations is below. For details on these specific vaccines, see the next section. Note: If you want to know what shots your baby is due for, use the CDC's free Immunization Scheduler. Go to: www2a.cdc.gov/vaccines/childquiz/ and just type in your baby's birth date!

Disease And Vaccine Specifics

Let's talk specifics—here is a breakdown of the vaccines and the diseases they are designed to stop. View our website at Baby411.com for a visual library of these diseases (click on "Bonus Material").

Diphtheria, Tetanus, Pertussis

◆ **Diphtheria**: This is a *bacteria* that causes a serious throat infection. It invades the tonsils, kills the tissue, and creates a thick pus lining that can block off the airway. It also produces a toxin that enters the blood and injures the heart, kidneys, and nerves. It is spread by respiratory droplets (coughs and sneezes). There is a 10% mortality rate from infection, even today. Before the vaccine, up to 20,000 Americans died per year. If you want some entertaining historical perspective about this disease, read about the 1925 anti-toxin serum run led by heroic sled dogs (Balto and Togo) to save infected children in Nome, Alaska.

◆ **Tetanus**: This is a *bacteria* that causes wound infections. It is not contagious person to person. Tetanus bacteria produce spores that are found in the soil and dust around the world. These are resilient little germs, so we will never eliminate them. Tetanus spores can enter open wounds (especially puncture wounds, animal bites, and umbilical cord stumps) and make a toxin that

VACCINATION SCHEDULE

Birth	1 month	2 months	4 months	6 months	12 months	15 months	18 months	19–23 months	2–3 years	4–6 years
HepB	HepB			HepB						
		RV	RV	RV						
		DTaP	DTaP	DTaP		DTaP				DTaP
		Hib	Hib	Hib	Hib					
		PCV	PCV	PCV	PCV					
		IPV	IPV	IPV						IPV
				Influenza (Yearly)*						
					MMR					MMR
					Varicella					Varicella
					HepA§					

attacks nerves. The affected nerves cause muscles to spasm (called "tetany"). These spasms prevent breathing and swallowing (lockjaw). There is a 30% mortality rate from infection.

◆ **Pertussis (Whooping Cough):** This *bacteria* causes irritation and inflammation of the throat. This swelling prevents mucous from being coughed up and creates a blocked airway, particularly for those with the smallest airways (infants). Pertussis infection initially looks like the common cold. Over time, infected people have coughing fits or spasms. As a person tries to get a breath in, they make a characteristic "whoop." Infants, who have smaller airways, are unable to breathe at all. So instead of whooping, they stop breathing and their faces turn red or purple. Children often throw up during a coughing fit. This illness is known in some parts of the world as the "100 Day Cough." The infection is spread by respiratory droplets. Prior to vaccine development, there were 200,000 cases a year in the U.S. There were 10,000 deaths annually, mostly in infants. In the last major outbreak in 2012, there were over 42,000 cases reported in the U.S. and 20 deaths. Over 75% of the hospitalizations were in infants under six months of age and most of the deaths were in babies.

DTaP: The vaccine

This is the vaccine that protects against **D**iphtheria, **T**etanus, and **P**ertussis (whooping cough).

The combination vaccine has been around since the 1940's. The original vaccine (DTP) was called a "whole cell" vaccine because the vaccine was derived from a whole dead whooping cough germ. This vaccine was effective, but caused a significant number of high fevers and convulsions. A newer, safer formulation (called the "acellular" vaccine or DTaP vaccine) came out in 1991. The immune response is formed to a piece of the bacteria (its signature).

The primary vaccination series is five total doses. The primary doses are given at two, four, and six months of life. The fourth and fifth booster doses (given to toddlers and before kindergarten) are more likely to cause a fever or redness at the injection site because our bodies recognize it and have an immune response ready to go. After the fifth dose of DTaP, a single Tdap booster is given to 11-12 year olds and anyone else who has never received it. And as of 2012, pregnant women should get Tdap with each pregnancy primarily to provide passive immunity to their baby. The tetanus and diphtheria booster (Td) is then given every ten years.

Here is the tricky thing about pertussis protection—it is short lived, whether you endure the actual disease or get the vaccine. Immunity wears off after about five years. That leaves susceptible teens and adults as reservoirs of infection to expose infants who aren't fully protected yet. So it's important for moms, dads, and other adult caretakers (under age 65) to get their Tdap vaccine!

Q. Is it true that whooping cough epidemics still occur?

Yes. In fact, whooping cough is alive and well. In 2012, there were almost 42,000 cases and 20 deaths, most of them babies. Washington state, a hub of anti-vaccine sentiment, experienced 11% of these cases. In 2019, there were 18,617 cases in the U.S.

Here are some things you should know:

1. Whooping cough epidemics occur about every three to four years.
2. Immunity to whooping cough wanes in teens and adults despite vaccination during

childhood. The good news: a whooping cough vaccine for teens and adults is available. The bad news: protection from the vaccine only lasts about five years.

3. Many cases of whooping cough are undiagnosed and untreated in older people. Have you ever had a cough that just "hung on" for several weeks? You may have had whooping cough and not known it.

4. Dropping immunization rates allow the disease to spread quickly through a community.

5. Infants are given their first whooping cough (pertussis) vaccination at two months of age. But, they don't have effective protection against the disease until they have received three doses of the vaccine (at six months of life). Yes, it is the youngest children who are the most susceptible and unfortunately, they also have the highest risk of serious illness and death.

BOTTOM LINE: If you or anyone in the family has a chronic cough, get it checked out. It's important for you and your baby. And please get your baby vaccinated.

Polio

This *virus* attacks the spinal cord and brain. It has particular affinity for the nerves that control leg muscles and the diaphragm muscle (that helps you breathe). Polio infections leave people paralyzed, or needing a machine to breathe for them. Prior to our modern day ventilators, people survived the illness by living in iron lung machines. The virus spreads through the stool of infected people. This was a common summertime epidemic, and whole households would get the infection. Before the vaccine, there were 20,000 cases of paralysis per year in the U.S. Since 1979, there have been no cases of naturally occurring polio infection in the U.S. We still give the polio vaccine because the infection is an airplane flight away.

The top two countries where polio virus is still actively circulating (endemic) are: Pakistan, and Afghanistan. There are 28 countries with current polio outbreaks and 7 countries at-risk due to low immunization rates. But thanks to the extraordinary effort of the Global Polio Eradication Initiative, we may be able to eradicate the disease, like smallpox. Efforts were put on hold during early pandemic lockdowns, though.

While this may happen in our lifetime, polio is still a threat.

Polio: the Vaccine

In the U.S., we give the inactivated form of the vaccine (a shot). The vaccine that was given from 1963-1996 was a live vaccine (a drink) that carried a small risk of acquiring vaccine-associated polio disease.

There were a few cases annually of vaccine associated polio disease when the live (oral) vaccine was used. In 1997, doctors switched to an all-inactivated vaccination series (IPV; that is, not live). IPV does not cause polio disease.

Polio vaccine is a four-dose series. The first doses are given at two and four months of age. The third dose is given at 6-18 months. The final dose is given before entering kindergarten.

Haemophilus Influenza B (Hib)

This is a *bacteria* that causes a potentially fatal throat swelling (epiglottitis) and **MENINGITIS** (infection of the brain lining). Despite the name, there is no relationship to influenza, the flu virus—yes, we realize that is confusing. HIB is spread by respiratory droplets (sneezing, coughing). Prior to vaccine development, there were 20,000 cases of HIB infection annually in the U.S. and 500 deaths. Most infections occurred in children less than five years old. Survivors of meningitis may be permanently deaf, blind, or intellectually disabled. About 5% of children with HIB infections die, and 20% suffer permanent disability.

HIB: The vaccine

The development of the HIB vaccine is a true success story of modern-day medicine. The vaccine was licensed in 1985. By 1992, HIB infections were virtually eliminated (less than 200 cases per year). Doctors who were in training or practice prior to 1992 literally watched this disease disappear. Younger doctors have never seen a case of HIB in their careers!

The HIB vaccine can be given either individually (in three or four doses) or in a combination product. Children form a good immunity with either of these products.

According to the CDC immunization schedule, babies complete a primary series of vaccinations for HIB at two, four, and six months of age. A HIB booster dose is given to toddlers at 12-15 months.

Measles, Mumps, Rubella

◆ **Measles:** This is a *virus* that infects the entire body. Infected people start out with cold symptoms and pink eye. It causes a dramatic head-to-toe rash, then the infection spreads to other organ systems. These include the intestines (diarrhea), lungs (pneumonia), and brain (encephalitis). The highest rate of these complications is in children under age five.

The virus is highly contagious and is spread through respiratory droplets (coughs and sneezes). The virus is so hearty, it can remain alive and infectious in the air and on surfaces for up to two hours.

Measles was as common as chickenpox used to be. Before the measles vaccine, there were an amazing four million cases per year and 500 deaths per year in the U.S. Today, measles is more common in other countries (particularly England, Germany, Austria, Italy, Australia, Switzerland, Israel, China, Vietnam, Thailand, Philippines), and international travel easily brings it to America.

Before the Great Measles Reboot of 2019, 2015 saw one of the largest U.S. measles outbreaks that began with an unvaccinated, measles-infected person visiting a mecca for children worldwide—Disneyland. Other visitors and Disney employees contracted the illness from this incidental exposure. There were 188 cases in 24 states, and 30% of patients had to be hospitalized for complications. Hollywood could not have written a better script! It served as a chilling reminder that unvaccinated people do not wear nametags and may unknowingly spread potentially fatal diseases. It truly is a small world after all.

But let's face it, the Disneyland-measles fiasco was nothing compared to 2019. There were 1282 cases of measles in the U.S., in 31 states. 90% of the infections occurred in unvaccinated

vaccinations

? ?

VACCINES

people or those with unknown vaccination status.

◆ *Mumps*: This is a *virus* that attacks the salivary glands. Mumps infect the glands located along the jaw line and causes a marked swelling. It also infects other body parts that swell up, including the testicles, ovaries, and brain. Mumps attacks the brain (meningitis) about 15% of the time. It can cause deafness and intellectual disability in survivors. Like measles, mumps is spread through respiratory droplets. Before the mumps vaccine was developed, there were up to 200,000 cases per year. We usually see fewer than 600 cases a year in the U.S. However, there were almost 3500 cases in 2019. The current vaccine is about 88% effective in preventing mumps disease. *(CDC)*

DR B'S OPINION

Even today, there is no treatment for measles. If you'd rather let your child get the measles than give them the shot to prevent it, you've never seen measles!

◆ *Rubella* (**GERMAN MEASLES**): This is a highly contagious *virus* that causes mild infection in children, but fatal or disabling infection in unborn fetuses. Rubella spreads through respiratory droplets and causes a runny nose, swollen glands, and a rash in children. If a pregnant woman gets rubella, the fetus can die in the womb (miscarriage) or be born with severe intellectual disability, deafness, or blindness (called congenital rubella syndrome). An epidemic in 1964 (prior to the rubella vaccine) affected 20,000 babies. The good news: For a decade now, there have been less than ten cases per year in the United States, and all people were infected during travel or living outside the U.S. We need to continue vaccinating since this disease is not eliminated worldwide.

MMR: the vaccine

The vaccines for measles, mumps and rubella are given together as the MMR vaccine. In the past, these vaccines were also manufactured separately. Since 2009, the only vaccine product on the market is the combination MMR vaccine.

Because the MMR vaccine is a live-attenuated vaccine, your child may develop a rash that looks like measles (red pimples) and/or a fever, one to four weeks after being vaccinated. There are two shots in the MMR vaccination series. The first dose is given at 12-15 months of age. A booster dose is given before entering kindergarten.

About 90-95% of people mount a lifelong immune response to the first dose of the vaccine. The second dose is given to protect 5-10% of people who did not mount a great response with the first dose. That said, the second dose of MMR vaccine can be given just four weeks after the first dose in times of an outbreak.

The MMR vaccine can also be given to infants from 6-11 months of age if they will be visiting a country where measles is more prevalent. Any MMR vaccine given prior to one year of age does not count as part of the two dose series.

Babies under one year of age do not mount a very good immune response to the MMR vaccine, which is why the standard recommendation is to administer it between 12-15 months of age. However, some protection is better than no protection during an outbreak. If there is a significant risk of exposure, the CDC/local health department may advise early and additional vaccination.

Hepatitis A

This *virus* attacks the liver. And there is a vaccine to prevent it. It's spread through infected poop, contaminated water and food. It spreads rapidly in childcare centers due to all the kids in diapers. Fortunately, children infected with Hepatitis A have a relatively minor illness. Some children don't even have symptoms. Adults, however, get very sick. Prior to the Hepatitis A vaccine, there were over 100,000 cases per year in the U.S.

In 2017-18, the homeless population of San Diego experienced a Hepatitis A outbreak with over 600 cases and 20 deaths.

Hepatitis A: the vaccine

The Hepatitis A vaccine was approved in 1995 and became part of the routine childhood immunization series in 2005. Vaccinating toddlers against Hepatitis A not only protects them but also prevents the spread of the disease to others in childcare centers. The vaccine is very effective: Israel saw a 98.5% reduction in disease since they began Hepatitis A universal vaccination.

Kids get the vaccine starting at age one. It is a series of two doses given at least six months apart.

Hepatitis B

This is another *virus* that attacks the liver. There are various types of Hepatitis. The most note-worthy are A, B, and C. Each type of virus is spread differently. Hepatitis B is spread through blood and body fluid (saliva, vaginal discharge, and semen) contact. It is extremely contagious. Yes, it is spread primarily by sexual contact and by exposure in the healthcare field. However, children are most at risk of exposure to Hepatitis B during birth if their mother has the disease.

The infection causes skin to turn yellow because the liver is unable to metabolize bilirubin as it should (see earlier in this book for a discussion of bilirubin). It causes stomach upset and lack of appetite. Some people with Hepatitis B recover quickly, while others die. Others have a chronic infection that goes on for 20 years until they die. And some people become carriers of the disease once they survive the infection.

Don't think of this disease as one that only happens to IV drug users or people with several sex partners. Of people who get Hepatitis B, 16% have neither of these risk factors.

Reality Check

There are over *1 million* Hepatitis B carriers walking around the U.S.

If this isn't enough to convince you to protect your child, Hepatitis B also is a known cause of liver cancer. Yes, the Hepatitis B vaccine is the first cancer vaccine. Before the vaccine became part of the childhood immunization series in 1991, 30,000 children were infected with Hepatitis B annually in the U.S.

Hepatitis B: The vaccine

Giving the vaccine as a part of the childhood immunization program ensures that your child gets immunized and has lifelong protection. Babies born to mothers who have Hepatitis B need to get the vaccination and immunoglobulin shot within 12 hours of birth to prevent infection. If they don't get these shots, newborns who get infected by their moms have a 90% chance of getting Hepatitis B.

The Hepatitis B vaccine is a three-dose series. The first dose is routinely given before hospital discharge. The second dose is given one or two months later. The third dose is given six to 18 months after the first dose.

Varicella (Chickenpox)

Before routine use of chickenpox vaccine in 1995, about four million people got chickenpox every year in the U.S. Some of you reading this book probably remember having this illness. *What most of you don't know is that chickenpox also led to 10,000 hospitalizations and 100 deaths annually.*

The varicella virus spreads by respiratory droplets and by the fluid found in the skin lesions. It is incredibly contagious. The virus attacks the whole body via the bloodstream. Infected people feel tired and run a fever, then break out in classic clear fluid-filled blisters that arrive in clusters. The average number of skin lesions is 350. Does it make you feel itchy just thinking about it? People are contagious for seven days, on average.

The virus itself can cause pneumonia and encephalitis. Even more problematic is that Strep bacteria have a field day with the open wounds when the blisters pop. These secondary infections can be deadly.

The vaccine has prevented 95% of severe chickenpox infections. And in kids under nine years of age, death from chickenpox is down by a whopping 90%. And vaccinated people who get chickenpox despite the vaccine have a very mild illness (less than 50 pox; occasional fever; lasts for just a few days).

Varicella (Chickenpox): The vaccine

The varicella vaccine is a live-attenuated vaccine. Hence, it contains a weakened form of the germ that causes chickenpox. As a result, some children will get a rash that looks like chickenpox one to four weeks after being vaccinated.

Some parents wonder if a recently vaccinated child can spread chickenpox to someone else (particularly someone who has an immune deficiency). Since the chickenpox vaccine came out in 1995, millions of people have been vaccinated. There have been *three* documented cases of vaccine-associated chickenpox. The risk is so low that even if your child develops a rash after their shot, they can still attend daycare. (*Pickering*)

There is a small risk of getting shingles (reactivated chickenpox) later in life. Evidence suggests that you are more likely to get shingles if you get the actual disease than if you have been vaccinated.

Parents also wonder if the vaccine will provide lifelong protection. While we don't have an entire generation's worth of data, we do have data on people who participated in the original studies of this vaccine dating back to 1975—and yes, those people have shown good immunity.

The American Academy of Pediatrics and Centers for Disease Control recommend two doses of vaccine for the most complete protection. The first dose is given at 12-15 months and the booster dose is given at 4-6 years, in preparation for kindergarten. Can adults get the

DR B'S OPINION:
CHICKENPOX CAN BE DEADLY

During my residency, I cared for a patient with chickenpox who came to our emergency room with a secondary Strep infection—the child died two hours later. That experience has left an impact on me. When parents perceive that chickenpox is just a minor illness, I tell them that story.

chickenpox vaccine? Yes, the varicella vaccine should be given to anyone over a year of age who has never had chickenpox.

Strep Pneumoniae

This is a *bacteria* that is in the Strep family. It is not the Strep that causes Strep throat. It's a distant cousin. This bacteria causes meningitis, pneumonia, blood infections (sepsis), sinus infections, and ear infections. The Prevnar vaccine protects against the top 20 strains of Strep pneumoniae (there are 90 total) that cause serious infection.

Respiratory droplets spread the bacteria. Once the bugs get in, they head for the respiratory system (ears, sinuses, lungs) or the brain. They travel via the blood en route to these places. Infected people run a high fever when the bacteria are in the bloodstream. Fortunately, many infections are treated before meningitis occurs. Prior to the Prevnar vaccine, there were over 16,000 cases of serious Strep pneumoniae infections a year in American children under age five. In babies, Strep pneumoniae is the #1 cause of bacterial meningitis. The highest risk groups for serious infection are infants and the elderly.

There are antibiotics to treat Strep pneumoniae, however, doctors are seeing more drug-resistant strains. It's survival of the fittest for germs—and these germs are some of the smartest around. Twenty percent of the Strep pneumoniae strains in the vaccine are resistant to Penicillin. Ten percent are resistant to three OR MORE types of antibiotics. Daycare children are at higher risk for Strep pneumoniae infection, particularly the drug-resistant strains.

Strep pneumoniae (Prevnar or PCV 20): The vaccine

Prevnar is recommended as part of the routine immunization schedule by the American Academy of Pediatrics. There has been an 87% reduction in serious Strep pneumoniae disease (meningitis, blood and pneumonia infections) since the immunization program began in 2000. Interestingly, we have also seen a 50% reduction in pneumonia in the elderly since there is less Strep out there.

Prevnar is a four dose series. The first three doses are given at two, four, and six months of age. A booster dose is given at 12-15 months.

Insider Secret

There are three vaccines that protect against different causes of bacterial meningitis: Prevnar/PCV 20 (20 strains of Strep pneumonia), HIB (Haemophilus influenza B), and

Vaccinations

MCV 4 (4 strains of Neisseria meningitides). Babies receive Prevnar and HIB vaccines as part of the routine immunization series. Preteens (11-12 year olds) routinely receive MCV 4, but babies with compromised immune systems can also get this vaccine starting at nine months of age.

Rotavirus

Rotavirus is a *virus* that comes to visit every winter.

Doctors always know rotavirus has arrived in a community. The littlest patients come into the office with so much watery diarrhea that parents cannot keep up with diaper changes. The vomiting part is pretty miserable, too. Because there is so much water lost in the poop, infants are at high risk of becoming dehydrated.

Before widespread vaccine use in 2006, Rotavirus infection caused about 50,000 hospitalizations of young American children every winter. There were also about 30 deaths per year in the U.S. from rotavirus. Worldwide, rotavirus kills 440,000 kids every year.

You can see why docs have long wanted a vaccine for this disease! Looking at data on diarrhea season (that's a fun job, eh), it's clear that rotavirus vaccine has made a significant impact in reducing the number and severity of cases. (*CDC*)

Rotavirus: The vaccine

The FDA approved the rotavirus vaccine (called Rotateq) back in 2006. It's a live, attenuated vaccine given in the form of oral drops at two, four, and six months of age. Rotarix, another FDA approved rotavirus vaccine, is a two-dose oral drops series.

The most common side effect of the rotavirus vaccine is mild diarrhea within a week. Past rotavirus vaccines had a very rare, nasty side effect: bowel obstruction (intussusception). However, since the vaccine came out, tens of millions of doses been given worldwide and results are promising—the risk of bowel obstruction is no greater in vaccinated babies than in the general population. Nonetheless, parents should be looking out for severe abdominal pain/irritability or blood in the poop/grape jelly poop after vaccination.

One word of caution: rotavirus vaccine is a live vaccine. Babies cannot receive the vaccine if they have a rare immune disorder called Severe Combined Immune Deficiency (SCID). And if any caretaker is immune-compromised (for example, on chemotherapy) there is a theoretical risk of an adult getting the disease from exposure to the vaccinated baby's stool. About 9% of babies will shed the weakened virus in their poop four to six days after the first dose of the vaccine. Less than 0.3% shed it after the second or third doses. Let your doc know and you can discuss your individual situation.

Influenza (Flu)

This is another *virus* we see every winter. It is an infection that attacks the respiratory tract. Worse than the common cold, flu causes higher fevers, body aches, headaches, and a crummy feeling in general. The runny nose and cough arrive later and last longer than a typical cold. Secondary bacterial infections (ear infections, sinus infections, pneumonia) occur more often with the flu than with your garden-variety cold virus.

Besides being generally unpleasant to endure, the flu can be deadly. The highest risk groups for serious health complications from the flu are children under two years of age and adults over age 65.

Influenza: The vaccine

Seven states currently require flu vaccine for preschool. You can find that list here: immunize.org/laws/flu_childcare.asp. Yep, you can't go to preschool there without proof of being vaccinated against the flu. Considering flu is the most common vaccine-preventable disease, and kids under age five are at risk for severe illness, it makes sense.

The Centers for Disease Control's recommendations for "Who should get flu vaccine?" are: EVERYONE who is six months old and up. But here are the people who are most at risk:

1. 50-years or older.
2. Immune-compromised (weak immune systems)
3. Suffering from chronic illness (asthma, heart disease, diabetes), age six months old or older.
4. Health care workers.
5. Pregnant women during flu season (November-March).
6. Children ages six months old to 18 years old.
7. Household contacts and caretakers of any child aged birth to five years.

The flu vaccine currently used for kids under two years of age is an inactivated vaccine, in the form of a shot. They won't get the flu from it. It provides immunity two weeks after getting the vaccine. The vaccine is effective for one year. The particular influenza virus strains that show up every year is different, so we have to get vaccinated for the new bugs in town each autumn.

Kids under nine years of age who get the flu vaccine for the first time need two doses given one month apart.

Currently, there is only one flu vaccine that is "preservative free" and allowed for use in infants as young as six months old. It's called Fluzone (Aventis Pasteur). The other flu vaccines contain a trace amount of thimerosal (0.025 milligrams per dose). However, the acceptable limit of exposure is over 12 times this dose (0.2-0.4mg). See the section "Controversies" later in this chapter for more information on thimerosal.

Reality check

Every spring, the World Health Organization determines the three or four strains of influenza virus that are most likely to show up in the Northern hemisphere in the upcoming winter flu season (based on those circulating in the Southern hemisphere). So each year, the seasonal flu vaccine protects against three or four different types of flu. That's why the flu vaccine is slightly different every year.

Q. I'm pregnant. Is it safe for me to get the flu vaccine?

YES! And, it will protect both you and your unborn baby.

The flu shot (not the nasal spray) is FDA approved for pregnant women during ANY trimester of pregnancy.

Pregnant women are at greater risk of complications from the flu because their bodies are in a functionally immune-compromised state (which allows the body to let a fetus with foreign DNA grow inside of her). So protection via vaccination is pretty important.

Moms-to-be who get their flu vaccine also protect their babies, once they are born. In fact, newborns and infants whose moms got flu vaccine during pregnancy have a 40% lower chance of being hospitalized for flu. (*Eick*)

Reality check

This advice also applies to the COVID-19 vaccine. Protect yourself and your unborn baby.

COVID-19

This virus really needs no introduction but . . . a novel type of coronavirus, called severe acute respiratory syndrome coronavirus 2 (SARS-CoV-2) or its nickname, COVID-19, entered our world for the first time in China in late 2019.

Shortly after the first positive case was identified in the U.S., the World Health Organization declared "a public health emergency of international concern" on January 30, 2020. There are many other viruses in the coronavirus family which infect humans as well as other animals. But COVID-19 is unique in how incredibly contagious and easily transmissible it is to others and just how serious the infection can be. The virus is spread via respiratory droplets that stay suspended in the air for a period of time. Infected people are contagious two days prior to symptoms—this then declines over a period of several days.

As of press time, it is difficult to quantify how many cases have occurred worldwide as more people are doing home COVID-19 testing. But there are over 464 million cases worldwide and over 6 million deaths in the record books due to this nasty virus. There are likely far more cases than that.

Children generally have milder cases of illness, but severe cases and deaths do occur. See Chapter 13, Common Infections, for more information on the COVID-19 disease.

COVID: The vaccine

As this book goes to press, there are two mRNA vaccines (Pfizer-BioNTech and Moderna brands) and one nonreplicating viral vector vaccine (Johnson and Johnson) which the FDA has approved for use in the U.S. The Pfizer-BioNTech mRNA pediatric vaccine is currently approved for use in children ages 5 and up. Studies are still underway for children ages 6 months and up. Stay up to date on the latest information at our online community.

Because mRNA vaccine is the only type approved for use in children, we will limit discussion to that vaccine.

Q. How does the mRNA vaccine work?

The mRNA is a tiny code or recipe that gives the body instructions to produce one very specific part of the COVID-19 virus called the "spike protein." Once our body produces that protein, our immune system sees that protein and mounts antibodies to it. The mRNA then gets broken down very quickly in the human body and is eliminated. That is the unique part of this particular vaccine. Like all other vaccines, our body makes antibodies before seeing an actual threat of virus/bacteria, so when we do encounter it, we recognize it, and prevent it from causing infection at all or causing serious infection.

Q. Can someone get COVID-19 infection from the vaccine?

No. There is no virus in this vaccine. You do not become infected by getting the vaccine and you cannot spread infection to others by receiving the vaccine.

Q. How long will vaccine immunity last and will it prevent infection entirely?

Great questions. We know the vaccination series (2-4 doses currently, depending on the age group and at-risk groups) offers excellent protection against severe disease. It keeps people out of the ICU—or the morgue, as vaccine expert Dr. Paul Offit would say. How long does the immunity last? How many doses of vaccine are optimal? Do we need a pan-coronavirus vaccine that covers multiple types of spike proteins? We don't know. More study is needed.

Q. Is it better to get natural immunity?

No. Getting vaccinated is a safer way to build your immunity. If you do get the infection, yes, you will have some immunity after recovering from the disease. The amount of immunity varies with the severity of the illness. And it appears that immunity wanes over time with either natural or vaccine-induced immunity. Either way, people don't seem to get a lifelong immunity card.

Q. Should I worry that a mRNA vaccine has never been used before?

No. This technology has been used for over a decade as a cancer treatment. It is just new to the infectious disease space. The initial concern (prior to the formal vaccine research studies)was whether it would provide an adequate immune response—it was already felt to be very safe after a decade of experience with it.

Q. If someone had COVID-19 infection, can they still get the vaccine?

Yes. Natural infection will not lead to lifelong immunity, but it may provide a few months of protection. There is no need to test for prior infection before getting the vaccine. You should not get the vaccine while you have an active infection with COVID-19 or if you have been recently exposed and in a period of quarantine.

Q. If my child is eligible to get the COVID-19 vaccine, should they get it?

Yes. The way I view it: the virus is the wild card, not the vaccine. There is more risk and uncertainty about COVID-19 disease than the side effects and very rare adverse reactions to the

? ?

VACCINES

vaccine. While most cases of COVID-19 infection are milder in children than in adults, over 1000 children have died in the pandemic thus far. COVID-19 infection can also lead to a serious complication called multisystem inflammatory syndrome (MIS-C) and long-term health issues, even when the initial illness seems minor.

It is true that we don't have a decade or two of experience with this new vaccine. But, since December 2020, over 11 BILLION people have gotten the vaccine. (*Bloomberg*) If there was a significant safety issue, we would have already seen it. And adverse reactions to any vaccine primarily occur within a 60-day window after receiving it--not months or years later. Despite what you may hear, the mechanics of the mRNA technology have no plausible way to cause infertility!

Controversies

Let's face it, controversy drives TV ratings, web traffic, and Spotify subscriptions. No one is interested in hearing about things that work as they should—and vaccines are a good example. Vaccines have been a hot topic for the last two decades. Unfortunately, rare adverse events and theoretical concerns tend to make more headlines and clickbait than the remarkable success story of vaccinations. These problems are then seized on by vaccine opponents and spread online through the web like a, well, virus.

So, let's address this head on. We have compiled the hit parade of controversies you might hear about with vaccines:.

Let's begin with the most recent ones related to the COVID-19 vaccine:

COVID-19 Vaccine

Q. Does COVID-19 vaccine cause infertility?

No. There is not a plausible way for this to occur.

The fear mongering began when a couple of research scientists in Europe speculated out loud that a protein on the surface of the placenta called syncytin-1 was similar to the COVID-19 spike protein. The hypothesis: if someone mounted an immune response to the spike protein, the immune system would also attack the placenta and lead to a miscarriage.

But there are several flaws with this hypothesis. First, the two proteins are not that similar! Next, the animal studies done on COVID-19 vaccine before the human trials began showed no impact on the reproductive system. And when women of childbearing age participated in the COVID-19 vaccine studies and accidentally became pregnant (oops), the miscarriage rate between vaccinated and unvaccinated participants was no different. Finally, natural infection with COVID-19 also creates an immune response to the spike protein. There has not been a decrease in the birth rates since the pandemic began.

Q. Will the mRNA alter our genetic code?

No. The mRNA is basically a self-destructing recipe for our bodies to make what looks like the coronavirus spike protein. The mRNA is very unstable—meaning it disintegrates quickly,

? ?

VACCINES

which is why it needs to be so darn cold and packaged in fat (lipid nanoparticle) to remain stable and enter your body. But once it has done the job, it is gone. To take you back to 7th grade science class, the mRNA enters the cytoplasm of our cells, not the nucleus where our DNA resides. It is not even remotely capable of entering our DNA and altering our genes.

Q. Is it possible to implant a microchip through a vaccine syringe?

Um, no. We won't even try to tackle the disinformation narrative behind this question! But, suffice it to say that a COVID-19 vaccine is injected with a 22-gauge needle that has an internal diameter of 0.41 millimeters. A 5G microchip is significantly larger than that. Now, a tiny RFID chip might fit, but the coil antenna (that makes it functional) is also significantly larger than the needle diameter. Bottom line: if you don't want anyone to track you, get rid of your smartphone!

Does MMR Cause Autism?

Q. I've heard that the MMR vaccine might cause autism. Is this true?

No.

Spend a little time online and you'll find theories that vaccinations cause autism . . . as well as multiple sclerosis, diabetes, asthma, and SIDS. None of these are caused by vaccination. The government operates a safety monitoring system (VAERS, FDA, CDC)—watching for any possible adverse effects from vaccines. *No one wants to increase autism rates.*

One small case report of only eight patients in 1998 led a research group to feel that the combination MMR vaccine might cause autism. (*Wakefield*) But don't try to find the article online because the journal that published the article later retracted it when a former member of the research lab revealed that the data reported in the study was fabricated! (*Newsweek.com*) Twelve years later, the lead author lost his license to practice medicine in England and was accused of fraud. The whole thing was a hoax.

Before this came to light, several reputable scientists tried to replicate the findings of this now discredited researcher. No one ever could—and now we know why!

Unfortunately, frightened parents chose to skip the MMR vaccine and measles epidemics occurred both in England and the U.S. as a result of these unfounded claims.

Bottom line: Talk to your child's doctor about any vaccine safety concerns.

Q. If the MMR vaccine doesn't cause autism, why is the diagnosis made around the same time as the vaccination?

One of the criteria used to make a diagnosis of autism is a language delay. Because children do not have significant expressive language under a year of age, doctors have to wait until 15 to 18 months to confirm a language delay and make the diagnosis. That's about the same time as the MMR vaccination, which leads some parents to wonder about autism and vaccination.

DR B'S OPINION: TIME TO MOVE ON

Vaccines have received intense scrutiny over the past twenty years in the search for a cause of autism. The best scientific minds, worldwide, have looked for a link and none has been found. We want you to realize that a) science has devoted much brainpower, time and money to this concern and has concluded there is no link and b) many families with a child who has autism do not feel that vaccines have anything to do with their child's disorder.

Rotavirus

Q. I've heard about a vaccine that was taken off the market. What was the problem with it? It makes me nervous about other new vaccines.

The original rotavirus vaccine was approved in August 1998 after a study was done on 10,000 individuals. It looked like a safe vaccine. That vaccine was then given to 1.5 million children over a period of nine months. During this time, there were 15 reports of bowel obstruction (intussusception) that occurred within a week of being vaccinated. There were no deaths. The CDC immediately pulled the vaccine off the market and initiated an investigation.

Although this was certainly a setback for new vaccinations, it proves that the adverse events reporting system (VAERS) works. Modifications have been made to the license process as a result of the rotavirus vaccine. This was the first vaccine recall in over 20 years.

As we mentioned earlier in the chapter, a newer rotavirus vaccine debuted in 2006—it was studied in 70,000 infants in Latin America and Europe before getting the nod by the FDA. After several years of use, this vaccine has clearly proven to be very safe. But given the history of the previous rotavirus vaccine, the FDA still closely monitors for any cases of bowel obstruction.

The Thimerosal (Mercury) Controversy

Q. I've heard there is mercury preservative in the vaccines. Is this true?

Not anymore. It was removed from all required childhood vaccines 20 years ago. This deserves repeating: *YOUR baby will not be getting required vaccines that contain mercury (thimerosal) as a preservative.*

Despite the fact that vaccines have been mercury preservative-free for about 20 years, speculation persists about vaccines *previously* containing mercury and links to autism. This speculation continues even after the Institute of Medicine published a conclusive report in 2004 negating any association between vaccines and autism. (The IOM spent four years studying both the mercury question and the MMR combo vaccine question and published a series of eight reports on the subject).

Q. Should I still ask my doctor if the vaccines for my baby are thimerosal-free?

We think you should ask as many questions as you need to feel comfortable. Remember that the entire childhood vaccine series went thimerosal (mercury) preservative-free 20 years ago. If your doctor has a 2001 vintage vaccine vial sitting on the shelf (which would be long expired by now), I'd have bigger concerns about your doc than their vaccine supply.

Here are the specific rules regarding thimerosal use in vaccines: the FDA requires manufacturers of *routine* childhood immunizations to no longer use thimerosal as a *preservative*. This rule does NOT apply to flu vaccine because (technically) this vaccination is optional (except in seven states) and not "routine."

Why does flu vaccine need thimerosal or any other preservative? First, understand the flu vaccine is reformulated every year to reflect the anticipated flu strains. Since millions of doses of flu vaccine are needed every year, the most efficient way to produce the shot is in multi-dose vials, which require a preservative.

Hence, *some* flu shots (not the flu nasal spray) contain the preservative thimerosal. However, there are single-dose preparations of flu vaccine that are mercury preservative-free. These can be given to young children and pregnant women. Ask your doctor for a thimerosal-free flu vaccine if you are concerned.

Q. Are there other additives in the vaccines?

Yes. And you should know about them.

As we have already discussed, vaccines contain the active ingredients that provide immunity. But there are inactive ingredients that improve potency and prevent contamination. Below is a list of additives and why they are there. These products are present in trace amounts and none have been proven harmful in animals or humans. (*Offit*)

◆ Preservatives: Prevent vaccine contamination with germs (bacteria, fungus). Example: 2-phenoxyethanol, phenol, (thimerosal, prior to 2001).
◆ Adjuvants: Improve potency/immune response. Example: aluminum salts.
◆ Additives: Prevent vaccine deterioration and sticking to the side of the vial. Examples: Gelatin, Albumin, Sucrose, Lactose, MSG, glycine.
◆ Residuals: Remains of vaccine production process. Examples: Formaldehyde, Antibiotics (Neomycin), Egg Protein, Yeast Protein.

See our web site (Baby411.com, click on "Bonus Material") for a list of ingredients for the routine childhood vaccination series.

Reality Check

If vaccines contain ingredients like aluminum or formaldehyde, wouldn't it be better if vaccine makers got rid of these additives? Shouldn't vaccines be "greener"?

This is a red herring argument against vaccines—current vaccines are safe, even with tiny/trace amounts of preservatives or additives like aluminum. And your baby is exposed to many of these ingredients every day . . . simply by eating or breathing.

Q. Why is formaldehyde in vaccines?

Small amounts of formaldehyde are used to sterilize the vaccine fluid so your child doesn't get something like flesh-eating Strep bacteria when they get their shots.

We know when you think of formaldehyde, that ever-present smell wafting from the anatomy lab in high school comes to mind. But what you probably don't know is that formaldehyde is also a naturally occurring substance in your body. And if you use baby shampoo, paper towels or mascara, or have carpeting in your home, you've been exposed to formaldehyde. The small amount used in vaccines is not a health concern. (*Dept of Health and Human Services*)

Q. Is it true that anti-freeze is used in vaccines?

No.

There is a chemical used in some vaccines (called polyethylene glycol) that is also found in antifreeze, as well as toothpaste, lubricant eyedrops and various skin care creams.

ALUMINUM 411

Now that the mercury (thimerosal) saga is coming to an end, anti-vaccine crusaders have come up with a new bad guy: aluminum. Yes, trace amounts of aluminum salts are used in some childhood vaccines. Here's all you need to know (and more) about aluminum. Bottom line: we are not worried about it. Here's the 411:

Aluminum is everywhere. It's one of the most common metals in our earth's crust. So it is naturally present in our water, soil, and even in the air. Fruits, vegetables, nuts, flour, cereal, dairy products, and yes, even baby formula and breast milk… all contain some aluminum. Do you wear antiperspirant? It's in there, too. To avoid aluminum exposure, you'd have to quit wearing antiperspirant . . . and basically leave the planet.

Why is aluminum used in vaccines? Aluminum enhances the immune system's response to the vaccine. It's been used safely for several decades. By using aluminum salts, some inactivated vaccines require fewer booster shots for the body to mount an adequate immune response.

Are there any health concerns with aluminum in vaccines? No. There is significantly less aluminum in vaccines than what babies are exposed to in the environment. Both the National Vaccine Program Office and the World Health Organization have determined that the aluminum content in the childhood vaccination series is safe. Humans rapidly eliminate aluminum salts from the body. The small amount of aluminum that accumulates in human brains (about 50-100 mcg in an adult brain) comes from food sources. (*Mitkus*)

Does aluminum poisoning cause autism? No. People with aluminum poisoning have bone problems (osteomalacia) and anemia, as well as neurologic issues. These include memory loss, fatigue, depression, behavioral changes, and learning impairment. Aluminum has also been proposed as the cause of Alzheimer's Disease. To date, however, there is little evidence that aluminum causes that disorder. (*Dept of Health and Human Services*)

? ?

VACCINES

Polyethylene glycol is used in the production process to purify vaccines (it is used in one flu vaccine, and mRNA COVID-19 vaccines, among others).

Q. Is it safer to delay vaccines or space them out?

Easy answer: no. Any "alternative" vaccination schedule is more appropriately termed "delayed vaccinations"—because it truly is a delay in getting protected.

The CDC publishes a recommended vaccine schedule for American children. Many, many doctors, scientists, and researchers work together with the CDC to decide what is the best timing to give shots. The goal: protect babies as soon as it is safe and effective to do so. This schedule was not created out of thin air.

How much aluminum is in vaccines? Very little. If your baby follows the standard immunization schedule, they is exposed to about **four to six mg** of aluminum at six months of life. By comparison, they are also exposed to **10 mg** of aluminum if they are breastfed, **40 mg** if they are fed cow's milk-based formula, or **120 mg** if they are fed soy formula. None of these are very large amounts, by the way. To put things in perspective, there's about 200mg of aluminum in a standard antacid tablet. In fact, the average adult ingests seven to nine mg of aluminum everyday. Here's a look at how much aluminum is in breast milk/formula, compared to vaccines:

Amount of aluminum exposure (milligrams per liter) (*Vaccine Education Center*)

	AMOUNT OF ALUMINUM
Breast milk	0.01–0.05 mg/L
Cow's milk based infant formula	0.06–0.15 mg/L
Soy based infant formula	0.46–0.93mg/L
Prevnar vaccine	0.125 mg/dose
DTaP vaccine	0.17–0.625 mg/dose
HIB vaccine	0.225 mg/dose
Hep A vaccine	0.225–0.25 mg/dose
Hep B vaccine	0.25–0.5 mg/dose
DTaP/IPV/HIB vaccine	1.5 mg/dose

Is it a good idea to space out vaccinations that contain aluminum salts? No. Since aluminum-containing vaccines do not cause any health risk, separating or spacing out these vaccines has no benefit. In fact, there is a risk to spacing out the vaccines—your baby will go unprotected against real vaccine-preventable disease.

Sketchy anti-vax online influencers, collectively called The Disinformation Dozen, often cry "too many shots, too soon." They also conveniently sell vitamin "immune-boosting" product lines as an alternative to vaccinations, by the way. But it makes new parents wonder if it would somehow be safer to wait on shots altogether or stagger them out.

Here's a nasty little truth about spaced-out vaccination schedules: they are all fantasy. There is absolutely no research that says delaying certain shots is safer.

In fact, studies have shown there is absolutely no difference in children's development whose vaccinations are delayed compared to children who receive their shots on time. *(Smith)* Studies also show that giving numerous shots at the same time and giving the recommended vaccination schedule has no impact on a child's risk of autism. *(DeStefano)*

I'd much rather follow a schedule that has been extensively researched for both safety and effectiveness by experts in the field of infectious diseases.

What we do know about alternative vaccination schedules is that delaying shots is playing Russian Roulette with your child. The simple truth is that you are leaving your child unprotected, at a time when they are the most vulnerable.

We realize that parents who choose to delay or opt out on vaccines are not bad parents. They are scared parents. What we are trying to help you realize is that the fear you *should* have is for the diseases that vaccines prevent. If you are on the fence about vaccinations, please take the time to research the diseases—see earlier in this chapter for details.

Q. If I want to do space out my baby's shots, how should I do it?

I suggest setting up a consultation with your own pediatrician to discuss what both of you feel comfortable with doing. Remember, the ultimate goal is to have your child vaccinated in a timely manner.

More pediatricians are increasingly adamant about protecting their littlest patients. Many refuse to deviate from the recommended schedule just to appease a nervous parent. It may be difficult to find a board-certified pediatrician willing to modify or delay shots. It's our job

DR B'S OPINION:
ASK YOUR DOC ABOUT THEIR KIDS

As parents, our job is to protect our kids as best we can. I get it. I am a parent, too. And I certainly understand, after browsing the internet and hearing parent chatter, that you may have more questions and concerns about vaccinations.

At the end of the day, you've got to put your trust in someone to help guide you in some of those decisions. I hope you and your baby's pediatrician have a good relationship and this person can answer questions that concern you on any topic. Our job is to advocate for and protect your child. If I ever had any doubt about vaccines, or anything else that might harm your child, I guarantee that I would be the first to stop doing it. I treat my patients like my own children. So I suggest asking your doctor the most important question you can ask regarding vaccines: Did you (or would you) vaccinate your own children?

I vaccinated both my children, and would do it again without hesitation.

to protect kids. Following the recommended schedule is the best way to do that.

Helpful Hints
Where to get more information
Our advice: don't type in "vaccinations" in a Google search. You will end up with inaccurate information from concerned groups who do a great job of creating parental anxiety. The following sites will provide *accurate* information:

- ◆ *CDC's National Immunization Program* cdc.gov/nip
- ◆ *American Academy of Pediatrics:* aap.org
- ◆ *Immunization Action Coalition* immunize.org
- ◆ *Vaccine Education Center, Children's Hospital of Philadelphia* vaccine.chop.edu

> ## DR B'S OPINION
>
> *"We have spent a lot of money studying vaccines. Now let's spend our research dollars on finding a cause for autism.*
>
> *A colleague of mine, Dr. Jill Nichols, said it best: 'This is not the case of two sides to every story. It is a case of fact vs. opinion.'"*

Feedback from the Real World
Vaccination Revealed, by Ginny Butler, Pregnancy & Newborn magazine March 2009:

"We live in an Information Age. We mothers can become experts in digital photography, gourmet cooking and up-to-the-minute runway fashion, merely by spending some time online. However, when we're making decisions that may be critical to our children's health and our communities' stability, obtaining correct information is vital."

Ryan's Story
Frankie Milley, a founder of Meningitis Angels (meningitis-angels.org), offered up this heartbreaking story about vaccines:

On June 22, 1998, a vaccine preventable disease called Meningococcal meningitis took the life of my only child, my son, Ryan. Thousands of children will develop meningitis each year and many will die. But death isn't the only outcome: children who survive are often left with limb amputations, organ damage, and the list goes on.

The two types of meningitis that are most common are meningococcal and pneumococcal (Strep pneumoniae). There are vaccines for both.

This vaccine preventable disease took away my identity, my right to ever be the parent at a wedding, to hold a grandchild, and to have the comfort of a child in my old age. We must work together in the United States to protect our children from epidemics which other parts of the world see everyday. Because epidemics are a plane ride away. And vaccinations save lives.

Yes, vaccines prevent sickness—but you can't be vaccinated against every infection. Up next, the infection hit parade, including a special focus on ear infections, when your child can go back to day care and more!

COMMON INFECTIONS

Chapter 13

"A family is a unit composed not only of children but of men, women, an occasional animal, and the common cold."

~ Ogden Nash (1902-1971)

WHAT'S IN THIS CHAPTER

◆ **WHAT ARE VIRUSES?**
◆ **WHAT ARE BACTERIA?**
◆ **ANTIBIOTIC RESISTANCE**
◆ **WHAT YOU ALWAYS WANTED TO KNOW ABOUT THE COMMON COLD**
◆ **WHEN YOUR CHILD CAN RETURN TO CHILDCARE OR PLAYGROUP**
◆ **GERM HIT PARADE**
◆ **COVID-19**
◆ **SPECIAL FEATURE— EAR INFECTIONS**

This chapter answers that age-old parent question: "So, when can my child go back to child care/playgroup?" Yes, it's time to take a look at the germs that like to invade us. We have a special shout out to the germ we all love to hate, COVID-19. But there are plenty of other bugs to discuss here, because infectious diseases are a large part of pediatrics. FYI: diseases that are not caused by infections are covered in the next chapter, Common Diseases.

Common infections are usually caused by one of two things—viruses and bacteria. We'll cover both in this chapter.

Most infections that your child will get are viruses. These are infections that go away on their own, without medication. One of the advantages of being a pediatrician is that in the case of viruses we do nothing, and our patients usually get better! In the pre-pandemic area, many parents did not understand what viruses are and doctors had to explain that their child would get better without a prescription. The only treatment was time. Now, thanks to COVID-19, we all pretty much get that concept. But as parents, it's normal for us to feel compelled to DO SOMETHING when our child feels miserable

You will be an honorary microbiologist after reading this chapter. It will prepare you for the numerous infections coming your way. We'll go over viruses and bacterium since those are the biggies. Fungi, mites, lice, and parasites are discussed in "Things that make you itch just thinking about them" in this chapter. Fun, no?

Viruses

Q. What is a virus?

These are tiny germs that need our body cells (called the "host") to survive and prosper. Viruses are like little copy machines. Their genetic coding allows the virus to reproduce quickly in the host.

Most viruses enter our bodies, reproduce for a few days, then leave to infect someone else. Examples include the cold virus, COVID-19 and hand/foot/mouth diseases (see the table at the end of this section for a complete run-down of viruses with their common and scientific names). A few viruses like to stick around, lie dormant, and then reactivate to torture us again, such as herpes and chickenpox. Rarely, a virus kills their host—one example is HIV.

Here's some cocktail party trivia for you: according to the International Committee on Taxonomy of Viruses (7th Report, 2000), there are more than 1550 virus species, divided into 56 families. Within each family, there are sometimes thousands of relatives for each virus. These identified viruses are just a small portion of what is actually out in the world.

Q. Where do viruses live when they aren't infecting someone?

Viruses can be airborne or live on surfaces for a period of hours to days. Germs live on surfaces called **FOMITES.** Fomites include door handles, grocery carts, gas pumps, changing tables, shared toys, etc. In other words, there is a "biofilm" that is living on items that you and your child touch every day.

BOTTOM LINE: Your mother was right—WASH YOUR HANDS!

Q. Is antibacterial soap a good defense against infections?

Hand sanitizers that use *at least* 60% alcohol as the active ingredient are a convenient alternative to soap and water if hands are not full of dirt. The only controversy related to these popular hand gels is that some products contain far less than 60% alcohol—which means they won't work.

We suggest using 60% alcohol-based hand sanitizer for when you are out and about or at the diaper changing table. But in most other circumstances regular soap will do just fine.

Denise's opinion: On a personal note, we have found that in the Fields' household, anti-

NEW PARENT 411: WHY EVERYONE IN THE HOUSE GETS SICK WHEN A CHILD HAS A VIRAL ILLNESS

Everyone gets sick because of what families do in their own homes. We hug, kiss, share drinks, touch door handles, touch hand towels, etc. We also wash our hands less in our homes than when we are out in public.

BOTTOM LINE: Think twice before you decide to finish what is left over on your child's plate. Is that half-eaten chicken nugget really worth it?

INFECTIONS

bacterial soap aggravates our chronic dry skin (we live in a very arid climate) and eczema. We stick to regular Dove soap and wash frequently. Also those alcohol based hand sanitizers like Purell are very painful if you have cracks from eczema. We avoid them as well.

Q. Do we pass viral infections back and forth in our house?

No. Once everyone is infected, everyone is immune to that particular germ, at least for a little while since immunity can wear off over a period of months or years for some infections.

Q. Why is my child always getting sick?

Because they are being exposed to infectious germs they have no immunity to.

There are literally millions of germs out there. Every time your child gets an infection, they make antibodies to a specific bug. But until your child has a large immune memory in their body's "hard drive," they will get almost every illness that comes down the pike. Most infections are spread through respiratory droplets (snot and cough secretions), saliva, and poop. Babies don't have good manners. They cough and sneeze on each other. They also explore toys in their mouths, leaving the germs behind for someone else.

Reality Check

Babies begin to get sick when they start venturing out in the world. Here are some astounding statistics:

◆ The average number of viral infections per year for kids under age five is EIGHT. Yes, you read that right.
◆ Each illness lasts seven to ten days.
◆ Most infections occur between October and April.
◆ That's 80 days of illness packed into six months of the year.

BOTTOM LINE: That's right, expect an infection every other week in the winter. And that's just the AVERAGE. If you win the sick kid lotto, you could be in for more. Astounding, eh?

Q. Why is my second child sicker than my first?

Because your older child is bringing home infections to share.

Firstborns often live in a bubble for their first year of life (unless they are in childcare). Second babies don't have that luxury. They get carted around to big brother or sister's activities. And big bro/sis share whatever infections they have acquired with the little ones. So, it is natural for a second child to get more illnesses earlier in life than the first.

Q. Why do we only see the flu virus in the wintertime?

Viruses prefer certain times of year to attack.

When a virus arrives in a community, it spreads in an epidemic fashion for a period of weeks, then disappears. Doctors know what virus has arrived because every patient has the same illness for a few weeks. Yep, it's a fact of life—viruses are always coming to town, it's just a matter of when they arrive every year. Here are the seasonal patterns of viral epidemics:

Summer: Coxsackievirus (hand/foot/mouth), Enteroviruses (stomach, skin, respiratory, eye)
Fall: Parainfluenza (croup), Rhinovirus (common cold)
Winter: Influenza (the flu), Rotavirus (stomach virus), RSV (bronchiolitis)
Spring: Parainfluenza again, Varicella (chickenpox)

What causes these seasonal patterns? There are various factors that influence the annual epidemics of these viruses. Scientists have been studying this for years. It seems to be a combination of atmospheric conditions and host (that's us) behaviors that lead to the perfect conditions for a virus to attack. Interestingly, viruses can be found infecting people in their "off-season," but not at epidemic levels. *(Dowell)*

Reality Check

At the time we went to press, COVID-19 seems to lack a seasonal pattern. It's the gift that just keeps on giving! However, infectious disease experts anticipate it will become a fall/winter virus with more predictable surges every year.

Q. How do viruses cause infection?

Remember, viruses need us to survive. Flash back to high school science class (or Ms. Frizzle and the Magic School Bus): viruses are just a collection of genetic material (DNA or RNA) wrapped in a protein coat. They invade a host (like, us) to use the host's cell machinery to reproduce more little viruses. They jump at the chance to enter any body orifice (eyes, nose, mouth, anus, vagina, urethra). Most often, they are spread via the nose or through cough droplets, saliva, poop, or sexual relations.

Garden-variety viruses enter our body, replicate, and leave. This makes it hard to detect a virus or use a medicine to stop a viral infection—by the time you realize you have been attacked by a virus, the virus itself may have moved on.

The symptoms we experience are due to our immune response to the infection. For example, the common cold virus (rhinovirus) attacks the nose. Our immune system sends white blood cells there to fight the infection. The result of the bug/white blood cell battle is mucous production.

Once we have symptoms, the virus has already replicated numerous times in our body. It's usually too late to do anything. Fortunately, most viral infections are not serious and our bodies recover from the invasion.

BOTTOM LINE: Think of a virus as a speedboat. It zips in and out of our body.

Q. How do doctors know that a child has a viral infection?

Your baby's doctor will usually make a diagnosis based on symptoms (the problems/complaints you describe) and the signs of infection (the abnormal findings on physical examination). *Most experienced physicians are able to accurately make the diagnosis of a typical viral infection on this information alone.*

Reality Check

COVID-19 is truly fascinating (among other adjectives!) from a physician standpoint. We are pattern readers and our skills have been put to the test with this virus. COVID-19 looks like everything (Strep throat, flu, common cold, croup, seasonal allergies) and it looks like nothing (no symptoms at all). It is difficult to predict which patients have COVID-19 based on symptoms and physical examination alone. But, when COVID-19 surges occur, it is the pervasive germ in the community and most of our patients who have symptoms do have COVID-19 infection confirmed by testing.

Q. Are there any tests that can detect a viral infection?

Yes. Most of the time, though, knowledge of which virus your child has is simply for knowledge's sake. It does not change the treatment, since there is no medication to treat most viral illnesses.

But the pandemic changed all that. It suddenly became important to know who was infected to prevent the spread of COVID-19 and to start treatment for those at risk of severe illness.

The problem with viruses is that they are extremely small. We can't see them with a regular microscope. And often, the virus is already out of the body so it can't be caught.

Here is an overview of tests available for COVID-19 and some other unpleasant viruses. Depending on the complexity (and cost) of the test, some can be done at home, at outpatient medical offices (called "point of care" tests), sent to an outside lab facility, or done in an emergency department or hospital setting.

1. PCR (polymerase chain reaction) accurately detects the presence of genetic material (DNA or RNA) of some viruses, bacteria, fungi, and parasites that cause infection. The technology amplifies even the smallest amount of infectious material present so a PCR test can identify and produce a positive test very early in illness.* PCR testing is generally done at outside lab facilities, emergency departments, or hospital settings.

Testing has a 1-8 hour turnaround for results. (The prolonged times during the pandemic varied due to collection, transport, and how many tests could be run on a machine at a time.)

PCR tests for: Influenza A and B, Rotavirus, COVID-19, RSV

*In the case of COVID-19, a PCR test can remain positive for several weeks after a person is no longer contagious or actively shedding virus.

2. Multiplex PCR tests (example: Biofire brand) uses the same PCR technology but can simultaneously screen for multiple viruses (and some other germs) that cause respiratory and gut infections. Few pediatric practices perform these tests because they are incredibly expensive and not universally covered by insurance plans...which means the patient gets stuck with a big bill. Unless the price goes down, it is impractical to test every child. And remember, there is no treatment for most of these infections.

Testing has a one-hour turnaround for results.

Respiratory PCR panel tests for:

—Viruses: Influenza A and B, several coronavirus strains, COVID-19, Parainfluenza strains, RSV, adenovirus, rhinovirus, enterovirus, human metapneumovirus

—Bacteria: Bordatella pertussis (whooping cough), Bordatella parapertussis, Chlamydia pneumoniae, Mycoplasma pneumoniae (commonly referred to as "walking pneumonia" or "bronchitis")

Gastrointestinal PCR panel tests for: 22 viruses, bacteria, parasites that cause severe gastroen-

infections

teritis (vomiting and diarrhea). These include norovirus, rotavirus, E.coli, Salmonella, C. difficile, and Giardia as well as several others.

3. Molecular assay NAAT (nucleic acid amplification test) detects the nucleic acid (DNA or RNA) of the virus, but it is less accurate than PCR technology. It is most accurate and useful when someone has symptoms. A positive test confirms an active infection. Medical offices offer NAAT testing.

Testing has 15-30 minute turnaround for results.

NAAT tests for: Flu A and B, COVID-19

4. Rapid Antigen tests detect a protein or toxin that is made by the virus. It is most accurate and useful when someone has symptoms. A positive test is accurate in confirming infection. A negative test does not rule out infection because it depends on the quality of the specimen (for example, a poor swab with a squirmy patient) and how much virus is actively being shed at the time. Medical offices offer rapid antigen testing. Home COVID-19 tests are also rapid antigen tests.

Testing has a 15-30 minute turnaround for results.

Rapid antigen tests for: RSV, COVID-19, Flu A and B

Other ways to test for viral infections include rapid testing for infectious mononucleosis ("mono"), antibody tests, and viral cultures for herpes virus.

Most of the time, your doctor can't just do a blood test to see if your baby has a virus. If a complete blood count is done on a child with a viral infection, the results are usually normal. The white blood cell count does not rise in response to a virus. In fact, some viruses cause a decrease in the number of cells that fight infection (termed *viral bone marrow suppression*). Influenza is classic for causing a low white blood cell count. White blood cells can be further differentiated by their shape under a microscope. The types of white blood cells that mount an immune attack to viruses are predominantly *lymphocytes*. Seeing a high number of lymphocytes is one of the only useful bits of information in a blood count to diagnose a viral infection.

BOTTOM LINE

Lab work and x-rays are rarely necessary to diagnose a run-of-the-mill virus in your baby. If a child does not improve as expected, though, doctors need you to call or follow up to explore things further.

Q. Are there any anti-viral medications?

Yes. There are a few available. But all of these medicines must be given within the first 24 to 48 hours of symptoms because they act by inhibiting the replication of the virus. It is useless to take an anti-viral medicine more than three days into a viral illness.

For most viruses, there is no anti-viral medication available to clear the infection. The ones that ARE available include:

1. Tamiflu (Oseltamivir) for Influenza A and B
2. Zovirax (Acyclovir) for chickenpox, shingles, or Herpes virus
3. AZT, Abacavir for HIV infections

4. Formvirisen for CMV eye infections
5. Remsdesivir for severe COVID-19 infections, Paxlovid (Nirmatrelvir) for patients over age 12 and risk of mild to moderate COVID-19 infection

Q. How long do most viral infections last?

You can expect a typical virus to cause symptoms for seven to 14 days.

Usually a fever is present for the first two to four days of illness. While there is a fever, your child is contagious. The virus is actively growing/replicating. The fever stops when the virus stops replicating. But our bodies will feel the impact of the infection for about a week.

Q. Is there any way to prevent a viral infection?

Yes—with vaccination.

We are fortunate to have vaccinations to prevent some of the most serious viral infections known to civilization: smallpox, polio, COVID-19, Hepatitis A, Hepatitis B, measles, mumps, rubella, Rotavirus, chickenpox and Human Papilloma Virus (HPV).

The Common Cold

Q. What is the common cold?

Answer: a viral infection usually caused by our friend, rhinovirus ("rhino" is the Latin word for nose.)

Here is what you need to know:

1. The virus enters the host body through the nose and goes to work.

So, how long with cold and flu symptoms last?

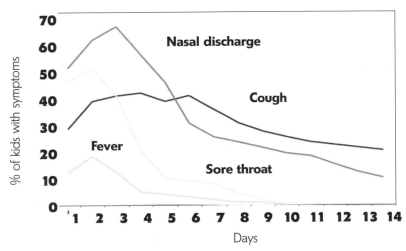

Source: Dr. S. Michael Marcy & Kaiser Permanente from data presented in JAMA

2. Fever and body aches occur when the virus starts reproducing.
3. Snot (mucous production), cough, with or without sore throat follows.
4. Symptoms last for up to 14 days, with day three or four being the worst.
5. The snot can change from clear to green and still be just the same old virus (not a sinus infection, which we'll discuss later in this chapter).

Q. How is the common cold diagnosed and treated?

A cold virus or upper respiratory infection is diagnosed based on the symptoms that the patient has. Yes, COVID-19 can look like the common cold so sometimes testing is needed to rule out other things.

For babies, the best treatment is to use saline nose drops as much as needed. Saline is salt water. (See home remedies in Medications, Appendix A.) A mist or two in each nostril before feedings and bed helps loosen the mucous and often makes babies sneeze. The beauty of saline is that it is safe and nearly impossible to overdose on it!

Remember, antibiotics will not cure a cold.

Top Remedies to Treat a Cold

◆ Saline nose drops.
◆ Running a humidifier in baby's room to help loosen the mucous.
◆ Having baby sleep in car seat or with head of mattress elevated (place a pillow or wedge *under* the mattress).

Reality Check

There are over 100 rhinoviruses. Once your child has a rhinovirus infection, they are immune to that one. But there are 99 more that they are not immune to. Get the picture?

Q. I can feel a rattling in my baby's chest. Are you sure the infection isn't in their lungs?

Yes. It's air moving through snot that you hear and feel. See transmitted upper airway noise

DR B'S OPINION:
COLD MEDS AND INFANTS

The Food and Drug Administration prohibits the sale of over-the-counter cough and cold meds for kids under age four. I never recommended them anyway. Infants under six months of age can have a paradoxical reaction to antihistamines (instead of sedating a baby, these medicines can leave your child wired). The decongestants used in most of these medicines can act similarly to caffeine. I personally would rather deal with a snotty sleeping baby than a snotty awake baby.

DR B'S OPINION: VAPO-RUBS

Some parents love to use this stuff. But here's what you need to know: it is not approved for use in children under two years of age. Camphor, one of the active ingredients, gets absorbed through the skin and can potentially cause seizures in babies. See Appendix B Complementary Medicine for information on menthols/peppermint oil.

info in the section on breathing problems in Chapter 15, First Aid.

Q. How long is a baby contagious with a cold virus?

In general, the first three days of illness.

With viruses in general, people are contagious while they have a fever. The infection is spread via hand-to-hand contact with snot (mucous). It is also spread from cough and sneeze droplets.

Q. When my baby has a cold, they have a runny nose for almost two weeks. I'm afraid to go back to playgroup because the other moms seem upset. How long is a cold contagious?

With the common cold virus or upper respiratory infection, the virus is spread in the first three or four days of illness (usually when kids have a fever). After that, it's just snot. You can return to playgroup. We have a handy table later in this chapter to go over other illnesses and their period of contagiousness.

Q. My baby has swollen glands. What is that?

Lymph nodes. Our bodies have chains of lymph nodes that look like a string of pearls. These chains are located throughout the body, but mostly in the neck, armpits, and groin. Each area works to protect a particular body area. For instance, the neck nodes are dedicated to

HUMIDIFIERS & VAPORIZERS: COLD VS WARM MIST DEBATE

A humidifier and vaporizer both do the same thing—they add humidity to dry air. Vaporizers have a place to add medicine to the mist but this feature is rarely used today. Kids who have asthma and need breathing treatments have a high-tech machine called a nebulizer.

Warm mist humidifiers are unnecessary and they make the nursery feel like the Bahamas. There is also a risk of an older baby burning their hand on a warm mist machine.

BOTTOM LINE: Buy a cheap, cool-mist humidifier. It loosens up mucous so babies can sleep when they have a cold. Just be sure to clean it every few days.

For a discussion of which humidifier models are best, ratings and buying advice, see the web site for our other book *Baby Bargains* (BabyBargains.com).

the head, ears, nose, and throat. These tiny glands are jam packed with the cells that fight off infection. When there is an active infection in the body, these glands rise to the occasion, swelling to several times their normal size. They can be tender and can remain enlarged for up to six weeks after the infection is gone. Swollen lymph nodes point us in the direction of where an infection is located.

Q. What is the significance of green snot? I always thought that it meant a bacterial infection.

Bacterial sinus infections cause green nasal secretions, but green snot alone does not diagnose sinusitis. The nasal secretions are a result of our immune system (white blood cells) fighting with either a virus or bacteria. The discoloration tells us that the battle has been going on for a while.

The change from clear secretions to yellow/green secretions WHEN ACCOMPANIED by fever, headache, fussiness, or prolonged symptoms (over two weeks of illness) is suspicious for a bacterial sinus infection.

The difference between a cold and a sinus infection

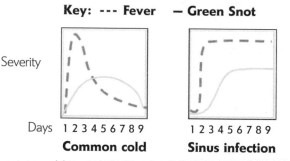

Key: --- Fever   — Green Snot

Severity

Days 1 2 3 4 5 6 7 8 9   1 2 3 4 5 6 7 8 9
      Common cold   **Sinus infection**

*The common cold causes a short lived fever with several days of snot.
A sinus infection causes prolonged fever and prolonged snot.*

Bacteria

Q. What are bacteria?

These are much larger germs than viruses. These bugs can live on their own without a host. Most bacteria do not cause illness, and live in harmony with us. Some bacteria cause infection only in susceptible humans (those that are "immune compromised"), or when they end up in places they don't belong (e.g. intestinal bacteria in the urinary tract causes a bladder infection). And there are only a few bacteria that live to hurt us.

Q. I have heard about "good bacteria." What are they?

The bacteria that live in and on our bodies are called *normal flora*.

These bacteria live on our skin, and in our mouths, nostrils, vagina, and intestines. Babies are born relatively sterile (bacteria free). But it only takes a day or two in the real world to become colonized with bacteria. Here are the typical bacteria that are in you and your baby's body:

- *Skin bacteria:* Staph and Strep
- *Nostril bacteria:* Staph and Strep
- *Gut bacteria:* Lactobacillus and E coli, among many others
- *Vagina and gut bacteria:* Group B Strep
- *Mouth bacteria:* too numerous to mention here

Q. How do bacteria cause infection?

They enter through any body opening under favorable conditions. These conditions include open wounds, mucous in the nose from viral infection, fluid in Eustachian tubes with a common cold virus, poop and bacteria pushed into the urethra/bladder opening. Other bacteria get in via respiratory secretions, saliva, or sexual activity.

Then they grow and fester in our bodies. Unlike viruses, they like to stick around.

Bacteria either invade our body tissues or produce a toxin (poison) that injures our bodies. Each bug has a particular body part they prefer to hang out in (throat, intestine, bladder, eye, etc.).

Q. I have heard the term "secondary bacterial infection." What does it mean?

Bacteria often capitalize on a person who already has an active viral infection.

The viral infection is the *primary* infection. The bacteria that come in later are termed *secondary* infections. This is an important concept to understand why a) you are at risk for bac-

HOW A DOC CAN TELL A BACTERIAL INFECTION FROM A VIRUS

1. **Your child is sicker.** Bacterial infections, in general, make people sicker than viruses.
2. **Your child's fever lasts longer than four days.** Viral illnesses usually cause fever for three to four days maximum (except influenza which last up to a week).
3. **Your child's fever is really high (over 105).** Viruses cause high fevers, too. But there is a greater chance it's a bacterial infection when you could fry an egg on your child's back.
4. **Your child has a localized area of infection.** Bacteria pick a body part to live in. The most common bacterial infections in childhood include: ear, sinus, throat, eye, lung, bladder/kidney, lymph node, intestine, blood, or the brain.
5. **Your child has abnormal lab work.** If there is not an obvious source of infection on examination, and they look really sick with or without prolonged or high fever, some tests will be done. A complete blood count shows an elevation of the cells that fight infection (total white blood cell count over 15,000, and a high percentage of **NEUTROPHILS**—see lab section in Appendix C for details). Or, white blood cells in urine, spinal fluid, etc. indicate that infection is there (white blood cells are never found in normal urine or spinal fluid).

? ?

INFECTIONS

terial infections when you have a cold or flu, b) you don't often get bacterial infections when you are well, and c) why many bacterial infections are not contagious to others.

BOTTOM LINE: Think of bacteria as tugboats. They are slower moving than viruses. Their lack of speed and tendency to stick around make them susceptible to antibiotics.

Old Wives Tales

◆ **Going out in the rain causes pneumonia. False!**
The truth: Having a viral infection (cold or flu virus) predisposes a person to getting a secondary bacterial infection (pneumonia is a bacterial infection in the lungs). The weather has nothing to do with it.

◆ **The wind or ceiling fans cause ear infections. False!**
The truth: If your baby has a cold (or any viral infection), they are more susceptible to getting an ear infection (or another bacterial infection). Like the old wives tale about the rain and pneumonia, the wind has nothing to do with ear infections.

Q. Are bacterial infections contagious?

It depends on the bug and the host.

Not all bacteria jump from person to person. Some just set up shop in one body and grow until they are killed off.

And some bacteria will only cause infection in people who are susceptible (either because they already have a viral infection or their immune systems are compromised—such as premature infants, the elderly, people on chemotherapy, AIDS patients).

As a general rule, assume your child is contagious if they have a fever. The fever tells you that the body's immune system is actively fighting the bug.

But your doctor can tell you if the particular bacterial infection is contagious to others (or read the final section of this chapter) For example, Strep throat (Group A Strep) infection IS contagious. An ear infection caused by Strep pneumoniae is NOT contagious.

Q. Can you find out which bacterium is causing an infection?

Yes.

Because bacteria don't leave the body, doctors can potentially catch the bacteria and identify them under a microscope or grow them on a culture plate. Blood, urine, stool, spinal fluid, eye discharge, ear discharge, throat pus, sputum (mucous coughed up), and vaginal discharge to name a few, can be examined. Bacteria living in our bodies can grow on a culture plate in about 48 hours.

The only problem is that we can't always get a specimen from the location of the infection (like an ear infection). Fortunately, a limited number of bacteria cause certain infections. Once the source of the infection is identified (eye, ear, sinus, lung, etc.), doctors have a pretty good idea which bacterium is wreaking havoc.

Q. How do doctors know which antibiotic will kill a bacterial infection?

Doctors select an antibiotic that kills the bacteria most likely causing the infection. Antibiotics are not all the same. They are each potent against specific families of bacteria. (See Appendix A, Medications.)

If bacteria grow on a culture plate (from an available specimen), doctors get exact information for antibiotic selection. The growing bacteria are placed on several "sensitivity" plates. These plates contain a growth medium and an antibiotic. If the bacteria can't grow on a particular antibiotic plate, the right medication to keep the infection from growing in the body is found.

DR B'S OPINION

"If you can get a child over three months old to smile at you, they aren't that sick. There is a scientific study that has proven this. In practice, I can tell you it's true."

Antibiotic Resistance

Q. I've heard a lot about drug resistant bacteria/antibiotic resistance. What is it?

Darwin's Survival of the Fittest.

Bacteria adapt to survive. There is a constant challenge to create more anti-microbials (antibiotics) to kill off the smart drug-resistant bugs.

Many people don't understand the concept of antibiotic resistance. They think that a *person* who is taking antibiotics will develop a drug resistance. *Drug resistance refers to the bugs.* When so many antibiotics are being used in the community, the bugs know our ammunition. Those that survive are drug resistant. The idea is that we can't overuse our weapons— otherwise we will be left with no defense. We need to use our antibiotic weapons judiciously.

Reality Check

Penicillin resistant strains of bacteria, particularly one called Strep pneumoniae (see Prevnar in the last chapter on vaccines) began emerging in 1991. Now 20% of Strep pneumoniae strains are resistant to Penicillin and 10% are resistant to at least three types of antibiotics. Strep pneumoniae cause five to seven million ear infections annually.

Q. What can be done to stop drug-resistant bacteria?

◆ Give the Prevnar vaccine to children at high risk of getting Strep pneumoniae infection (children under age five).
◆ Use a higher dose of the first-line antibiotic (amoxicillin).
◆ Save the big gun, broader spectrum antibiotics for persistent infections.
◆ Only use antibiotics when it is really necessary.

Q. When should antibiotics NOT be prescribed?

1. The common cold or "upper respiratory infection."
2. A sore throat caused by a virus (as opposed to Strep throat which is caused by a bacteria).
3. Green snot (see the common cold section earlier in this chapter).
4. Because someone else in the house is on antibiotics.

INFECTIONS

? ?

NEW PARENT 411: ANTIBIOTICS

Just because YOU are on an antibiotic, does not mean your child needs to be on one. Whole families can get infected with a virus. But not everyone gets a secondary bacterial infection from the virus. Remember that secondary infections are not contagious. So, even if you now have a sinus infection, your baby most likely will still have just a cold.

The abuse of antibiotics

Here are a couple of startling stats: In 1980, U.S. healthcare providers wrote four million prescriptions for amoxicillin (a popular antibiotic) for children. By 2010, that number jumped to 18 million.

In fact, amoxicillin was the most prescribed medication to kids under age two.

It is clear that doctors over-prescribe antibiotics. Want to know the number one reason doctors site for over-prescribing? Parent expectation that an antibiotic will be prescribed!

Truth be told, it's not just the parents' fault. One study showed that doctors often misperceive what a parent expects at an office visit (and try to satisfy them). (*Mangione-Smith*)

Old Wives Tale
I am on an antibiotic for an upper respiratory infection. My child is sick, too. They need antibiotics.

The truth: Not everyone with a cold develops a sinus infection. That is probably why you are taking an antibiotic. Your child should be checked for a secondary bacterial infection if he has a fever, crankiness, or prolonged symptoms (beyond ten to 14 days). It was common 15 to 20 years ago that if one person in a house had a Strep infection, then doctors prescribed antibiotics for the ENTIRE family. Now, we realize that is NOT the answer. Giving antibiotics to healthy folks only strengthens the bugs' resistance to drugs.

Reality Check
If a bacterial infection is diagnosed, an antibiotic is in order. Viruses are not cured by antibiotics. Your child will get better on their own.

Putting it all together...

Now you know the usual suspects. Here is how doctors put it all together. When a child has a fever, your doctor looks for infection. (There are other causes for fever, but infection tops the list). The symptoms IN ADDITION TO the fever are what lead to the diagnosis. (Vomiting, diarrhea, cough, runny nose, decreased appetite, rash...) The constellation of symptoms and findings on physical examination are often enough information to make the call. Lab work and x-rays are sometimes needed to help figure out the source of infection.

Viral infections for the most part do not require any medication and are fought off by our body's immune systems. Bacteria, fungi, mites, and parasites respond to medication, which helps eliminate the infection. The medication selection is often based on the usual suspects for

? ?

INFECTIONS

a particular illness. If an infection doesn't clear up or the patient is pretty sick, cultures can help identify the particular bug and the right medication.

Bacterial infections are frequently secondary infections that capitalize on a weakened immune system that is fighting a virus (ear infections, sinus infections/adenoiditis, pneumonia). Doctors worry about secondary infections when a child with a viral infection suddenly gets worse (i.e. new fever, new green snot, new irritability, new respiratory distress).

Viral Infections

And now, here's an overview of the viral infections that most impact babies, here's an overview of the viral infections that most impact babies, including that trendy one, COVID-19.

I. Respiratory Viruses

The Flu (Influenza)

Disease: Respiratory illness caused by either Influenza A or B. A different strain causes epidemics every year. Influenza causes more severe respiratory illness than the common cold. There is a higher risk of secondary bacterial infections in infants, people with chronic lung disease, or other chronic diseases.

Symptoms: High fever, body aches, and chills. Then runny nose, cough and sore throat.

Diagnosis: Based on symptoms. White blood cell count is low (less than 4,000) with mostly lymphocytes. Rapid flu assay is available, but it is only about 50% accurate in identifying the flu.

Treatment: An anti-viral medication can be given to babies over two weeks old if diagnosis is made within 48 hours of becoming ill.

Contagious: From 24 hours before symptoms start, and while person has symptoms. Spread via respiratory droplets, fomites.

Incubation period: 1-3 days after exposure

Season: Winter

Prevention: Annual flu vaccine offered each fall season. Recommended for everyone, starting at six months of age. (*Pickering*)

Bronchiolitis (RSV)

Disease: RSV stands for Respiratory Syncytial Virus. (Or, as one of my patient's dads says, "Really Sucky Virus".) It can infect anyone, but causes more severe illness in infants, especially babies born prematurely. As opposed to the common cold or upper respiratory infection, RSV attacks the tiny branches of the lower lung airways (bronchioles). Swollen bronchioles make the air flow turbulent through them, creating a wheeze with inspiration, similar to the mechanism of asthma. RSV infection can be serious enough to require hospitalization.

Symptoms: Fever, runny nose, breathing faster than normal and wheeze, but no "distress." Infants and premature babies may have more "respiratory distress" (see glossary). About 30% of children who wheeze with an RSV infection will have asthma. The cause is debatable. Does the RSV infection cause long term damage to the airways, predisposing to asthma; or are the kids who wheeze with RSV really asthmatics with sensitive airways?

? ?

INFECTIONS

Regardless, damage to the bronchioles from RSV takes a long time to heal. Symptoms can go on for weeks.

Diagnosis: Based on symptoms. A rapid assay test is available, but it is not always performed. Testing is only useful if it will affect treatment decisions.

Treatment: Some kids respond to asthma medication (Albuterol) via a nebulizer machine to aerosolize the medication. Some kids need oxygen, which requires hospitalization.

Contagious: 3 to 8 days, but sometimes up to 3 weeks. Spread by fomites (biofilm), respiratory droplets.

Incubation period: 2 to 8 days.

Season: Winter, early spring

Prevention: For children under 12 months of age who were born prematurely (less than 29 weeks gestation), those born less than 32 weeks of age who have chronic lung disease, and those with significant heart disease or severe immune system defects, RSV-Antibody (Synagis) provides immunity for one month. The medication is a shot given monthly through RSV season. (It's about $1000 a shot, and the series is usually six injections). (See Appendix A "Medications" for details on Synagis.) (*Pickering*)

COVID-19

Disease: A viral infection that attacks the respiratory tract (lungs, throat) but can attack multiple other organ systems affecting the heart, blood vessels, gut, brain, nerves, skin, blood, kidneys, and pancreas. Children with obesity and other health conditions (asthma, diabetes, chronic lung disease, sickle cell disease, immunocompromised) are at greater risk of severe illness. Complications of infection include Multisystem Inflammatory Syndrome in Children (MIS-C), diabetes, myocarditis, long COVID-19.

Symptoms: None to severe illness. ***In young children:*** fever, cough—sometimes croup (Omicron variant), sore throat, body aches, fatigue, vomiting, diarrhea, shortness of breath, rash. ***In multisystem inflammatory syndrome in children:*** Fever + severe stomachache, lethargy/confusion/difficulty staying awake, red eyes, red/swollen cracked lips and tongue, red/swollen hands and feet, rash, vomiting, diarrhea, headache, rapid breathing, rapid heart rate

Diagnosis: PCR is the gold standard; rapid antigen testing

Treatment: Fever control, hydration. Antiviral treatments for severe illness.

Contagious: On average, 2 to 3 days before symptoms and for 8 days*. Spread via respiratory droplets.

Incubation period: 2 to 14 days. The mean is 5 days after exposure.

Season: Currently year-round with periodic surges as new variants arise.

Prevention: Vaccination. Recommendations for infants are pending at time of this writing. *Quarantine and isolation recommendations are evolving. When the CDC shortened the isolation period to 5 days, they also acknowledged that one-third of people still shed virus until day 8. It is rare to shed infectious virus after 10 days of symptoms, except for those who have severe illness or are immunocompromised. (*Kimberlin*)

Croup

Disease: A viral infection that attacks the voice box area. The smaller the child, the smaller the airway tube, the more problematic when the airway is swollen.

Symptoms: Fever. Cough is a classic "bark", like a seal. Always worse at night when lying down. This is a three night illness. With babies, significant swelling can occur. A squeal is heard. Persistent squealing (stridor) more than five to ten minutes is a medical emergency. Adults with croup have laryngitis instead of a bark because adults' airway tubes are larger.

Diagnosis: The bark is usually enough to prove it. A neck x-ray is occasionally done to identify the swollen area.

Treatment: Turn on the shower in a closed bathroom. The steam works well. Humidifier in room. For more severe cases, steroids (taken by mouth or a shot) help reduce the airway swelling. A breathing treatment (racemic epinephrine) also relaxes the airway for kids with stridor.

Contagious: 4 to 7 days. Spread via direct contact, fomites, respiratory droplets.

Incubation period: 2 to 6 days.

Season: Fall. (*Pickering*)

2. Mouth And Tonsil Viruses

Hand-Foot-and-Mouth (Coxsackievirus)

Disease: A virus that causes ulcers in the back of the mouth and tongue, and sometimes a rash on the palms, soles, and around the anus/genitals.

Symptoms: Fever, lack of interest in eating. Rash can be flat red dots or raised like pimples. Ulcers in the *back of mouth and sometimes tongue*.

Diagnosis: The ulcers in the back of the mouth are classic. No diagnostic testing is done. See Rash-o-Rama on Baby411.com for a picture.

Treatment: Avoid citrus and salt. Acetaminophen (Tylenol) or Ibuprofen (Advil) for discomfort. Make up a concoction of liquid Benadryl and Maalox (1 tsp of each), then give about 0.8 ml of the mixture before feedings. This coats the ulcers.

Contagious: Up to 7 days. Spread through saliva, poop, and fomites.

Incubation period: 3 to 6 days.

Season: Summer, fall. (*Pickering*)

Fun fact: The nails can also be affected by this virus. Your child's nails may peel off a few months after this virus. No worries--they will grow back normally.

Oral Herpes Stomatitis

Disease: Viral infection caused by HSV Type 1. (Type 2 is genital herpes— a completely different infection). Once a person is infected, the HSV-1 lies dormant for life and can re-activate as a cold sore. Cold sores appear on the outer lip and last for a week. Cold sores spread HSV-1 to others. The worst case scenario is a newborn who contracts HSV infection (75% of these are from genital herpes type 2, but 25% are HSV-1). These babies are at high risk of getting an infection of the brain (**ENCEPHALITIS**) from HSV.

Symptoms: Fever over 102 for a week. VERY poor fluid and food intake (at risk of dehydration). Numerous ulcers in mouth, gums, tongue called **GINGIVOSTOMATITIS.** The pain is so severe, some children avoid swallowing their saliva. These kids feel awful.

Diagnosis: Can be made just by looking at the mouth lesions (very impressive looking). Can also be grown (takes 3 days) in a culture by taking a specimen from the ulcer base. It's not always cultured because by the time the culture grows out, it's too late to treat the infection.

infections

Treatment: FLUIDS. Acyclovir, an antiviral, is used if the diagnosis is made within 48 hours. Gingivostomatitis is usually diagnosed too late (after two days of illness) to use an antiviral medication. Cold sores can be treated with anti-virals.

Contagious: VERY! For 7 days. Spread via saliva and direct contact with the lesions.

Incubation period: 2 to 14 days.

Season: Year round.

Prevention: Avoid contact with child if someone has an active cold sore. (*Pickering*)

Reality Check

If Great Aunt Suzy has a cold sore, kindly ask her not to hold your newborn. If you have a cold sore, don't touch your lips and don't kiss your family members.

3. Viral Sore Throat

Disease: A viral infection that causes the tonsils to be swollen. Caused by many different viruses. Adenovirus often causes pink eye (viral conjunctivitis), runny nose, and ear infections in addition to a sore throat.

Symptoms: Fever, decreased appetite, redness or pus (white patches) on tonsils.

Diagnosis: Based on age group and associated symptoms. No lab test. Strep test rarely done because it is rare for babies under age two. It is extremely rare for babies under age two to get Strep (bacterial) throat.

Treatment: To treat the symptoms only. Acetaminophen (Tylenol) or Ibuprofen (Advil), lots to drink.

Contagious: While child has a fever. Spread by direct contact, respiratory droplets, fomites.

Incubation period: 2 to 14 days.

Season: Winter, spring, summer. (*Pickering*)

4. Gastrointestinal Viruses

There are many types of viruses that are known collectively as the "stomach virus." They are all treated the same way—lots of fluids to prevent dehydration. Stomach viruses come every winter. You've been warned.

Viral gastroenteritis (Rotavirus)

Disease: Rotavirus enters the stomach and intestines. Prior to routine vaccination in 2006, almost all kids got this infection by three years old. (And people can get it more than once). The kids at greatest risk are infants. They lose so much water in the diarrhea that it's hard to keep the fluid intake greater than the losses. That's why some babies get admitted to the hospital for IV fluids.

Symptoms: Fever, vomiting, and extremely watery diarrhea (often more than 20 times a day). This lasts for about a week.

Diagnosis: Usually obvious by the volume of diarrhea! Assay test is available.

Treatment: Lots of fluids. See Diarrhea section in Chapter 15, First Aid.

Contagious: VERY. FOR THE WHOLE TIME YOUR CHILD HAS DIARRHEA. Spread via contact with infected poop, fomites. Spreads like wildfire through childcare centers and households.

Incubation period: 1 to 3 days.

Season: Winter (starts southwest and moves northeast every year—the opposite of birds)
Prevention: Rotavirus vaccine, given at two months of age, with one or two doses to complete the series.

Viral gastroenteritis (Norovirus)

Disease: Another common stomach virus that prefers group settings like cruise ships, nursing homes, and child care centers. The cause of up to 30% of all gastroenteritis in the U.S.
Symptoms: Nausea, vomiting, abdominal cramps, non-bloody diarrhea, occasionally fever.
Diagnosis: Health department does testing when there are a large number of people affected in an outbreak.
Treatment: Lots of fluids. See Diarrhea section in Chapter 15, First Aid.
Contagious: VERY. FOR THE WHOLE TIME YOUR CHILD HAS DIARRHEA. May return to childcare when symptom free for 48 hours. Spread via contact with infected food, water, poop, fomites (contaminated surfaces), and person-to-person contact.
Incubation period: 12 to 48 hours.
Prevention: Good hand washing with soap and water for at least 20 seconds. Alcohol based hand sanitizers are not an acceptable substitute for this resilient little virus. (*MMWR*)

5. Viral Exanthems (viruses that cause rashes)

See rashes section in Chapter 15, First Aid for more info on treatment.

Roseola (Herpes virus 6)

Disease: A virus that the entire world population over one year of age has had. Because it is a Herpes virus (this is NOT genital herpes HSV-2), it stays in our bodies forever. We all shed this virus in saliva and respiratory droplets daily. Mom's antibodies (immunity) are passed to baby and provide protection against illness for 9 to 12 months. When immunity wanes, babies get this infection. The only time you see a roseola "epidemic" is if you hang out with a bunch of one year olds.
Symptoms: Fever over 102 for about four days with no other signs of infection. Kids are usually in good spirits. *When the fever breaks, the rash comes out.* The rash can be subtle or dramatic. It is mostly flat, with some raised areas. Red, blotchy. On chest, back, arms. Not itchy, goes away within hours to a few days.
Diagnosis: Obvious after the rash comes out. The fever often prompts lab work (CBC, urinalysis) to prove that there is not a bacteria causing the fever.
Treatment: None. Acetaminophen (Tylenol) or Ibuprofen (Advil) for the fever.
Contagious: We are all contagious because we shed the virus for a lifetime once we are infected.
Incubation period: Ten days.
Season: When is your baby's first birthday?

Chickenpox (Varicella)

Disease: Caused by Varicella-Zoster virus, another type of Herpes virus. Like all Herpes viruses, it lies dormant forever in previously infected people. Because chickenpox can cause serious infection and death, vaccination became the standard of care in 1995. The vaccine is given to all children at one year of age and anyone (including adults) who has never had chickenpox. The vaccine is not 100% effective in preventing infection. But people who get infection despite vaccination have a very mild form of the disease. Babies under three months of age are usually protected via Mom's immunity (as long as Mom had chickenpox). Both immunized and infected kids can get Zoster (shingles) infection later in life (reactivation of Varicella). Shingles infects only one group of nerves (called a dermatome). A group of lesions come up in one patch. These blisters are more painful than itchy. They contain the virus and are contagious.

Symptoms: A full blown case causes fever, body aches, and a rash of tiny fluid filled blisters (called **VESICLES**) that appear in crops. New crops come up over a period of 3 to 4 days. The average number of pox is 350. Very itchy. Secondary Strep skin infections can occur. Watch for red areas surrounding pox, or a new fever after the initial fever breaks.

Diagnosis: Classic rash. Virus (found in vesicle fluid) will grow in culture in 2 to 3 days.

Treatment: Acyclovir, an anti-viral, can be given within 48 hours of illness. It will shorten the course of illness by a couple of days and reduces the total number of lesions (not dramatically though)

Contagious: VERY. FOR ONE WEEK. Child is contagious for 24 hours before the rash comes out and until all lesions (which contain the virus) are crusted over. Spread via respiratory droplets and direct contact.

Incubation period: 10 to 21 days. If you know when your child has been exposed, look for infection 10 days later and for the next 11 days. If you make it out of that window, you are safe.

Season: Winter, early spring

Prevention: Vaccination.

Slapped Cheek (Parvovirus)

Disease: Also known as **FIFTH DISEASE** or **ERYTHEMA INFECTIOSUM**. Occurs more in school age children. Questions arise more with exposure in pregnancy than anything else. The biggest problem with this infection is that it can cause miscarriage. If a pregnant woman (usually in the first 20 weeks) is not immune to Parvovirus and gets the infection, her fetus is at risk. Unfortunately, by the time we know a child has had Parvovirus (i.e. the rash appears), they have has already exposed everyone. Note: If you are pregnant and have been exposed to any child with parvovirus, notify your obstetrician.

Symptoms: Mild or even undetectable when a child is contagious. Low fever, body aches, or headache. Ten days after the infection is gone, a classic rash erupts. The red cheeks look as if someone slapped them plus a lacy, mostly flat, red rash on chest, arms, and legs. The rash can last several weeks. When older kids and adults get infected, they may get joint pains that last for weeks.

Diagnosis: Easy once the rash has erupted. Antibody levels can be checked for evidence of recent infection.

Treatment: None.

Contagious: Hard to know when contagious because often there are no symptoms. Spread via respiratory droplets, blood products.

Incubation period: 4 to 21 days.

Season: Winter, spring.

6. Mosquito born viral illness

Zika Virus
Disease: Caused by virus carried by Aedes aegypti mosquitos living in mostly tropical and sub-tropical locations. Congenital infection causes most severe disease. When a pregnant woman becomes infected with Zika virus, the virus can cause neural tube (brain and spinal cord) defects, eye abnormalities, deafness, and bone and joint problems (high tone, club-foot, developmental dysplasia of hips) in the baby. When a child is infected, illness is typically minor. There have been no confirmed cases of Zika virus disease in the U.S. since 2019 *(CDC, 2022).*
Symptoms: Congenital infection causes small head and severe brain defects (microcephaly), vision defects, hearing loss, muscle and joint problems, thyroid and liver abnormalities. Children and adults who are infected have fever, rash, pink eye (conjunctivitis) and joint pains.
Diagnosis: Blood, urine, or spinal fluid testing for PCR and IgM antibodies confirm infection.
Treatment: Supportive. There is no cure.
Contagious: Spread via sexual contact (semen, vaginal fluids), blood, urine.

Reality Check
Beware of mosquitoes. There were over 2600 cases of West Nile Virus reported in 2021. About 1 in 150 WNV-infected people suffer from more serious illness called viral encephalitis. Before you pack your bags to Antarctica (the only place in the world that is mosquito-free), know that very few mosquitoes carry WNV and 70-80% of people with WNV infection experience no symptoms at all. Just remember the 3 D's of prevention:
- ◆ Drain any standing water near your home.
- ◆ Dawn and dusk are peak mosquito feeding hours. Stay indoors.
- ◆ Defend and protect your family with DEET or Picaridin-based insect repellants. *(CDC)*

7. Enteroviruses

This is a big family of viruses (64 different types) that love to infect humans. The good news is that most of the time, we do not even know we are infected as there are few to no symptoms. The bad news is that some of these little viruses can be very serious. Some of the noteworthy viruses in this family are poliovirus (yes, it causes polio), coxsackievirus A (hand, foot, and mouth disease-see earlier in this section for more info), coxsackievirus B (a potentially more serious strain than A), echovirus (viral meningitis), enterovirus D71 (polio-like illness more common in Asia/Pacific) and enterovirus D68 (implicated in acute flaccid myelitis or AFM).

Bacterial Infections

1. Sinus Infections
Disease: Caused by the same bacteria that cause ear infections. Sinus infections are a second-

ary bacterial infection after a person has a common cold or flu. The virus sets up fluid in the sinus cavities behind the cheeks and above the eyes. More common in older children.

Symptoms: Prolonged runny nose over 14 days. New onset of discolored nasal secretions (snot) after 10 to 14 days of illness. New fever. Nighttime cough.

Diagnosis: Mostly by examination. Occasionally sinus x-ray is helpful.

Treatment: Same antibiotic choices as for ear infections, but often needs longer course.

Contagious: No.

2. Lung Infections (pneumonia)

Disease: Lung tissue inflammation that can be caused by bacteria or a virus. Bacterial pneumonia is a secondary infection after a viral illness (cold or flu).

Symptoms: High fever, wet cough, respiratory distress, vomiting. Child is getting worse instead of better with an illness, or new fever after initial fever resolved from an upper respiratory infection.

Diagnosis: Abnormal lung exam, chest x-ray, elevated white blood cell count

Treatment: Antibiotics. Rarely hospital admission—for labored breathing, need for oxygen.

Contagious: Depends on the bug.

3. Skin Infection (Impetigo and cellulitis)

Disease: Skin infection caused by bacteria that normally live on the skin that get under the skin. Bacteria capitalize on open wounds (bug bites, raw nostrils, burns).

Symptoms: Wound gets red with a golden, crusty, weeping discharge over it with impetigo. The skin is red, warm, and tender with cellulitis.

Diagnosis: Based on symptoms. Bugs can also grow in a culture if drainage from wound is obtained.

Treatment: Impetigo can be treated with prescription antibiotic cream. Extensive impetigo and cellulitis are treated with antibiotics given by mouth.

Contagious: Impetigo—yes. Spread by direct contact with wound. Not contagious after 24 hours of antibiotic therapy. Cellulitis is not contagious.

Incubation period: 7 to 10 days.

Season: Year round.

Special alert: Drug-resistant Staph infection. "MRSA" (Methicillin Resistant Staph Aureus) is a bacterial skin infection that is a real problem to treat.

Disease: Skin infection caused by Staph (bacteria) that is resistant to several antibiotics and can spread through the whole household.

Symptoms: Infections look like spider bites, boils, or red, tender areas.

Diagnosis: Suspicious looking lesions can be lanced to drain as well as obtain culture to check for the germ and its susceptibility to antibiotics.

Treatment: Topical or oral antibiotics, IV antibiotics for serious infections. People who are carriers (not infected) may harbor MRSA in their noses. They can be treated with topical antibiotics to the nose.

Contagious: Yes. Spread via carriers of MRSA, or those infected with it spread to another person's skin.

Prevention: Wash hands thoroughly with soap and water or alcohol based hand sanitizer. Keep

? ?

INFECTIONS

cuts/scrapes clean and covered with a bandage until healed. Avoid contact with other people's wounds or bandages. Do not share personal items like towels, washcloths. (CDC)
Season: Year round.

4. Eye Infections "Pink Eye" (Bacterial conjunctivitis)

Disease: Infection of the eye lining. Can be caused by either viruses or bacteria. Bacterial infections usually cause yellow or green eye discharge. Viral infections usually cause watery eye discharge. One bacteria, Haemophilus influenza, causes pink eye, sinus infections, and ear infections at the same time. About 30% of babies under age two with bacterial pink eye will also have an ear infection to go with it.
Symptoms: Red, itchy eyes with discolored thick fluid draining or matting the eyes shut.
Diagnosis: Based on exam. Occasionally, a culture is done of the fluid.
Treatment: Antibiotic eye drops if infection is bacterial. No treatment for viral pink eye.
Contagious: VERY. Spread by direct contact with eye discharge. Use separate hand towels.
Incubation period: Varies. For viral pink eye, 2 to 14 days.
Season: Year round.

5. Food Poisoning (E. coli, Salmonella, Shigella, and others)

Disease: Bacterial infection spread through contaminated food (and infected people's mouths and poop). Salmonella bacteria is the most common cause of food poisoning (80% of the time). E. coli Type 0157: H7, although less common, can be particularly serious. This bug releases a toxin/poison that causes **HEMOLYTIC UREMIC SYNDROME** (HUS). HUS causes severe anemia, low platelet count, and kidney failure. It is a reversible condition, but can be fatal. These kids are *really* sick with abdominal distention, pain, bloody diarrhea, and **PETECHIAE.** E. coli 0157 comes from cow and deer poop. Ground meat can have bacterial contamination throughout. Because of that, the meat needs to be cooked thoroughly to kill any of these bugs. Whole muscle cuts are only contaminated on the surface of the meat, which are always cooked well. (The poop gets spread to the meat during hide removal or evisceration). (*Pickering*)
Symptoms: Vomiting, diarrhea mixed with blood or mucous. Fever. Body aches. Abdominal pain.
Diagnosis: Stool culture, blood and white blood cells in poop, some blood test abnormalities.
Treatment: FLUIDS to avoid dehydration. Some bacterial infections need antibiotics to clear. Some bacterial infections should NOT be treated with antibiotics as it causes the person to remain a "carrier" of the infection.
Contagious: Spread through contaminated food/water (poultry, undercooked eggs, alfalfa sprouts, unpasteurized milk, undercooked hamburgers), breast milk, fomites (e.g. raw meat on countertop), direct contact with infected poop, saliva. Salmonella is also spread via pet iguanas and turtles, who are carriers. People, especially infants, who get Salmonella will often remain carriers for months after the infection.
Incubation Period: Varies on the bug, usually 6 to 72 hours.
Season: Year round.
Prevention: Never eat a hamburger that can moo back at you (it needs to be well done). Avoid fresh fruit/vegetables and water when traveling to developing countries. Drink only pasteurized milk and apple cider. Be careful in the kitchen. Food preparation should be separated from baby products (bottles, nipples, etc.). Avoid pet iguanas or turtles.

BOTTOM LINE

Yes, we know it is trendy in some circles to drink unpasteurized or raw milk. People who prefer this product believe that the pasteurization process takes out some of the "natural" ingredients ... like bacteria that can cause serious illness or death. Please purchase pasteurized milk and dairy products!

Reality Check

There was an E. coli outbreak a few years ago blamed on a petting zoo. Kids touched animals that had rolled around in cow manure. The kids later touched their mouths with their contaminated hands. Note: wash your child's hands thoroughly after going to a petting zoo.

6. Bladder Infections or Urinary Tract Infections (E. coli and others)

Disease: A bacterial infection caused by intestinal bacteria that get into the bladder. Bacteria (e.g. E. coli) routinely come out in our poop. They only cause infection when they creep into our bladders. Babies who are in diapers are susceptible to bladder infections (especially girls) because the poop collects where the opening to the bladder sits (urethra). Some babies are prone to bladder infections because of an abnormality called **VESICOURETERAL REFLUX.**

Symptoms: Fever, fussy mood, lack of other symptoms to explain fever

Diagnosis: Abnormal urinalysis, urine culture grows bacteria. Certain children with bladder infections have an evaluation done of their urinary tract system to rule out abnormality.

Treatment: Depends on the age and severity of infection. Babies under three months of age are hospitalized because of a higher risk of kidney infection and meningitis from infection.

Contagious: No.

Prevention: Clean poopie diapers as soon as possible. Wipe girls front to back.

7. Meningitis

Disease: Inflammation of the tissues that line the brain. This can be caused by viruses or bacteria. Bacterial meningitis is a life threatening illness. There are different bacteria that cause meningitis in various age groups. Meningitis can be caused by more than one type of bacteria. The top two that you need to know about are discussed below:

Group B Strep

Disease: With a newborn, the bacteria you will hear the most about is **Group B Strep**. This bacteria is normal flora in the intestines, bladder, and the vagina of mothers. It uniquely causes infection in newborns as they pass through the birth canal. Pregnant women are routinely screened at 35 to 37 weeks to check for the presence of Group B Strep (GBS). If Mom is a carrier, they are given IV antibiotics during labor to suppress the growth of this bacteria. If Mom goes into labor before 37 weeks, has broken their water more than 18 hours, or has a fever greater than 100.4, they also get IV antibiotics because of the risk of Group B Strep infection. (Women who have planned C-sections don't have to worry about this stuff.) Doctors watch all newborns closely, but those with GBS-positive Moms get watched even more closely. A standard protocol is to get a complete blood count and blood culture on a newborn if Mom is GBS-positive and didn't get pretreated with antibiotics (i.e. a quick labor), baby is born less than 35 weeks gestation, or if a baby starts misbehaving (temperature instability, respiratory distress). There is also potential for a late onset GBS infection up to three months after delivery.

Diagnosis: Bacteria can be seen in blood or spinal fluid under a microscope (see Gram stain in lab section). Blood or spinal fluid cultures give the definitive answer in 2 to 3 days.

Treatment: IV antibiotics. Penicillin works well.

Contagious: Spread via birth canal.

Incubation period: 0-3 months.

Season: N/A.

Prevention: Prophylactic antibiotics to Mom while in labor.

Strep pneumoniae

Disease: This type of Strep is also known as *pneumococcus* (very confusing). This bacteria has been the top cause of bacterial meningitis in infants. (It also causes ear infections, blood infections, sinus infections and pneumonia). Strep pneumoniae has developed resistance to many antibiotics. This is why the Prevnar vaccine (for Strep pneumoniae) was a welcome arrival back in 2000. Since then, we have seen an 87% disease reduction in bloodstream (bacteremia) infections and meningitis.

Symptoms: High fevers (usually more than 103), *without obvious symptoms*, irritability. If the infection is caught early while it is in the blood, treatment prevents travel to the brain (meningitis).

Diagnosis: Blood infections (bacteremia) by an elevated white blood cell count over 15,000 (often over 20,000) and a blood culture which may grow the bug. Meningitis is diagnosed by an abnormal spinal fluid (white blood cells in it) and a culture that grows bacteria.

Treatment: Blood infections get treated with an antibiotic shot initially, then oral antibiotics. Meningitis requires IV antibiotics and hospitalization.

Contagious: Spread by respiratory droplets. Strep pneumoniae lives everywhere. Some people are carriers. Children get infected when they already have a viral upper respiratory infection.

Incubation period: 1 to 3 days.

Season: Winter mostly.

Prevention: Prevnar (PCV-20 strains) vaccine for infants and children under five who are high risk. There is also a Pneumococcus vaccine (23 strains) for high risk children and elderly people. High risk: sickle cell disease, children with no spleen, kidney disease, immune compromised, HIV. (*Pickering*)

Things That Make You Itch Just Thinking About Them

Note: We will also discuss some of these lovely germs in Chapter 15, First Aid in the section on rashes. Go to our online Rash-o-Rama at Baby411.com (click bonus material) to see pictures.

Fungal Infections

Disease: Fungi are plant relatives (yeast, mold) that don't need light to live. Fungi prefer places where there is little competition (i.e. low bacteria levels). And, some fungi thrive on people whose defenses are down (i.e. immune compromised). We get infected in the following ways:

1. Fungus infestation. These are the accidental tourists. These fungi thrive on our skin, but

infections

don't go any deeper than that (**RINGWORM, ATHLETE'S FOOT, JOCK ITCH**). They are passed from person to person, or via a pet. These fungi just happen to be at the right place at the right time.

2. Opportunistic infection. These fungi grow when other factors alter our body defenses to fungi. Infants are susceptible to fungal infections (**THRUSH, YEAST DIAPER RASH**) because their bodies are relatively free of bacteria flora. Kids are also at risk for yeast diaper rash after having a course of antibiotics because the antibiotic not only kills the bad bacteria, but also the good normal flora. Other fungal opportunities include people on chronic steroids or with diabetes.

3. Invasive infection. This virtually never happens to normal, healthy people. A fungus invades the blood or lungs after its spores are inhaled.

Diagnosis:
Ringworm. Classic circular area with raised red border, and central scale. Fungus visible under microscope. Culture will grow in 2 to 3 weeks.
Ringworm of scalp. Patch of hair loss with overlying scale, or dots of hair loss with stubs of broken hair, or big ugly pus pockets (kerion) in the scalp. More in black kids (fungus likes the hair texture). Culture grows in 2 to 3 weeks.
Thrush. Classic white plaques on a red base in the cheeks, gums, tongue. Looks like milk you can't wipe off. Diagnosis based on examination.
Yeast diaper rash. Raw meat red area with satellite pimply dots. Won't improve with Desitin. Found often when thrush is present in the mouth.

Treatment:
Ringworm. Anti-fungal cream for 2 to 4 weeks.
Ringworm of scalp. Anti-fungal medicine by mouth for 1-2 months (cream won't kill it). The fungus imbeds in the hair follicle and is very hardy. We see some drug resistant strains.
Thrush. Anti-fungal mouthwash for 1 to 2 weeks. Sterilize all nipples, pacifiers.
Yeast diaper rash. Anti-fungal cream for 1 to 2 weeks.
Contagious: Until treated for 24 hours with anti-fungal medicine.
   Ringworm. Direct contact with infected person or animal (itchy dogs). Fomites too.
   Ringworm of scalp. Direct contact with combs, hairbrushes, bed sheets.
   Thrush. Direct contact with infant's mouth (spreads to Mom's nipples).
   Yeast diaper rash. Opportunistic infection. Not particularly contagious. (*Pickering*)

Scabies (Mite Infection)

Disease: An infestation caused by mites, tiny bugs that are somewhere between parasites and ticks. The female scabies mite burrows into our skin and lays her eggs. She lays 200 eggs in eight weeks. When the eggs hatch, the babies burrow into our skin and start eating. This is the ITCHIEST rash ever. Even after treatment, people are itchy for weeks afterwards.
Symptoms: The mites usually burrow between our fingers, elbow creases, armpits, belly button area, and genitals. In infected kids under two years old, they prefer the neck, palms, and soles. What you will see is a streak made out of tiny bumps—they start out gray, but are

usually red by the time a person seeks medical attention.

Diagnosis: If the rash is classic, diagnosis is made on examination alone. For unclear cases, a scraping of a burrow can be done. It may reveal the mite, mite egg, or mite poop under the microscope.

Treatment: A scabicidal body wash (Elimite-5% Permethrin) is available by prescription. ALL FAMILY MEMBERS GET TREATED. Clothing and bedding used for four days before treatment need to be washed and dried on the hot cycle. Disinfecting the house is a waste of time.

Contagious: Until treated with Elimite. Spread by direct contact, especially by holding hands. Co-sleeping is also an easy way for the whole family to get infected with scabies. Mites cannot survive off of humans for more than 24 hours.

Incubation period: 4 to 6 weeks.

More mite facts:

Chiggers are mites who like pores and hair follicles of people. These are self-limited infestations, but are also very itchy.

Dust mites do not cause infection. They feed off of the dead skin that we slough off on a daily basis. Some people are allergic to dust mite poop and have chronic nasal congestion as a result of it (see environmental allergies). (*Pickering*)

Lice

Disease: Infestation by a human louse. Head lice enjoy feeding on us via human hair. They don't have wings. They migrate from one head to the next by crawling over. They can't survive away from hair for more than 24 hours. The adult females lay eggs in the hair shafts (less than 1/4 inch from the scalp). Adults live about one month. The eggs become thriving nymphs in about one week. Head lice prefer straighter, thinner hair. Outbreaks happen more in school age children, but younger kids can acquire lice at childcare centers.

Symptoms: Itchy scalp, white flakes that are firmly adherent to the hair shaft.

Diagnosis: Adult lice are brown and visible with the naked eye—but they move quickly. The diagnosis is made most often by finding white nits (empty eggshells). Nits stick firmly to the hair shaft close to the scalp. Dandruff is rubbed off easily, nits are not.

Treatment: An over-the-counter shampoo called Nix (1% permethrin) kills adult lice and the eggs. Two treatments, one week apart (to kill any baby lice that survived the first round). Since the nits are empty eggshells, removing them is more of a cosmetic issue than a therapeutic one. The phrase "nit-picking" comes from the tedious task of removing the sticky nits that are close to the scalp. Many little lice are resistant to current over-the-counter treatment.

Contagious: Until treated. "No-nit" policies in childcare facilities are not necessary.

Incubation period: 6 to 10 days.

Creative treatment for resistant head lice: If living *adult* lice are found (not nits), then re-treatment is in order. The list of alternatives include prescription Sklice (ivermectin), Natroba (spinosad), 5% Permethrin (Elimite), Ulesfia (benzyl alcohol), and Malathion (a pesticide). A combination of tea tree oil, eucalyptus oil, and olive oil (1 teaspoon of each mixed together) applied to the scalp may also prove effective for kids over age three.

infections

INFECTIONS

? ?

For more information on lice: www.headlice.org

Pinworms

Disease: Pinworms live in our intestines and lay eggs on the outside of the anus. Infection is spread when a worm-ridden Child #1 scratches their bottom and plays in the sandbox. Child #2 plays in the sandbox later and picks up the eggs on their fingers. Those little fingers go in their mouth, and voila! Child #2 has pinworms too!

Symptoms: The female pinworm comes out to the anus at night and lays her eggs. This causes a symptom called pruritus ani (Latin for "itchy tushie"). Itchy vagina also happens from pinworms.

Diagnosis: Often based on symptoms alone. Parents can go on a worm hunt. The female comes out of the anus about two hours after a child is sleeping. Put clear Scotch tape on a toothpick and obtain a specimen.

Treatment: Two doses of over-the-counter Pyrantel (brand name Pin-X), given two weeks apart. Alternative: prescription strength Emverm (mebendazole). Doctors often treat the whole family. Bathing in morning helps remove the eggs.

Contagious: Until treated. Infected people often re-infect themselves by scratching their anus and ingesting more eggs.

Incubation period: 1 to 2 months (egg is ingested, then matures into an adult egg-laying female in 1 to 2 months). (*CDC*)

Parasites

Another stomach infection is called Giardia. This is a parasite spread via water. Yes, this includes swimming pools, hot tubs, and area lakes. Someone with the infection who is swimming in the water can share it. It frequently haunts childcare centers. Prolonged or foul-smelling diarrhea deserves to be tested for parasites.

Special Feature: Ear Infections

Is your child earning frequent flier miles at the doctor's office? Are you exhausted by the constant ear infections your poor baby has had to endure? Then this section is for you.

Q. Why is my baby prone to getting ear infections?

Thanks to your baby's facial structure, their Eustachian tubes are not working right. The Eustachian tubes equalize pressure changes in the ear and clear the fluid created from infection or allergies. Babies are born with round heads to get through the birth canal. As a result, the Eustachian tubes (connection between the ears and the back of the nose) *lie horizontally* in kids until three years old. This keeps the tubes from draining effectively. As a child grows, their head and face elongates. The Eustachian tubes ultimately slant downwards (and work better).

When a child gets a cold or upper respiratory infection, the virus causes the lining of the Eustachian tubes to swell, making the tubes even more inefficient. Bacteria like to grow if the fluid sits there long enough. The body's immune response to the bacteria creates pus, and that is the definition of a middle ear infection (**ACUTE OTITIS MEDIA**). Older children and adults rarely get ear infections because their Eustachian tubes drain more effectively.

Inner ear
Middle ear
Adenoids (in back of nose)

Ear canal   Eardrum   Eustachian tube

Your Baby's Ear, in a nutshell
Notes:
1. The ear is divided into three parts—the inner, middle, and outer areas.
2. The Eustachian tubes attach to the middle part of the ear.
3. The eardrum (tympanic membrane) is a piece of tissue that separates the middle and outer ear.
4. The eardrum protects the delicate middle ear bones and nerves.

TOP 7 RISK FACTORS FOR EAR INFECTIONS

Parents often ask if there is anything that can be done to prevent an ear infection from happening. Here are the risk factors:

1. **The common cold/upper respiratory infection.** By definition, fluid must be present in the Eustachian tubes to allow bacteria to grow. Having a cold is the perfect set up for fluid accumulation in the sinuses and Eustachian tubes.

2. **Daycare.** Children get more cold viruses when they are around other kids. Naturally, kids in daycare will get more colds, thus more ear infections. And the bacteria that live there are more likely to be drug resistant bacteria.

3. **Second hand smoke.** Smoke is irritating to the whole respiratory tract, from the nose down to the lungs. Irritation of the Eustachian tubes causes swelling of the tissues and inefficiency in clearing fluid.

4. **Pacifier use.** Constant sucking seems to create a backup of fluid in the back of the throat and Eustachian tubes.

5. **Bottle propping.** Babies who lie down and hold their own bottles allow fluid from the back of the throat to end up in the Eustachian tubes. The fluid is a set up for infection.

6. **Native American.** The facial structure of this ethnic group predisposes them to Eustachian tube dysfunction.

7. **Cleft lip/palate.** This facial structure predisposes them to Eustachian tube dysfunction.

infections

Ear Infection Facts

◆ By the age of three, 75% of all children have had at least one ear infection.
◆ 40% of all antibiotics prescribed for children are for ear infections.
◆ The peak age of ear infections is six to 18 months of age.
◆ 90% of ear infections are caused by bacteria; 10% by viruses.

Q. What is the difference between an ear infection and swimmer's ear?

An "ear infection" generally refers to a *middle* ear infection (**ACUTE OTITIS MEDIA**). The pus/infection sits behind the eardrum (see diagram on the previous page). A "swimmer's ear" (**OTITIS EXTERNA**) refers to an infection of the skin lining the *outer* ear (the canal where Q-tips don't belong!).

Middle Ear Infection (Acute Otitis Media)

A normal looking eardrum is grayish and translucent. The bones that control hearing (the ones you learned about in junior high science class) are visible behind it. An infected eardrum has pus behind it and is swollen and red. The pus and swelling obscure the view of the middle ear. *Think of the infection as being a zit.* It has to drain before it gets better. It can either rupture the eardrum and drain (undesirable) or drain down the Eustachian tube (desirable). The use of antibiotics taken by mouth clears the pus and decreases the chance of the zit bursting (**PER-FORATED EARDRUM,** see more on the next page).

Swimmer's Ear (External Otitis)

This is a skin infection caused by either pooled water that collects in the ear canal of kids who swim under water or skin irritation from being scratched (from a Q-tip). Both situations

NEW PARENT 411: EAR TREATMENT GUIDELINES

Here are the American Academy of Pediatrics treatment guidelines for ear infections:
Infants under six months of age with acute middle ear infections should be treated with antibiotics. They are more likely to suffer complications from ear infections.

Kids ages six months to two years with *clear cut infections* are also treated, but when the diagnosis is in question, a wait and see approach is in order. Your doctor may ask you to return for a follow-up visit or have you fill a prescription in a couple of days if your child's symptoms don't improve.

The guidelines attempt to limit antibiotic use in kids with mild to moderate symptoms and avoid use when the diagnosis itself is in question (not all ear infections are so black and white).

Ask your doctor for their opinion about this issue. Record their thoughts here:

? ?

INFECTIONS

allow bacteria to penetrate the skin and cause infection. *Swimmer's ear causes extreme pain with touch or movement of the outer ear* (the part you can see). There is swelling, redness, and sometimes debris in the canal. The eardrum is normal. These infections usually clear up with antibiotic eardrops.

Q. My baby's eardrum popped! Will they have permanent hearing damage?

No. Perforated eardrums heal like a piece of skin that has been cut.

Remember the zit analogy? The eardrum is under pressure with all that pus behind it. When the pimple pops, it lets the pus drain out. The perforation hole is usually small and not completely ruptured. The ear feels better if this happens. The infection still needs to be treated, though. The doctor may prescribe antibiotic drops and oral antibiotics if this occurs. It should heal up without any long-term consequences as long as the infection is treated.

Q. Will my child get an ear infection from lying in bath water?

No.

Bath water is fairly clean and very little collects in the outer ear canal. But it's a good idea to wipe the water out of the ears. It's not a major player in causing swimmer's ear. And it has absolutely nothing to do with middle ear infections (which happen on the other side of the eardrum).

Q. My child was just in the doctor's office two days ago. Now they have an ear infection. Didn't the doctor see it then?

Back to the zit thing. Ears can go from normal to bulging with pus in a matter of hours.

Q. Can I buy one of those ear scopes (otoscope) and examine my own child's ears?

Sure. But you might not know what you are looking at.

An acute middle ear infection may present itself in one of several ways. The obvious bulging red ear is one you'd be able to diagnose. But not all of them look like that. Some infections are more subtle. It doesn't just take the light of an otoscope to make the diagnosis. It takes the experience of looking at thousands of ears for comparison.

One positive outcome of the pandemic is that primary care providers offer telemedicine in their practices. Newer digital otoscopes allow us to see your child's eardrum from your living room. You can buy one at Amazon.com for about $45.

Q. I've heard that not all ear infections require antibiotics to go away. Do we have to treat every ear infection with antibiotics?

Not all middle ear infections require antibiotics.

A small percentage (10%) of ear infections are caused by viruses. And up to 60% of bacterial ear infections will clear on their

DR B'S OPINION

"I always pick the least potent antibiotic that will work in a given situation. The only way to have the 'big gun' when you need it is to avoid using it when you don't need it."

own without any consequences. However, bacterial ear infections clear more quickly with antibiotics.

A study in the *New England Journal of Medicine* looked at the standard recommendations for treating ear infections in children ages six to 23 months of age. Their conclusion: little kids feel better faster when they are treated with antibiotics. (*Hoberman*)

That said, the American Academy of Pediatrics guidelines advise healthcare providers to be judicious about diagnosing ear infections based on stricter criteria and only treat true infections. Their message to parents: be patient. Every illness does not improve with antibiotics.

And for kids over age two, a provider might diagnose an ear infection and send a child home without a prescription. They might tell the parent to give the child a pain medication and come back the next day for a re-check. If the ear looks worse or unchanged, she prescribes antibiotics. If the ear is improved, no therapy is required.

Q. What happened in the days before antibiotics when children had ear infections?

Some children did just fine. Others did not.

Untreated bacterial infections can lead to *hearing loss* (from chronic fluid accumulation, chronic infection, and chronic ear drum perforations), *mastoiditis* (infection invades the skull bone), and *brain abscesses/meningitis* (infection extends to brain and spinal fluid). In the old days before antibiotics, 80% of ear infections would go away on their own. But the last 20% of ear infections that were untreated led to these significant complications. (*Rosenfeld*)

Q. What antibiotics are typically used to treat ear infections?

The right drug for the bug.

The most common bacteria that cause middle ear infections are:

◆ Strep pneumoniae (now less common thanks to Prevnar vaccine).
◆ Moraxella
◆ H. Influenza *non-typable* (a cause of pink eye with an ear infection)
◆ Group A Strep

There are basically four antibiotic classes that kill all of these bugs. As a general rule, doctors prescribe amoxicillin (in the Penicillin class) as their first choice. It is a broad-spectrum antibiotic that is well tolerated by most kids, has been around for a long time, and is relatively inexpensive (about $10 for generic). It works about 85% of the time, depending on the amount of drug resistant bacteria living in your neighborhood. That's a pretty good track record.

If it has been *less* than 30 days since a previous ear infection, doctors may select a different class of antibiotics because the bacteria may be resistant to the amoxicillin (that is, the same bug may have grown back after being off medication).

If there is pink eye associated with an ear infection, there is a good chance that H. influenza is the bug. This bug is resistant to amoxicillin about 50% of the time (again, depending on your neighborhood). So, a doctor may choose a different antibiotic in this situation.

Q. My child was on amoxicillin before and it never works.

Your child is not resistant to amoxicillin—the bacterium causing the infection is resistant. Children in daycare settings tend to have more ear and sinus infections with drug-resistant bacteria. That does not mean that amoxicillin will *never* work. For instance, Group A Strep (which causes Strep throat) is almost always cured with amoxicillin.

Q. My child is pulling on their ears. Should I be worried about an ear infection?

No. It's not a reliable indicator.

Parents frequently rely on ear pulling as a sign of an ear infection. There was an excellent study done on this suspicious behavior that showed ear pulling predicted ear infections only 5% of the time; 95% of the time, babies pull on their ears because they can! (*Baker*)

Q. Why do I have to bring my child back for an "ear check" after they have been treated?

Because infants can't tell you that their ears are better.

The antibiotic prescribed should kill the bacteria. But there are smart, resistant bugs that will survive. That's one reason why the doctor wants to see your child back two to three weeks after the diagnosis.

The other reason is that residual sterile fluid (**SEROUS OTITIS MEDIA**) can remain for a long time after the bacteria is gone. This is basically pus that is dissolved, but not dried up. The fluid is not infected, but can create two problems:

◆ It puts a child at risk for getting another middle ear infection down the road.

◆ It inhibits sound waves from getting through the middle ear (**CONDUCTIVE HEARING LOSS**). It's like walking around with earplugs in all day long. Chronic fluid (more than three months duration) is a problem for a child who is trying to learn his native lan-

---

RESIDUAL EAR FLUID

The pus from the ear infection gradually dissolves and gets reabsorbed by the body. The name for this sterile (bug-free) fluid is called **SEROUS FLUID** or serous otitis. 70% of children will still have serous fluid two weeks after an ear infection. Up to 40% of kids will still have serous fluid one month later, and 10% have fluid three months after infection. (*Peter*)

The serous fluid does NOT need to be treated with antibiotics to clear up. However, kids with residual fluid need to be re-evaluated to make sure the fluid goes away. As mentioned earlier, chronic fluid in the ears interferes with language development (in the short term).

If a child has chronic fluid in the ears, over three months duration, an Ear/Nose/Throat specialist may want to drain the fluid by popping the eardrum with a needle. Frequently, if the drum is popped, a PE tube is inserted to prevent further accumulations of fluid.

guage (**EXPRESSIVE LANGUAGE DELAYS**). As Dr. Nina Shapiro, Director of Pediatric Otolaryngology and Professor at David Geffen School of Medicine at UCLA, points out, hearing loss is *temporary* and *reversible* when it is due to fluid behind the eardrum. She comments, "As long as the fluid eventually resolves by either PE tubes or time, there are no long-term speech or language deficits." We will discuss PE tubes in detail later in this section.

Q. My child feels better after just a couple of days taking amoxicillin for his ear infection. Why do we have to continue the medicine for ten days?

Antibiotics start to clear an infection within 48-72 hours. However, it can take five to ten days to kill off all of the bacteria. Stopping an antibiotic early allows a germ to re-grow and cause infection (and pain) to return.

Q. We are flying with our baby tomorrow and they were just diagnosed with an ear infection. Should we cancel our trip?

No. Go have fun.

As anyone who's traveled on a plane knows, the pressurized air in the cabin requires you to "clear" your ears (by chewing gum, yawning, etc). Babies have the same needs—their middle ear must accommodate to the pressure change. When a child has an acute ear infection, pus fills in the middle ear space and the eardrum cannot move. The ear won't hurt. In fact, the pressure change might make the drum pop to release the pressure (and that's okay—see perforated eardrum earlier in this chapter).

It is more problematic when an ear infection is starting to clear up. Then there is both air (normal) and fluid (not normal) in the middle ear. The eardrum will try to accommodate to the pressure change and will be only partially successful. This HURTS. Don't cancel your trip; just be prepared for some discomfort on take off and landing. Nursing, feeding your child a bottle or sucking on a pacifier can help relieve the pressure.

DR B'S OPINION:
WHEN TO CALL IN AN ENT

Here is how I would approach making a referral to an Ear/Nose/Throat (ENT) Specialist for a child with recurrent ear infections (other than the "too many" criteria above).

Scenario 1: If a child already has had three ear infections by Thanksgiving, that doesn't bode well for the rest of the season (cold and flu season will continue through March). Refer now to an ENT.

Scenario 2: If a child gets ear infections sporadically through the winter and gets a fourth infection in April, wait and see if the ear infections stop as the season ends.

Scenario 3: If a child gets two ear infections during the summer months and a third in September, the child gets one more chance before referring. But I prepare the family for the possibility.

THE INFECTION HIT PARADE: VIRUSES AND BACTERIA

So, let's sum up this chapter. Here is a list of the top infections, as caused by viruses and bacteria:

Viruses That Cause Infection

The most common VIRUSES that cause infection in babies ages birth to age one.

Viral Respiratory Infections
1. The Common Cold or upper respiratory infection (Rhinovirus)
2. The Flu (Influenza)
3. Bronchiolitis (RSV)
4. COVID-19
5.. Croup (numerous viruses)

Viral Mouth And Tonsil Infections
1. Hand-Foot-and-Mouth (Coxsackievirus)
2. Herpes Stomatitis (Herpes Type-1)
3. Sore throat virus (Adenovirus)

Gastrointestinal Viruses
1. Stomach virus, or "stomach flu" (Rotavirus, Norovirus)

Viral Exanthems (Viruses That Cause Skin Rashes)
1. Roseola (Herpesvirus-6)
2. Chickenpox (Varicella)
3. Slapped Cheek or Fifth Disease (Parvovirus)

Bacteria That Cause Infection

Here are some of the bacterial infections in babies birth to age one. For details, please see earlier in the chapter.

1. **Ear Infections** (Strep pneumoniae, H. Influenza, and others)
2. **Sinus Infections** (Strep pneumoniae H. Influenza, and others)
3. **Eye Infections** (H. Influenza, Strep pneumoniae, and others)
4. **Throat Infections** (Group A Strep)
5. **Lung Infections** (Strep pneumoniae, Staph, and others)
6. **Food Poisoning** (E. Coli, Salmonella)
7. **Bladder Infections** (E. Coli, and others)
8. **Meningitis** (Group B Strep, Strep pneumoniae)
9. **Skin infections** (Staph, MRSA, Strep)

Things That Make You Itch Just Thinking About Them

1. **Fungus:** Ringworm, Thrush, Yeast diaper rash
2. **Mites:** Scabies, Lice
3. **Parasites:** Giardia
4. **Worms:** Pinworms

Q. How many ear infections are too many?

Great question. For this answer, we've recruited Dr. Mark Brown, an Ear, Nose, and Throat specialist for some advice:

"Most kids outgrow the problem of ear infections by about three years of age. (See earlier for information on why this is). So theoretically, we can all wait until your child turns three. But there are some important considerations that compel doctors to take a more active approach." Here are some key questions:

1. **How many courses of antibiotics are too many?** Antibiotics can have unpleasant side effects like diarrhea and yeast infections. Being on antibiotics frequently leaves a child susceptible to bacteria that are smarter (the drug-resistant strains) and allows bacteria in the community to see our weapons. From an economic standpoint, every ear infection costs parents a visit to the pediatrician, missed work, and another round of antibiotics.

2. **How old is the child?** If a child is in the midst of language acquisition (nine months to age two), it's critical to hear what people are saying. Otherwise, the infections can contribute to short-term expressive language delays. In the long run, these kids do catch up and have normal language skills.

3. **How miserable is the child?** Ear infections hurt. That leads to disrupted sleep for the whole family. This important point tends to get overlooked by both parents and doctors.

Reality Check

It's important to look at what is in the best interest of the child. There is some variability amongst doctors, but a reasonable answer to what is "too many" is the following:

◆ Four infections in the peak (winter) season
◆ Three infections in the off peak (summer) season
◆ Three months of persistent residual fluid (serous otitis media)
◆ Three back-to-back courses of antibiotics for the same ear infection.

Too many ear infections buy your child a trip to see the Ear, Nose, and Throat specialist. These doctors assist in decision making for children with recurrent ear infections. If necessary, they can place pressure equalization tubes in the eardrum to reduce the number of ear infections (we'll discuss this more in detail later in this chapter).

Ear infections occur mostly in cold and flu season. (Remember, bacteria are secondary infections for a child with fluid in his ears already). So, it's expected that more infections will happen then. Kids who get middle ear infections in the off-season are time bombs for the winter.

Q. How can I prevent ear infections from happening?

There are a few things you can do:

1. **Feed your baby in an upright position.** Milk can get into the Eustachian tubes if a baby is lying horizontally while eating.

2. **Avoid pacifiers after six months of age.** There is some data to suggest this is a

risk factor for ear infections. (*Post*)

3. **Don't smoke.** Smoking is a respiratory irritant—both to the smoker and their family. It causes swelling of the Eustachian tubes, which can lead to infection.

4. **Infection control during the cold and flu season.** Good hand-washing and flu shots for the family are helpful. The Prevnar vaccine for your child helps limit some (not all) infections.

5. **Reconsider your childcare options.** There is no question that children in daycare settings get more infections (and with drug-resistant bugs). When families have reached the end of their ropes, doctors may discuss this subject.

Q. Can we just start an antibiotic when my child has a cold? What about preventative antibiotics through the winter months?

Doctors used both of these methods in the past. And to a certain degree, they worked. However, the price paid is too great. This approach created drug-resistant bacteria.

Q. Can I prevent an ear infection from happening by using a decongestant or antihistamine to dry up all that snot?

No.

You would think that if you got rid of the fluid, the ear infection could be prevented. This idea was studied about 30 years ago and it didn't prevent ear infections. There is a reason it doesn't work. When there is infection, the Eustachian tubes are full of fluid *and* get swollen. This prevents them from draining effectively.

Q. What are "tubes"?

The official term is Pressure Equalization (PE) Tube.

The alternative to antibiotics for recurrent ear infections is to insert PE tubes into the eardrums. These tubes are the length of a pencil point and the diameter of angel hair pasta (i.e. really small). The procedure is relatively simple. An ENT Specialist makes a tiny hole in the eardrum, cleans out any fluid/pus, and inserts the tube. The tube falls out on its own after a lifespan of 6-18 months. The eardrum heals beautifully 99% of the time.

Children have this procedure done in a day-surgery facility. They do require anesthesia, but don't require an IV, breathing tube, or ventilator. Why anesthesia? It's helpful not to have a squirming child when someone is poking a hole into the eardrum. The procedure takes about five minutes. Kids are usually back to themselves again later that day.

Many parents are incredibly fearful of having PE tubes placed. They are afraid of the procedure, the anesthesia, or the risk of having an opening in the eardrum (you have to keep water out of the ear). Most of these concerns should be clearly addressed by your ENT doctor.

Helpful Hints: Understanding PE Tubes

Think of PE tube placement as a *procedure* and not surgery. I think the word surgery really freaks people out.

◆ This is a simple, quick procedure. For adults, it could be performed in an office setting.

◆ The risk of anesthesia is no greater than the risk of all the antibiotics your child has been taking.

◆ You'll no longer need to see the pediatrician every week. My frequent fliers stop visiting my office after they have PE tubes placed. I always enjoy seeing my patients, but I see some kids too often.

BOTTOM LINE

As a general rule, PE tubes are a life changing experience for the whole family. Even the most anxious parents report how "easy" the experience is, how much better their child feels, and wonder why they waited so long to do it. I've never had a family tell me they regretted the decision to get tubes!

When can Johnny go back to childcare/playgroup?

DISEASE	TREATMENT	RETURN TO CHILDCARE?
COVID-19	None	5 days after positive test & symptom free.
Common cold	None	When fever is gone.
Influenza	+/- Anti-viral Rx	When fever is gone.
Croup	+/- Steroid Rx	When fever is gone.
Hand-foot-mouth	None	When fever is gone.
Herpes stomatitis	None	When lesions are healed.
Conjunctivitis/Pink eye	None if viral infection	When eyes are clear.
Bacterial conjunctivitis	Antibiotic eye drops Rx	After 24 hrs. of treatment.
Stomach virus	None	When poop is formed.
Viral rashes	None	Depends on the infection.
Chickenpox	+/- Antiviral Rx	When all lesions crusted (1 wk).
Fifth disease	None	Not contagious once rash appears.
Impetigo	Antibiotic Rx	After 24 hours of treatment.
Food poisoning	Depends on the bug	When poop is formed.
Giardia	Anti-parasitic Rx	When poop is formed.
Ringworm	Anti-fungal Rx	After 24 hours of treatment.
Scabies	Body wash Rx	After 1 treatment.
Head lice	OTC shampoo	After 1 treatment.
Pinworms	OTC Anti-parasitic	After 1 treatment.

KEY—Rx: prescription medicine; OTC: over-the-counter medicine. (*Donowitz*)

Whew! That was a load of viruses and bacteria. Now, it's on to other medical problems that are NOT caused by infectious bugs. The next chapter explores the most common diseases that affect babies.

COMMON DISEASES

Chapter 14

"Sooner or later we all quote our mothers."
~ Bern Williams

WHAT'S IN THIS CHAPTER

◆ EYES: LAZY EYE
◆ LUNGS: ASTHMA
◆ HEART: MURMURS
◆ BLOOD: ANEMIA,
    SICKLE CELL DISEASE,
    IRON DEFICIENCY,
    LEAD EXPOSURE
◆ SKIN: ECZEMA
◆ MUSCLES/BONES:
    INTOEING, BOWED
    LEGS, FLAT FEET,
    TORTICOLLIS, HIP
    DYSPLASIA
◆ ENDOCRINE: DIABETES
◆ ALLERGIES: SEASONAL,
    ENVIRONMENTAL
◆ GENITALS: PENILE,
    LABIAL ADHESIONS
◆ WHAT'S THAT SMELL?
    UNUSUAL ODORS

This chapter is devoted to the most common medical problems in infants ages birth to one. Some topics have been discussed in other chapters. (See the index if you can't find the disease you are looking for in this chapter). The common thread of these medical problems is that they are not caused by an infectious bug.

We've organized this discussion by body system—first up, it's the eyes.

Eyes

Q. I'm worried my baby has a lazy eye. How do you check for that?

By examining the eyes every time you visit your doctor.

Under three months of age, babies can look cross-eyed occasionally. The muscles of both eyes aren't working together yet.

After three months, both eyes should move together. There are two medical reasons for why they don't:

1. **Strabismus.** The muscles that move the eye are weak.
2. **Amblyopia.** The eye itself is weak or injured.

Often a parent will notice this at home. Doctors check by covering up one eye and checking that the other eye can focus on an object. A child looks away or tries to remove the examiner's hand when the unaffected eye is covered. Cool trend: high-tech vision screening devices (Pediavision, iScreen, Spot, etc.) for the pediatrician's office.

These handheld gadgets interpret images of the eyes and detect vision problems—even in squirming toddlers. While the American Academy of Pediatrics supports early vision screening, major insurance plans have not embraced this technology yet. In other words, you may need to pay out of pocket for it. Our advice: it's worth it.

Children who fail a screening test should see an eye specialist (ophthalmologist). If a lazy eye goes untreated, permanent problems can occur. Eye doctors prefer to assess these problems before three years of age.

Helpful Hint

There is a benign condition called **PSEUDOSTRABISMUS** where kids just have narrowly set eyes. This is not a medical problem.

RED FLAG

If your child has a dramatic new problem with an eye turning in, go see your doctor ASAP. This can be a sign of a brain tumor. Don't panic yet, just get it checked out.

Lungs

Q. What is asthma?

In short, it's like hay fever in the lungs.

Asthma is a process of swelling, muscle tightening, obstruction, destruction, and mucous production in the big and little airways of the lungs. This chain of events occurs due to a revved up immunologic/allergic response to *infections, allergies, weather, and emotions*.

The narrowed airways interfere with the air exchange (getting clean air in and dirty air out) that occurs with each breath. As a result, children are "air hungry." Their bodies try to get more air in by breathing fast and pulling the rib muscles in when breathing. The characteristic wheeze comes from air traveling through a narrowed passageway.

Asthma attacks (termed exacerbations) occur intermittently depending on what a child is hypersensitive to. Often, kids with asthma have flare ups with upper respiratory infections. This makes for a very long, bad winter.

Q. How do you diagnose asthma?

Asthma is a diagnosis made by physical examination.

If a child is caught wheezing three or more times in their life, they carry a diagnosis of asthma. The first and second time a child wheezes, it might be bad luck. The third time, it's a trend.

There are reasons other than asthma that make children wheeze. Babies can get RSV bronchiolitis (see more below) or another infection that results in wheezing. Older babies can get a raisin (or other small object) stuck in their airway and wheeze, too.

Your doctor can get a chest x-ray to rule out an infection or a foreign body in the airway. Blood tests aren't particularly helpful. Probably the best information to confirm a diagnosis is a child's response to asthma medication. If their lungs clear up with asthma medication, they likely have the diagnosis.

DISEASES

Q. My doctor said my child has "Reactive Airway Disease." Is that asthma?

Basically, yes. It's just a nicer term to use for a younger child who has not been diagnosed asthmatic.

Doctors tend to hedge on the diagnosis of asthma in a child before the first birthday. Some infants get hit really hard with an RSV infection and wheeze for what seems like months. By definition, they have airways that are "reacting" to infection–by getting swollen and full of mucous.

Still other babies with severe acid reflux (**GERD**) will wheeze when the airway gets irritated. This type of wheezing resolves when they outgrow their reflux.

Doctors use this term for little ones who haven't proven themselves to be true asthmatics yet.

Q. My husband had asthma as a child. What are the chances that my baby will have it?

There is definitely a genetic predisposition to asthma and other allergic disorders. There is probably a 25% chance your child will have asthma. That means there is a 75% chance he won't. Given the odds, it doesn't pay to worry.

Q. My baby had RSV bronchiolitis this winter. What are the chances that they will have asthma?

Thirty to forty percent.

It is true that kids who wheeze with RSV tend to wheeze again (asthma) in their lifetimes. This is a chicken or the egg dilemma. We just don't know which came first.

Interestingly, not all kids who get RSV wheeze. And of the kids who do wheeze with RSV, not all of them respond to asthma medication. So, there may be just a subset of kids who would have wheezed anyway who have trouble with RSV infection. See the RSV section in Chapter 13, Infections, for more details.

Q. Are there any other factors that cause asthma?

Besides genetics, there's nothing else that is solidly proven to predispose a child to asthma. However, a few interesting studies have recently been published on this subject. Research suggests babies who are born four months before peak cold and flu season seem to be at higher risk of developing asthma later in life. One study points to RSV, while others point to the common cold (rhinoviruses) as the culprits. (*Stein*)

Other studies have found correlations with using the European equivalent of acetaminophen (Tylenol) in babies or exposure in the womb and development of allergies and asthma later in life. None of these studies prove that acetaminophen causes asthma. It's an age-old rule of science: correlation does not prove causation. (*Beasley, Allmers, Persky, Bakkeheim*)

But, considering that several studies have found similar results, it makes sense for babies and pregnant women to only take acetaminophen when they absolutely need it.

There is one major risk factor that is totally preventable, though: smoking. If you can't quit for your own health, hopefully your child's health and wellbeing can motivate you.

Q. How do you treat asthma?

◆ *For immediate rescue:* A **BRONCHODILATOR** (albuterol) very quickly relaxes the airways. This is usually inhaled via an inhaler device or a nebulizer machine (a souped-up vaporizer). For infants, the nebulizer provides the most immediate, effective relief. This medication can be given for prolonged periods in an office or emergency room setting. It can be administered every four to six hours at home.

◆ *For prevention of attacks:* Kids who wheeze more than twice a week or one night a month need a medication to keep their asthma in check. Persistent symptoms mean chronic destruction to the lungs, which we now know, can be permanent. An **INHALED STEROID** (Budesonide/Pulmicort) is administered via nebulizer daily for these high-risk kids. (*Expert Panel Report II*) Children with severe, persistent wheezing may need a round of steroids given by mouth. An oral medication called Singulair is also used to prevent flare-ups (see Appendix A, Common Medications for more info.)

Asthma is categorized by the severity of symptoms into *Intermittent, Mild Persistent, Moderate Persistent,* and *Severe Persistent*. The National Asthma Education and Prevention Program created standardized guidelines for asthma management. The treatment plans are divided by the severity of the symptom categories. See below:

SEVERITY	SYMPTOMS DAY/NIGHT	RX TO MAINTAIN CONTROL
Intermittent	2 or less days/week Uses rescue meds < 2 days/week	No daily medications Use rescue meds as needed Daily inhaled steroid at the start of a respiratory infection
Mild Persistent	>2 days/week but not daily 1-2 nights/month Uses rescue meds >2 days/week	Daily low-dose inhaled steroid 2nd choice: Singulair
Moderate Persistent	Daily symptoms 3-4 nights/month Uses rescue meds daily	Daily medium-dose inhaled steroid or daily low-dose inhaled steroid and long-acting rescue
Severe Persistent	Continual symptoms >1 night/week Uses rescue meds several times a day	(see below)

Treatment for severe persistent asthma:

1. Daily medium-dose inhaled steroid plus long acting rescue
2. Alternative: Daily medium-dose inhaled steroid plus Singulair

? ?

DISEASES

Q. What are the chances my child will outgrow asthma?

50/50.

Those odds aren't bad for a chronic illness. Unfortunately, no one can predict if and when your child will outgrow it. As a general rule, kids who have asthma before the age of five tend to outgrow it. Children who are diagnosed with asthma when they are older are more likely to have it in adulthood. (*Behrman*)

Q. What are the long-term consequences of asthma?

Asthma can cause permanent airway damage.

Kids who have *occasional* asthma flare-ups do fine in the long term. If a child has *chronic* wheezing, normal parts of the lung can be damaged—and don't recover. So, doctors are more aggressive about treatment for a child with persistent symptoms. Chronic obstructed airways also decrease the amount of oxygen getting to the body on a daily basis.

Q. My child has eczema. Does this mean they have a higher risk of developing asthma? Why?

Because allergic diseases can occur as a group. This particular problem is called **ATOPY.**

Atopy or atopic disease refers to a classic triad of asthma, eczema, and seasonal allergies. Of the kids who have eczema, 30% get either asthma or seasonal allergies (but 70% won't get either). (*Behrman*)

Q. My child wheezes. Could it be Cystic Fibrosis?

Yes, but it is very unlikely. Cystic Fibrosis (CF) is a genetically inherited disorder that affects one in 1600 children. It causes an abnormality in body cells that impair absorption of chloride. The result of this is that the lungs pull in too much sodium. Normal airway secretions get thick and don't move. Chronic lung infections develop. Other body systems are affected by this cell abnormality, particularly the intestines, pancreas, and reproductive system.

If your baby wheezes chronically, and especially if they have trouble gaining weight, a screening test for cystic fibrosis may be in order. A simple assessment of a baby's sweat will give the answer. (*Behrman*)

Interesting fact: all 50 states include cystic fibrosis on their newborn metabolic screening tests. While not 100% (some children with CF may have a negative or equivocal newborn screen), many babies are diagnosed now before they have any symptoms. And, those children may have better nutritional and developmental outcomes as a result. Bottom line: if your wheezing baby passed their newborn metabolic screening test, the odds are very low for having CF.

Heart

Q. What is a heart murmur?

A murmur is an extra noise that is heard when your doctor listens to the heartbeat with a stethoscope. The normal heartbeat is actually a series of sounds best described as "lub-dub." A murmur is an extra noise that may sound like rushing water ("p-ssh") or a squeak ("eek"). The quality, duration, and location of that noise help your doctor determine what is producing it.

If the cause isn't obvious by simply listening, your doctor may recommend that a heart specialist (pediatric cardiologist) see the baby. Tests, such as an electrocardiogram (EKG) or echocardiogram ("echo" or ultrasound examination of the heart), may be recommended to gain additional information about your baby's heart.

Q. My doctor heard an "innocent" heart murmur in my baby. I'm freaking out.

No.

We recruited one of our favorite pediatric cardiologists, Karen L. Wright, M.D., to field this one: "An innocent murmur is the sound of normal blood flow passing through the heart chambers and blood vessels. These sounds are commonly heard in infants, and are no cause for alarm. If your baby is doing well and an innocent murmur is detected, your baby's doc will let you know and make a note to check on this during future visits. If there is any concern, or reassurance is needed, your baby's doctor can arrange for you to see a pediatric cardiologist."

Q. My baby has a heart murmur and is going to see a specialist. Should I be worried?

Be appropriately concerned, but not alarmed. Most heart murmurs are innocent (see above) and are not a problem.

Doctors err on the side of checking things out to be sure everything is okay. The term for a murmur caused by a defect in the heart is a **PATHOLOGIC MURMUR**. Most pathologic murmurs are caused by a problem with the way the heart developed before a baby was born (**CONGENITAL HEART DISEASE**). A congenital heart defect occurs in about one in 100 newborns.

Normal heart

According to Dr. Wright, "The vast majority of those defects are pretty mild, and do not significantly interfere with a child's life. In fact, some of these defects truly go away on their own. A common type of congenital heart defect is a hole between the pumping chambers of the heart, called a **VENTRICULAR SEPTAL DEFECT (VSD)**. Most of these holes are small, and will often close as the baby's heart grows."

VSD

Other, less common defects may require either a procedure or surgery to correct.

DISEASES

Q. Are there other types of heart problems seen in babies?

SUPRAVENTRICULAR TACHYCARDIA (SVT) is an abnormally fast heart rhythm and it can make babies pretty ill. Fortunately, it's rare.

A baby's normal heart rate is already fast (up to 180 beats/minute), so it can be difficult to tell what is *too* fast. But if a baby is unusually fussy, feeding poorly, or breathing rapidly, SVT is one thing to think about. Get it checked out by your doc.

Blood

Q. What is anemia?

Let's discuss what red blood cells are first.

Red blood cells (which come from bone marrow) carry oxygen to our body tissues and remove carbon dioxide. Hemoglobin is the name of the protein that performs this function in each red blood cell. The key ingredient of hemoglobin is iron.

"Anemia" means there are not enough red blood cells circulating in the bloodstream. The causes of anemia are either *excessive destruction* or *inadequate production of red blood cells*.

Examples of *excessive destruction* of red blood cells include:

◆ More blood is being lost than made (such as menstruating women).
◆ Abnormal red blood cells are made and destroyed (such as sickle cell disease).

Examples of *inadequate production* of red blood cells include:

◆ Bone marrow production slows (such as bone marrow suppression by virus).
◆ Iron deficiency limits production due to lack of a key ingredient (that is, iron-deficiency anemia).
◆ Lead poisoning (technically, this is competition for iron's place in the red blood cell).
◆ Poor nutritional intake of key vitamins like B12/Folate.

The number one cause of anemia in childhood is iron deficiency. Kids who are severely anemic are pale and fatigue easily. Anemia sometimes presents with odd symptoms, like breath-holding.

Q. My baby had an abnormal newborn screen. We found out they have "sickle cell trait." What does that mean?

Let's be geneticists for a moment. Babies get one set of genes/DNA from each biological parent. Some diseases require one defective gene to affect someone (**AUTOSOMAL DOMINANT**). Some diseases require *both* genes to be abnormal to manifest themselves (**AUTOSOMAL RECESSIVE**).

Sickle cell disease is an autosomal recessive disease. People with one defective gene and one normal gene are called carriers. They carry the trait (gene) for the disease but are typically not affected by it. About 8% of the U.S. black population are sickle cell carriers. Sickle cell trait is also more common in people with Mediterranean, Middle Eastern, sub-Saharan Africa, and Indian ancestry.

Both sickle cell trait and disease can be detected by that first newborn blood test sent to the state laboratory (see Newborn Screening Tests in Chapter 1). It's detected by the type of protein

diseases

chain that makes up red blood cells.

Elite athletes with sickle cell trait have a slight risk of muscle breakdown or a ruptured spleen if they exercise rigorously at high altitudes where there is less oxygen. (FYI: this is why the NCAA requires sickle cell testing for all college athletes, but this is a highly controversial policy amongst medical experts.) But, for everyone else with sickle cell trait, just stay hydrated and enjoy that ski trip. (CDC)

Sickle cell trait is potentially a problem if your adult child decides to become a parent someday. If both biological parents have sickle cell trait, their children are at a high risk for having sickle cell disease. This is routinely addressed in preconception counseling and screening tests. (*Behrman*)

Q. My baby has sickle cell disease. Can you explain what that means and what I should worry about?

Sickle cell disease is caused by abnormal protein (hemoglobin) in red blood cells. This protein causes the red blood cell shape to be deformed. Instead of an oval shaped cell, these cells look like half moons (like the "sickle" on the old Soviet Union flag).

Sickle cells die more quickly, have trouble carrying oxygen, and clog up blood vessels. This blood vessel clogging kills the tissues that the blood vessel supplies (muscle, bones, spleen, lung, kidney, intestine).

The consequences in infancy and early childhood are the following:

1. **Chronic Anemia:** This shows up by age three months. Folate supplements are given to promote red blood cell formation.
2. **Dactylitis:** Infants get hand and foot swelling from clogged blood vessels.
3. **Non-functional spleen:** The spleen filters red blood cells as well as white blood cells (infection fighters). Because of the spleen's job, it takes the greatest hit as far as clogged vessels. We can't rely on the spleen being a functional organ in a child with sickle cell disease. This leaves children prone to infection, particularly with Strep pneumoniae and H. influenza bacteria. These kids need Prevnar vaccine, flu vaccine, and the Pneumonia (pneumococcal) vaccine that elderly people get.
4. **Failure to thrive:** Because of a chronic lack of oxygen to the tissues, these children are shorter and smaller than their peers.

There are a variety of medical problems associated with sickle cell disease as a child gets older. For more information, see sicklecelldisease.org.

Q. My nine-month old's routine blood test identified iron-deficiency anemia. Is this common?

Yes, this is why we routinely screen older babies for anemia. Full term babies are born with a full tank of iron from their moms. They gradually use up that iron over the first four to six months of life. Then, they are on their own and need a daily source of iron in their diet. That said, there are two preventable reasons why iron-deficiency anemia occurs at this age:

1. **Exclusively breastfeeding** without introducing iron-rich foods or supplements by four to six months of age and beyond. (Don't do this!)
2. **Replacing breast milk or iron-containing formula with regular cow's milk**

before the first birthday. (Don't do that!)

Q. How is iron deficiency anemia treated?

With a high iron diet and an iron supplement (we discuss this in detail in Chapter 7, Solids).

If your child is diagnosed with iron-deficiency anemia, your doctor will prescribe an iron supplement. Don't try to treat anemia by yourself without professional help. Why? Because iron, in high doses, can be toxic.

As a result, although vitamins containing iron are available without a prescription, the infant drops are located at the pharmacist's counter. The pharmacist dispenses these medications so they can counsel you on the correct dosage.

Also: there is a difference between the recommend daily allowance for iron (*maintenance iron dosage*) and the dose required for *replacement therapy* for those with low iron stores (iron-deficiency anemia). Doctors usually treat a child with iron-replacement therapy and then recheck their blood counts in three months.

Helpful Hints
Getting your child to take an iron supplement.

◆ Iron supplements universally taste bad.

◆ It's okay to mix the medicine in juice. Just make sure your child drinks *all* the juice. Vitamin C actually helps the iron get absorbed into the bloodstream.

◆ DO NOT MIX WITH MILK. The calcium in milk competes with iron and can block absorption.

◆ Iron can cause a temporary gray/brown stain on the teeth. You can use baking soda on a toothbrush to remove it.

◆ Iron can make poop look black. It's not blood. Don't worry.

Q. We live in an old house. I'm worried about lead exposure. When should I get my child tested?

The appropriate time to get tested depends on when your child becomes mobile.

Most children who have lead poisoning live in homes built before 1978. These older homes have lead paint and lead pipes. Chipping paint is a very popular item for kids to pick up and eat. There is also lead in the soil surrounding these homes.

As we have learned from Flint, Michigan, corrosion of lead and iron water pipes can also lead to lead-contaminated water. This catastrophic event, where 10% of Flint's children experienced lead intoxication, has focused more attention on the dangers of lead exposure.

Screening for lead exposure is usually performed at nine to 12 months of age. In high-risk areas (urban, older homes), all children have a blood test done routinely. In low-risk areas, doctors will screen with a risk-factor question list. If there is a possible exposure, a blood test is performed.

For more information, check out the Environmental Protection Agency's website at epa.gov/lead/index.html or call the National Lead Information Center (NLIC) at 800-424-5323.

While the Environmental Protection Agency recommends consumers turn to professionals to have their homes tested for lead, there are also a number of home tests available on the market. For under $10, you can purchase a lead test kit that includes swabs with a chemical that changes colors when it comes in contact with lead. Unfortunately, the accuracy of these tests has not been independently proven. And each $10 test kit only tests one area in your home (hence, you will end up buying several test kits.) If you're looking for a reputable professional testing lab in your state, check out the EPA's website at epa.gov/lead. Once you contact a certification officer in your state, they will be able to provide a list of certified labs.

 Feedback from the Real World

I cared for a family who carefully de-leaded their home built in 1910 before moving in with their young children. Unfortunately, a central air conditioning unit was installed AFTER the move and it spewed old dust from the attic into all of the children's rooms. The children required medication to remove the lead from their bloodstreams. They are all doing fine now.

Skin

Q. What is eczema?

This falls into the allergic disease category. Eczema is a broad term to describe dry, scaly, itchy skin that appears in patches. It is often referred to as "the itch that rashes." In other words, kids have particularly sensitive, itchy skin. The itching is what produces the rash that you see.

The sensitive skin flares up with *dryness, exposure to perfumes/dyes,* or *allergies to metals/plants*.

The rash appears in different places depending on the age of the child. Younger kids tend to get it on their elbows, knees, and face. Older kids get it in their elbow and knee creases. We have more on managing eczema in Chapter 4, Hygiene and below.

Head back to Chapter 7, Solid Foods, for a detailed discussion on eczema and its potential to sensitize babies to food allergies. For this reason, we strongly encourage you to be aggressive with using thick moisturizer cream/ointment several times a day to keep that skin barrier intact.

Q. How do you get rid of eczema?

It's a long battle. In fact, it's a more realistic goal to keep it under control than to get rid of it.

The key to managing eczema is to keep the skin moist. Eczema always flares up in the wintertime because of cold, dry air.

Q. My baby has severe eczema. Should I be worried about using steroids all the time to treat eczema?

No, these are not the dangerous steroids that some professional athletes use. Topical steroids are extremely good anti-inflammatory medicines. They act by reducing the irritation of the skin, thereby reducing the itching. Long-term use (for months or years), especially with high potency products, can cause unwanted side effects.

It's always a good idea to use the lowest potency steroid creams and ointments for the least amount of time. Doctors move up on the strength level until they find one that works, and taper back down when the eczema improves. Ointments work best, followed by creams and lotions. High potency steroids should *not* be used on the face. And always use the product as prescribed. More is not better.

There is another alternative to topical steroids (approved for use in kids over age two) called immunoregulators. They are sold under the brand names Elidel and Protopic. They are an alternative for short-term or intermittent use to treat eczema. Because any medication has potential adverse effects, ask your doctor their opinion. FYI: these two products have FDA black box warnings due to the potential for increased risk of cancer.

Then there are moisturizers/emollients available by prescription only (and they are pretty expensive). They act by repairing the skin's top layer and reducing inflammation and itching. For details, see Appendix A.

Finally, you may want to consider food allergy testing if your baby has
severe eczema—let your baby's doc decide as all eczema looks "severe" to parents! You may improve the skin by eliminating an allergenic food.

LIVING WITH ECZEMA: 7 TIPS & TRICKS

As a parent of a child with severe eczema, we've been there, done that. Here are our tips:

1. Moisturizing soap. The cheapest in this category is good old Dove soap. Other options are Cetaphil, Aveeno, and Neutrogena. Avoid alcohol-based hand gels—they sting cracked skin.

2. Avoid perfumes and dyes. If it smells good, don't use it on your child. That goes for laundry detergent too. Use All Free and Clear or an equivalent product.

3. The thicker and greasier the moisturizing cream, the better. Eucerin cream, Aveeno, CeraVe, and Cetaphil are popular choices among dermatologists. You need to lube your child up several times a day. As soon as you get your child out of the bathtub, apply the moisturizer (I'm serious—have the tube ready).

4. Apply 1% hydrocortisone cream to really red areas twice daily. 1% hydrocortisone cream is a low-potency steroid cream available without a prescription. It is very safe to use on a daily basis when flare-ups occur.

5. Give a sedating antihistamine like diphenhydramine (Benadryl) at bedtime, for babies over six months: it will help reduce the amount of scratching that goes on when you aren't watching your child.

6. No bubble bath—most contain dyes and perfumes that can aggravate eczema. Instead, consider oatmeal bath treatments (Aveeno makes one). If you bathe your child every night, do it in lukewarm water. Consider bathing every other night in winter. The combination of frequent baths and dry heated air can cause flare-ups.

7. If you have tried all of this and your child is still miserable, it's time to check in with your pediatrician. They can recommend prescription products that are safe and effective. Don't hesitate to see a dermatologist if you and your pediatrician can't keep your baby's eczema under control.

Q. Is there a link between eczema and asthma?

Yes, for some people.

Eczema is an allergic disorder. About 70% of kids who have eczema have a parent, brother or sister who has some type of allergy (hay fever/seasonal allergies, eczema, asthma).

About 30% of kids with eczema will have the classic triad of **ATOPY** (eczema, seasonal allergies, and asthma). But 70% of kids have eczema without any other type of allergic disease. (*Behrman*)

It's just something to pay particular attention to.

Q. Will my baby outgrow eczema?

Chances are, yes.

About 70% of kids will outgrow eczema. But no one can predict if and when your child will outgrow it. Chances are better if your child gets eczema as a baby. Kids who get eczema later in life have a greater chance of having it into adulthood.

Muscles/Bones

Q. My baby's feet turn in. Will they need to wear special shoes or a brace?

No.

The official term for this is called **INTOEING**. This is very common and usually corrects itself as your child becomes a good walker.

Old Wives Tale

Pigeon toed children need to wear corrective shoes.

The truth: It was trendy 40 to 50 years ago to have kids wear corrective shoes or braces (for example Forrest Gump) if they turned their feet in while walking. Since then, doctors discovered feet get better whether a child wears this apparatus or not—so why put a child through the trauma of special shoes or braces.

Q. My one year old is bow-legged. Will they always walk like this?

No.

Kids have some trouble finding their center of gravity. When they first start walking, they bend their knees to support their body weight. As they get older, they often go the opposite direction and look knock-kneed. It's nothing to worry about unless one leg is misshapen or both legs look severely deformed.

Q. My baby seems to have flat feet. Do we need to see a podiatrist?

No, you don't need to see a podiatrist yet.

The term "flat feet" refers to a lack of a natural arch in the bones of the feet. Some flat feet are flexible (the arch is seen when standing on tip-toe) and some are rigid (always flat). The feet that are always flat can cause some discomfort when kids become teenagers and adults. But placing a shoe insert (**ORTHOTIC**) into a toddler's shoes is not going to change the results down the line. The American Academy of Pediatrics feels orthotics are not necessary for kids with flat feet.

Q. My doctor says my baby has TORTICOLLIS. What is it and what do I do about it?

Here we go with the Latin again. This term literally means "twisted neck." It is caused by a tightening of a neck muscle (**STERNOCLEIDOMAS-TOID MUSCLE**) on one side of the neck. This neck muscle tightening occurs while the baby is still in the womb. The fetus may get stuck in one position for several weeks, forcing the baby's head to tilt towards the shoulder.

The muscle tightening gets worse after birth if babies sleep in the same position all the time. You may notice that your baby prefers to turn or tilt his head to one side. Babies who are at greater risk for this are boys, large birth weight babies, twins/multiples, breech, moms with uterus abnormalities, and first pregnancies. (*Stellwagen*)

If your child has torticollis, their head and neck movements will be limited. And if you don't

EXERCISES FOR TORTICOLLIS

Here are two exercises you can do at home to fix this problem.

It's easiest to remember if you do the exercises after each daytime diaper change. Your baby will respond best if they are relaxed and have a full tummy. You can do the exercises on the changing table or on your lap.

1. *Tilt the head, ear to shoulder, stabilizing the chest with one hand.* Hold for 10 seconds and repeat on the other side. Repeat three times on each side.

2. *Turn the baby's head, chin to shoulder, while stabilizing the chest with one hand.* Hold for 10 seconds. Then repeat in the other direction and hold for 10 seconds. Repeat three times on each side. (*Stellwagen*)

actively do something about it, the head and facial shape may be affected. See the previous box for home exercises to work on. Do the exercises at each diaper change, if you can.

Here are a few other practical tips (warning: your baby will not like any of them) (*Barrow Neurological Institute*):

◆ Place your baby to sleep on alternating ends of the crib.
◆ Place your baby's head on alternate ends of the changing table.
◆ Put toys on the side of the stroller/swing/crib where your baby's neck rotation is most limited. This forces him to work to see those toys.
◆ When carrying your baby, alternate which hip or arm used.
◆ Try to interact with your baby on the side where their neck movement is limited.
◆ Tummy time. Tummy time. And more tummy time.

If you do not see improvement in six to eight weeks, it's time to call in a physical therapist to help you.

Physical therapy is very effective in treating more severe cases of torticollis. For the few kids who fail that intervention, BOTOX injections and minimally invasive endoscopic surgery have both been used to release the affected muscle.

Q. My baby was born breech and the doctor wants to do a hip ultrasound. Should I worry?

No, but you should do the test. The concern: developmental dysplasia (dislocation) of the hips or DDH. In some babies, the hip joint forms abnormally and so the top of the thighbone does not stay in the joint. The result is that the bone is either loose or entirely out of the joint. The dislocation may be apparent at birth, or be identified as the joint loosens with time and activity.

There are certain babies who are at increased risk of this deformity: girls who are born in a breech presentation have the highest risk. First-born children and those with a family history of hip dysplasia are also at risk.

If DDH is diagnosed in infancy (the earlier the better), it is fairly easy to treat and correct. If DDH is not diagnosed or not treated, it can cause joint pain and arthritis. That's why pediatricians carefully examine a baby's hips and order a simple ultrasound test on babies who are born breech, who have a family history of DDH, or who have a concerning hip examination. Radiologists suggest doing a hip ultrasound at six weeks of life for these babies. A follow up x-ray of the hips may be in order at six months of life for some at-risk babies.

Reality Check

Notify your baby's doctor if your baby:
◆ Has uneven leg creases on the thighs.
◆ Has legs that are a different length.
◆ Seems to use one leg less than the other.
◆ Limps or waddles when walking.

FYI: Experts are increasingly concerned that tightly wrapping a baby's legs while swaddling (aka the baby burrito wrap) may increase the risk of DDH. So it's a good idea to leave some wiggle room for the legs. Allow the legs to bend up and out at the hips.

DISEASES

Endocrine

Q. Diabetes runs in my family. How can I get my baby tested for it?

Let's discuss diabetes first.

Diabetes mellitus is a chronic disease due to impaired sugar metabolism. There are two types (Type 1 and Type 2). They are divided by the cause of the disorder and the treatment. Although both can be inherited diseases, Type 2 tends to "run in families" more often.

Here is a brief explanation of the malfunction:

Since a person with diabetes doesn't breakdown sugar properly, the sugar ends up in vast quantities in the bloodstream. The body tries to eliminate the sugar by filtering it through the kidneys and into the urine. The sugar pulls excessive amounts of water with it into the urine. The result?

- ◆ Elevated blood sugar level.
- ◆ Excessive urination (with sugar found in the urine).
- ◆ Excessive thirst to keep up with fluid loss in the urine.
- ◆ Weight loss (from poor metabolism and fluid losses).

Type 1 Diabetes is also known as *Juvenile Diabetes,* or *Insulin Dependent Diabetes.* This is an autoimmune disease—that means the cells in the pancreas that make insulin get killed off by a person's own body. Insulin is the chemical in our body that metabolizes sugars.

There are some genes that have been identified in people with Type 1 diabetes and genetic defects can be passed on to offspring. Treatment is life-long with insulin injections and dietary modifications. Onset of Type 1 Diabetes is usually around school age (six to seven years old). It is extraordinarily rare to be diagnosed with diabetes while a child is still in diapers.

Type 2 Diabetes is also known as *Adult Onset Diabetes.* This type of diabetes is caused by the body's impaired response to insulin—this impairment is related to obesity.

As you can tell by the name, this USED to be an adult disease. Unfortunately, there is a virtual "epidemic" today of Type 2 Diabetes in pre-teens and teens. Children at risk are obese (defined as a Body Mass Index greater than 85%—see Chapter 5, Nutrition and Growth for details on the BMI) as well as other family members with Type 2 diabetes. Treatment includes dietary modifications and medications taken by mouth. FYI: There is a higher risk of developing this disorder among non-Hispanic blacks, Hispanics, and Native Americans. *(Behrman)*

Interestingly, there seems to be an increased risk of developing diabetes if babies are exposed to wheat and barley *before* four months or *after* six months of age. The theory is that introducing these foods too early or too late can trigger an autoimmune response that damages the body's insulin-making islet cells. *(Snell-Bergeon)*

BOTTOM LINE

Diabetes is not a disorder of infancy. But, offering wheat and barley between four and six months of age may prevent diabetes later on.

If you have a family history of diabetes it's a good idea to watch your child's growth. Eating a healthy diet and avoiding obesity is even more important in your family.

As your child gets older, a screening test for diabetes can be done by obtaining a urine and blood sample. For more information, check out this web site: diabetes.org.

Allergies

Q. My partner and I both have seasonal allergies. What are the chances that our baby will have allergies?

50%.

For each parent who has allergies, a child has a 25% risk of developing some form of allergic disease. This refers to seasonal allergies, asthma and eczema. Some doctors might also put food allergies on this list, too. The earliest manifestations of an allergic child are eczema and food allergies. Asthma is usually diagnosed after a year of age. Seasonal allergies come even later.

Reality Check

The hereditary patterns of allergies do *not* apply to *drug* allergies. Just because you have an allergy to Penicillin doesn't mean your child will have one too.

Q. My baby seems to have a runny nose all of the time. Is it due to seasonal allergies?

No.

Allergies ("hay fever") that cause a runny nose can be divided into perennial (all year long) or seasonal categories.

◆ *Perennial allergies.* These are year round allergies caused by something a child is exposed to on a daily basis. This is something inside your house, not outside your house. The most common causes are dust mites or cat dander. Molds are found both inside and outside the house year round.

◆ *Seasonal allergies.* These are allergies caused by something that's in the air outside of your house. These pollens include weeds, trees, and grasses that come in seasonal pat-

Allergies over the years

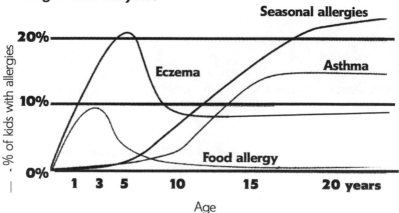

Source: *Contemporary Pediatrics, August 2007*

FELINES ARE OUR FRIENDS

Although most people have heard that having a cat causes allergies, research shows that early exposure (first year of life) to cats and dogs may actually prevent allergies. Kids who grow up on farms have significantly less problems with allergies, presumably due to their constant exposure to animals and the germs they carry.

---

terns. Most children under one year of age do not get *seasonal* allergies. Allergies, by definition, are a body's hyper-response to an allergen they have seen before. In the first year of life, a child has never seen these pollens before so there is no response.

BOTTOM LINE

Newborns do not have seasonal allergies when they are congested for the first six weeks of life. Nor does a nine month old have a ragweed allergy.

Most of the time, a chronic runny nose is caused by one viral upper respiratory infection after another. Although there are conflicting viewpoints, some doctors feel that perennial allergies or food allergies may cause a chronic runny nose year round in kids under age two.

Helpful hint

For perennial allergies (for example, dust mites), allergists often recommend plastic bedding covers, air filters, etc. These products are available through medical supply companies. Check out the following resources for a product catalog: National Allergy Supply, Inc. (800-522-1448, natlallergy.com) or Allergy Asthma Technology Ltd. (800-621-5545, allergyasthmatech.com).

Genitals

Q. My son is circumcised, but the penis doesn't look circumcised anymore. What do I do?

See Chapter 4, Hygiene for a frank discussion on **PENILE ADHESIONS.** Some parents will comment that they see a white blister (called a bleb) on the skin, or a red swollen area, or that the penis just doesn't look right. These are usually all the same problem. The white blister is dead skin that has collected and is allowing the skin to stick together. The red swollen area may be the penis trying to unstick on its own. The penis doesn't look right because you can no longer see the helmet part.

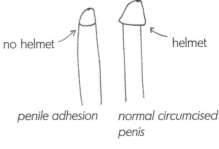

no helmet · helmet

penile adhesion · *normal circumcised penis*

Q. The skin of my daughter's genitals is sticking together. My doctor said not to worry about it . . . but I am worried.

? ?

DISEASES

Don't worry. This is a common problem called **LABIAL ADHESIONS**. The labia and vaginal areas stay lubricated and open when estrogen is being produced. Young women

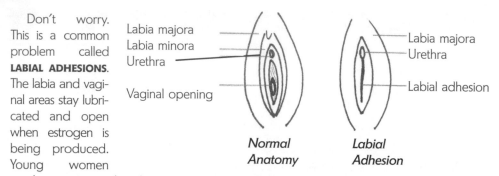

Normal
Anatomy

Labial
Adhesion

produce estrogen when they start menstruating. So pre-pubertal girls are prone to labial adhesions until they go through puberty.

The only time this is a problem is when the labia are so fused together that the urethral opening is blocked too (that's where the urine comes out). See the nearby graphic to understand what we're talking about.

Labial adhesions are treated by using a prescription estrogen cream twice daily on the area for a couple of weeks. After that, apply petroleum jelly (Vaseline) on a daily basis to keep the area moist and open. Very rarely, a surgical procedure is necessary to open the area.

What's that smell?

Have you ever gone to a wine tasting and tried to describe the "nose" of a wine? When babies smell unusual, parents go to great lengths to come up with adjectives to explain the odor to their doctor.

We hesitate to explain this category of disorders in a chapter entitled "Common" diseases. But there are some very rare metabolic disorders that are associated with unusual body odors. It is important that you are aware of them, and seek medical care if you notice any of the following smells:

- ◆ *Body odors:* Barn-like, mousy, musty, horsey, wolf-like, sweaty socks, cheesy.
- ◆ *Breath odors:* fruity/sweet, fishy, ammonia-like, clover, musty fish, raw liver, foul.
- ◆ *Urine (pee) odors:* mousy, musty, horsey, wolf-like, barn-like, maple syrup, caramel, boiled Chinese Herbal medicine, yeast, celery, malt, brewery, sweaty feet/socks, ripe cheese, tomcat urine, dead fish, cabbage.
- ◆ *Stool (poop) odors:* foul, vile. (*Fleisher*)

Note that other problems may cause you to turn your nose: poisonings and infections.

BOTTOM LINE: Bad odors are worth checking out.

Now that you've been briefed on the most common diseases that affect children, let's talk safety. The next chapter covers top safety concerns, including food, water, air quality, home and outdoor environment, and more.

SAFETY
Chapter 15

WHAT'S IN THIS CHAPTER

◆ TOP HEALTH CONCERNS
◆ FOOD
◆ HOME
◆ AIR
◆ BABY PRODUCTS
◆ 28 TIPS TO REDUCING ECO-HAZARDS

Let's talk about safety and your baby–specifically how the environment might affect your baby's health. Before having a baby, you might have given only this a passing thought. Like many things in your life, however, a baby changes everything . . . including your perspective on this topic.

Just because folks are paying more attention to the environment doesn't change the rather stark facts about eco hazards: babies born today are exposed to more environmental pollutants than any previous generation in history. And babies are more susceptible than adults to adverse health effects from these pollutants.

Eighty thousand chemicals have been used in commerce since the 1960's. Three thousand are used in high volume production of consumer products and foodstuffs. Most of these chemicals were invented in the past 40 years. MANY of them have never been tested for their effect on your health.

Even more scary: we don't know basic toxic info on more than HALF of these chemicals . . . and even less is known about how these chemicals affect the development of young children. (*Goldman*) The Toxic Substance Control Act of 1976, designed to protect pregnant women and children who are particularly vulnerable to toxic chemical exposure, finally got revamped "for the 21st Century" in 2017. The EPA is now required to compile and regularly update a list of chemicals that may have an impact on our health. You can access that list here: epa.gov/chemicals-under-tsca

Warning: This chapter may be hazardous to your *mental* health. Environmental health is an emerging science. Many factors contribute to certain diseases . . . so we cannot necessarily say exposure to pollutant X causes disease Y. There are also more questions than answers, and more shades of grey than pure black and white. As you know, we are fairly non-alarmist folks who make recommendations based on solid scientific evidence. However, when solid science is lacking, it's more challenging to offer advice.

Bottom line: we'll try not to freak you out.

What's important is that you weigh the evidence (or lack thereof) so you can make a more educated decision if you are concerned about reducing your child's exposure to environmental hazards.

Our key goal: this chapter should help you consider the HEALTH risks of various eco decisions (Organic versus regular milk? Should I get my home radon tested?). Of course, many of these decisions have other environmental factors (sustainability, etc.)—we'll leave that discussion to the numerous platforms out there dedicated to living a green life.

We will also tackle more ubiquitous safety tips in this chapter—water safety and drowning prevention, home safety hazards, as well as dangerous toys and baby products.

So, let's get rolling. First, let's talk about why babies are vulnerable to eco toxins.

Q. Why are children vulnerable to environmental toxins?

Babies and children are not little adults—their growing bodies work differently. And while they may live in the same macro-environment as their parents, they live in a completely different micro-environment (that is, the carpeted floor of a home in Hometown, USA). This can make a significant impact on what environmental hazards babies are exposed to on a daily basis.

Here are the top nine reasons why the environment can be hazardous to your baby's health:

1. **Breathing:** Babies breathe at faster rates than adults, so they take in more air. They also breathe lower to the ground where chemical matter settles.
2. **Fluid intake:** For their body weight, babies drink the adult equivalent of 1.75 gallons of fluid a day.
3. **Food intake:** For their body weight, babies eat three times more food than adults.
4. **Oral exploration:** Babies stick stuff in their mouths—and it's not always food. So they are at risk of ingesting pollutants, like lead in the soil.
5. **Gut absorption:** To add insult to injury, a baby's gut absorbs more toxins than an adult's. Case in point: lead. A baby's gut absorbs 50% of lead that's been ingested, whereas the adult gut only absorbs about 10%.
6. **Surface area:** Compared to adults, babies have twice the surface area per pound to absorb chemicals.
7. **Location:** Babies spend many more hours on the floor, grass, carpeting, and wood decking. These offer more opportunities for exposure where chemical matter settles.
8. **Developing bodies:** Embryos, fetuses, babies, and young children are uniquely sensitive to environmental exposures that can permanently interfere with how organs and body systems develop.
9. **Lifetime burden:** Babies born today have a longer lifespan, giving them a longer opportunity for adverse health effects from exposures to arise. (*AAP*)

Q. Where are these pollutants?

Well, they are lurking everywhere. That's encouraging, huh? Sometimes we think ignorance may be bliss. But seriously, it's important to know where the greatest potential health hazards lie, so you can limit your baby's exposure where possible in a practical way.

- **Food:** Additives, antibiotics, hormones, arsenic, methylmercury, Polychlorinated Biphenyls (PCB's), contaminants.
- **Water:** Lead, methylmercury, industrial chemicals.
- **Home:** phthalates, bisphenol-A (BPA), lead, arsenic, flame retardant.
- **Air:** Radon, carbon monoxide, second hand smoke, radio frequency/electromagnetic fields, industrial chemicals.

Q. What damage can they do?

Some exposures have very defined health risks. Others are a bit murkier, or have only been proven to have adverse effects in animal studies—not humans. Environmental health is a very young scientific field. Compared to other fields, scientists have only just started to look at the effects of natural and man-made environmental exposures. And while some health risks are obvious (for example, smoking increases your risk of lung cancer) there are very few long-term studies that have been able to tease out one individual exposure as a direct cause of one particular disease.

Here is how the major categories of health risks are divided:

- **Carcinogens:** These agents are known to cause cancer. (Examples: arsenic, tobacco, solvents like benzene).
- **Mutagens:** These agents increase the rate of change ("mutation") in genetic material. This can lead to defective cells and cancer. (Example: ionizing radiation).
- **Teratogens:** These agents alter a fetus during development in the womb. Abnormalities are present at birth. (Example: alcohol).
- **Neurotoxins:** These agents damage or interfere with nerve/brain function. (Example: lead, methylmercury, Polychlorinated Biphenyls or PCB's, organophosphate pesticides). The scary part: there is a spectrum of neurotoxicity. Severely affected people will have obvious symptoms. Those with lower amounts of exposure may have more subtle symptoms such as a shorter attention span or slightly lower IQ.
- **Endocrine disruptors:** These agents mimic the body's natural chemical messengers (hormones) and can potentially interfere with body responses in the reproductive system and thyroid gland. (Example: phytoestrogen).
- **Irritants and allergens:** These agents cause allergic responses in the airway and/or the skin. (example: Volatile Organic Compounds or VOC's).

Q. What are the top health concerns?

Certain disease rates are on the rise. While we can't blame the environment for everything, these diseases are currently hotbeds of research for the possibility of environmental triggers. These Include:

- *Asthma.*
- *Leukemia.*
- *Male reproductive system problems* such as an increase in testicular cancer (up

60% in the past 30 years), hypospadias (abnormal penis development has doubled in the past 30 years), and falling sperm counts.
- ◆ *Neurodevelopmental disabilities* such as dyslexia, ADHD, and Autism Spectrum Disorders.
- ◆ *Obesity*.

Q. If I can't avoid these pollutants, how much exposure is acceptable and how much is "too much"?

Unfortunately, the threshold of "acceptable limits" of exposure changes as more research is done. For instance, 40 years ago experts used to think that some lead exposure (levels under 40 mcg/dl) was perfectly safe. We now know that *any* level of lead exposure can have subtle, but permanent effects on the brain. (*Canfield*) And for some pollutants, it also depends on *when* the exposure occurs.

Food: Additives, Contaminants, Facts and Fables

Formula

Q. Does soy formula cause early puberty or breast cancer?

Soy formula has been through some controversies. Some researchers think soy formula may interfere with reproductive or immune functions when given in high doses to infants.

Why? Soy formula contains isoflavones, which is a plant version of estrogen. It's possible that exposure to this hormone-like substance could adversely impact a baby's reproductive development.

One recent study showed that infant girls who were fed soy baby formula had subtle body changes typically seen with estrogen exposure. That said, there are no studies to date that prove long-term harm and soy formula has been around for over 40 years. For now, the AAP advises soy formula for specific situations—when a baby has a metabolic disorder (galactosemia) or a family desires a milk-free formula. (*Adgent*)

Q. Is powdered baby formula safe? I heard about a huge formula recall after some babies died from contaminated formula.

Yes, it is safe. But as we discussed in back in Chapter 6, powdered formulas are heat-treated but cannot be commercially sterilized like ready-to-feed formula. Thus, powdered formulas contain low levels of microorganisms. One particular germ, Cronobacter sakazakii, can cause serious infections in babies who are low birth weight, born pre-maturely, or immune compromised.

In 2022, the Abbott Nutrition manufacturing plant in Michigan produced several batches of powdered baby formula (Similac, Alimentum, Elecare) contaminated with Cronobacter. Two babies became seriously ill and two babies died.

That's why we recommend boiling bottled water before mixing with powdered formula and avoiding powdered formula if you have a baby with one of the aforementioned medical risk factors.

Organic Food

Q. Which fruits and vegetables contain the most pesticides?

The Environmental Working Group (ewg.org) has compiled the "dirty dozen" list of produce that contains the highest pesticide load. If you have an organic food budget (let's face it, going organic is very expensive), these would be the top organic foods worth the splurge.

Here is the list, in order of the most to least contaminated:

#1 Strawberries	#7 Cherries
#2 Spinach	#8 Peaches
#3 Kale	#9 Pears
#4 Nectarines	#10 Bell and Hot Pepper
#5 Apples	#11 Celery
#6 Grapes	#12 Tomatoes

Fun Fact: no authoritative medical organization supports avoiding these produce items or paying the price for the organic version of them. Why? There is not enough evidence to prove the risk is worth the price tag.

Hence, your family can eat non-organically farmed spinach and not worry about it. It's more important to eat spinach!! We share this list with you to let you decide.

Reality Check

It is widely accepted knowledge that children are more sensitive than adults to many pollutants. When it comes to pesticides, children are about ten times more sensitive. (AAP) The question that remains is if the pesticide exposure in foods has significant adverse health effects. At the moment, there is no major evidence of that. (Forman)

Q. Is it worth it to buy organic formula, milk and dairy products?

Organic milk and dairy products claim to be free of pesticides, antibiotics, and hormones. But organic milk can cost almost twice the price. Is it worth the cost? As we've already discussed, children today are exposed to more environmental pollutants than past generations. Is it worth it to limit these exposures when it comes to milk?

First, let's discuss the three questionable ingredients consumers are concerned about in their milk and dairy products:

◆ *Pesticides*: Pesticides are in both water and soil. So there will be some in just about anything our children eat or drink (including breast milk and yes, organic products). Organic milk promises to be chemical free, but because chemicals remain in the soil for so long, even organic milk may contain pesticides. Organic farmers may also use organic pesticides. *Bottom line: compared to say, apples, the pesticide residue in all milk products is rather low.*

◆ *Antibiotics*: All milk products are screened for antibiotic residues. If residue is detected (which happens in about 1 in 1000 tankers of milk), the milk is rejected for sale. Hence,

safety

SAFETY

? ?

conventional milk should also be antibiotic-free. Our concern here: even though the finished product is antibiotic-free, antibiotic use in livestock is contributing to antibiotic resistance. Doctors have tried to limit antibiotic overuse in humans; it is time to reduce use in animals too. Your grocery store purchases drive the marketplace. *Bottom line: while there is probably no antibiotic residue in milk, buying organic milk encourages milk manufacturers to avoid using antibiotics.*

◆ *Hormones*: Even in "juiced" cows, all milk has about the same composition (see below for more discussion on bovine growth hormone.).

So, is organic worth almost twice the price? If you look strictly at health risks, organic milk doesn't have much advantage over conventional milk (with the possible exception of the antibiotic issue discussed above).

To us, the main argument for choosing organic when it comes to formula, milk, and dairy products is this: when it comes to young children, dairy is their biggest food group. If you are going to spend your organic dollars somewhere, this would be the most cost-efficient for the volume your child consumes.

Q. Is it worth it to buy organic baby food?

First and foremost, we want babies to eat what you are eating. So, you should decide if it is worth it for your entire family. Without strong scientific evidence to justify the cost, we advise being very selective on how much money you spend on organic food.

But yes, baby food jars and pouches are very convenient and it's likely you will probably buy some of them. And, eating conventional baby food is NOT hazardous to your baby's health.

Processed food (including jarred/pouched baby food) is actually subject to *stricter* federal regulation than fresh produce. So, baby food should have *less* pesticide residue than what you might find in the regular (conventional) produce aisle. And some baby food manufacturers make their products pesticide-free even if they are not labeled as "organic." (*AAP*)

Bottom line: there isn't much difference between regular and organic baby food. If you decide to go organic, we advise you make your own baby's Food using organic fruits and vegetables (see the discussion earlier for the fruit that's most likely to have pesticide residue).

SIX WAYS TO REDUCE PESTICIDE EXPOSURE FROM FOODS

Don't want to spend your entire paycheck on organic groceries? Here are some tips to reducing pesticide exposure:

1. Scrub produce with a brush under running water to get rid of any obvious residue.
2. Peel whatever produce you can. (FYI: this often removes the fiber benefit, though).
3. Don't eat the outer leaves of leafy vegetables (e.g. lettuce, kale).
4. Grow your own garden and don't use pesticides.
5. If you are buying imported produce, only purchase produce that can be peeled.
6. Buy produce that is in season. (*AAP*)

Unfortunately, that doesn't eliminate all the pesticides, but it helps.

Q. Should I buy organic meat?

There are plenty of reasons to choose organic meat, but the key health issue is antibiotics.

Antibiotics are given to healthy animals to prevent disease and improve growth. In fact, at least 40% of the antibiotics used in the United States are used in animals that are destined to become our next meal. Antibiotics used in the food industry are indirectly a problem for humans because they allow antibiotic resistant bacteria to evolve.

So while there is no direct health hazard from eating conventional meat, there is an indirect health risk. If you want to buy antibiotic-free meat simply on principle, look for meat labeled USDA Organic.

Q. I've heard rice cereal contains arsenic and it's dangerous. True?

Yes, arsenic has been found in baby rice cereal, as well as in brown and white rice and other rice-containing products like rice milk and rice cakes.

Inorganic arsenic is a potentially harmful chemical that is all over our universe, thanks to natural causes (like being part of the earth's crust) as well as human causes (like burning coal). Because of its ubiquitous nature, it is in our air, water, and soil…and thus in our food supply. The arsenic levels in a particular food can vary widely, depending on its origin.

Inorganic arsenic is known to cause cancer. It's also possible that fetuses and young children who are exposed to arsenic may have lower IQ scores. *(Centers for Disease Control)*

The FDA sets industry standards for acceptable levels of inorganic arsenic in infant cereals. Their limits are similar to European Commission regulations.

Bottom line: Like all environmental health issues, it's wise to limit exposures whenever possible. It's fine to give your baby products made out of rice. But providing a varied diet consisting of other grains will reduce your baby's arsenic intake.

RBGH

Q. Will my baby go through puberty early if they have milk or yogurt with bovine growth hormone?

No.

Some dairy farmers give bovine growth hormone to lactating cows to increase their milk production. There are no direct associations to early puberty or cancer. All cows, in fact, make this hormone naturally. Even though these cows are "juiced," the composition of conventional milk vs. organic milk is almost the same. Pasteurization destroys 90% of the bovine growth hormone. Additionally, bovine growth hormone is species-specific. So even if there is some bovine growth hormone in commercial milk, it does not affect humans. *(Forman)*

Despite the lack of scientific evidence, consumer demand drives retail decisions. Wal-Mart, Kroger, and Safeway brands are now all synthetic bovine growth hormone-free. And Starbuck's only uses hormone-free dairy products at their stores.

Reality Check

Northern American girls have had earlier menstrual cycles since 1840 when nutrition improved. Some experts think early puberty these days is due to the obesity epidemic—which turns on hormones earlier than it should. So, if milk is to blame at all, it's because kids over age two are drinking whole or 2% when they should be drinking skim! Also: puberty standards have also changed over the years in the US to reflect the normalcy of earlier puberty in our racially diverse population.

Q. Is it safe for my baby to eat genetically-modified foods?

This is a hot topic in parenting circles. A quick primer on GMO's: humans have been genetically modifying foods since the beginning of time. As technology has advanced, scientists have been able to splice genes of seeds to make plants resistant to drought, disease and so on. This has provided an abundance of food at a very low cost. That's the good news. Opponents of genetically modified foods (GMO's), however are concerned with the potential long-term health impacts of GMO foods and want mandatory labeling of GMO's in foods. The battle over "Frankenfoods" rages on.

So what does the science say? The FDA and the American Cancer Society both say there are no concerns about potential health risks from bioengineered foods. Meanwhile, baby food companies are responding to consumer concerns by only using non-genetically modified ingredients.

And, all the major American and European infant formula companies tout their non-GMO premium products.

Here's our take: so far, there is no science to support fears that GMO's are dangerous. No child has become sick from eating baby food made from genetically modified organisms. So avoiding GMO foods is a personal preference—if you go this route, look for "non-GMO" or "100% certified organic."

Nitrates

Q. I've heard it's not safe to make your own baby food out of carrots, beets, and spinach. Is this true?

No, that is false.

It is safe to make your own baby food out of root and leafy vegetables. Just don't offer those food items to babies *under three* months of age because their guts are too immature to appropriately breakdown a chemical called nitrates. (This should be a non-issue, because we don't recommend starting solid food until at least four to six months of age).

Nitrates are the product of nitrogen fertilizer and animal waste breakdown that ends up in our water supply and soil. Nitrates aren't toxic, but the bacteria in a baby's gut converts them to *nitrites*, which can be a health hazard. Nitrites interfere with the oxygen carrying capacity of red blood cells, and can cause Blue Baby Syndrome (**METHEMOGLOBINEMIA**).

Bottom line: You can make your own baby's food out of beets, broccoli, cabbage, carrots, and spinach as long as your baby is at least four months old.

FYI: If you have well water and a septic system, be sure to get it tested for nitrates. You don't want to give this to a baby under three months of age for the same reasons outlined above!

High fructose corn syrup

Q. Is high fructose corn syrup safe?

Yes, it's safe.

High fructose corn syrup (HFCS) is found in many processed foods, from soda to pancake syrup. Over the years, HFCS has replaced many other types of sugar in foods for one simple reason: it's cheap.

At the same time, however, concerns have been raised about HFCS: is it contributing to our nation's obesity epidemic?

Here's the latest science: high fructose corn syrup does not cause obesity or any other malady.

However, like natural sugar, you should limit how much HFCS you offer to your baby. And since HFCS is found mostly in processed foods, it is more nutritious to stick with fresh foods for overall health reasons.

Reality Check

A recent study found that countries with HFCS-containing food supplies have 20% higher rates of Type 2 Diabetes. In short, processed-food-loving Americans have the highest rates of Type 2 Diabetes. It's not necessarily the HFCS that is the problem, but the types of diets that are rich in HFCS.

Artificial sweeteners

Q. Do artificial sweeteners cause cancer?

No. The U.S. National Toxicology Program says that consumption of Splenda, Nutrasweet, Equal, and Saccharin has no increased risk of cancer. Saccharin can cause bladder stones that lead to cancer in rats, but not in humans.

Food coloring

Q. Does food coloring cause Attention Deficit Disorder?

Several years ago, scientists looked at a possible link between food coloring and attention problems. The "Feingold Hypothesis" failed to pan out and the theory basically died. About ten years ago, researchers resuscitated this theory in a study published in the journal Lancet. Children who drank beverages with red or yellow dye, or sodium benzoate (a common preservative) had more hyperactive behavior than their peers. Kids who drank sugary drinks had no change in their behavior, by the way.

The FDA looked at this question a few years ago and did not find an association between artificial food coloring (AFC) and ADHD, but noted that a small number of children are intolerant to AFC and exhibit behavioral changes. We don't recommend changing your life on the basis of one study, but it's not a bad idea to limit processed foods (which usually contain food coloring and preservatives).

Grilling

Q. Is it okay for my baby to eat grilled foods? Does BBQ cause cancer?

Cooking foods quickly at high temperatures—by grilling, frying, or broiling—produce heterocyclic amines (HCA). HCA's are on the National Institutes of Health's list of chemicals "reasonably anticipated to be carcinogens."

However, we believe it is okay to enjoy BBQ *in moderation*. Here are a couple of tips:

◆ Certain foods produce more HCA's than others. Chicken produces the most, hamburgers the least.

◆ Fat drippings on the grill create (warning: big chemical word ahead) polycyclic aromatic hydrocarbons (PAH). These are also carcinogens. Charred meat has more PAH's . . . so, it's wise to limit fat drippings and scrape off any charring.

Sodium nitrate

Q. I've heard that lunchmeats and hot dogs processed with nitrites/nitrates are dangerous. Is it worth it to buy preservative-free meats?

Sodium nitrite keeps you from getting botulism from a frankfurter or other processed meats like lunch meat, bacon, ham, and smoked fish. It also makes the meat look more appetizing (otherwise your hotdog would look sickly grey).

The health concern: nitrites can convert to nitrosamines, which are known animal carcinogens (but only *potentially* carcinogenic in humans). U.S. food manufacturers now add ascorbic acid or erythorbic acid to nitrite-containing meat products, which prevents that chemical conversion to nitrosamines. So the health concern is much lower now than twenty years ago.

However, processed meats like hot dogs and lunchmeats contain more salt (and often more fat) than unprocessed, preservative-free products. For that reason alone, we recommend limiting them in your baby's diet. (*CSPI*)

Fish

Q. I've heard there is mercury in certain types of seafood. How can I reduce my baby's exposure?

Yes, fish can absorb methylmercury from coal-fired power plant waste that ends up in nearby rivers, lakes, and oceans. And excessive methylmercury intake during brain development of a fetus or young child can lead to language, attention, and memory problems. In addition to

SAFETY

methylmercury, seafood can also be contaminated with polychlorinated biphenyls (PCB's).

However, fish is also a very healthy food choice and contains Omega 3 Fatty acids that promote brain development.

So, how do you avoid toxins in fish? Stick with the safest fish and avoid risky varieties:

Safest fish:
◆ Butterfish, catfish, domestic crab, crawfish, shrimp, fresh or canned salmon, pollock, tilapia, whitefish.
◆ Freshwater trout.

Risky fish:
◆ Freshwater fish (with the exception of trout) are more likely exposed to industrial waste products.
◆ Predators (shark, swordfish, tuna, king mackerel, tilefish) who live a long time build up methylmercury.
◆ Fatty fish (mackerel, carp, catfish, lake trout) are more likely to contain PCB's.

If you are really interested, you can see how much methylmercury is in fish at this website: www.fda.gov/food/consumers/eating-fish-what-pregnant-women-and-parents-should-know

Here are some specific recommendations on fish for both your baby and you if you are breastfeeding:

◆ Completely avoid eating shark, swordfish, mackerel, and tilefish.
◆ Eat less than 12 oz. a week of shellfish, canned fish, small ocean fish, or farm-raised fish.
◆ Eat six ounces or less a week of white albacore tuna. Canned light tuna, and specifically Carvalho Fisheries and King of the Sea are lower in methylmercury.
◆ Eat six ounces or less of local fish if you are unsure of local water contamination. (*FDA*)

Water

Q. Is it worth it to get a water filtration system?

It depends on the type of system. Those little filters that attach to faucets aren't going to do very much. Tap filters may remove lead and other toxins, but not excessive fluoride. And if you don't take care of them properly and replace the carbon filters regularly, bacteria will end up growing in the filters.

Our advice: It's cheaper to merely run your tap water for two minutes in the morning before you use it—that flushes any lead out.

Reverse osmosis filters do remove both toxins and fluoride—but these are much more expensive and need to be installed house-wide.

Here's our recommendation: get your community's water quality report (most are posted online on water company home pages). If your community has a serious problem with contamination, then a whole-house reverse osmosis filter would be a useful investment. The same is true if you are relying on well water: get it tested and treat it if necessary.

Home

As your baby becomes more mobile, safety will be a constant priority. We'll try to cover the basics on eco hazards and injury prevention here.

Lead

Q. Is it safe to decorate with holiday/Christmas lights?

Yes.

Readers have asked about this after seeing holiday lights sold in the state of California plastered with a warning label about lead. So is the lead in holiday lights dangerous? And why is it there in the first place?

Lead is used in the manufacturing process of holiday lights to stabilize the plastic bulbs (so the plastic doesn't burn and set your tree on fire). The lead acts as a flame retardant—which is a good idea.

Bottom line: unless your baby is eating or chewing on holiday lights, they are NOT in any danger of lead poisoning.

WATER SAFETY 411: HOW TO PREVENT DROWNING

Drowning is the leading cause of injury-related death in children one to four years old. Half of these drownings occur in backyard swimming pools. Others occur in public pools with a certified lifeguard on duty, or under an adult's supervision. Yes, surprising, but true.

Drowning can be sudden and silent. Unlike the movies, kids don't scream for help and flail around when they are struggling.

Take these simple steps to protect your children.

1. Be a Water Guardian. Even if there is a lifeguard on duty, a designated adult should actively supervise children who are near or around water…without distractions. No talking, texting, drinking a margarita. Just watching.

2. Teach your child to swim. Preschoolers who take formal swimming lessons reduce their risk of drowning by 88 percent. That's why the AAP advises children as young as 12 months old to take formal swim lessons if they are physically and emotionally ready to do so.

3. Never leave your child unattended near water, including bathtubs and kiddie pools. You hear the phone while you are bathing your baby or toddler? Just let it ring.

Q. Are there any other sources of lead exposure I should know about?

Yes.

Here's a surprise: your garden hose most likely contains lead. Lead is used to stabilize the hose material (which is made of polyvinyl chloride).

If water has been standing for a while in the hose, the lead concentration in the water is higher. If you are filling up a baby pool in your backyard with that garden hose, you should let the water run for a minute before you start filling. Yes, your baby will probably play *and* drink that water. If you are in the market to buy a new garden hose, buy one that is labeled "safe for drinking".

We discuss lead exposure in old homes in Chapter 14, Diseases.

Cleaning products

Q. Are cleaning products safe to use?

Home cleaning products have been scrutinized in recent years, as an entire industry has grown around eco alternatives to conventional cleaning chemicals.

4. Set up four-sided barriers to backyard pools and hot tubs. Fence off the water area from your house and the rest of the yard. If you have an inflatable baby pool, always be sure to drain the water out after playtime is over.

5. Life jackets. Children who cannot swim need a proper life jacket around water. We're not talking about "water wings" or "floaties"—we mean certified life jackets.

6. If you've got a pool or hot tub, install anti-entrapment drain covers. Water safety advocates suggest using VGB-compliant drain covers, named after a 7-year-old girl who died after becoming stuck by the suction force of a hot tub drain. Check out pool-safely.gov for more info.

7. Have a phone nearby. Always call 911 in an emergency.

8. Learn CPR. In drownings, every second counts. The faster a person on the scene begins resuscitation, the better chance a child has of surviving and not suffering serious brain damage.

Check out colinshope.org for more information. This website was created by parents who have dedicated their lives to educating families about water safety after losing their four-year-old son, Colin, in an accidental drowning.

safety

SAFETY

? ?

So is there a health risk here? Well, if your baby accidentally inhales, drinks, or bathes in a cleaning product, that's a real problem. Yes, they are toxic and, in some poisoning situations, fatal.

As for other potential health hazards from everyday, appropriate use . . . that's a bit more difficult to say. At this point, there's no scientific evidence linking everyday use with health problems.

If you'd prefer to go the green route, check out web sites like EarthEasy.com for extensive lists of eco alternatives and homemade recipes for cleaning products.

Carpeting

Q. Is it safe to install new carpeting in our home?

New carpeting, as well as the padding and adhesive that goes with it, can release Volatile

---

THE MOST DANGEROUS HOUSEHOLD PRODUCTS

Here is a list of childhood favorites to keep out of reach. (Place items in high cabinets out of reach or in places with cabinet locks).

Chemicals
◆ cleaning products
◆ paint thinner
◆ dishwashing detergent
◆ gasoline

Medications
◆ Especially Mom's prenatal vitamins (iron)
◆ Especially visiting grandparents (heart or blood pressure medications)

Plants (some of these are common houseplants).
◆ Christmas favorites: poinsettias, mistletoe, holly
◆ wild mushrooms
◆ hyacinth, narcissus, daffodil, elephant ear, rosary pea, larkspur, Lily-of-the-Valley, iris, fox-glove, bleeding heart, daphne, wisteria, golden chain, laurels, azaleas, jasmine, lantana

Hygiene products
◆ mouthwash
◆ nail polish remover
◆ rubbing alcohol
◆ hair dye

Food and wine
◆ liquor
◆ pottery from foreign countries (lead)

? ?

SAFETY

Organic Compounds (VOC's). VOC's can irritate eyes, nose and/or throats as well as cause coughing or trouble breathing.

Also: carpeting is a nice place for pesticide residue, molds, and dust mites to settle. This is the same place your baby will be crawling and rolling for several hours a day. Our advice: considering putting down a playmat or washable area rug over the carpeting in rooms where baby plays.

Q. Is it safe to get my carpets cleaned?

Yes. Although there is no specific health risk, it's still a good idea to wait until your carpets are completely dry before your baby plays there. You may also want to use a no- or low-solvent cleaner.

Pesticides

Q. Is it safe to use pesticides in our home?

Here is what we know for certain, according to the Centers for Disease Control: "Home pesticide use overall has been linked to childhood cancers such as soft tissue sarcomas, leukemias, and cancer of the brain." Some studies have specifically linked organophosphate pesticides to lymphoma and leukemia, but the study results are controversial and inconclusive. (*CDC*)

We've got some tips to reduce your child's exposure: If you have to use pesticides, set traps or treat the *outside* of the house first. This should be done BEFORE use of any an indoor insecticide spray or "bombs." The pesticide residue will collect on upholstery, rugs, carpeting, and even stuffed animals. And only treat for pests when there is a problem. Skip scheduled or routine pesticide applications.

It's also a good idea to avoid doing routine pesticide treatments on your lawn—only treat your lawn when there is a problem.

Q. Is it safe to use insect repellent on our baby?

Yes, we cover this answer in detail in Chapter 4, Hygiene.

Radon

Q. Should I have my home tested for radon?

Yes.

Radon is an odorless, colorless, tasteless radioactive gas formed from the decay of naturally occurring uranium in the earth's rocks, soil, and water. Radon gets into homes from cracked foundations, granite walls, and porous cinderblocks. Exposure is usually more of a problem in homes with basements.

Because radon exposure is a known carcinogen, you should get your home tested. For

SAFETY

? ?

more info, check out the Environmental Protection Agency's website at epa.gov/radon or call 800-767-7236. (*AAP*)

Q. Do you have a checklist to help me baby-proof my house?

Yes, we do!

Now is the time to make your home safe.

Children start to explore their world as a natural part of their development. Make their world safer so they can accomplish their goals. Here are the Top 20 Safety Tips:

1. *Safety gates need to be at the top and bottom of the stairs.* The best and safest option is to permanently install gates (instead of using pressure gates).
2. *Electrical outlets need to have plastic safety covers.*
3. *Do not place nightlights in lower electrical outlets.*
4. *Get down on the floor and look at the world through your child's eyes.* Electrical cords need to be moved behind furniture.
5. *Toxic cleaning products in lower cabinets need to be moved.*
6. *Cabinet locks on cabinets with knives, glass containers, china, and alcohol.*
7. *Unplug appliances when not in use.*
8. *Install stove knob covers if they are within a child's reach.*
9. *Make trashcans inaccessible by storing in a locked cabinet or closed pantry door.*
10. *Coffee tables and fireplace hearths with corners need safety bumpers.*
11. *Anchor bookshelves, TV stands, and large furniture to the wall.*
12. *Get toilet lid locks so your baby cannot fall in.* Better yet, make it a habit of keeping the bathroom door closed.
13. *Set your hot water heater to 120 degrees or less.*
14. *Empty the bath tub water immediately after use.* Do not leave water in buckets.
15. *Get cord shorteners, wall brackets, or cordless blinds to avoid dangling drapery cords.*
16. *Remove houseplants altogether or move them to a room inaccessible to your baby.* Some plants are poisonous, some pots are heavy and can be pulled over, and yes, kids will eat dirt.
17. *Remove any toys hanging over the crib by the time your baby is five months old.*
18. *Keep medicine out of reach. Be especially watchful of grandparents who come to visit.* They are more likely to be taking a medication and leaving it out on a bathroom counter or in an open purse on the floor or couch.
19. *If you drop something, pick it up.* Otherwise, your baby will do it for you and stick it into their mouth.
20. *If you are a gun owner (remember I live in Texas, y'all), lock 'em up.* Guns should never be accessible to children. Store ammunition elsewhere and lock it up, too.

Air

Carbon monoxide

Q. Should I install a carbon monoxide detector?

Yes.

Carbon monoxide poisoning can be quite serious. The health effects can range from headaches and dizziness to coma and even death. People are exposed to carbon monoxide from woodstoves, fireplaces, charcoal grills, poorly ventilated combustion appliances, motor vehicle exhaust, and tobacco smoke. (*AAP*)

Bottom line: it's wise to have a detector in your home, since carbon monoxide is odorless and invisible. Be sure to get one that is UL certified. Good brands include American Sensors and Kiddie; check ConsumerReports.org for the latest ratings.

Tobacco smoke

Q. If I smoke outside the house, my baby will not be exposed to second-hand smoke, right?

Wrong. Sorry to ruin the fantasy here but . . . your baby is very likely to be a secondhand smoker unless you wear a towel over your head and clothing while you are smoking outside. The smoke is pervasive and will settle on your hair and clothing. Once you re-enter your house and pick your baby up onto your chest or shoulder, your baby will be breathing in the particulate matter from the smoke.

Besides the obvious long-term health hazards to a child, the immediate health consequence is often wheezing. Babies and young children exposed to tobacco smoke are more likely to have symptoms of asthma.

Factoid: Poor air quality has a direct link to asthma. Air pollution can cause new cases of asthma—and can trigger symptoms in people with existing asthma. Clearly, there is a genetic susceptibility (that is, you have a greater chance of having asthma if other family members have asthma/allergic disorders). But environmental pollutants don't help.

Electric and magnetic fields

Q. I worry about exposing my baby to electric and magnetic fields. Should I worry?

Electro magnetic fields (EMF's) are invisible lines of force created by electric charges. Power lines, electric appliances, cell phones (and towers), the earth's magnetic field, and even humans, emit these EMF's.

Low frequency fields don't have enough energy to cause damage to you or your baby's DNA or body organs. (*NIH*) Hence, your hair dryer, coffee maker, and microwave are probably safe. But researchers continue to look at possible connections between EMF's (including cell phone use) and brain tumors and certain types of leukemia. At this time, many experts believe that cell phones do not emit enough energy to damage human DNA. The greatest concern is the distance of the body organ (example, the brain) from the EMF source (say, the cell phone).

One suggestion to avoid EMF exposure via cell phones: use a hands-free device or Face Time grandma instead. It's not a bad idea for you to do this as well. (*American Cancer Society*)

Ionizing Radiation

Q. My baby hit their head and the ER doc wants to do a head CT scan. Is there a health risk from the radiation?

Short answer: yes.

Long answer: While the risks from ionizing radiation are low, we know that children are more radiosensitive than adults. Studies show that a child who has two to three head CT scans has a three times greater risk of developing a brain tumor later in life.

Clearly, doctors should only recommend an imaging study that involves ionizing radiation when it is absolutely necessary. And they should lower the radiation settings or opt for non-radiation imaging (ultrasound, MRI scans) if possible. In this scenario, the head CT scan is the right thing to do if your child has sustained a significant head injury or has an abnormal neurologic examination.

Baby Product and Toy Safety

Bisphenol-A (BPA)

Q. Are plastic baby bottles safe? Do I still need to worry about BPA?

Prior to 2009, all the best-selling clear, hard plastic baby bottles were made of polycarbonate, which contained a chemical called Bisphenol A (BPA). It is the BPA that makes the hard, clear plastic bottles . . . well, hard and clear. BPA is also used in the linings of cans for liquid foods (more on that later).

BPA's chemical bond with polycarbonate breaks down over time, especially with repeated washing or heating of the bottle. As a result, BPA leaches out of the plastic and ends up in the liquid—that is, the breast milk or formula.

BPA is an endocrine disruptor. It can mimic the natural female sex hormone, estradiol. While most data about BPA comes from animal research, these studies show even low level exposure of BPA *may* be linked to everything from early puberty and breast cancer, to attention and developmental problems.

We don't know all the answers about BPA—the research is evolving. But, the FDA banned BPA in baby bottles and sippy cups in 2012 over potential health concerns. When you go bottle shopping today, the plastic bottles you see in major chain stores are all BPA-free. As long as you don't use hand-me-down baby bottles, you should be in the clear.

Q. How do you lower your exposure to BPA?

The National Toxicology Program has these recommendations to reduce BPA exposure:

◆ Avoid plastic containers with #7 on the bottom (some—but not all—that have a #7 recycling number may have BPA).
◆ If you own polycarbonate plastic containers, do not wash them in the dishwasher with harsh detergents.
◆ Do not microwave polycarbonate plastic food containers. BPA may break down from repeated use at high temperatures.
◆ Eat less canned food. Opt for fresh or frozen foods.
◆ Use glass, porcelain, or stainless steel containers, particularly for hot food or liquids.

Q. Are plastic baby bottles made out of polypropylene safe?

Maybe.

Most plastic baby bottles are now made with polypropylene. A recent study published in *Nature* showed that babies who drink from plastic baby bottles ingest 1.5 million tiny pieces of plastic, called microplastics, on a daily basis! The good news is most of that also comes out in their poop on a daily basis...but it is concerning, nonetheless. (Li) The World Health Organization says there is not enough evidence at this point to prove there is any health risk.

The microplastics flake off into liquid when the plastic is hot, and especially if the bottle is shaken. If you want to minimize risk, prepare baby formula in a glass container and then transfer it to the plastic baby bottle when cooled. Or, opt for glass baby bottles.

Phthalates

Q. Are there any other harmful plastics? What should I know to protect my baby?

The other big plastic issue you should be aware of: phthalates.

Phthalates are plasticizers that make plastic soft and durable. The health concern? Phthalates are considered endocrine disruptors (weak estrogens and androgen-blockers) and animal carcinogens. While there is much controversy about phthalates, there is still no scientific consensus that they are dangerous to humans.

Phthalates are used just about everywhere. For example, you'll find them in plastic cooking wrap, plastic food packaging, baby shampoos, diaper rash creams, and toys. Phthalates can be both ingested and absorbed through the skin. Babies have been found to eliminate the breakdown products of phthalates in their urine.

The good news: both the U.S. and Canada require toys and products that are intended for use in the mouth (pacifiers, teething toys, bottles) to be phthalate-free. And newer U.S fed-

safety

eral legislation has tighter restrictions on phthalate use.

The Consumer Product Safety Commission is in charge of enforcing this ban, and for the record, do not find a significant health risk to young children. According to the CPSC, a child would have to suck/mouth a phthalate-containing toy for at least 75 minutes a day to have any significant health consequences.

Our advice: If you want to reduce phthalate exposure, use a napkin or paper towel when you heat food in the microwave and do not use second-hand soft plastic toys.

Baby Gear

Q. Are infant recliners, loungers, and bassinet swings safe?

Let's talk about these products. There are potential concerns about all of them, so we don't love them.

Why? It's risky for a baby to relax (or let's be honest, snooze) at an angle. There is a risk of suffocation and Sudden Infant Death Syndrome (SIDS).

Before 2022, recliners, loungers, and swings did not have strict regulations like bassinets and cribs because they were technically not designed to be a sleep space. They are supposedly used for "supervised awake time."

DR B'S OPINION

"Just because a product is for sale on the market does not mean it is safe."

Despite this intended use, parents put their babies in these devices all the time and yes, babies do sleep in them. The Consumer Product Safety Commission (CPSC) has recalled numerous products in this category over the years and is finally closing the loophole for products that do not "fit" in the infant sleeper category. Bottom line: products that place an infant under five months of age at a 30 degree angle (known as "inclined sleepers") are no longer allowed to be marketed as a place for baby to sleep.

Our advice: avoid all loungers (also called nests) and other products—only put your baby to sleep in a crib or bassinet.

Q. Are slings safe to use?

Yes, but make sure your baby's body does not end up in a C-shape position where their chin is slouched into their chest. You need to be able to see your little one's face. It should not be smothered in the fabric.

Q. Are hand-me-down cribs safe?

It's probably a safer choice to buy a new one. Safety standards changed in 2011, when cribs with drop sides were prohibited. Yet cribs often lack manufacture dates. As a result, we don't recommend using a hand-me down.

Also remember: the safest crib is a naked crib. All you need is a mattress with a fitted sheet. No bumper pads, fluffy bedding, sleep positioners, pillows, or stuffed animals. Position the crib away from any cords.

Crib mattresses

Q. Are organic crib mattresses safer than traditional mattresses?

In short, no.

Yes, conventional crib mattresses do utilize synthetic ingredients such as polyurethane foam, polyvinyl chloride (aka vinyl), phthalates, and flame retardants.

Rumors have circulated the Internet for years that sleeping on a conventional crib mattress was related to Sudden Infant Death Syndrome (SIDS). The theory: inhaling all the fumes from a traditional mattress caused SIDS. Scientific research has debunked this theory: SIDS is NOT caused by foam or coil crib mattresses.

However, we understand why parents would want to limit exposure to these chemicals—and let's face it, your baby will spend a good amount of time on his mattress.

An entire alternative crib mattress industry has sprung up in recent years to fill this demand—companies are now selling "organic" mattresses filled with soy-based foam, latex, coir (coconut husks) and more. Most of these mattresses are covered with organic cotton covers or food-grade polyethylene plastic. And, of course, these mattresses are much more expensive than traditional crib mattresses: $300 to $600, compared to conventional mattresses that start at $100.

One major negative to some organic mattresses: some have covers that are NOT waterproof. As you probably can guess, diapers leak, babies spit up (and more) in their crib. A waterproof cover is critical to keep bacteria from growing inside the mattress. Hence some folks buy an all-organic mattress but then use a waterproof protector that contains many of the same "bad" chemicals they were trying to avoid in the first place.

So where's the science that says organic is better for mattresses? There isn't much. Most of the "proof" circulating around the web comes from a company in New Zealand, which is selling its own special mattress cover which it claims protects against SIDS.

Our opinion: we don't think an organic mattress is going to reduce the risk of SIDS. If you buy an organic mattress and don't have a waterproof cover, the occasional pee that escapes the diaper will enter your organic mattress and leave a nice nesting ground for bacteria. (*Sherburn*)

Bottom line—here's what we'd recommend:

◆ Get a mattress with a vinyl cover that is triple-laminated (basically thicker). The cover should be listed as waterproof, not just water resistant.
◆ Use a waterproof pad over the mattress. Some "quick change sheets" (Ultimate Crib Sheet) have waterproof backing that would provide extra protection to keep liquid out of the mattress.
◆ Don't use a hand-me-down mattress, since it might have not been water-protected.
◆ Consider changing out the mattress with each child (new baby, new mattress). No matter how hard you try, some leakage might happen.
◆ If you want to limit chemical exposure, look for mattresses that are GREENGUARD certified. These mattresses are tested to meet strict standards for low chemical emissions.

Car Seats

Q. What tips do you have about using a car seat safely?

Installing it properly is a good first step! Some basics:
- ◆ Use a new car seat.
- ◆ Do not use if it has been in an accident (even if it looks undamaged).
- ◆ Read (and follow) the instructions.
- ◆ Make sure the seat is at the correct angle for positioning.
- ◆ Never add padding or pillows under the harness straps.
- ◆ Car seats belong in the back seat. The front seat airbag is a health risk if it deploys.

Q. When do I turn my baby around to face forward?

Children should be rear-facing as long as possible in a car seat—yes, you can turn them forward-facing after age two if you wish. But rear-facing is safer. Why? A child under two lacks neck support to avoid injury in a car accident when forward-facing. Hence, rear-facing is safer. That's the official advice from the American Academy of Pediatrics—a child should ride rear-facing until age two or longer if the car seat allows. The good news: most car seats (both infant and convertible) work rear-facing to 30 or 40 lbs.—some even higher!

Toys

Q. Is it safe to buy toys from resale shops? How can I be sure they have not been recalled and are lead free?

You can't be sure.

Yes, the Consumer Product Safety Improvement Act requires toys and products intended for use by children under 12 years of age to contain less than 0.009% lead. The law also requires testing for lead and other heavy metals.

Any children's products (including toys) made in the past decade are required to be certified to meet this new standard—this includes both American made and imported items.

The best course: buy NEW toys, certified to meet the current standards. All toys sold in major chain stores would qualify. Avoid hand-me-downs from friends, relatives or older siblings.

Q. Where can I get information about toy safety?

The U.S. Consumer Product Safety Commission is at cpsc.gov or toll free at 1-800-638-2772. They post product recall information.

You can also check out the advocacy organization, Safe Kids Worldwide. Head over to SafeKids.org and sign up for their newsletter. They curate news about child-related products as well as product recalls and deliver it to your inbox.

Q. Is it safe to have a sandbox for my baby?

Here's the health concern for sandboxes: synthetically-made play sand can contain asbestos-like fibers. Asbestos is a known carcinogen (exposure can cause cancer later in life). Real sand from the beach is fine.

Except for the state of California, manufacturers do not have to list whether or not the sand is real or synthetic, and whether or not it is asbestos-free. Our advice: buy only natural river, beach, or silica-based products for your baby's sandbox. If you know where the sand is coming from, go for it. (*AAP*)

 ### Helpful Hints

◆ *Take a CPR course* and have any caregivers who are taking care of your child take one, also. The biggest potential problem for a child after nine months is choking. Kids this age do not get the famous Heimlich maneuver— they get back blows to force out the foreign object. You'll want to find out how to perform this if you don't know already.

 DR B'S OPINION

"I know, I know, pediatricians are such buzzkills. I promise we don't hate fun. But full disclosure—none of us own trampolines! My daughter plans to buy one for her own kids someday just to get me back."

◆ *Have Poison Control's phone number in your favorited contact list.* The national number is: 1-800-222-1222. You can find your local Poison Control number from the American Association of Poison Control Centers' web site at aapcc.org. Always call poison control first if your child has ingested something.

28 tips for reducing eco hazards

We know that going green can sometimes be impractical and costly. Here are some easy, common sense things you can do to reduce your family's exposures to environmental pollutants.

1 **HAVE FORCED AIR FURNACES, FUEL-BURNING APPLIANCES** (gas water heaters, stoves, clothes dryers) **PERIODICALLY CHECKED** by a professional as the manufacturer recommends.

2 **PILOT LIGHTS PRODUCE CARBON MONOXIDE SO MAKE SURE THEY ARE WORKING PROPERLY.**

3 **DON'T USE GAS STOVE TOPS OR OVENS AS A HEAT SOURCE.**

4 **VENTILATE SPACE HEATERS PROPERLY.**

5 **DON'T USE HIBACHIS OR BBQ GRILLS INDOORS.**

6 **DON'T LEAVE A CAR RUNNING IN THE GARAGE**, even when the door is open.

7 **LIMIT THE AMOUNT THAT YOUR BABY TALKS/LISTENS DIRECTLY ON YOUR CELL PHONE.**

8 **LIMIT THE TIME/INCREASE THE DISTANCE BETWEEN YOUR BABY AND SMALL APPLIANCES.**

9 **IF YOU HAVE TO USE PESTICIDES,** set traps or treat the outside of the house instead of using an

? ?

SAFETY

indoor insecticide spray or "bomb" indoors. The pesticide residue will collect on upholstery, rugs, carpeting, and even stuffed animals.

10 **TREAT FOR PESTS ONLY WHEN THERE IS A PROBLEM.** Skip scheduled or routine pesticide applications in your home and on your lawn.

11 **SCRUB PRODUCE WITH A BRUSH** under running water to get rid of any obvious residue.

12 **PEEL WHATEVER PRODUCE YOU CAN.** (FYI: this often removes the fiber benefit, though).

13 **DON'T EAT THE OUTER LEAVES OF LEAFY VEGETABLES** (for example, lettuce, kale).

14 **GROW YOUR OWN LITTLE GARDEN, AND DON'T USE PESTICIDES.**

15 **IF YOU ARE BUYING IMPORTED PRODUCE, ONLY PURCHASE PRODUCE THAT CAN BE PEELED.**

16 **BUY PRODUCE THAT'S IN SEASON.**

17 **COMPLETELY AVOID EATING SHARK, SWORDFISH, MACKEREL, AND TILEFISH.**

18 **EAT LESS THAN 12 OUNCES A WEEK** of shellfish, canned fish, small ocean fish, or farm-raised fish.

19 **EAT SIX OUNCES OR LESS A WEEK OF WHITE ALBACORE TUNA.** Canned light tuna, and specifically Carvalho Fisheries and King of the Sea are lower in methylmercury.

20 **EAT SIX OUNCES OR LESS OF LOCAL FISH** if your community's fishing advisories are unknown.

21 **AVOID PLASTIC CONTAINERS WITH #7 ON THE BOTTOM** (some—but not all—that have a #7 recycling number may have BPA)

22 **IF YOU OWN POLYCARBONATE PLASTIC CONTAINERS, DO NOT WASH THEM IN THE DISHWASHER WITH HARSH DETERGENTS.**

23 **DO NOT MICROWAVE POLYCARBONATE PLASTIC FOOD CONTAINERS.** BPA may break down from repeated use at high temperatures.

24 **EAT LESS CANNED FOOD.** Opt for fresh or frozen foods.

25 **USE GLASS, PORCELAIN, OR STAINLESS STEEL CONTAINERS**, particularly for hot food or liquids.

26 **CONSIDER USING MORE ECO-FRIENDLY CLEANERS.**

27 **RUN YOUR TAP WATER FOR A COUPLE OF MINUTES IN THE MORNING BEFORE USING IT.**

28 **DON'T SMOKE.**

We dedicate this chapter to Michael Shannon, M.D., FAAP. Thank you for your sage advice and guidance. You are missed.

Section 5

First Aid

Top 12 Problems & Solutions

FIRST AID

PROBLEMS & SOLUTIONS

Chapter 16

*"It's no longer a question of
staying healthy. It's a question
of finding a sickness you like."*
~ Jackie Mason

WHAT'S IN THIS CHAPTER

1. YOUR FIRST AID KIT
2. TAKING VITAL SIGNS
3. THE TOP 12 PROBLEMS
   & SOLUTIONS
   ◆ ABDOMINAL PAIN
   ◆ ALLERGIC REACTION
   ◆ BLEEDING AND
     BRUISING
   ◆ BREATHING PROBLEMS
     (RESPIRATORY
     DISTRESS)
   ◆ BURNS
   ◆ DIARRHEA AND
     VOMITING
   ◆ FEVER
   ◆ POISONING
   ◆ RASHES
   ◆ SEIZURES
   ◆ DOES IT NEED STITCHES?
   ◆ TRAUMA (ACCIDEN-
     TAL INJURY)

Are you afraid your pediatrician will fire you for calling too much? Although doctors entertain this thought occasionally, we never act on it (well, almost never). Phone calls (portal messages, and other forms of communication) are a part of the job. Most panicky questions come from new parents. You are not alone.

The purpose of this chapter is to help you troubleshoot the most common problems you will encounter on the front line of your baby's medical care. It should help you determine when to contact the doctor. It also prepares you for what the doctor will ask when you connect.

This chapter does not replace the need to check in with your doctor. But learning these basics helps you worry less and trust your instincts more. Pick up the phone if you are worried. Yes, most offices still prefer to speak to patients on the phone for urgent medical concerns. Technology offers other ways to communicate remotely, so find out what the office's preferred method is before an emergency arises. You may be meeting with your doctor in the Metaverse soon.

Helpful Hints
On Call Etiquette

How can you make the most of a call to your baby's doctor? As a doctor who has spent one third of her life on call, here are some important points to consider:

1 **THE ON-CALL DOCTOR IS NOT IN THE OFFICE.** Doctors leave the office at the end of the workday and carry a cell phone for after hours calls. Doctors also go to sleep. If you call about your child's diaper rash at 2 am, the doctor won't be as perky as when you call during office hours. (FYI: Many offices utilize nurse call centers to handle minor middle-of-the-night questions and save the more pressing emergencies for the physicians.)

2 **TELL THE ON-CALL DOCTOR/NURSE ABOUT PAST MEDICAL PROBLEMS.** Most pediatric and family doctor practices have SEVERAL doctors on staff. After hours, there is usually one doctor (who picks the short straw) that is on-call. This may or may NOT be your regular doctor. As a result, the on-call doctor may not know your child. If the practice participates in a multi-practice on-call group, the on-call doctor may not have access to your child's electronic health record. As a general rule, assume that they don't. (Nurse call centers don't have access to your child's chart either.) Explain any previous medical problems, surgeries, or hospitalizations. It might have a bearing on the particular problem at hand.

3 **TELL THE ON-CALL DOCTOR/NURSE ABOUT ALLERGIES TO MEDICATIONS.** If your child has an allergic reaction to a medication, put it in YOUR family medical records. Don't rely on an on-call doctor or your pharmacy to know this information.

"The pink medicine" or "some antibiotic" is not adequate. Most doctors inquire about drug allergies before any medicine is prescribed—but we appreciate it if you tell us.

4 **HAVE A PHARMACY PHONE NUMBER READY.** Yes, doctors have smartphones and can Google a pharmacy phone number—but it is helpful if you have your preferred pharmacy phone number available for us. Often, there is more than one Walgreen's on a major street, so being as specific as possible is helpful. That way, we can call in your prescription after we talk with you.

5 **DON'T CALL FOR REFILLS, REFERRALS, OR APPOINTMENTS AFTER HOURS.** Universal doctor rule—we don't do these things without patient charts or schedules available. Medical emergencies are the only exception to this rule.

6 **BE PATIENT.** During cold and flu season, it may take a while for the doctor/nurse to return your call (the on-call doctor or nurse call center may get several calls per hour). We appreciate it if we can get through to you when we call you back. Keep your phone within reach and be ready to answer an unknown call or "no-caller ID."

7 **DON'T USE CALLER ID TO CALL THE ON-CALL DOCTOR BACK WITH ANOTHER QUESTION.** Okay, for the doctor, this is just creepy. If you call back through the appropriate answering service or voicemail system, you will always get your call returned. There is a protocol for a reason, folks—there is often a queue of patients who may need callbacks. If your caller ID shows the doctor's home or cell phone number, don't use it.

8 **DON'T EXPECT OR DEMAND THAT ANTIBIOTICS BE PRESCRIBED OVER THE PHONE.** There is a good reason why antibiotics aren't available over the counter. A child needs to be seen to make a diagnosis of a bacterial infection. Remember the drug-resistant bacteria problem. (This is mentioned in Chapter 13, Infections). Doctors usually prescribe "supportive relief" (such as acetaminophen (Tylenol)) until your child can be evaluated.

FIRST AID

9 **IF YOU HAVE A QUESTION ABOUT A MEDICATION, HAVE THE BOTTLE IN HAND WHEN YOU CALL.** Just common sense here. We will probably ask you to read the information on the bottle to us.

Q. What should I have in our first aid kit at home?

Here is your grocery list:

◆ Band-Aids (lots of them—they become badges of courage)
◆ sterile, non-stick dressing and tape
◆ "butterfly" bandages or thin adhesive strips
◆ Ace wrap
◆ a roll of gauze dressing
◆ rectal thermometer
◆ petroleum jelly
◆ acetaminophen (Tylenol)
◆ ibuprofen (Motrin, Advil)
◆ antibiotic ointment (Neosporin)
◆ diphenhydramine liquid (Benadryl)
◆ saline nose drops (home made or store bought)
◆ decongestant nose spray (Afrin)
◆ 1% hydrocortisone cream
◆ baking soda
◆ tweezers
◆ measuring spoon, cup or dropper; you'll want one with cc/ml measurements for those tiny infant doses. (See Chapter 5, Nutrition & Growth for a list of common measurements)
◆ Add the National Poison Control Center 800-222-1222 to your favorite contacts list.

Q. Should I take a CPR course?

Yes!
Learn how to handle emergencies before they happen. Even if you can't remember exactly what to do, you will be more prepared to take action if something bad happens.

It's also helpful to learn how to take your child's vital signs. This information is very useful for when you call your doctor for advice.

Q. How do I take my child's vital signs?

Vital signs include the heart rate (pulse), respiratory rate (breaths per minute), and temperature. You can assess your baby's vital signs at home with the instructions below. You can also easily measure your child's oxygen saturation (how effectively oxygen is flowing to the body) with a simple, painless pediatric pulse oximeter. You can buy one on Amazon for about $30. Pediatric blood pressure cuffs for home use also exist, but trust us, those are difficult to use on an infant and not worth the cost. Despite that caveat, vital signs are very useful to share when you speak with the on-call provider or do a telemedicine visit.

1. **Temperature:** Know how to take a rectal temperature. (See fever section later in this

first aid

chapter for details.)

2. **Pulse:** Feel your baby's pulse in the inner part of the elbow or in the groin. Count the number of pulsations for 15 seconds and multiply by four. This gives you the beats per minute. Below is a list of average heart rates for your baby's age:

Average heart rates for babies, birth to three years of age:
>Birth to one week: 95–160
>One week to six months: 110–180
>Six to 12 months: 110–170
>One to three years: 90–150
>(Compare these to an adult's heart rate of 60–100 beats per minute.)
>*If you own a pulse oximeter, the device will also assess your child's heart rate. Bonus!

3. **Respiratory Rate:** Watch your baby's chest as it moves in and out. Count one breath for each time they breathe in for 30 seconds and multiply by two. This gives you the number of breaths per minute. Babies have very erratic breathing, so you won't get an accurate count if you only look for ten or 15 seconds. Below are the details.

Average respiratory rates by age:
>Newborns: 25–50
>One week to one year: 24–38
>One to three years: 22–30
>(Compare to an adult's respiratory rates of 12–16 breaths per minute.) (*Gunn*)
>**Pulse oximeter**
>Normal oxygen saturation 95-100%.

HOW CAN DOCS MAKE A DIAGNOSIS OVER THE PHONE WITHOUT EXAMINING A CHILD?

Your doctor will rely on you to provide the signs and symptoms (the clues).

Doctors are very systematic in the way they make a diagnosis. A professor once told me that 90% of the time, a diagnosis can be made purely on the history of the problem. Only 10% of the time will the physical examination of the patient be necessary to make the diagnosis. It's true. I usually know what I will find when I examine the patient just by listening to the story. But this requires some detective work. I always ask the same questions for each complaint to get a history of signs and symptoms (that is, location/type of pain, length of fever, appetite or lack of, sleep disruption, runny nose, cough, vomiting, etc.) When you contact your doc, expect to be interrogated.

We know you are anxious and worried about your baby. That might make you focus on one particular symptom, like a fever. (See fever section later in this chapter). Doctors are trying to figure out the big picture and we need to know about various symptoms to put the puzzle together. Let the doctor guide you in the right direction to determine what is going on with your baby!

Insider Tip

A pulse oximeter also measures the heart rate. A baby's heart rate may vary from 90–180 beats per minute. If the heart rate is less than say, 85, the device is probably not accurately detecting the pulse. And then the oxygen saturation is also not accurate. So, do not freak out if your baby's heart rate is 40 and the oxygen saturation is 50–it's probably the device and not the baby. Just keep your baby calm and their finger from squirming and try again.

Helpful Hint

When a child runs a fever, all the other vital signs are elevated, too. Don't worry about the heart racing when children run a fever. That is to be expected and normal.

The Most Frequent Emergencies

First, here's some doctor lingo: ever heard the guys on Grey's Anatomy say a patient was "in triage?" Triage just means to sort out by severity of the condition. The point: the doctor triages medical problems into the following categories:

◆ **Priority 1:** Needs immediate evaluation and treatment–NOW.
◆ **Priority 2:** Needs appointment the next day.
◆ **Priority 3:** Watch and wait. Needs appointment if there is no improvement or worsening of symptoms.
◆ **Red flags:** Denote symptoms that are medical emergencies.

We've adopted this system in this chapter to give you a general idea of how problems are managed. But every problem is unique. If you have concerns, the right answer is to call your doctor.

Abdominal Pain

Q. My baby has a stomachache. When do I need to worry?

It's hard to tell when an infant has a stomachache, unless they are vomiting or have diarrhea. Some reliable signs include irritability during/after feedings, pulling up of the legs, or a tense, full belly. There are also medical problems that have nothing to do with the stomach that cause abdominal pain (such as bladder infections).

Abdominal pain is divided into acute (a new event as of yesterday or today) or chronic pain (the problem has been going on for over a week). Acute issues *only* are discussed below.

Priority 1: Needs immediate evaluation and treatment—NOW:

The most serious problems are called surgical emergencies or an "acute abdomen." A piece of bowel may be kinked, blocked, or infected. Babies with these problems look sick and are often inconsolable. Concerning symptoms include: swollen and/or tender belly, lack of interest In eating, persistent vomiting, unusual looking diarrhea, and difficulty settling down. These problems need to be addressed quickly. See the Red Flags on the next page. Diagnoses include: **INTESTINAL OBSTRUCTION, INTUSSUSCEPTION, INCARCERATED HERNIA, APPENDICITIS, PYLORIC STENOSIS.**

Priority 2: Needs appointment the next day.

Most problems fall into the non-urgent category. These symptoms are less severe and babies are consolable. Symptoms include: gas, trouble settling after a feeding, crying/straining while attempting to poop, and one or two episodes of vomiting. Observation and medical evaluation is in order if things are not improving. NOTE: In babies under a year of age, it's better to be cautious and contact your doctor if you are worried.

Diagnoses include: **GAS, CONSTIPATION, EARLY VIRAL GASTROENTERITIS**

Helpful Hints

What the doctor will ask you about ABDOMINAL PAIN:
1. Does your baby have a fever?
2. Is your baby vomiting? What does the vomit look like?
3. Does your baby have diarrhea? Is it watery, bloody, mucousy, look like grape jelly?
4. Does your baby's tummy look like they are pregnant? Does it hurt to touch?
5. How long has the pain/vomiting/diarrhea been going on?
6. Does your baby have at least three wet diapers (urine) a day?
7. Is your son's scrotum swollen?

RED FLAGS

Call your doctor immediately if you see the following symptoms with abdominal pain:

♦ Fever and pain without diarrhea.
♦ Projectile vomiting or bright green/yellow vomit.
♦ Diarrhea that is bloody/mucousy/grape-jelly like.
♦ Tense, distended belly.
♦ Pain more than two hours in duration.
♦ Prolonged vomiting (see vomiting section later in this chapter).
♦ Prolonged diarrhea (see diarrhea section later in this chapter).
♦ Less than three wet diapers a day.
♦ Swollen scrotum.
♦ Crying with urination.

Feedback from the Real World

My four-year-old daughter slept for 12 hours once and awakened with the tensest belly I had ever seen. She was very uncomfortable and was having difficulty walking. She screamed when I tried to touch her belly. She had no interest in eating. Being quite convinced that she had an acute abdomen, I called one of my pediatric surgeon friends to evaluate her in the ER. As we drove to the hospital, she proclaimed that she needed to pee NOW. I pulled off the highway onto the shoulder. She urinated in my portable car trashcan. She had a full bladder. She felt much better and asked if we could go out to lunch after visiting the doctor. We sheepishly walked into the ER together. She skipped to the exam room. I apologized for calling my friend to look at my perfectly normal child. His comment was, "Well, she does have a *cute* abdomen!"

Lessons learned here:

1. Sometimes benign processes (like a full bladder, constipation, etc.) can look like an acute abdomen. Doctors prefer to check out suspicious patients rather than wait.
2. It's hard to be objective when dealing with your own child.

Allergic Reaction

Q. I think my child is having an allergic reaction. Do I need to go to the ER?

Clarify the reaction. Do you see a rash or is your baby having difficulty breathing?

Priority 1: Needs immediate evaluation and treatment—NOW:

RED FLAGS
Anaphylactic Reaction
Call 911 for a child who is drooling, anxious, having obvious labored breathing (stridor), lip swelling, sweating. Another serious allergic reaction is called Stevens-Johnson Syndrome. This is an extensive rash accompanied by mouth ulcers. This requires immediate medical attention.

If your child is having an anaphylactic reaction, do not attempt to drive to the hospital. Call 911 and get immediate help. Most ambulances are equipped with medicine to handle these reactions immediately.

Diagnoses: **ANAPHYLACTIC REACTION, STEVENS-JOHNSON SYNDROME**

Priority 2: Needs appointment the next day.

Most rashes are less of an emergency. (See details of other rashes in the rash section later in this chapter). Allergic reaction rashes can have various configurations. They are all itchy. Rashes (except Stevens-Johnson Syndrome, see above) can be evaluated by a doctor when the office is open. These include:

- *Hives:* raised mosquito bites with flat red circles around them or large flat red areas with raised edges (for example, a drug allergy).
- *Erythema multiforme:* extensive, small, flat, red patches with raised edges (for example, a drug allergy).
- *Eczema:* red plaques with a scaly rough appearance overlying it (for example, a food allergy).
- *Contact dermatitis:* red pimples or blisters in a patch or streak (for example, poison ivy).

See our web site at Baby411.com for a visual library of common rashes.

Reality Check
Have your child in front of you when you speak to the doctor on the phone. You will be asked to describe what you see over the phone. The same goes for

telemedicine visits—the beauty of telemedicine is being able to see the patient!

What the doctor will ask you about ALLERGIC REACTIONS:
1. Is your baby having any trouble breathing?
2. What does the rash look like? Where is it on the body?
3. When did you first see the rash?
4. Is the rash itchy?
5. Is your baby currently taking any medication?
6. Has your baby been exposed to any new foods, laundry detergents, clothing, or soaps?

Helpful Hints
◆   Unless your child is having an anaphylactic reaction (see above), give diphen-hydramine (Benadryl) and schedule an appointment. Take a picture of the rash in case it disappears at the time of the appointment.
◆   Stop any other medication until a doctor sees your child.
◆   Try to think of any new medication or food your child may have had recently.

Reality Check
FYI: An allergic reaction is caused by a release of a chemical called histamine. Diphenhydramine (Benadryl), an ANTI-histamine, effectively clears the results of histamine (the rash) until the medicine wears off (about six hours). Histamine levels stay elevated for several DAYS. So, don't be surprised to see the rash "come back" after the medicine wears off. You will need to use the antihistamine medicine for a few days.

Diphenhydramine (Benadryl), cetirizine (Zyrtec), and loratadine (Claritin) are all antihistamines approved for babies ages six months and up. Benadryl can be used in babies under six months of age, if necessary, to treat an allergic reaction.

Causes of allergic reactions: Food allergy, medication allergy, bug bites, poison ivy (rhus dermatitis).

Bleeding And Bruising

Q. My child bruises easily. Should I be worried?

No, not usually.

Bruising in high trauma areas is not worrisome (shins, knees, elbows, forehead). We worry much more about bruising on the torso—most falls do not cause bruising to this area.

Easy bruisability can be a sign of low platelet count (platelets help your blood clot). Bruising is much more worrisome when it is seen with **PETECHIAE**. (pe-teek-ee-eye). See box on the next page. Bruising accompanied by excessive bleeding can indicate a blood clotting disorder.

See our web site at Baby411.com (click on Bonus Material) for a picture.

Common Diagnoses include: Trauma/injury, temporary bone marrow suppression from a viral infection.

Uncommon Diagnoses include: Hemophilia, von Willebrand's disease

NEW PARENT 411: ALL YOU EVER WANTED TO KNOW ABOUT PETECHIAE BUT WERE AFRAID TO ASK

Petechiae are flat, purplish, pinpoint dots that almost look like freckles. When you push down on them, they remain colored (that is, they do not blanch). Petechiae are caused by broken blood vessels. They arise for the following reasons:

1. *Pressure*: Straining while pooping, giving birth, coughing, or vomiting forcefully.
2. *Infection*: Strep, meningitis, Rocky Mountain Spotted Fever.
3. *Low platelet count:* Leukemia, Idiopathic Thrombocytopenic Purpura, temporary bone marrow suppression from a viral infection.

If there is a good reason to have petechiae (such as repeated coughing), and they are located above the level of the chest only, you can relax a bit, but still call your doctor.

If there is not a good reason, your baby needs to be seen quickly to rule out the serious medical problems on this list.

Leukemia, Idiopathic Thrombocytopenic Purpura, Immunoglobulin A Vasculitis, Meningitis.

Priority 1: Needs immediate evaluation and treatment—NOW:

1. A fever with petechiae rash
2. Petechiae AND bruising, with or without a fever
3. Bruising and lethargy
4. Excessive bruising (beyond the knees/elbows)
5. Uncontrollable bleeding

Priority 2: Needs appointment the next day.

1. Bruising with no other symptoms
2. Recurrent nosebleeds

What the doctor will ask you about BRUISING OR BLEEDING:
1. Where are the bruises?
2. Are there any other rashes on their body?
3. Does your baby bleed excessively? Does anyone in the family have bleeding problems?
4. Has your baby been unusually tired or been running a fever with no explanation?

Q. My child is having a nosebleed. What do I do about it?

Lean your child's head *forward*, not backwards. Apply pressure to the base (soft part) of the nose for ten minutes. If this doesn't work, you can spray some medicated decongestant nose drops into the nostrils (Little Remedies for Noses or Children's Afrin are two brand names). This causes the blood vessels to shrink and stop bleeding.

Most nosebleeds stop in about ten minutes. If it goes beyond that, call your doctor.

first aid

Q. My child just vomited blood. Where is it coming from and should I be worried?

If it looks like fresh red blood, it can't be coming too far from the mouth. Blood that comes from the stomach is partially digested and will look like coffee grounds. Be prepared to describe the vomit. Lack of an obvious explanation for the blood needs an evaluation.

What the doctor will ask you about VOMITING BLOOD:
1. How old is your baby?
2. Are you breastfeeding? Are your nipples cracked and raw?
3. Have you been suctioning your baby's nose with a bulb syringe?
4. Has your baby been vomiting forcefully?
5. What does the vomit look like? Are there streaks of blood? Coffee grounds? Mucous?

The most common cause of *Upper GI Bleeding* (official term for vomiting blood) in a newborn is Mom's cracked nipples. The blood in the spit up is really Mom's. There is a test to prove it, but one look at Mom's nipples is a dead give-away.

The next likely culprit is that dreaded bulb syringe we told you to throw away in Chapter 4. It causes an irritation in the lining of the nose, making it raw to the point of bleeding. Nasal secretions are swallowed and then spit up.

As your baby gets older, they will explore their body parts. Kids pick their noses and cause trauma. The number one cause of bloody vomit in an older child is a nosepicker's nosebleed.

Now, for more serious causes. Forceful vomiting can cause a small tear in the lining of the esophagus. A child with persistent blood in vomit needs to be examined.

Vomit that looks like coffee grounds also needs to be evaluated. In older babies, doctors worry about a toxic ingestion/poison that irritates the esophagus or stomach, ulcers, gastritis, or esophagitis. If the vomit looks like Folger's coffee, call your doctor.

Diagnoses of an upper GI bleed include: Mom's cracked nipples, esophagitis, toxic ingestion/poisoning, gastritis, ulcers

Priority 1: Needs immediate evaluation and treatment—NOW:

1. No obvious source for bleeding.
2. Vomit that looks like Folger's coffee.
3. Persistent bleeding.

Q. My baby has blood in their poop. Should I worry?

No, but Lower GI bleeding *always needs to be evaluated by a doctor*. If you see blood in the diaper, save the diaper. It's helpful to bring a fresh specimen to the office visit. If your baby doesn't cooperate, doctors have other ways to get what they need (via a rectal exam).

You will describe every detail of that poop to the On-Call Doctor. If the blood looks red and fresh, the source is close to the anus. If the blood looks darker or the poop looks like meconium, it comes from further up the pipes (small or large intestine). The age of the child partially determines the cause of the problem.

◆ *Newborns:* Bad *diaper rash* is often the explanation. Blood is usually found on the diaper wipe more than in the poop with an obvious raw bottom. Babies under four months of age with streaks of blood often have a *milk protein allergy*. Even exclusively breastfed babies can encounter this because the cow's milk protein can enter the breast milk. It often takes six weeks for the blood to clear once babies eliminate the cow's milk from their diets. Even if this is what the working diagnosis is, bacterial stool cultures are in order to rule out infection.

Diagnoses include: diaper rash, milk protein allergy, food poisoning (Bacterial gastroenteritis).

◆ **Older babies:** Babies who have started solids often get constipated. If your baby looks like they are giving birth when pushing out a solid poop ball, they might bleed with it. An *anal tear or fissure* can be seen if you look for it. This is not serious. Put some petroleum jelly (Vaseline) on the area and check out fiber facts in Chapter 8, The Other End.

Now for more serious causes. Babies can get *food poisoning*—even those who aren't eating off the Chinese buffet line yet. Where do babies get it? Human carriers, pets, and food exposure. Babies in daycare are at higher risk of parasite infections. Your doctor can test for all of these bugs with cultures (see bacterial infections and parasites in Chapter 13, Infections). Symptoms include diarrhea with streaks of blood and mucous.

Finally, poop that looks like grape jelly (currant jelly stool) is a medical emergency. The diagnosis is *intussusception*, where the bowel telescopes on itself and creates an obstruction. Symptoms include abdominal pain (pulling up of the legs), irritability, and grape jelly stool.

Diagnoses: Anal fissure/tear (caused by constipation), food allergy, food poisoning (bacterial gastroenteritis), parasite infection, antibiotic induced colitis (C difficile infection), intussusception

What the doctor will ask you about BLOOD IN POOP:

1. How old is your baby? Was your baby premature?
2. What did you see in the diaper? Streaks of blood mixed in poop? Solid poop with blood on the diaper wipe? Explosive bloody diarrhea? Mucous also? Grape jelly?
3. Is there a diaper rash?
4. What is your baby eating?
5. Has anyone in the house had diarrhea?
6. Does your baby look sick or well? Fever?
7. Is your baby's belly full and distended?
8. Is your baby interested in eating? Any vomiting?
9. Has your baby been on antibiotics recently?

Priority 1: Needs immediate evaluation and treatment—NOW:

◆ Bloody diarrhea
◆ Grape jelly poop
◆ No obvious diaper rash or anal tear
◆ Former premature baby

Priority 2: Needs appointment the next day.

◆ Streak of blood with normal looking stool and well appearing child

Priority 3: Watch and wait. Needs appointment if there is no improvement or worsening of symptoms:

FIRST AID

? ?

HOW TO AVOID FOOD POISONING

Steer clear of the following foods and remember to clean cutting boards, knives, and countertops when dealing with these products. Keep a spray bottle of bleach handy in the kitchen to clean these tools. Here is what to avoid:

◆ unpasteurized dairy products
◆ unpasteurized juices (fresh squeezed OJ, apple cider)
◆ alfalfa sprouts
◆ raw shellfish
◆ oysters
◆ undercooked and raw meat or seafood
◆ unwashed fruit and vegetables
◆ undercooked eggs* (sunny side up, raw cookie dough, fresh Caesar salad dressing, homemade ice cream, homemade mayonnaise)

We highly advise buying pasteurized eggs to limit the risk of food-borne illness, especially if you are using undercooked eggs in a recipe.

Natural food warning: While it doesn't seem likely that you and your baby would come across the above items, think for a moment about unpasteurized juices. These are common in health food stores and some vegetarian/vegan restaurants. It can be easy to pick up a bottle of such juice without thinking about it. The same goes for unpasteurized dairy products—gourmet cheeses at health food stores sometimes fall into this category. While adults might be able to eat these products without a problem, they are much more dangerous to infants and children. Check the labels: raw milk cheese, for example, should be clearly labeled as such.

◆ Obvious constipation
◆ Obvious diaper rash

Feedback from the Real World
Dr. Brown's TRUE STORIES about food poisoning:

1. One mother was a short order cook who discovered she was a carrier of Salmonella when her newborn had it. She truly was "Typhoid Mary" (named for a woman who was a cook and a carrier of typhoid fever—a cousin of Salmonella). Sometimes parents are carriers who have had a previous infection and don't know it.

2. Unusual pets can be carriers of Salmonella. One of my patient's uncles had a pet iguana that roamed freely on the family's kitchen counter.

3. Raw eggs and chicken are also known to have Salmonella. I had a patient who acquired Salmonella when Grandma was preparing chicken gizzards next to Mom preparing a bottle for the baby.

Feedback from the Real World

There was an outbreak of the deadly E. coli 0157 bacteria (Hemolytic Uremic Syndrome) on the East Coast several years back. It was traced to an apple cider producer in New Hampshire. It had been a bad apple season, so the producer used apples that had already fallen off the trees to press for cider. Unfortunately, the cows that lived on the farm pooped on those apples and contaminated them with the E.coli. There are new regulations for cider production now. Moral of the story: Never drink unpasteurized apple cider.

A similar outbreak happened with Odwalla apple juice—a small batch of unpasteurized juice contained E.coli bacteria, sickening more than a dozen children. This juice was blended with other products as well. Be sure to look for these products—make sure ALL the ingredients in a blended juice product are pasteurized.

Burns: Water, Sun, Hot Drinks, Appliances, BBQ

Q. My child got a burn from _____. What do I do? Does this need an appointment?

Don't get out the butter . . . and yes, you may need a doctor visit.

First rule: If it blisters, it should be looked at.
Second rule: Apply cool water, not butter.
Third rule: Don't pop a blister.

Any type of burn damages the top layer of skin. This causes redness (first degree). Burns that go deeper than that create blisters (second degree) or damage to the full thickness of the skin. Your skin is your body's protection from foreign invaders such as infection. Without the skin, the body is defenseless. To help combat infection, it's always a good idea to use an antibiotic ointment (such as Neosporin) on a burn and cover it with a non-stick dressing.

For second-degree burns, a prescription product called Silvadene may be needed. Second degree burns (or worse) need to be seen by your doctor to assess the damage, look for infection, and clean away any dead skin (this debris inhibits healing and promotes infection). Any burns on the hands, genitals, and on large areas should also be seen.

Priority 1: Needs immediate evaluation and treatment—NOW:

◆ Extensive areas burned.
◆ Area looks infected (red, weeping pus, fever)

Priority 2: Needs appointment the next day.

◆ Second degree burns (blisters).
◆ Burns on the hands or genitals.

Priority 3: Watch and wait. Needs appointment if there is no improvement or worsening of symptoms:

◆ First degree burns.

first aid

Breathing Problems (Respiratory Distress)

Q. My baby is having trouble breathing. What do I do?

Knowing what true respiratory distress looks and sounds like is very important. Read the section below first. Then understand how calls like this are triaged. The short answer is—if your child is having labored breathing, call your doctor immediately.

Understanding the Respiratory System

Think of the respiratory system as one big tube. The opening of the tube starts at the nose. The bottom end branches into tiny tubes in the lungs. Air goes in and out of this tube with each breath.

What is an UPPER respiratory infection?

The common cold or flu viruses live in the top of the tube (nose and sinuses). The body forms mucous or snot as a result of it. A person coughs because the mucous drips down the tube towards the lungs. Coughing protects our lungs. The cough brings the mucous up so it can be swallowed (into the stomach) instead of collecting in the lungs. Upper respiratory infections rarely cause labored breathing. They do cause noisy breathing, though, as air travels through the snot in the nasal passages.

Diagnoses include: Common cold, the flu (influenza)

What is a LOWER respiratory infection?

Bronchiolitis (RSV), bronchitis, or pneumonia are infections (viral or bacterial) that invade the tubes in the lungs or the air sacs (alveoli). Because there is swelling or mucous in the tiny tubes and lung tissue, it is hard to exchange air effectively (remember that oxygen/carbon dioxide thing you learned about in science class). A person with a LOWER respiratory infection may become air hungry. We'll discuss this more in detail later in this section.

Rattling in the chest or ***hearing wheezing*** are NOT usually signs of a lower respiratory infection.

Diagnoses include: RSV Bronchiolitis, bronchitis, pneumonia

Any others?

There are also infections that attack the middle of the airway tube (larynx and trachea)

WHAT AN AIR HUNGRY CHILD LOOKS LIKE: A MUST READ

The diagnosis of an air hungry child can be made without a stethoscope. It's not what is heard—it's what is seen. A baby or child who is air hungry breathes rapidly and shallowly *(elevated respiratory rate)*, sucks in their rib cage (retractions), and flares their nostrils (flaring). A child may also make a grunting noise at the end of each breath. These are the body's way of using every muscle to pull in more air with each breath. The number of breaths taken per minute (respiratory rate) is much higher than normal. (See guide to vital signs earlier in this chapter). If a child is air hungry, call your doctor immediately.

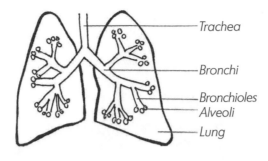

The Lungs

where the voice box (vocal cords) is located. The tube swells in this area. Because a child's tube is smaller in diameter than an adult's tube, they are more compromised by these infections. The younger the child, the more problematic.

Diagnoses include: croup, whooping cough (pertussis)

Now that you understand the tube analogy, here's the scoop.

Think about the tube. You know how your pipes are all attached in your home? When you flush your toilet upstairs, you can hear it in the kitchen. Here is the analogy: nose is to toilet as lung is to kitchen. The water is in the nose, not the lung—but it can be heard and felt down there. This is called ***transmitted upper airway noise.*** The wheezing noise is ***air passing through snot—it whistles.***

A child who is really wheezing enough to be audible to the naked ear is in such severe distress that you will *see* it in his chest (**AIR HUNGRY**).

Helpful Hints

◆   Sometimes your doctor can tell what the problem is just by listening to the baby breathing on the phone. They can also watch your baby breathe on a telemedicine appointment. So, have your baby handy for the call or videochat.

◆   When a person lies down, the snot from the nose drips down the back of the throat. Our body's job is to cough and keep it out of the lungs. The cough is likely coming from nasal secretions when it seems to be worse at night.

EVERYTHING YOU EVER WANTED TO KNOW ABOUT CROUP

A virus causes croup. It appears in epidemics every winter. A croup cough has a characteristic bark that sounds like a seal. Although impressive, this can be managed by quality time spent in your bathroom with a steamy shower running for twenty minutes. When the airway tube is markedly swollen, the bark changes to a high-pitched squeal, called stridor. Stridor requires an emergency breathing treatment and steroids to reduce the swelling or the airway. Croup is always worse at night. FYI: COVID-19 is one of several viruses that can cause croup.

FIRST AID

? ?

Red Flags

◆ Air hungry.
◆ Croup under age two. (See below).
◆ Repeated coughing spasms, followed by reddening of face, possibly a "whoop," or vomiting.
◆ Episodes of not being able to catch one's breath.

What the doctor will ask you about RESPIRATORY DISTRESS:
1. How long has your baby been having trouble breathing?
2. Could they have swallowed something?
3. Any fever?
4. Are they barking like a seal? Any high-pitched squeals?
5. Look at your baby's chest. Do you see sucking in the ribcage with each breath (retractions)? Any panting or breathing fast? Are the nostrils flaring? Is there grunting at the end of each breath?
6. Has your baby wheezed before? Ever stayed in the hospital overnight for it?
7. Are there coughing spasms? Any gasping for breath? Vomiting or turning red with cough?

Priority 1: Needs immediate evaluation and treatment—NOW:

◆ Signs of air hunger.
◆ Any stridor noise (see croup box nearby).
◆ Trouble catching breath.
◆ Child who has asthma.
◆ Child who is a former premature infant.
◆ Choking (see choking emergencies on the next page).

Priority 2: Needs appointment the next day.

◆ Barking like a seal, but no squeal.

Priority 3: Watch and wait. Needs appointment if there is no improvement or worsening of symptoms:

◆ Chest rattling.
◆ Intermittent wheezing noises WITHOUT labored breathing.

Red Flag

When your child stops breathing. Call 911 immediately if your baby has any episode of true apnea (lack of breathing over 15 seconds).

Reality Check

There is a difference between apnea (not breathing) and **PERIODIC BREATHING**. Newborns frequently pause for several seconds between breaths. It is your child's job in life to give you grey hairs. Adults breathe 12 times a minute at a nice regular rate. Newborns breathe 30-60 times per minute at an irregular rate. *Newborns can pause for up to ten seconds and be feeling just fine.* To monitor the respiratory rate of a newborn, count the breaths for a whole minute.

What the doctor will ask about APNEA:

1. Is your child breathing okay now or is does breathing seem labored?
2. Any fever?
3. Any problem with acid reflux?
4. Was your baby born prematurely?
5. Any recent trauma or injuries?

Babies with apnea get admitted to the hospital to be evaluated.

Diagnoses include:

1. Near Sudden Infant Death Syndrome (SIDS) event or acute life threatening event (ALTE).
2. Gastroesophageal reflux.
3. Infection (whooping cough, RSV bronchiolitis).
4. Metabolism problem.
5. Head trauma.

Choking Emergencies: 4 Tips

1 **DO NOTHING IF YOUR CHILD IS ALERT AND MAKING NOISES (CRYING, GAGGING, COUGHING).** Your child is effectively attempting to clear their airway.

2 **IF YOUR CHILD IS IN DISTRESS AND NOT MAKING ANY NOISE,** try to dislodge the object by putting their belly on your forearm, face down (hold your baby like a football). Push forcefully between the shoulder blades with the lower part of your palm five times (called back blows). *Do not perform the Heimlich maneuver on infants under one year of age.* If back blows are unsuccessful, try performing five chest thrusts: place two or three fingers in the center of the infant's chest just below the nipple line and compress the breastbone about 1½ inches. Repeat the five back blows and five chest thrusts until the object comes out or the baby becomes unconscious. Call 911.

3 **DO NOT BLINDLY SWEEP YOUR FINGER IN THE MOUTH AS IT MAY PUSH THE OBJECT FURTHER INTO THE AIRWAY.** Call 911 if the foreign body does not come out.

4 **IF YOUR CHILD BECOMES UNCONSCIOUS, CALL 911, AND BEGIN CPR.**

Feedback from the Real World
Another True Story from Dr. Brown

I was on-call and answering a page. While I was on the phone, my nine month old son crawled over to our dog's food bowl and did a taste test. In my panic, the first thing I did was to blindly put my finger in his mouth to pull the food out. I ended up pushing it down and he swallowed it whole. After that scary (and painful) experience, he never touched the dog's food again! And I never made the mistake again of ignoring my own advice.

FIRST AID

? ?

CPR for Infants (Age <1)
If you are alone with the infant give 2 minutes of CPR before calling 911.

1. Shout and Tap

Shout and gently tap the child on the shoulder. If there is no response and not breathing or not breathing normally, position the infant on his or her back and begin CPR.

2. Give 30 Compressions

Give 30 gentle chest compressions at the rate of 100-120/minute. Use two or three fingers in the center of the chest just below the nipples. Press down approximately one-third the depth of the chest (about 1 and a half inches).

3. Open The Airway

Open the airway using a head tilt lifting of chin. Do not tilt the head too far back

4. Give 2 Gentle Breaths

If the baby is not breathing or not breathing normally, cover the baby's mouth and nose with your mouth and give 2 gentle breaths. Each breath should be 1 second long. You should see the baby's chest rise with each breath.

CONTINUE WITH 30 PUMPS AND 2 BREATHS UNTIL HELP ARRIVES

Cough And Congestion

Q. My baby's nose is so congested that they can't eat or sleep. What do I do?

This is the second most popular phone call. (Fever is number one). Nasal congestion happens for many reasons:

◆ Newborns all have nasal congestion for the first four to six weeks of life. They ALL sneeze and snort and snore. They do not have allergies (and rarely have a cold).

◆ Babies with acid reflux can have congestion from the milk that heads upwards behind the nose.

◆ Mucous pouring out the nose suggests an upper respiratory infection.

Diagnoses include: Common cold, the flu (Influenza), RSV bronchiolitis, COVID-19

Tricks of the trade: How To Make (And Use) Saline Nose Drops

The most safe and effective way to clear the mucous is to flush the nostrils with saline nose drops. Saline is just a salt-water solution. You can't overdose on it. You can make your own concoction (1/2 tsp salt to eight oz water). Or you can buy it for about a dollar at the grocery store. Shoot several drops in each nostril before feedings. *You don't need to suck it out with a bulb syringe.* The saline will either make your baby sneeze or loosen the mucous enough to swallow it. Babies are usually not big fans of this maneuver, but it is effective.

There are other methods of reducing the amount of mucous, but doctors always suggest saline first. Over the counter cough and cold medicines are *not recommended* under four years of age.

Yes, new parents seem to really love the Nose Frida (snot sucker). If you are one of these folks, just be careful not to get overly zealous with your sucking as it can irritate the lining of the nose and cause a nosebleed.

What the doctor will ask you about NASAL CONGESTION

1. Has your baby ever breathed through their nose?
2. Any fever?
3. Is anyone else in the house sick? Is your baby in childcare?
4. Is your baby fussy or having disrupted sleep?
5. Any goopy eyes and/or green snot?

Helpful Hint

If a baby under age two has an upper respiratory infection, the flu, or especially RSV, they are at risk of getting an ear infection. Nasal discharge with fever, goopy eyes, and/or fussiness deserves a visit to the doctor to check for an ear infection.

Priority 1: Needs immediate evaluation and treatment—NOW:

◆ Has labored breathing or appears air hungry.
◆ Under four weeks of age and has a fever of 100.4 or greater (see fever section later in this chapter).
◆ Irritable and inconsolable.

Priority 2: Needs appointment the next day.

◆ Never breathes through the nose.
◆ Under four weeks of age, WITHOUT fever.
◆ Four weeks old to six months old, nasal congestion with or without fever.
◆ Fussy mood or disrupted sleep.
◆ Goopy eyes or red eyes.
◆ New appearance of green nasal discharge after clear discharge for at least one week.

Priority 3: Watch and wait. Needs appointment if there is no improvement or worsening of symptoms:

◆ Over six months of age with nasal congestion, runny nose, and cough for less than one week's duration (see fever section for other reasons to call).

FIRST AID

? ?

Q. My child is keeping up the whole house with a cough! Make it go away.

We know it stinks. We are parents, too. Nighttime coughs cause sleep deprivation for the child *and the parent*. Take a moment to review the respiratory system lecture. Coughing is a protective mechanism to keep the nasal discharge from collecting in the lungs. The cough is worse at night because your baby is lying down. Always try saline nose drops first.

If the cough is keeping baby awake, the only "natural" product I can recommend is Zarbee's baby cough syrup. The active ingredient is agave nectar (not honey!). It has more of a placebo effect on the parents than actual effect on the baby, but it is safe to try. *(Paul, I).*

If the cough is keeping YOU awake, turn off the baby monitor!

What the doctor will ask you about COUGHING:

1. How long has your baby had the cough? (Over three weeks deserves an appointment).
2. Is it worse at night or in the daytime?
3. Any breathing difficulties? (See that section).
4. Any barking like a seal? Squealing?
5. Any panting or breathing shallowly?
6. Any apnea (no breathing for 15 seconds or more)?
7. Any concern for having swallowed a foreign body?
8. Any new fever?

Priority 1: Needs immediate evaluation and treatment—NOW:

◆ Breathing appears labored—grunting, flaring, retractions, stridor, or elevated respiratory rate.
◆ Trouble catching breath with coughing episodes.
◆ Foreign object known to be swallowed.
◆ Known asthma and not responding to medication.

Priority 2: Needs appointment the next day.

◆ Persistent cough.
◆ Cough sounds productive (wet or juicy).
◆ Vomiting or turning red with coughing episodes, but no apnea.
◆ Barking like a seal, but no squeal.
◆ New fever with a cough and NO labored breathing.

Priority 3: Watch and wait. Needs appointment if there is no improvement or worsening of symptoms:

◆ Cough under three weeks duration.
◆ Exposure to someone with a chronic cough.

Chronic Coughs

Not all coughs are caused by infection. Prolonged coughing (over three weeks) should be evaluated. Occasionally, we discover something interesting that has ended up in a branch of the lung airway. Ear, Nose, Throat specialists removes toy jacks, beads, peanuts, teeth, and popcorn kernels in the airways of small children on a regular basis.

The major causes of chronic cough include: foreign object in airway asthma, sinusitis, adenoiditis, whooping cough, tuberculosis (rare).

Red Flags
◆ Cough with breathing difficulties.
◆ Chronic cough over three weeks.
◆ New fever with worsening cough.
◆ Possible foreign body (swallowed object).

Diarrhea

Q. My baby has diarrhea. What do I do ? When do I worry?

Most of the time, diarrhea is a sign of a *stomach virus* (**VIRAL GASTROENTERITIS**). Some people call it the stomach flu. It's not THE flu. (The flu that we can get vaccinated for is influenza—a respiratory virus.) At best, your baby vomits once and the diarrhea continues for three to five days. At worst, your child vomits for 12-18 hours and has diarrhea 25 times a day for ten days (see rotavirus infection in Chapter 13, Infections). Those "24 hour bugs" don't really exist.

Food poisoning (**BACTERIAL GASTROENTERITIS**) is a concern when there is mucous or streaks of blood in the diarrhea. (See abdominal pain section earlier for details). Bacteria will cause only 10% of intestinal infections. Of those 10%, the most common culprit is **SALMONELLA**. *Other diagnoses include:* Shigella infection (bacteria), Yersinia infection (bacteria), Campylobacter infection (bacteria), C. difficile (bacteria, after an antibiotic) Giardia (parasite), Cryptosporidium (parasite), food allergy.

FYI: Chronic diarrhea (over two weeks duration) is a different problem More on this next.

Diarrhea for more than two weeks

If the diarrhea has been going on this long, your baby needs to see the doctor. Most commonly, chronic diarrhea is the result of an acute stomach virus.

Stomach viruses tear up the intestine's normal "flora" of good bacteria that help digest food. Stomach viruses can also break up a digestive enzyme called lactase, which helps the body digest milk sugar (lactose). Occasionally, infants and children can get a temporary lactose intolerance for up to six weeks after a stomach virus. Diarrhea results from repeated dairy intake and inability to digest it.

Another culprit is high juice intake. This is more of a problem with toddlers who become juice-a-holics. The high sugar content pulls water into the poop, causing increased frequency and watery stools.

Causes of chronic diarrhea include: Lactose intolerance (post-stomach virus), high juice intake, food intolerance, celiac disease, parasite infection, Inflammatory Bowel Disease.

What the doctor will ask you about DIARRHEA:
1. How old is your baby?

2. How long has the diarrhea been going on?
3. Has there been vomiting or fever?
4. What does the diarrhea look like? Watery, bloody, mucous or blood streaked?
5. Is your baby still urinating?
6. Has your baby eaten any new foods?

Priority 1: Needs immediate evaluation and treatment—NOW:

◆ Under three months of age.
◆ Blood or mucous in diarrhea.
◆ Grape jelly diarrhea.
◆ Not urinating at least three times in 24 hours.
◆ Unsure about frequency of urination.
◆ Lethargy.

Priority 2: Needs appointment the next day.

◆ Diarrhea more than one week.

HOW TO TELL IF YOUR BABY IS DEHYDRATED—A MUST READ

1 **Urine output:** When our body needs fluid, less water is released as urine. If your baby pees (urinates) at least three times in 24 hours, he is doing okay. It's sometimes hard to tell if there is pee in the diaper, though, when there is explosive poop in it. (See helpful hint on the next page).

2 **WEIGHT LOSS:** If your baby has lost 10% of their body weight, they are severely dehydrated. This is an emergency.

3 **SUNKEN FONTANELLE:** Babies under a year still have a soft spot in their skull. That is their oil gauge equivalent. If the tank is low, the soft spot is sunken. That's the first place a doctor will touch when we examine your baby.

4 **SKIN TURGOR:** You know what your skin looks like when you have been in the bathtub too long? That prune like appearance is a clue to dehydration. Nice doughy skin has plenty of water in it.

5 **DRY LIPS AND MOUTH:** When you're dry, you stop making saliva.

6 **CAPILLARY REFILL:** Press down gently on your fingernail. You will see the pink color turn white. When you release the pressure, the pink color returns in less than two seconds. In severe dehydration, that refill will take more than two seconds because the blood supply is sluggish.

7 **LETHARGY:** This is a difficult one to assess. If your baby looks like a wet noodle, it's time to visit the doctor.

◆   Age over three months and fever more than three days.

Priority 3: Watch and wait. Needs appointment if there is no improvement or worsening of symptoms:

◆   Watery diarrhea for less than one week, with frequent wet diapers, and over three months of age.

Q. I'm worried about my baby getting dehydrated. Should I be?

Yes.

Babies under a year old are at higher risk of getting dehydrated. *Contrary to popular belief, dehydration is caused more by diarrhea than vomiting.* The vomiting part of an illness usually stops within about 12 hours. There is only a limited amount of fluid lost from vomiting (once the stomach is empty, there's not much left to throw up). As long as the vomiting is short lived, dehydration is not a problem. Diarrhea is another story. Frequent, explosive, watery diarrhea for a week causes a tremendous amount of water loss. Your baby needs to keep up with these losses with fluid intake.

BOTTOM LINE: Although vomiting is scary, persistent diarrhea is more likely to cause dehydration.

Helpful Hint
How to tell if there is urine in the diaper:

Put a tissue in the front part of the diaper. The urine looks yellow on the tissue because it is concentrated. You can also just opt for those disposable diapers with built-in wetness sensors.

Q. What can I give my baby to eat and drink to prevent dehydration?

Start with liquids, then slowly add solids.

Presuming that vomiting has come first in this scenario, make sure that fluids stay down before going back to solid food (if baby is over four months old). *Liquids are much more important than solids.* It's the fluid that replaces the losses. Babies make up for lost time and will eat when they are feeling better.

Your doctor may recommend a rehydration electrolyte drink (Pedialyte) to treat dehydration—see the vomiting section later for details. Once your baby has kept the rehydration drink down, return to regular formula or breast milk.

Here are some other suggestions:

1. Try Isomil DF formula for severe or prolonged diarrhea. (see formula section in liquid nutrition, Chapter 6) The DF stands for Diarrhea Formula. But it also stands for Dietary Fiber. The formula is lactose free and has a high fiber content that helps bulk up the poop.

2. Try a high fat, high fiber diet for babies over four months old. Resume solids when a baby is interested in food again. Depending on the age and what foods your baby has tried, look for high fiber foods (prunes, oatmeal, beans) and high fat foods (whole milk

FIRST AID

? ?

yogurt, avocados) to feed your baby.

3. Try yogurt or probiotics. Stomach viruses kill off the "good germs" that live in the intestines and help digest food. Replenishing the gut with good germs improves digestion. If your baby is over six months, offer yogurt daily during the illness. Another option: probiotics with Lactobacillus GG (Culturelle and others) may reduce the diarrhea by a day or so.

4. Try a lactose (dairy) free diet for diarrhea lasting over one or two weeks. If the diarrhea is prolonged, a secondary lactose intolerance may be the culprit (see chronic diarrhea section earlier).

BOTTOM LINE: Liquids are the priority in re-hydration. Your baby will eat solid food again when they are well.

Old Wives Tales

1. Avoid milk when your baby has diarrhea.

The truth: Your baby will have diarrhea no matter what they are eating or drinking. Give them what they are willing to drink. If the diarrhea has been going on for *over a week*, however, dairy restriction may be in order to avoid a lactose intolerance (see earlier section on chronic diarrhea).

2. Use the BRAT diet for a baby with diarrhea (Bananas, Rice, Applesauce, Toast).
The Truth: Fat and fiber are more effective in bulking up the poop than these foods. The *old* school of thought was called the BRAT diet. It was thought that a bland, carbohydrate diet was best for infants with diarrhea. The latest research suggests that fat and fiber are actually more effective in reducing water loss in diarrhea.

Q. Can I give my baby any anti-diarrhea medications?

No.

There are a couple of concerns here.

Concern #1: Infant deaths have been reported from products containing loperamide (Imodium). The medication can bring intestinal movement to a screeching halt. While it is nice to stop the diarrhea, stopping the intestines from moving entirely can be life threatening.

Concern #2: Using products containing bismuth subsalicylate as an active ingredient (Pepto- Bismol, Kaopectate) when a child has a flu-like illness or chickenpox has a theoretical risk of causing liver failure (Reye's Syndrome). These products are okay for toddlers and older kids, with that caveat.

Vomiting

There is spit up, and then there is vomit. All babies spit up (see acid reflux in Chapter 8, The Other End). Vomiting is the forceful elimination of food and fluid that is in the stomach.

There is only a fixed amount of stomach contents. So, if a child is vomiting repeatedly, eventually they have "dry heaves" (vomiting with nothing coming out). If a child is vomiting *bile* (fluorescent green/yellow fluid), that is coming from the small intestine and may be a concern for an intestinal blockage.

In the strictest sense, repeated vomiting causes dehydration. If your child is vomiting more than 18 hours straight, they may be unable to maintain adequate fluid intake. *This rarely happens*. With most garden-variety stomach viruses, the vomiting stops within 12 hours and kids are drinking again. The greater risk of dehydration is the water lost in the diarrhea that accompanies the vomiting. Dehydration usually occurs later in the course of the illness.

All vomiting is not due to stomach upset. Babies and young children have active gag reflexes. *Forceful coughing* can result in vomiting (see **POST-TUSSIVE EMESIS**). So a baby with a common cold might vomit after coughing. Headaches can also be accompanied by vomiting. This category includes ear infections, head injury, brain tumors, or meningitis. That's why unexplained vomiting needs to be checked out.

BOTTOM LINE: Persistent vomiting with no obvious cause should be evaluated.

Causes of vomiting include:

Gastroesophageal reflux	Early viral gastroenteritis
Pyloric stenosis	Intestinal obstruction (rare)
After coughing (post-tussive emesis)	Ear infection
Head injury	Brain tumor (rare)
Meningitis	Metabolic disorders (rare)
Bladder/ kidney infections	Food poisoning (bacterial gastroenteritis)

What the doctor will ask you about VOMITING
   1. How old is your baby?

WHAT TO DO WHEN YOUR BABY VOMITS

1. While your baby is actively vomiting, DO NOT GIVE THEM ANY FOOD OR DRINK. Parents are often so afraid that their baby will get dehydrated, they offer fluids immediately. And it comes right back at them. Don't give fluids on an unsettled stomach.

2. If it has been at least one hour since your child has vomited, offer a few sips of Pedialyte (see below). The goal is one teaspoon every five minutes for an hour. Do not offer a whole bottle to your child. Your baby is thirsty and will drink the whole thing—only to vomit again because their stomach isn't ready for that much. If this plan fails (that is, your baby vomits again), call your doctor.

3. If the Pedialyte stays down, you can add to the volume one to two ounces every time your baby wants to drink. If this plan fails, call your doctor.

4. If your child has four hours vomit free, return to breastfeeding or formula.

5. After eight hours of success, babies who are already eating solid foods can return to eating again.

2. How long has your baby been vomiting?

3. Is it projectile (Exorcist-like) or just coming up effortlessly?

4. What does the vomit look like? Any fluorescent green or yellow color? Any blood or coffee grounds?

5. Any fever?

6. Any diarrhea?

7. Is your baby around other children/anyone sick in the house?

8. Does it seem like your baby's stomach hurts?

9. Is your baby still urinating?

10. Any recent head injuries?

Priority 1: Needs immediate evaluation and treatment—NOW:

◆ Vomiting with a head injury.

◆ Vomiting bile (bright green or yellow).

◆ Vomiting over 12 hours straight.

◆ Projectile vomiting more than three times in a row.

◆ Vomiting only in the mornings.

◆ Vomiting blood or coffee grounds.

◆ Appears dehydrated (see section earlier on this topic).

Priority 2: Needs appointment the next day.

◆ Large volume spit ups frequently.

◆ Recurrent vomiting.

Priority 3: Watch and wait. Needs appointment if there is no improvement or worsening of symptoms:

◆ Isolated episode of vomiting in well appearing child.

Q. What is Pedialyte?

Pedialyte, conceptually, is kind of like Gatorade for babies*. It's a rehydration electrolyte drink made especially for babies ages birth to one year. While the Pedialyte package information says "for age one and up," the product is actually intended for infants from 0-12 months of age and pediatricians recommend it for babies. It has a high salt and moderate sugar content and tastes like salt water. Usually babies under a year don't mind the flavor. (Kids over a year are pretty smart and will refuse it.) If you want to make your own Pedialyte, check out Appendix B for a recipe you can make at home.

Do NOT give plain water to babies when they have vomiting or diarrhea. Their body salts are already depleted and giving plain water messes up the delicate electrolyte balance even more.

For older kids, try Pedialyte popsicles, flat ginger ale, or clear chicken broth.

*Note: The "oral rehydration" solutions (brand names Pedialyte or Ricelyte) have the perfect concentration of salts to replenish body electrolytes. Gatorade and other sports drinks actually have a higher salt concentration and can lead to increased diarrhea—so don't use them interchangeably.

? ?

FIRST AID

Reality Check

Regular Pedialyte is a clear fluid. But it also comes in "flavored" varieties—which contain food coloring. Stick with the clear version. Why would you give a child who is vomiting a purple drink?

Eye Problems

Q. My newborn has goop draining from their eyes. Is it pink eye?

No. It's a blocked tear duct.

Babies are born with narrow canals that let the tears flow out of them. Until the canals widen, the tears can get clogged. This can happen intermittently through the first year of life. (See glossary for **NASOLACRIMAL DUCT OBSTRUCTION**). Just wipe away the goop with warm water.

Call your doctor if the white of the eye is red, or if the eyelids are swollen.

Q. My nine month old has goop draining from their eyes and has a cold. Is it pink eye?

Probably.

When the eye goop is accompanied by other symptoms (runny nose, cough, fever), it's more likely to be an infection called conjunctivitis or pink eye.

Conjunctivitis can be caused by either a virus or bacteria. Bacterial infections cause goopy eye discharge (eye boogers) and viral infections cause watery eye discharge. Both are extremely contagious. Bacterial infections can be treated with antibiotic eye drops or oral antibiotics. Viruses cannot be treated and can last up to a week.

Children under age two years with bacterial conjunctivitis (goop) should see a doctor. About 30% have an ear infection or sinus infection to go along with it. The bug is usually Haemophilus influenza non-typable (a cousin of the HIB we vaccinate against). This is a smart bug often resistant to first line antibiotics.

BOTTOM LINE: A child under age two with goopy eyes needs to be seen by a doctor. There is an association of pink eye with ear infections and sinus infections.

Q. My baby's eye is red. Is it allergies?

Unlikely.

HOW TO AVOID HAVING THE WHOLE FAMILY GET PINK EYE

Pink eye is spread by the sick person touching the infected eye and leaving the germs for someone else to touch (doorknobs, hand towels, toys). The best approach if you have pink eye in your house is to wash hands frequently and make a concerted effort not to touch your face.

first aid

FIRST AID

? ?

As a general rule, babies under one year do not have seasonal allergies. A red eye is either caused by *trauma, irritation,* or *infection.* If just one eye is red, consider trauma (corneal abrasion—see below, foreign body) or irritation (soap, sun block). If it is bothersome to your baby, try flushing the eye with some lukewarm water.

If your baby looks uncomfortable, he needs to be evaluated.

Causes of red eyes: trauma, irritation, infection—viral or bacterial.

Q. My baby's eye is swollen shut. Should I worry?

Yes—if they have a fever.

Usually the cause of impressive swelling is a local allergic reaction. If a bug bite or poison ivy occurs on an eyelid, the reaction can be impressive. Proof of a bite or rash is helpful.

The concern is a serious infection called **ORBITAL CELLULITIS**. This is a sinus infection that extends into the area where the eye rests in the skull (orbit). It happens in stages, and the prognosis is obviously better if caught early. The first sign is redness and swelling of the eyelid. It then progresses to a bulging eye, with limited motion of the eye itself.

If you see this, call your doctor NOW. This is a medical emergency. See our web site at Baby411.com for a visual library picture (the picture titled "eyelid swelling" is the example you're looking for).

Q. My baby's eye is tearing constantly today. What is wrong?

Probably a corneal abrasion.

Babies can scratch their eyes accidentally. This is a superficial scratch that takes a day or two to heal. Foreign bodies (dust, etc.) can also cause similar symptoms. Doctors check for abrasions using a purple light and fluorescent dye. If a scratch is found, antibiotic eye drops are prescribed. If a foreign body is found, it can be flushed out.

What the doctor will ask you about RED EYES
1. How old is your baby?
2. Is there eye discharge? Is it watery or goopy?
3. Is there fever, runny nose, or fussiness?
4. If the eyelid is swollen, is there any bug bite or rash visible? Any fever?

Priority 1: Needs immediate evaluation and treatment—NOW:
- Eyelid swollen shut with fever.
- Question of foreign body in the eye.
- Very uncomfortable child with a red eye.

Priority 2: Needs appointment the next day.
- Goopy eyes with a cold, with or without fever

Priority 3: Watch and wait. Needs appointment if there is no improvement or worsening of symptoms:
- Newborn with eye that waters frequently, without redness.

FIRST AID

Fever: Special Section

Fever is the number one reason pediatricians get called at night. At some point in your baby's life, they will have their first fever. And like every new parent that has come before you, you will have some anxiety. So, let's go over our advice. Note: please read this section in its entirety! If you only read a portion, you may miss key details. (Note: all temperatures are in degrees Fahrenheit).

Q. What is the definition of a fever?

Fever is an elevation of the body's regular temperature.

Contrary to what you learned in junior high science class, our body temperature is not 98.6 for 24 hours a day. It varies on a daily rhythm based on hormone levels. Our body is the coolest at 7 am (as low as 97.6) and the hottest at 7 pm (as high as 100). *The true definition of fever is a body temperature of 100.4 or higher taken rectally.*

When an infection (most common reason for fever) enters the body, the body mounts a defense via the immune system. The immune system revs up all other body systems into attack mode. This raises all vital signs (temperature, heart rate/pulse, respiratory rate, blood pressure). A warmer body temperature actually helps fight infection. FEVER IS NOT BAD.

Because the normal body temperature is lowest in the morning and highest at night, our fever will be lower in the morning and higher at night. With a typical viral infection, we may have a temperature of 99 in the morning and be 102 at night. This is why pediatricians get phone calls about fever at night. *The fever doesn't go away and come back. It's always there. It's just lower in the morning. Fevers often last for three to four days for a viral infection.*

Fever, in and of itself, does not do any harm to the body. But it is an indicator that something (usually infection) is going on in the body. *Parents tend to worry about the fever. Pediatricians worry about what the diagnosis/infection is.* Body temperatures over 108 cause brain damage. Infections do not cause body temperatures over the 106 range. (Hyperthermia, the term for body temperatures over 107, are usually caused accidentally—for example, someone locked in a

first aid

DR B'S OPINION: FEVER-PHOBIC PARENTS

Here is a typical phone encounter on fevers:

Parent: "Doctor, my baby has a fever."
Doctor: "Yes, but tell me what else is going on?"
Parent: "But, doctor, he has a fever."
Doctor: "I understand, but can you tell me if there are any other symptoms?"

You get the picture. I heard you. I know your baby has a fever. I need to figure out WHY they have the fever. *The fever is not the problem—it's a clue for the real problem.* Be a good detective and help me look for clues. It will make for a much more productive conversation!

car in the middle of August).

Fever is often the first sign of illness. It can take several hours to see the other symptoms blossom from the infection. So, unless a baby is under three months of age (see protocol below), you may need to watch and see how things evolve.

Fever Phobia

A study looked at parent misconceptions of fever: (*Crocetti*)
* 91% believed fever could cause harmful effects (death, brain damage).
* 44% believed that a fever over 102 was a "high" fever.
* 7% believed that a fever could rise to 110 if left untreated.
* 25% gave fever reducing medicine for temperatures less than 100.
* 85% said they awaken their child to give fever-reducing medicine.
* 44% dosed the fever reducing medicine incorrectly.
* 52% said they checked their child's temperature at least every hour when they had a fever.

BOTTOM LINE

The body is coolest at 7 am (as low as 97.6) and hottest at 7 pm (as high as 100). So, the true definition of fever is a body temperature of 100.4 or higher taken rectally.

Fever is the body's immune response to infection. The immune system revs up all other body systems and raises all vital signs. A warmer body temperature actually helps fight infection. Therefore, fever is *not* bad.

Remember, fever is not the problem, rather it is a clue to finding the problem. And fever is often the first sign of illness.

Don't be fooled that your child is fever-free in the morning if they had a fever the night before. It's just naturally lower in the morning. If you send your baby to childcare, you will get called to take them home when their fever spikes in the afternoon. Prepare to stay at home next day if your child has a fever at night.

Reality Check

Most of the time, newborns have a virus they picked up from a family member. But your doctor doesn't want to take any chances. Now you know why the standard advice is to limit visitors during the first four weeks after birth.

Helpful Hint

Newborns can also have problems if they have LOW body temperatures. If your newborn has a persistently low body temperature (under 97.6 taken rectally), it's best to check in with your doctor.

Q. At what temperature should I be worried?

Below is the protocol for fever in infants. The management plan is based on a child's age. The protocol is fairly universal for all babies under three months.

FIRST AID

Priority 1: Needs Immediate Evaluation And Treatment—NOW:

◆ *Age zero to 28 days: any fever in this age group is an emergency!*

Newborns have a unique risk of serious bacterial infections due to delivery and congenital urinary tract defects (Group B strep meningitis, pneumonia, sepsis, urinary tract infections/kidney infections). They are tested for all of these potential infections as fever may be the only symptom of serious infection in this age group (see sepsis workup in Appendix C, Lab Tests).

1. A rectal temperature of 100.4 or greater requires a medical evaluation ASAP. Newborns (0-28 days old) are routed to a children's hospital emergency department for urgent assessment and lab work to test for serious infections. Babies who are 0-21 days old are hospitalized for 48 hours for IV antibiotics and observation until bacterial cultures are clear of growth. Babies who are 22-28 days of age still get the extensive lab work but a *few babies* may be able to go home and not stay overnight if initial labs are reassuring and their doctor can see them the next day. *(Pantell)*

2. ***Never give acetaminophen (Tylenol) to your feverish newborn. Call your doctor.***

◆ *Age 29-90 days: any fever in this age group is an emergency!*

1. A rectal temperature 100.4 or greater requires examination and lab evaluation.

2. These infants need to be seen either in the doctor's office or in an emergency room depending on the hour. They still run the risk of having those bacterial infections that newborns get.

3. If there is an obvious source of infection (e.g. a cold), and the baby's lab work looks reassuring, hospitalization is unnecessary.

4. ***Never give acetaminophen (Tylenol) without calling the doctor.*** Exception: If your two-month-old baby received their vaccinations, and then starts running a fever within 24-72 hours, it's not a problem unless there are other symptoms going on. We expect your baby to run a fever after getting their shots. Review Chapter 12, Vaccinations, for more information.

◆ *Age three months to six months: a fever AND these problems in this age group is an emergency.*

1. A fever over 102.

2. A fever lasting more than three days.

3. A new fever, after a recent illness.

4. No obvious symptoms of viral infection (cough, runny nose, diarrhea).

5. Fussy mood/inconsolable.

6. Petechiae rash (See bleeding section earlier).

◆ *Age six months to one year:*

1. A fever of 104 or above deserves a phone call. (We know—that's way beyond your comfort level.)

2. A fever lasting more than three days.

3. A new fever, after a recent illness.

4. No obvious symptoms of viral infection (cough, runny nose, diarrhea).

5. Fussy mood/inconsolable.

6. Petechiae rash (see bleeding section earlier in this chapter.)

Priority 2: Needs appointment the next day.

◆ *Age three months to six months:*
1. If everyone in the house has a cold and your baby has the same symptoms, make an appointment if the fever persists longer than three days (or something else is concerning—i.e. dehydration, labored breathing).
2. *You can give acetaminophen (Tylenol) for the fever. Just make sure you have figured out why your baby has the fever first.*

Priority 3: Watch and wait. Needs appointment if there is no improvement or worsening of symptoms

◆ *Age six months to one year:*
1. Obvious symptoms of a virus (cough, runny nose, vomiting, diarrhea), you can probably manage the infection without a doctor's visit.
2. *You can give acetaminophen (Tylenol) or ibuprofen (Motrin) when your baby has a fever. Just make sure you know why your baby has the fever.*

Reality Check

After six months of age, it's not the degree of the fever that is concerning, it's what the baby looks like. Everyone looks sick when they are running a fever. If a baby still looks sick after taking a fever reducing medicine, it's time to call the doctor.

Insider Tip: Roseola

Children usually get the common childhood infection, **ROSEOLA**, between nine to 12 months of age. It causes a high fever (103 to 104) for about three days with no other symptoms. These kids look perfectly happy and go about their daily routines. On day four, when they are fever free, the classic roseola rash (flat red patches on the chest and arms) comes out. They are not contagious with the rash. High fevers (104 or above) deserve to be evaluated, but roseola is often the culprit.

DR B'S OPINION: THERMOMETERS

Ear thermometers are not my friend. Their reliability is based upon the ability of the user to line the tip up with the eardrum. If you compare your own two ears and get two different readings, you will understand what I mean. Ear thermometers can also overestimate the degree of fever and create parent panic. I've received frantic calls regarding kids with fevers of 107 taken with an ear thermometer that turned out to be 102 or 103 when taken rectally.

Except for the ear thermometers (which OVER estimate fever), alternative methods to check temperature UNDER estimate the degree of fever. Parents often ask, "Do you add or subtract a degree from the non-rectal measurement?" My response is, "If you ever get an actual reading that is 100 or over, you know your child has a fever. That is all the information I need."

TREATING A FEVER: DR. B'S 10 COMMANDMENTS

1 IF YOU HAVE YOUR DOCTOR'S BLESSING, IT'S OKAY TO GIVE A FEVER REDUCING MEDICA-TION. (See age discussion earlier.)

2 BABIES FROM THREE TO SIX MONTHS CAN USE ACETAMINOPHEN (Tylenol). It's fine for two month olds to take acetaminophen after getting vaccinations. However, many docs suggest waiting until several hours later to give acetaminophen. Giving a dose too soon may blunt the appropriate response to the vaccination. Ask your doc for dosing instructions.

3 BABIES OVER SIX MONTHS OF AGE CAN USE IBUPROFEN (Motrin/Advil) OR ACETAMINO-PHEN (Tylenol).

4 I PREFER IBUPROFEN FOR OLDER BABIES BECAUSE THE MEDICATION LASTS FOR SIX HOURS INSTEAD OF FOUR. Since the fever will climb at night, this will buy everyone two extra hours of sleep.

5 ACETAMINOPHEN IS PREFERRED IF A CHILD IS DEHYDRATED or has a stomach virus (ibuprofen can upset an empty stomach).

6 BE FOREWARNED: THESE MEDICATIONS ARE CALLED FEVER REDUCERS NOT FEVER ELIMI-NATORS. At best, these medications will bring the body temperature down by two degrees. If your baby is cooking at 104, they will be feeling more comfortable at 102. That's as good as it gets.

7 I DON'T ROUTINELY INSTRUCT PARENTS TO ALTERNATE ACETAMINOPHEN AND IBUPROFEN. If a baby is old enough for the ibuprofen, stick with that. There is no proven benefit of alternating medicines.

8 DON'T BOTHER PUTTING BABY IN A TEPID BATH. If you had the chills, would you want to sit in cold water? This cooling technique is only necessary in an emergency sit-uation (such as extreme hyperthermia, a 107 temperature). Bringing your child's temper-ature down with this technique is not only unpleasant, but a waste of time and effort.

9 NEVER GIVE YOUR CHILD **ASPIRIN**. It can cause liver failure when given with par-ticular viral infections.

10 ALWAYS USE THE MEDICINE DROPPER THAT COMES WITH THE PACKAGE. The term "one dropperful" refers to the dropper that comes with the medicine.

FIRST AID

? ?

Q. My baby is running a "low grade" fever. Should I be worried?

What is a low-grade fever? It's not in the doctor dictionary. And no, don't worry. Many people think a body temperature of 99 to 100 is a fever. This is not, by definition, a fever. It has no association with an infection unless your baby is 100 at 7am when the body temperature should be at its lowest point. In that case, it does not bode well for what the night will bring as the body temperature rises throughout the day and there may, in fact, be a fever at night.

Q. My baby has had a fever "on and off" for several days. I thought the fever broke. Why does it keep coming back?

Let's review. A typical viral infection will cause a fever for three or four days.

Remember, it may look like your baby doesn't have a fever in the morning, but it always comes back at night. If there is a fever at any point in a 24-hour day, your child still has fever on a daily basis. This is helpful when you are reporting symptoms to the doctor. Doctors want a record of how many days in a row your child has had a fever. It helps make diagnostic decisions.

Fever reducing medicine, acetaminophen (Tylenol) and ibuprofen (Motrin), will help bring the body temperature down for four to six hours. But once the medicine wears off, the fever will return. The medicine does not make the infection go away. (See later questions on fever-reducing medications).

BOTTOM LINE: A truly NEW fever after being fever free for a period of at least 24 hours is concerning for a bacterial infection that has capitalized on a sick person (such as ear infection, sinus infection, pneumonia). Make an appointment to see your doctor.

Helpful Hint
On Fever Curves

Another important trend doctors watch is the fever curve over a period of days.

At the beginning of an infection, the fever is the highest. As the body effectively fights off the infection, the maximum fever spikes should be lower. If a fever curve trends up instead of down (fevers are getting higher on a day to day basis), this is more concerning and may prompt an evaluation.

Q. How do you recommend taking a baby's temperature?

For the target age of this book (birth to age one), you need to take the temperature with a rectal thermometer.

Most parents cringe just thinking about this task. Are you cringing? Don't. Babies really don't mind. It does not hurt or make them feel like you've invaded their space. In fact, it's a good trick to make them poop. But I digress.

Rectal temperatures are the most accurate way to check a human's body temperature. And for infants under three months of age, one tenth of a degree will make the difference between whether you stay at home in your nice warm bed or head out for an evening of fun at your local emergency room.

If you call the doctor or nurse at 2 am and tell them that your six week old has a fever, the first thing they will ask is, "How did you take the temperature?" If you took it any way other

? ?

FIRST AID

than rectally, we make you get a rectal thermometer and call us back. Invest in one now—digital rectal thermometers cost about $5.

After one year of age, there is more flexibility about how to take your child's temperature. Trendy products on the market for toddler temperatures include a pacifier thermometer, ear thermometer, temporal artery scanners, and plastic skin stickers. Using an oral thermometer in the armpit is also okay. None of these are as accurate as a rectal temperature. But after a year of age, the actual degree of fever is much less important to making a management plan for your child. That is, a child with 101 or 103 is managed based on the *other symptoms* they have in addition to the fever.

Mom Knows Best

There was a great study that tested Mom's method of temperature taking (placing the hand on the forehead). Guess what? Mom is usually right—at least 80% of the time—with this method. Some thoughts on this:

1. After six months of age, if you say your child "feels hot," that's often enough proof of fever.
2. Trust yourself! Parents think they need to take their baby's temperature periodically to make sure they are okay. You hold your baby 24 hours a day. You will know when they feel hot. Then you can get out the thermometer.

New Parent 411:
How to take a baby's rectal temperature.

Don't be embarrassed. You've never done this before. Get out your digital rectal thermometer. Place some petroleum jelly (Vaseline) on the tip. With one hand lift up your baby's feet, holding them together. With your other hand, insert the tip of the thermometer into their anus about one inch. Leave the thermometer in there for one minute (or until it beeps at you). See, you and baby did just fine.

Q. What is the correct dose of medication? It says on the box to consult a physician.

Ever wonder why it says this on the box? It's to make sure that you call the doctor when your newborn has a fever. Now that you know when you need to call, we will tell you how to dose these medicines. Both acetaminophen (Tylenol) and ibuprofen (Advil) are dosed at five milligrams per pound per dose. See the dosing chart on the following page.

How to avoid overdosing your baby

1. Acetaminophen is the generic name for Tylenol, Feverall, and Tempra.
2. Ibuprofen is the generic name for Motrin and Advil.
3. Both acetaminophen and ibuprofen are effective fever reducers and pain medications.
4. Acetaminophen is dosed every four hours. Ibuprofen is dosed every six hours.
5. As we've said earlier, always use the medicine dropper/syringe that comes in the

FIRST AID

? ?

package. To reduce dosing confusion, acetaminophen liquid now comes in only one standard concentration. However, ibuprofen comes in two different strengths—infant concentrated drops and a children's syrup.

6. Acetaminophen suppositories (medicine bullets inserted in the anus) are available for babies who resist taking medicine or are actively vomiting.

7. When you graduate to the syrup medicine, use a medicine cup to dispense. Silverware teaspoons are not an exact teaspoon measurement. They can be larger or smaller depending on your set. Medicine syringes are also helpful—they make it easier to measure and dispense medicine.

DR B'S OPINION

"I have too many stories about Tylenol overdoses to share in this book. It's just not as easy to figure these medicines out as it should be."

Dosing Chart

Acetaminophen:

BABY'S WEIGHT IN LBS.	6-11LBS	12-17LBS	18-23LBS	24-35LBS
Dose in ml	1.25 ml	2.5 ml	3.75 ml	5 ml
Dose in mg *(160 mg per 5 ml)*	40 mg	80 mg	120 mg	160 mg
Suppositories (80mg)	——	1 suppository	1 1/2	2
Suppositories (120mg)	——	——	1	1 1/3

Ibuprofen:

BABY'S WEIGHT IN LBS.	6-11LBS	12-17LBS	18-23LBS	24-35LBS
Dose in mg	*	50 mg	75 mg	100 mg
Infant drops *(50 mg per 1.25 ml)* 1.875 ml is a dropperful	*	1.25 ml	1.875 ml	2.5 ml
Children's syrup (100mg per 5 ml)	*	2.5 ml	3.75 ml	5 ml

* Note: Ibuprofen is NOT for babies under six months of age

Q. Is it safe to give a fever reducing medicine longer than five days? It says on the box to consult a physician.

The medicine itself is safe to give. This warning is a way to make sure you have checked in with your doctor if your baby has a prolonged fever. A child with a fever more than four days straight should be seen by her doctor.

Q. I have given my baby acetaminophen (Tylenol) and they still have a fever.

The most common reason this happens is that your child has outgrown the dose of medicine you have given them. Fever reducing medicines (as well as most other types) are dosed based on the weight of a child. A few pounds can make a difference for the correct dosing.

Look at the chart above. When your doctor tells you the dose of acetaminophen (Tylenol) at your child's two-month well check, don't think that the dose will never change.

The second most common reason: Acetaminophen and Ibuprofen are fever reducers (not eliminators). If your child has a high fever, it won't be completely eliminated by the medicine. The fact that the fever does not go down with medication has no implication on the severity of the illness.

Q. I've heard that fevers can cause seizures in babies. Is this true?

Yes, babies can have febrile seizures or convulsions.

A few children—less than 5% (ages six months to five years) are prone to having a seizure/convulsion as a fever is shooting up. "Febrile seizures" do not cause brain damage or lead to a seizure disorder such as epilepsy.

The seizure happens when the body temperature rises quickly. If your child's temperature is already at 104, they have most likely missed the window of having a seizure. So, you can relax now.

Yes, it is terrifying to watch a child have a full-blown seizure in your living room. Fortunately, febrile seizures last less than five minutes. And children are fine afterwards.

About 30% of children who are prone to febrile seizures have more than one episode in their lives. But after the first time, parents are much more comfortable about managing it. Unfortunately, giving fever-reducing medication around the clock will not necessarily prevent a child from having another seizure.

The first time a child has a febrile seizure, they need to be evaluated thoroughly. Once this diagnosis is determined, treatment focuses on the cause of the fever.

Old Wives Tales
Don't give your baby a bath while they have a fever.
Don't let your baby drink milk while they have a fever.
Fevers cause brain damage. Teething causes fever.

The Truth: None of these statements are remotely true. Keep feeding your baby breast milk or formula, go ahead and give them a bath, and unless their fever reaches the extreme temperatures mentioned earlier, relax a bit. Oh, and teething has *nothing* to do with fever.

What the doctor will ask you about FEVER:
1. How old is your baby?
2. How did you take the temperature?
3. What other new symptoms are you seeing?
4. Is anyone else in the household sick?
5. Is your child exposed to other children?
6. How many days has the fever been going on?
7. Any recent illnesses prior to the fever?
8. Any rashes?
9. Have you given any fever reducing medicines?
10. What dose of medicine did you give?
11. What does your baby look like after giving the medicine?

Red Flags

◆   Fever under three months of age.
◆   Fever over 102 in three to six-month-old.
◆   Fever of 104 or above in six months and older.
◆   Fever lasting over three days.
◆   Fever without obvious source of infection.
◆   Fever with petechiae rash.
◆   Fever with irritability or lethargy.
◆   Febrile seizure.
◆   Fever with a limp or limb pain.

Poisonings/Ingestions

If your child accidentally swallows a household product, call poison control immediately.

Have the phone number in your favorites contact list. Do NOT try to make your child vomit. Other treatments are more effective (and vomiting can, in some cases, causes MORE harm than good). Poison Control is an amazing resource of information on any product a curious child might ingest. They will tell you whether the product can do potential harm to the body or not. And they know the antidotes.

Occasionally, a parent is not even aware of the ingestion happening. They only know that their child is acting unusual. *Some clues to ingestion include: mouth burns, drooling, rapid or shallow breathing, vomiting without fever, seizures, extreme lethargy, or body/breath odor.*

Helpful hint

If Poison Control directs you to an emergency room, take the poison/medication with you if you have it. It helps determine the ingredients and amount that was swallowed.

Feedback from the Real World
Dr. B True Story

I cared for a patient once who ate part of a necklace a mother had brought back from traveling abroad. The beads were made of ricin, the active ingredient of poison darts (think Bond, James Bond).

Bottom Line: Be careful. Babies are programmed to taste everything.

What the doctor will ask you about POISONING:

1. Is the product toxic vs. non-toxic?
2. Do you have the bottle/container?
3. Is your child having trouble breathing?

When to call:

All poisonings and ingestions are Priority 1: Needs immediate evaluation and treatment—NOW!

Rashes

Trying to diagnose a rash over the phone is always a challenge. Your pediatrician may offer telehealth services, a patient portal, or health privacy compliant text messaging to help see that rash. But if not, you need to be the eyes for your doctor. Without actually seeing the rash, the best we can do is figure out whether the rash fits into the worrisome or the non-worrisome categories. Worrisome rashes need prompt attention. Non-worrisome ones can wait until the office opens the next day. Causes of rashes include:

- ◆ **Infection:** viruses, bacteria, fungi, mites
- ◆ **Allergy:** eczema, contact allergy (poison ivy, sensitivity to a skin care product), food/medication allergy
- ◆ **Newborn rashes:** due to hormonal changes
- ◆ **Blood cell abnormalities**

See our website at Baby411.com (Bonus Material) for a visual library of rashes.

What the doctor will ask you about RASHES:
1. How long has the rash been there?
2. Where on the body did the rash start? Is it spreading? Where?
3. Is there a fever?
4. Is it itchy? Really really itchy?
5. Anyone else in the house with a rash?
6. Is the rash flat or raised? (Can you feel it with your eyes closed?)
7. Is it scaly on top?
8. What color is the rash?
9. How big are the spots?
10. When you press on the rash, does the color turn white? Or, does it remain discolored?
11. Is your child taking any medications?
12. Has your child eaten any new foods?
13. Have you used any new skin products? (sun block, lotion, soap, detergents)
14. How old is your child?

Q. Which rashes are worrisome?

Petechiae with or without bruising. (See bleeding section earlier for details on petechiae). Petechiae are small flat freckle or pinpoint dots, purplish in color, that stay purple when you push on them.

This is really the only rash that needs immediate attention. Petechiae can be caused by forceful coughing or vomiting. But this rash can also indicate meningitis, Rocky Mountain Spotted Fever, idiopathic thrombocytopenia purpura (ITP), or leukemia. Petechiae are ***Priority 1: Needs immediate evaluation and treatment—NOW.***

RASH-O-RAMA: COMMON RASHES SEEN WITH

Viral exanthems: (rashes caused by viruses)

	Rash looks like	**Where?**
Chickenpox	fluid filled blisters; come up in crops	all over; avg. 350 lesions
Shingles	fluid filled blisters	1 patch
Measles	red, raised pimply	face to body
German measles	red, raised	face to body
Roseola	FLAT red ovals/ lace	chest, arms, neck, +/- face
Parvovirus (Fifth disease)	"slapped cheeks"; Flat, red, lacy on body	chest, arms
Coxsackievirus (hand, foot, and mouth)	red dots or blisters	palms, soles, +/- buttocks
Unilateral Latero-thoracic Exanthem	raised red bumps, scaly on top	one armpit
Pityriasis rosea	raised red streaks; a little scaly	back, angled, like a fir tree

Special viral rashes:

Herpetic Whitlow	blister, red around	thumb, finger
Molluscum Contagiosum	pinpoint blisters	anywhere

Bacterial infections:

Impetigo*	red, raised with weeping golden crust	anywhere
Scarlet fever* (usually over 2 yrs old)	red, sandpaper feel, rough raised dots	armpit, groin, neck, body
Meningitis*	petechiae (purple freckles)	spreads head to toe

Fungal infections:

Ringworm*	circle, red raised edge +/- overlying scale	anywhere
Yeast diaper rash*	raw meat red with surrounding pimples	diaper area

Tick borne illness:

Lyme Disease*	bullseye with bite in the center	bite site
Rocky Mountain Spotted Fever*	starts out flat, red then petechiae (purple freckles)	wrist, ankles palms, soles

Mites:

Scabies*	lines of red raised, bumps (burrows) blisters in babies	head, neck, palms, soles, armpits, finger webs

Other:

Kawasaki Disease*	red cracked lips, peeling skin on fingers flat/mildly raised red spots	lips, palms, soles of feet

*Denotes an infection that needs treatment

INFECTIONS, HOW LONG THEY LAST AND MORE!

Duration	Other symptoms
1 week	fever, itchy
1 week	painful
1 week	fever, pink eye
3 days	swollen glands
1 day	high fever that breaks then rash appears
2-40 days	mildly itchy, joint pains
1 week with ulcers	fever, sore throat
4-6 weeks	mildly itchy
6 weeks	mildly itchy
1 week	very painful
1-2 years	
gets worse until treated	very itchy
3-4 days	sore throat, fever
hours	fever, irritability, light sensitivity
gets worse until treated	very itchy
gets worse until treated	itchy
enlarging diameter	fever, fatigue
1-6 days	fever, vomiting, irritability, light sensitivity
worse until treated	**ITCHIEST RASH EVER!**
over five days	fever for more than 5 days, pink eye, swollen lymph nodes in neck

first aid

Q. What are hives and what causes them?

A rash that appears due to release of a chemical called histamine. 20% of the population will get hives once in their lives. But 75% of the time, the cause is never found. (*Fleisher*)

Hives look like mosquito bites with red circles around them. Or, they look like a flat red area with a raised border. Hives vary in size and shape. They are itchy and occur anywhere on the body. The individual lesions come and go. See Chapter 14, Common Diseases for causes of hives.

What to do if your child breaks out in hives

◆ *Relax.* If your child is not having any trouble breathing, this can be managed at home.
◆ *Try to figure out what caused the hives* (foods, medications, illness).
◆ *Stop any medications until you see the doctor.*
◆ *Give an antihistamine.* Liquid diphenhydramine (Benadryl) comes in 12.5mg per 5 ml syrup. A 20 lb. baby can have 4 ml. If your baby is smaller than 20 lbs., call your doctor before giving it. Babies six months up to two years of age can have 2.5 ml of liquid cetirizine (Zyrtec) or loratidine (Claritin), which are also available over the counter.

Q. What does a drug allergy rash look like?

True drug allergies will cause hives or **ERYTHEMA MULTIFORME.** Any other rash does not require avoidance of a particular medication.

Erythema multiforme basically means "redness in multiple forms." What you see is a full body rash of red flat patches and raised borders. Many of the patches run into each other.

If you see a concerning rash while your child is on medication, hold the dose of medicine and bring the child in to be seen. A particular medication class should not be avoided unless there is a documented allergy.

Q. What does a food allergy rash look like?

Food allergies can cause hives and lip swelling if the reaction is severe. But it can also cause a flare up of a rash called eczema. Eczema is an allergic skin disorder—the equivalent of hay fever. Eczema looks like a scaly plaque lying on top of a red base. With a food allergy, the eczema can cover huge body surface areas.

Food allergies do NOT cause mild diaper rash, a few patches on the face, or heat rashes.

Q. My child has a scaly rash on their elbows and knees. What is it?

Eczema. It is sensitive skin. In infants, it likes the elbows and knees because these areas get chewed up from crawling. It also ends up in the skin folds of the elbows and knees from rubbing. See Chapter 14, Common Diseases for more details on this.

Q. Which rashes are likely to be contagious due to infection?

Most of them. Kids have wonderful immune systems (much better than ours). And rashes are created from an immune response to a particular infection.

? ?

FIRST AID

The diseases listed on the previous pages are The Classics. There are also a variety of nondescript rashes that fit in the category of "viral and non-worrisome."

Q. I know that all newborns get rashes. Are there any I need to be worried about?

Yes. Herpes.

Moms with genital herpes have a chance of spreading it to their newborn during a vaginal delivery. (If Mom has an obvious outbreak a Caesarian section is performed.) A herpes rash in a newborn shows up within two weeks of life. The lesions look like little blisters either alone or in crops. This is *Priority 1: Needs immediate evaluation and treatment—NOW!*

Q. My four week old has a pimply rash all over their face and chest. What do I do?

It's acne, but don't break out the Oxy 10. This rash is caused by a hormonal change in the baby. Leave it alone and it goes away by eight weeks of age.

Feedback from the Real World
Dr. Brown True Story

My son woke up one morning with three distinct red circles on his chest. I thought he had ringworm until I realized the circles matched the snaps on his sleeper pajamas. He had an allergy to the metal snaps.

Necklaces, earrings, and snaps on jeans can cause a similar reaction in people with sensitive skin.

Q. Is it possible that my one year old has measles?

Theoretically, it's possible, but did they have their one year well check recently? That rash is the response to the MMR vaccination. (Kids also get a chickenpox-like rash with the chickenpox vaccine). Be happy. This means they have formed a good response.

These rashes usually appear one to four weeks after being vaccinated.

Q. My baby has a diaper rash. What do I do about it?

See Chapter 4, Hygiene for details on how to treat diaper rash.

Priority 1: Needs immediate evaluation and treatment—NOW:
◆ Hives that occur while taking medication or trying a new food.
◆ Hives with difficulty breathing *(Call 911).*
◆ Petechiae rash.
◆ Newborn with a blistery rash.
◆ Any rash with a fever.

Priority 2: Needs appointment the next day.
◆ Rashes that are scaly, without fever.
◆ Rashes that are not going away after being treated by a doctor.

Priority 3: Watch and wait. Needs appointment if there is no improvement or worsening of symptoms:

◆ Newborn (birth to eight weeks) with a non-blistery rash, acting well.
◆ Diaper rashes.
◆ One year old with rash after being in for their one year well check.

Seizures

Seizures are scary to watch. If your child has a seizure, **dial 911.** Once the episode is over, you can review this information.

Q. What is a seizure?

Involuntary muscle (motor) activity is the definition of a seizure. This is caused by an electrical brainwave that has fired incorrectly. In kids under age one, the most common type of seizure is associated with a fever that is rising quickly (See febrile seizure in the fever section of this chapter).

Causes of new onset seizures include: Febrile seizure (convulsion), head trauma/ injury, meningitis, poisoning/ingestion, metabolic disorder, seizure disorder

What To Do If Your Baby Has A Seizure

◆ *Call 911.*
◆ Put them in a safe place (a carpeted floor).
◆ Make sure they can breathe.
◆ Do not put anything in their mouth to hold their tongue.
◆ Start CPR if baby looks blue.

What the doctor will ask you about SEIZURES:

1. Has your baby ever had a seizure before?
2. How old is your baby?
3. Does the baby have a fever?
4. Anyone in the family prone to febrile seizures as a child?
5. Any history of head trauma?
6. Any history of poisoning or ingestion?

Priority 1: Needs immediate evaluation and treatment—NOW:

◆ Known history of febrile seizures, with another episode
◆ Has a known seizure disorder.

Stitches (Sutures)

The key point to remember: *Stitches (sutures) or Dermabond (surgical glue) must be placed within 12 hours of the injury. So they are always considered Priority 1.* Any later than that, the

? ?

FIRST AID

wound has a much higher chance of getting infected. If your child has a wound that might need stitches, call your doctor now.

What the doctor will ask you about NEEDING STITCHES:

1. **What happened?** For example, animal bites usually are not stitched because of infection risk.
2. **How long ago did the injury happen?** If over 12 hours, wound can't be sutured.
3. **Where on the body is the cut (laceration)?** Location of the wound makes a difference because of cosmetic issues (face) and potential nerve damage (hands).
4. **If on the face, is it crossing the lip/skin line or the eyebrow line?** It may need stitches for better cosmetic result.
5. **How deep is it?** If you can see fat, it needs stitches—anything deeper than 1/4 inch.
6. **Is the bleeding under control?** If not, it needs stitches.
7. **For older wounds: Is there any pus, redness around the wound, streaks of red from the wound, or fever?** Needs to be seen for possible wound infection.
8. **Are your child's immunizations current?** Needs tetanus shot if not up to date.
9. **Does your child have any bleeding disorders?** There is a risk of large volume of blood loss.

Q. Are there any body parts that always need stitches?

Yes. Eyebrows and lip lines. The lip line means the area where the lip meets the skin. If a wound crosses this line, the lip will not line up correctly without stitches. The same is true for the eyebrow line. Cosmetically, this is a big deal.

Q. Are there any body parts that never need stitches?

It is RARE to need stitches on the lip itself, tongue, or gums. The blood flow to these areas

first aid

HOW TO CLEAN AND CARE FOR MINOR WOUNDS

It's not what you use, it's how you use it. Plain old soap and water is fine. You don't have to get high tech here. The key is to flush the wound and repeat this several times. Wash the wound every day until it heals. Here's how to care for minor wounds:

1. Apply pressure to the wound with a gauze pad or towel for ten minutes.
2. Thoroughly clean wound with soap and water. The most important part of the cleaning process is flushing with water repeatedly—especially with puncture wounds (bites, sharp objects). Your doctor will use a mechanism much like a Waterpik to clean "road rash" scrapes.
3. Apply antibiotic ointment for two or three days. This prevents infection and improves cosmetic results.
4. Look for signs of infection. (Redness, pus, fever).
5. For cuts in the mouth or tongue, try popsicles or ice cream (if age appropriate) to help control bleeding.

is tremendous (which is why they bleed so much). This blood flow allows very rapid healing.

Feedback from the real world: Tongue injuries

One of our readers suggested we add some tips on tongue injuries (after her $74 adventure to the doctor's office). Her two-year-old daughter had bitten her tongue and there was a visible gap. So, Michele C., this one's for you!

As long as the tongue is not cut (lacerated) through, it usually does not require stitches and will heal up beautifully in one or two days. You don't need to visit your doctor or the ER.

Our reader recommends offering scrambled eggs, mashed potatoes, and ice cream to little ones with tongue injuries.

Q. How can I tell if the wound is infected?

Pus (white/yellow/green discharge) will start to ooze out of the wound. There will be red and tender skin around the wound site, and maybe even a streak of redness starting from the wound. There may also be a fever.

Q. Is my child's tetanus shot up to date?

If your child is receiving their immunizations regularly at well baby checks, they are well protected. Babies/children get a tetanus shot at two, four, six, fifteen months and again at five years old. Your child is probably better protected than you.

Q. Can I get water near the stitches?

YES!

This is a common misconception. Clean the wound, even if it has stitches in it. The not-cleaned ones have crust around them, making it a challenge for the doctor to remove the stitches.

Q. When should the stitches be removed?

It depends on the location. Skin heals at different rates on the body. The doctor who puts the stitches in will tell you when they need to come out. Try to do it when suggested— a delay in suture removal can not only impair the cosmetic result, but can also be very painful if the stitches are imbedded in the skin.

To give you an idea of the variability of suture removal, stitches on the face come out in four days. Stitches on the palm of the hand come out in 14 days.

Q. What is that glue used to close wounds? Can we use that instead of stitches?

The brand names are Dermabond or SurgiSeal, and they are fairly popular alternatives to stitches. It's like superglue. It dissolves on its own and does not need any removal. Sounds great, right?

Well, it can't be used for every wound. If the skin is under any tension (gets pulled frequently), the glue won't be able to hold the wound together. The glue is also not intended for use near the eyes.

Dermabond and SurgiSeal are products sold only to medical providers. There are some over-the-counter topical skin adhesives, but we cannot attest to their effectiveness.

Q. I've also heard about using staples instead of stitches. Is this better than stitches?

It's easier than stitches for placement, but they are painful to remove. For non-cosmetic areas such as the head, it is a reasonable option.

Helpful Hint
Cuts on the scalp and face bleed a lot. The blood flow to these body parts is much greater than any other areas. Don't be alarmed. It is only a problem if you can't get the bleeding under control.

Priority 1: Needs immediate evaluation and treatment—NOW:
◆ Any skin wound that you think might need stitches or surgical glue.
◆ Unable to control the bleeding after ten minutes of pressure to the wound.
◆ Wound in a cosmetically undesirable location.
◆ Looks like it is getting infected (redness, pus, fever).
◆ If immunizations are not current.

Priority 3: Watch and wait. Needs appointment if there is no improvement or worsening of symptoms:
◆ Make an appointment for suture removal.

Trauma (Accidental Injury)

No matter how good of a parent you are and how safety proofed your house is, your child will find a way to hurt themselves. Welcome to parenthood—this is only one of the many reasons that your child will give you grey hairs.

This section is body part specific. The section on skin trauma/injury is covered in the Stitches section.

What the doctor will ask you about TRAUMA / ACCIDENTAL INJURIES

1. What happened?
2. Any loss of consciousness or did they cry immediately?
3. With head injury: Any vomiting or confusion?
4. With head injury: How far did the child fall and what surface did they fall onto?
5. Any bleeding or fluid draining from the nose or ears?
6. Are there any obvious broken bones, sticking out of the skin?
7. Any pain with touching or movement of a body part?

8. Any bruising or swelling?

9. Can you check the eye pupils. Are they equal?

Helpful Hint

The mechanism of injury (that is, what happened) is the most reliable factor in determining the severity of a body injury.

1. Head injury

Once babies are mobile, they run into things like the coffee table and fireplace hearth. The result is a big bruise (a.k.a. "goose egg") on the forehead. It is an impressive bump because of that vast blood supply to the head and face. Despite the appearance, goose eggs are not too worrisome.

The mechanism of injury is much more concerning. Here are the red flags for head injuries:

Priority 1: Needs immediate evaluation and treatment—NOW!

For injuries for a concussion or bleeding in the head.

◆ Child falls a distance greater than their own height.

◆ Child falls onto hardwood floors, tile, or concrete.

◆ Child loses consciousness (blacks out) after the injury.

◆ Child vomits more than once after the injury.

◆ Baby's soft spot is bulging.

◆ Seizure after head injury.

◆ Acting abnormal or confused.

◆ Bruising behind the ear or bleeding from the ear.

◆ Clear fluid draining from the nose.

Priority 2: Needs appointment the next day.

◆ Child falls a distance less than their height, onto a padded surface, no loss of consciousness.

NEW PARENT 411: HANDLING MINOR HEAD INJURIES

◆ Put a bag of frozen vegetables on the goose egg, if your child lets you. It will be less swollen in the morning, but will change into a rainbow of colors for a week or two.

◆ Watch for signs of concussion for the next two days (vomiting, irritability from headache, confusion, lethargy)

◆ Let your child go to bed. Invariably, it's nap or bedtime when these events happen (probably because your child is tired and clumsy then). You can monitor your baby every few hours by watching their breathing and gently touching them to see if they stir. Vomiting or seizure activity happens whether they are awake or asleep.

Priority 3: Watch and wait. Needs appointment if there is no improvement or worsening of symptoms:

◆ Child has a minor accident resulting in a large bruise on the head (goose egg), no loss of consciousness, no vomiting, and is acting normally.

BOTTOM LINE

Every child who has rolled off a bed onto a carpeted floor does not need to be rushed to an emergency room. (And yes, this will happen to you!)

Which head injuries require a CT scan?

When there is a concern for a severe head injury (bleeding inside the skull), a CT scan (Computer Tomography) is helpful to check it out. However, because there is a significant amount of radiation involved, docs avoid ordering them for every kid who rolls off the bed. Here are the criteria:

◆ all kids under two years of age
◆ loss of consciousness for over one minute
◆ trauma (knife, bullet)
◆ abnormal neurologic examination (dizziness, weakness, abnormal reflexes.)
◆ vomiting
◆ seizures
◆ bulging soft spot (fontanelle)
◆ bruising behind the ear or bleeding from the ear
◆ clear fluid draining from the nose
◆ depressed skull fracture (i.e. a break in the skull detected on a plain x-ray)

Reality Check

Walkers cause over 6000 head injuries in the U.S. annually. Yes, the newer models have more "safety features" that keep them from rolling down stairs. But we say save your money or buy some other really cool toy.

2. Neck and back injuries

CALL 911 and do not try to move your child. They will be immobilized on a straight board until x-rays can prove that no spine damage has occurred.

3. Eye injuries

All eye injuries should be evaluated by a doctor immediately. Here are the most common problems:

◆ **Corneal abrasion:** surface of the eye is scratched. It heals in a day or two. Frequent tearing is a clue to this diagnosis.
◆ **Hyphema:** bleeding that occurs beneath the surface of the eye (a doctor sees it with special equipment). If the blood is not removed, vision can be lost. This is fairly uncommon, but it is the reason that all eye injuries need a medical evaluation.

◆ **Subconjunctival hemorrhage:** bleeding occurs on the surface of the eye. It can be seen on the white part of the eye. Although it looks dramatic, it's not serious.

4. Ear injuries

Outer ear: (the part you can see) can be bruised and cause permanent cartilage damage. If you see bruising, this is a *Priority 1: Needs immediate evaluation and treatment* call–the blood might need to be drained.

Inner ear: (the inside) can be injured when curious kids put things in their ears. Usually they don't get anywhere near the eardrum. If you see bleeding, it's likely from scratching the lining of the canal. Doctors need to see these kids, but it can wait until the office opens (*a priority 2 call*). The only emergency is if your child had a head injury and you notice blood draining out of the ear or a bruise behind the outer ear. This is a sign of a skull fracture.

5. Nose injuries

Priority 1: Needs immediate evaluation and treatment—NOW:

◆ A nosebleed after a nose injury increases the chances of it being broken.
◆ A clear drainage or bloody nose after a head injury increases the chances of a skull fracture.
◆ Inability to breathe through the nose after an injury may mean a severe bruise in the nose (septal hematoma)
◆ Nose is obviously crooked (displaced nose fracture).

Priority 2: Needs appointment the next day.

◆ Nose injury without bleeding or obvious fracture.

6. Mouth injuries

See stitches section for details. The bottom line: Very few injuries to the mouth require stitches. They bleed a lot but heal quickly and beautifully. Injuries that go through the inside of the mouth to the outside of the skin, or full thickness through the tongue need to be seen (*Priority 1: Needs immediate evaluation and treatment–NOW*).

7. Tooth injuries

Injuries to baby teeth rarely need intervention. Worry only if the tooth was "knocked out" and you can't find it anywhere. That is a sign of a tooth intrusion. The tooth can get pushed

---

HOW TO IMMOBILIZE AN INJURED LIMB

◆ Use a scarf or large towel and wrap it around the shoulder to keep an arm in place. Pinning a long arm sleeve to the shoulder also works.
◆ Use a piece of cardboard and an Ace wrap to form a makeshift splint for an arm or leg.

back into the gums *(Priority 1: Needs immediate evaluation and treatment—NOW; call the dentist)*.

FYI: You may know about the trick of placing a knocked out tooth in milk and rushing to the dentist to re-implant it. They only do this for permanent teeth, not baby teeth.

8. Bone injuries

Q. Is it BROKEN?

The best way to tell over the phone is to know the mechanism of injury and what your child is doing with the limb. The list of red flags is below.

If there is a break (fracture), your child needs a cast. Some specialists prefer to see kids with broken bones 48 hours after the injury so the swelling will be down before casting. As long as the bone is immobilized, it is fine. A temporary (splint) cast can be applied to keep the bone fixed and comfortable.

RED FLAGS
Does it need an x-ray?
All of these are *Priority 1: Needs immediate evaluation and treatment—NOW:*
1. Unable to move a limb without crying.
2. Limping or refusing to bear weight.
3. Impressive bruising or swelling.

BOTTOM LINE
Broken bones hurt. If you can distract your child and move or touch the area without pain, it may just be bruised.

Helpful hint
Kids have areas in their bones called growth plates. This area is located at the end of each bone that gives it growing room. These plates fuse when children go through puberty (hormone levels cause them to close). A normal x-ray of a child's bone shows a gap where the growth plate is. Occasionally, if there is a fracture along the line of the growth plate, it may not be seen when the x-ray is read. So, even if an x-ray is read as "no fracture," call the doctor if there is no improvement in your child's symptoms in five to seven days.

Q. My child was walking and put his hand out to break their fall. Is the wrist broken?

Probably. Your wrist joint is not intended to sustain your body weight. Your baby needs an x-ray.

Q. I was walking with my child and holding their hand. They pulled away from me and now they won't use their arm. Is it broken?

No—it's probably dislocated.

This is called a nursemaid's elbow. The elbow joint has gotten pulled out of its socket. Some children are repeat offenders. It can be easily fixed by your doctor in a matter of seconds. For frequent fliers, parents can learn how to do it at home. It's a good idea not to pull your kids up by their arms, or jerk their arms when they resist motion. And obviously, kids with frequent dislocations shouldn't play on the monkey bars!

9. Fingers and toes

The classic injury here is the finger that gets slammed in a car door. If there is bruising or swelling, it needs an x-ray (*Priority 1: Needs immediate evaluation and treatment—NOW*). If there is a blood blister/collection of blood under the fingernail (subungual hematoma), it may need to be lanced by a doctor to relieve the pressure (*Priority 1 or 2*).

The fingers and toes are an exception for casting of broken bones. Some of these breaks only require stabilization (buddy taping) to the finger or toe next to it.

So, how do you immobilize a finger or toe? Tape fingers or toes together (buddy tape) for an injured digit. The neighbor of the injured digit gets taped to it for support.

RED FLAGS

A recap:

◆   any true head injury in a child under two years of age

◆   head injury with loss of consciousness

◆   head injury with vomiting

◆   head injury with confusion

◆   significant height of fall or to a hard surface

◆   any eye injury

◆   head injury with nosebleed or ear drainage

◆   ear injury with bruising

◆   limb injury with swelling/bruising and discomfort

◆   fall onto an outstretched arm

◆   jerked elbow

◆   neck or spine injury—call 911

◆   bone injury with exposed bone

BOTTOM LINE

If you are ever in doubt, call your doctor.

Section 6

Reference Library

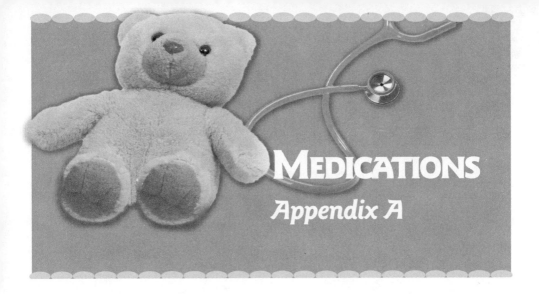

MEDICATIONS
Appendix A

Here's a look at the most common medications used by children. Obviously, with the huge universe of possible medications, this chapter is by no means comprehensive. Instead, we focus on the most popular and widely used meds in children. We will cover both over the counter products and prescription medications. (*Murphy*) Let's begin with some general questions regarding administering medicine to your child.

Q. If my child throws up right after I give them medicine, do I re-dose the medicine or wait until the next dose is due?

If your child throws up less than 20 minutes after administering medicine, give the dose again. It didn't have time to get through the stomach and be absorbed into the blood stream.

Q. Is a generic medication as good as a brand name?

For the most part, yes.

When a pharmaceutical company develops a medication, the company obtains a patent for it, which lasts for 17 years. Because it takes several years of research before a medication is approved for use, a medication may be on the market for an average of eight years before the patent runs out. Once the patent runs out, any pharmaceutical company can make their own product, which is a duplicate of the original brand.

The potency is the same, but sometimes the taste is not. And the cost is definitely not the same. Generic medications are often much cheaper than the brand name.

Q. If my doctor prescribes an expensive medication, can I ask for a generic brand at the pharmacy?

Good news. Most antibiotics used for children are available in generic form. However, some medications that need to be specially compounded for babies have no alternatives.

That said, making a medication from scratch can be costly and may not be covered by insurance.

Helpful Hint

If you are paying out-of-pocket for prescription medications, speak up! Don't be shy about inquiring about the cost of the medication. Your doctor may be able to prescribe a less-expensive generic drug if available.

Q. How do I get my baby to take medicine?

Here are a few tricks to getting all the medicine down:

1. Give small amounts over several minutes, instead of the whole dose at once.
2. It is okay to mix certain medications in with formula or expressed breast milk—but check with your pharmacist for the particulars. The only problem with this plan is that your child has to drink the whole thing. Be sure to mix the medicine in a small volume of fluid (less than an ounce).
3. For a small fee, some pharmacies will add flavorings to your child's prescription to make it more palatable.
4. Taking a prescription medicine is not optional. It may take two parents to administer medicine to one strong-willed child.

Reality Check

Just a spoonful of sugar makes the medicine go down. Here are some tips from Edward Bell, Pharm.D., BCPS:

1. White grape juice or chocolate syrup masks a medicine's after taste.
2. Graham crackers get rid of the leftover drug particles in the mouth.
3. Strawberry jam mixed with a crushed chewable tablet disguises the flavor.

Q. Is it okay to use a medicine if it is past the expiration date?

No.

For the most part, medications start to lose their potency after the listed expiration date. So the medication may be less effective (for example, Albuterol for an asthma attack).

Q. The prescription medicine was supposed to be given for ten days. We ran out of it after eight days. What happened?

This occasionally happens due to the thickness of the liquid suspension. Use a medicine dropper with milliliters (mls) to dispense it. Squeeze the rubber top to remove any air first, then slowly draw up the medicine to the appropriate line. That should help make the medication last for the correct number of days.

Q. I have some leftover antibiotic from a prescription. Can I save it and use it for another time?

No.

First of all, you should never have leftover antibiotics. Your doctor wanted your child to have a specific length of therapy for that medication. If your child stops taking an antibiotic "because they feel better," you run the risk of the bacteria growing back. This is particularly true of Group

A Strep (of Strep throat fame). Yes, people often forget to give all of the doses of antibiotic—we're human. But try to finish a prescription as it was intended to be used.

Second of all, antibiotics that are in liquid form will only stay potent for about two weeks. They come as a powder from the manufacturer and the pharmacist mixes it with water when they fill the prescription order. If you have any medicine leftover—toss it.

Q. Are all medications administered to children of all ages?

No.

Many medications are not approved for infants under six months of age. Doctors' choices are more limited for these patients. There are also some medications that are purely for adult usage (for example, Tetracycline).

Q. How do I know if there is a problem taking more than one medicine at a time?

The official term is "drug interactions."

Your doctor or pharmacist can answer this question. Don't assume that your doctor knows all the medications your child is taking. If your child received a prescription from another doctor/specialist, it might not be recorded in your child's chart.

Reality Check

Tell your doctor if your child is taking any herbal remedies. There can be overlap in effects of herbal and over-the-counter products. For instance, Sudafed (a traditional decongestant) and ephedra (an herbal decongestant) can cause heart rhythm disturbances when taken together. It pays to ask.

Q. Can you use acetaminophen (Tylenol) & an antibiotic at the same time?

Yes. It is okay to use a fever reducing medication like Tylenol/Motrin and an antibiotic simultaneously.

Q. What does the term "off-label" mean?

It means that a pharmaceutical company has not received FDA (Food and Drug Administration) approval for a medication to be used for a particular problem or age group.

Medications are approved for use based on research studies for particular medical problems. Once a drug is available for use, doctors may find it useful to treat other ailments. In this case, a doctor might prescribe a medicine to a patient and explain that it is being used "off label."

What frequently happens in pediatric medicine is that clinical research studies are done on adults, so a medication is approved for use only in adults. When it appears to be a safe product, the medication is used in pediatric patients as well. Pediatricians feel relatively comfortable using these medications for children, but your doctor should always explain to you if they prescribe a medicine that does not have FDA approval for use in a particular age group. Good news: There is now a law requiring pharmaceutical companies to test medications in kids as part of their research.

MEDICATIONS

? ?

Q. How can I find out if a generic equivalent is available for the medicine my doctor has prescribed?

Ask your doctor or pharmacist. For the medication tables below, generic availability is noted with an (*) asterisk. Note: while all medications have a generic name, not all of them are available to be purchased in generic form.

Q. How do I read a doctor's prescription? I've always wondered what they really mean.

It's written in medical abbreviations, so here's how to read it. You'll need this for the medication tables later in this appendix.

How often to take a medicine
QD or QDay: once daily
BID: twice daily
TID: three times daily (preferably every eight hours)
QID: four times daily (preferably every six hours)
QHS: once daily, at bedtime
QOD: every other day
PRN: as needed

How medicine is given
po: taken by mouth
pr: insert in rectum
ou: put into each eye
au: put into each ear

How medicine is dosed
1 cc (cubic centimeter): 1ml (milliliter)
tsp: teaspoon (1 tsp is 5 cc or 5ml)
T: tablespoon (1 T. is 3 tsp or 15cc or 15 ml)
tab: tablet
gtt: drop
cap: capsule

Q. How do I know which medications require a prescription?

We've included some handy tables later in this chapter with information on common medicines used for treating babies. In the tables, you'll note the following symbols.
◆ **Rx**: Denotes that a product is available with a doctor's prescription only. If nothing is designated, assume the product in question is prescription-only.
◆ **OTC**: Denotes that a product is available Over The Counter (that is, without a prescription).

MEDICATIONS

Q. How do I know if a medication is safe for me to take while I am pregnant or breastfeeding?

Great question! Several years ago, the FDA eliminated prescription drug labeling guidelines that helped determine safety in taking medications while pregnant or nursing. Nice. Now healthcare providers must decide the risk versus benefit for a breastfeeding mom who needs to take a particular medication. And unfortunately, that may lead moms to stop nursing unnecessarily.

Thank goodness for Thomas Hale, RPH, PhD. Dr. Hale is a nationally acclaimed pharmacologist who has spent the past twenty years reviewing medication safety for nursing moms. We use his indispensable website, InfantRisk.com, as well as the National Institute of Health's LactMed, as our source to provide guidance below.

Dr Hale's Breastfeeding Categories
L1: Compatible. Okay to use while nursing.
L2: Probably compatible. Okay, but use with caution. Limited studies show no adverse effects in the baby.
L3: Probably compatible. Unknown whether there is a risk. No studies or limited studies show minimal effects to baby.
L4: Potentially hazardous: Evidence of harm.

L4: Potentially hazardous.
Codeine (Tylenol #3)**

L3: Probably compatible.
Aripiprazole (Abilify)
Buspirone (Buspar)
Oral contraceptives

L2: Probably Compatible (Okay, But Use With Caution)
Acyclovir (Zovirax)
Cetirizine (Zyrtec)
Diphenhydramine (Benadryl)
Dextromethorphan ("DM" products-
    Delsym, Robitussin DM)
Erythromycin
Escitalopram (Lexapro)
Fluconazole (Diflucan)
Fluoxetine (Prozac)
Omeprazole (Prilosec)
Ondansetron (Zofran)
Prednisone (Deltasone, Meticorten, Orasone)
Sertraline (Zoloft)
Warfarin (Coumadin)

L1: Medications (Okay To Use While Breastfeeding)
Acetaminophen (Tempra, Tylenol)
Albuterol (Proventil, Xopenex)
Penicillin antibiotics like Amoxicillin (Amoxil, Augmentin)

medications

MEDICATIONS

? ?

Cephalosporin antibiotics (Cefzil, Keflex, Omnicef)
Ibuprofen (Advil, Ibuprofen, Motrin, Nuprin)
Loratadine (Claritin)
Teeth whiteners

**Use only if necessary, for breastfeeding woman.*

Note: Pseudoephedrine (brand names: Sudafed, Actifed), a popular decongestant, may reduce milk supply by up to 25%. Use this product with caution, especially if milk supply is already low. (Hale T, AAP Committee on Nutrition)

Herbal Remedies and breastfeeding
Fenugreek and Blessed Thistle are both L3 for breastfeeding. Per Dr. Hale, data is lacking for blessed thistle's effect on improving milk supply.
Herbal products that are unsafe while nursing include: Comfrey, Blue Cohosh, Sage, and Valerian Root.

Medication Index

1. Allergies
2. Dental/Mouth
   ◆ fluoride
   ◆ teething products
3. Ear Problems
4. Eye Problems
5. Fever and pain
6. Gastrointestinal
   ◆ antacids/gastroesophageal reflux
   ◆ constipation
   ◆ diarrhea
   ◆ gas/colic
   ◆ vomiting
   ◆ rehydration solutions
7. Infections
   ◆ antibiotics (for bacterial infections)
   ◆ antifungals (for fungal infections)
   ◆ antihelminthics (for pinworms)
   ◆ amebicides (for Giardia infection)
   ◆ antivirals (for viral infections)
8. Nutrition
   ◆ iron supplements
   ◆ vitamins
9. Respiratory
   ◆ asthma
   ◆ cough and cold preparations
10. Skin
   ◆ antibiotic creams
   ◆ antifungal creams
   ◆ scabies/ head lice medications
   ◆ steroids
   ◆ anti-inflammatory
   ◆ diaper rash creams

Medications

1. Allergy Medicines

These medications are used for allergic reactions, itching, and nasal congestion. For skin allergy products, see skin section (10).

Antihistamines have been around for decades. They are classified by their "generation." The first generation products are very effective but also have more side effects (drowsiness, dry mouth). Second and third generation products do not cause nearly as much sedation and can be dosed once every 24 hours.

Under six months of age, doctors use all medications with caution. Antihistamines, which are usually sedating, can result in excitability in infants. Consult your doctor before using any of these products.

GENERIC	BRAND	DOSE	RX?	AGE LIMIT
Cetirizine	Zyrtec*	QDay	OTC	over 6 months
Desloratadine	Clarinex	QDay	Rx	over 6 months
Diphenhydramine	Benadryl*	QID	OTC	over 2 years
Fexofenadine	Allegra*	BID	OTC	over 2 years
Hydroxyzine	Atarax*	QID	Rx	Infants ok
Loratadine	Claritin, Alavert*	QDay	OTC	over 2 years

KEY: Rx? Rx medications are available by prescription only; OTC is over-the-counter. * A generic is available for this brand-name medicine.

Side effects: Drowsiness, dry mouth, headache, paradoxical excitability
Serious Adverse effects: tremors, convulsions

Feedback from the Real World

You may be tempted to use diphenhydramine (Benadryl) as a sleep aid for your child. A study, appropriately called the TIRED study—Trial of Infant Response to Diphenyhydramine, showed there was no significant improvement in a baby's sleep when used in kids six to 15 months of age. Go back to Chapter 9, Sleep, if you need tips that will actually work!

2. Dental/Mouth

Fluoride Supplements

Fluoride is a mineral well known to prevent cavities. But as we discussed back in Chapter 5, Nutrition and Growth, the recommendations are confusing and a bit of a moving target when it comes to babies and young children.

Infants *under* six months of age should have little to no fluoride intake. Thus, the American Dental Association currently recommends that you prepare powdered or liquid concentrate formula with filtered tap water (reverse osmosis) or bottled water.

Infants *over* six months of age until age 16 years need a source of fluoride to significantly reduce cavities in both primary (baby) and secondary (adult) teeth. Fluoride is added to tap water in many cities and counties in the United States. Find out if your city has added fluoride to its water supply. Ideally, your water supply should have 0.7 ppm of fluoride. Once your baby is six months old, he should start drinking some water on a daily basis (about four to six ounces).

Who needs a fluoride supplement? There are just four specific situations where a fluoride supplement is recommended if baby is over six months of age AND:

1. In a household that has well water, and has no other source of fluoride-containing water.
2. Exclusively breast fed, and does not drink fluoride-containing water.
3. Formula is prepared with bottled water or uses ready-to-feed formula, and does not drink fluoride-containing water.
4. The local water supply does not contain added fluoride, and natural fluoride levels are less than 0.6ppm.

If you fall into one of the categories above, the American Academy of Pediatrics and American Dental Association recommends supplementation. This can be accomplished by applying a fluoride varnish or using a high fluoride toothpaste called Prevident.

Possible side effects: Overuse of fluoride can cause white spots on the teeth (fluorosis). This occurs in daily doses of greater than 2 mg of fluoride /day.

Q. Is fluoride safe? I've heard it can cause bone cancer in lab rats.

Yes it is safe. If you give toxic mega-doses of any product to rats, you will create medical problems. So just how much fluoridated water would you have to drink each day to equal the volume that the rats drank? Answer: 42 gallons a day!

Helpful Hint
Give fluoride drops on an empty stomach. Milk prevents the absorption of the medication.

Teething

The only medication we recommend for teething is acetaminophen (Tylenol), or ibuprofen (Advil) for babies who are at least six months of age or older. They are both safe and effective pain relievers.

The FDA advises *against* using topical numbing products that are rubbed on the gums to provide temporary relief. The active ingredient in all of these products is benzocaine, which can potentially cause a life-threatening blood disorder called methemoglobinemia. The brand names we are talking about are: Baby Anbesol, Baby Numz-it, Baby Oragel, and Zilactin Baby.

The FDA recalled homeopathic "Hyland's Teething Tablets" a few years ago. These tablets contained a small amount of belladonna, which is a known toxin to the nervous system. Because the tablets are homeopathic, they were not required to have FDA approval for safety or therapeutic benefit. (This is a convenient loophole in the lucrative complementary medicine industry. More on that in Appendix B, Complementary Medications). A newer version of

Hyland's is back on the market and these tablets are belladonna and benzocaine-free.

Reality Check

Teething gets blamed on fussy moods, disrupted sleep, runny noses, and diarrhea. RARELY is teething the cause of any of these maladies! If you want a natural teething remedy, try freezing a mini bagel or banana, and let your little one gnaw on that!

3. Ear Medication

Antibiotic Ear Drops

For swimmer's ear (otitis externa) or for children who have ear infections with PE tubes, antibiotic eardrops are used. Because the medicine is not absorbed into the bloodstream, there are more antibiotic family choices. Below are the most popular antibiotic eardrops. Note: most products also contain a steroid. The steroid reduces the inflammation and swelling of the ear canal so the antibiotic can work more effectively.

GENERIC	BRAND	DOSE	RX
Acetic Acid*		QID	yes
Acetic Acid + Hydrocortisone	Vosol-HC*	QID	yes
Ciprofloxacin + Dexamethasone	Ciprodex	BID	yes
Ciprofloxacin + Hydrocortisone	Cipro HC	BID	yes
Ciprofloxacin + Fluocinolone	Otovel	BID	yes
Fluocinolone	Derm Otic	BID	yes
Ofloxin	Floxin Otic*	BID	yes
Polymyxin B + Neomycin + + steroid	Cortisporin*	TID	yes

KEY: Rx? Rx medications are available by prescription only; OTC is over-the-counter.
* A generic is available for this brand-name medicine.

Side Effects: Irritation of the ear canal such as itching and stinging.

Swimmer's Ear Prevention Drops

These drops dry up any left over water in the ear canal after swimming. Drops are placed in the ears immediately after swimming. These are used primarily for older kids, not infants.

You can make your own concoction: 2 drops of rubbing alcohol and 2 drops of vinegar per ear.

Brand names: Auro-Dri, Swim Ear. Both products are OTC. Active ingredient: Rubbing Alcohol.

Ear Wax Drops

These drops help loosen or dissolve earwax. Earwax rarely is a problem unless it is hard and stuck in the canal (impacted). If the earwax is impacted, earwax drops loosen up and

medications

break down the earwax.

Brand names are: Auro, Debrox, and Murine eardrops. OTC Active ingredient: carbamide peroxide *Dosing: 3 drops per ear, TID, for 3 days*
   Colace, a stool softener, also works nicely to soften up earwax. It's available OTC.

BOTTOM LINE
We don't recommend routine cleaning with Q-tips. Q-tips can irritate the ear canal and push the earwax backwards, creating wax that is hard and stuck (impacted).

Helpful Hints
◆ Rub the eardrop bottle in your hands for a minute or two before administering the drops. Warm drops in the ear are less bothersome than cold ones.
   ◆ If a child has a perforated eardrum or PE tubes, many types of eardrops should NOT be used (exception: approved antibiotic drops). Check with your doctor.

Reality Check
ENT specialists frequently use antibiotic eye drops for the ears. If you get a prescription filled for your child's ear infection and it turns out to be eye drops, don't think we have lost our minds. One caveat here: It's okay to use *eye drops* for the ears, but you cannot use eardrops for the eyes!

4. Eye Problems

Antibiotic Eye Drops/Ointment
These are used primarily for conjunctivitis (pink eye) and corneal abrasions.

GENERIC	FAMILY	BRAND	DOSE	RX ONLY?
Azithromycin	Erythromycin	Azasite	Qday	yes
Besifloxacin	Quinolone	Besivance	TID	yes
Ciprofloxacin	Quinolone	Ciloxan*	BID/QID	yes
Erythromycin	Erythromycin	(many)*	BID/QID	yes
Gatifloxacin	Quinolone	Zymaxid*	QID	yes
Gentamicin	Aminoglycoside	(many)*	QID	yes
Levofloxacin	Quinolone	Quixin*	QID	yes
Moxifloxacin	Quinolone	Moxeza,* Vigamox*	BID	yes
Ofloxin	Quinolone	Ocuflox*	BID/QID	yes
Tobramycin	Aminoglycoside	Tobrex* Tobradex*	QID	yes

KEY: Rx? Rx medications are available by prescription only; OTC is over-the-counter. * A generic is available for this brand-name medicine.

Note: Although the quinolone based products are not FDA approved for under one year of age, your doctor may feel comfortable prescribing them.

Side effects: Burning, itching, local irritation

Insider Tip

Eye drops only work if they enter the eye. After the first attempt, your baby will be smart enough to close their eyes when they sees the eye drops coming! No worries--just place a drop on the eyelid in the corner of the closed eye near the nose. When they opens their eyes, the drops will go in.

5. Fever And Pain Medications

Please keep in mind the following points about fever medication:

1. If your baby is less than four weeks old and has a fever, do NOT give a fever reducing medicine—call your doctor immediately.
2. Never give aspirin to a child unless directed by a doctor. Aspirin use is associated with Reye's syndrome (liver failure) when taken during an influenza or chickenpox infection.
3. Ibuprofen is not recommended for babies under six months of age.
4. Tylenol is the brand name. The generic name is acetaminophen (other brand names include Tempra, Feverall)
5. Ibuprofen: brand names are Motrin, Advil
6. Do not use more than one fever reducing medicine at a time, unless your doctor specifically recommends it.
7. REMEMBER TO USE THE DROPPER THAT COMES WITH THE PACKAGE OF MEDICINE. See Chapter 15, First Aid, for details on fever and when to administer medication (as well as a dosing chart).

DR B'S OPINION:
ALTERNATING FEVER MEDS

I do not recommend alternating fever medications to keep the body temperature down. I also prefer to use acetaminophen (Tylenol) for children who are dehydrated or not eating. Ibuprofen is more likely to cause stomach upset when taken on an empty stomach.

6. Gastrointestinal Problems

Antacids/Gastroesophageal Reflux

GENERIC	BRAND	DOSE	RX?	AGE LIMIT
Calcium Carbonate Supreme	Mylanta	TID/QID	OTC	ask Dr.
Famotidine	Pepcid*	BID	Rx	over 1 yr of age
Lansoprazole	Prevacid*	QDay	Rx	over 1 yr
Metoclopramide	Reglan*	QID	Rx	severe cases only
Nizatidine	Axid*	BID	Rx	over 12 yr
Omeprazole	Prilosec*	QD/BID	Rx	over 2 yr
Omeprazole+ Sodium bicarbonate	Zegerid	QD	Rx	over 18 yr

KEY: Rx? Rx medications are available by prescription only; OTC is over-the-counter.
* A generic is available for this brand-name medicine.

Note: Despite the lack of FDA approval, gastroenterologists and pediatricians prescribe these medicines routinely.

Side effects:
◆ Aluminum hydroxide (Gaviscon, and others) is generally not recommended for use in babies due to possible side effects.
◆ Most common side effects are headache, constipation, or diarrhea.
◆ Metoclopramide (Reglan) can cause rare but significant neurological problems, sedation, headaches, and diarrhea. Because of these adverse effects, Reglan is only used in very sick babies.

Helpful Hints
◆ It is more effective to give these medications 30 minutes before a meal if you can.

◆ Prilosec liquid has to be specially compounded at a pharmacy. It will become inactive within about two to four weeks. You will need to refill it frequently.

◆ Prevacid solutabs are a popular option because they can be cut into halves or quarters for smaller kids and suspended in a few drops of water. Once a day dosing is also convenient.

◆ Zegerid is occasionally used by pediatric gastroenterologists because the combination product seems to improve symptoms when nothing else has worked. It can be extremely expensive, though.

◆ Medications in the "proton pump inhibitor" family such as Prilosec, Prevacid, and Zegerid carry an FDA warning. There is an uncommon, but potential risk of developing a diarrheal illness caused by C. difficile infection.

◆ As with other medications, dosing is based on a child's weight. Your baby may outgrow his therapeutic dose every few weeks/months. Ask your doctor to recalculate his dose based on his current weight.

Often times, medication isn't working because babies metabolize it at different rates at different ages. If your baby is not responding to medication and clearly has the diagnosis of acid reflux, ask your doctor to decide if your baby's medication should be adjusted.

Constipation

GENERIC	BRAND NAME	DOSE	RX?	AGE LIMIT
Glycerin	(suppository)	1 dose	OTC	None
Guar gum	Benefiber	QD	OTC	over 6 mos
Lactulose	Duphalac, Chronulac*	QD	Rx	Ask Dr.
Malt soup	Maltsupex	BID	OTC	over 1 month
Mineral oil	Kondremul	QD/ TID	OTC	over 5 years
Polyethylene glycol	Miralax*	QD	OTC	Ask Dr.
Senna	Senokot*		OTC	over 1 mo

Side effects: diarrhea, bloating, gas, body salt (electrolyte) disturbances with excessive or prolonged use.

Diarrhea

GENERIC	BRAND NAME	DOSE	RX?	AGE LIMIT
Lactobacillus	Lactinex,* Culturelle*		OTC	None

KEY: Rx? Rx medications are available by prescription only; OTC is over-the-counter. *A generic is available for this brand-name medicine.

Helpful Hint
Fat and fiber intake both help bulk up the stools.

BOTTOM LINE
If diarrhea has been going on more than a week, check in with your doctor. Doctors also want to know about blood or mucous in the stools. (See Chapter 15, First Aid for more).

Gas/Colic

GENERIC	BRAND NAME	DOSE	RX?	AGE LIMIT
Ginger-Fennel	Gripe Water	QID	OTC	None
Lactobacillus	Biogaia, Gerber Soothe	QD	OTC	None
Simethicone	Mylicon, Phazyme* Little Tummys	up to 12x day	OTC	None

Cool product alert: Biogaia Protectis drops contain both Vitamin D and L reuteri probiotic.

Reality Check

Remember, there is no miracle cure for either gas or colic. These products are okay to try, but they may not work.

Vomiting

GENERIC	BRAND	DOSE	RX?	AGE LIMIT
Dimenhydrinate	Dramamine*	QID	OTC	over 2 yrs
Diphenhydramine	Benadryl*	QID	OTC	over 2 yrs
Ondansetron	Zofran*	TID	Rx	over 1 mo
Phosphorated-Carbohydrate	Emetrol*	QID	OTC	Ask Dr.
Promethazine	Phenergan*	QID	Rx	over 2 yrs

KEY: Rx? Rx medications are available by prescription, OTC is over-the-counter.
* A generic is available for this brand-name medicine.

Helpful Hints

◆ Home remedy: The equivalent of Emetrol is to give 1-2 teaspoons of heavy fruit syrup (fruit cocktail juice) every 20-30 minutes. This occasionally works to relieve nausea.
◆ Phenergan has a black box warning from the FDA discouraging its use in kids under age two.
◆ Zofran is very popular for babies and kids under age two.

Rehydration Solutions

These products are the Gatorade equivalent for babies. They are designed to replace water, body salts, and sugar lost when a child has vomiting and diarrhea. They are most helpful in the early phase of a stomach virus when a child is just starting to take fluids after actively vomiting. Doctors prefer rehydration solutions instead of plain water, juice, milk, Gatorade/sports drinks, or soda for infants. Once a child is keeping down this clear fluid, we usually suggest that your child resume breastfeeding or formula. All products are available over the counter. See Chapter 15, First Aid, for more information on using this product. See Appendix B, Complementary Medicine, for a recipe you can make at home.

Brand Names: Enfalyte, Gerber Pediatric Electrolyte, Kao-electrolyte, Pedialyte.

7. Infections

Antibiotics (Bacterial infections)

This list contains the most popular choices of antibiotics (taken by mouth). There are basically four classes of medications approved for pediatric use. There are more classes available to adults. Take special note of the class or family each medicine belongs to. If a person develops an allergic reaction to a medication, ANY antibiotic that belongs to that class is to be avoided.

In this chart, we note what these medications are typically used for (usage): Ear and sinus infections (1), Pneumonia (2), Skin infections (3), Bladder infections-UTI (4), Strep throat (5).

Note: all products are available by prescription only.

GENERIC NAME	BRAND NAME	FORM	DOSE	USAGE
PENICILLIN FAMILY				
Amoxicillin	Amoxil, Polymox, Trimox, Wymox*	Liq/Chew	BID	1,2,4,5
Amoxicillin+ Clavulanate	Augmentin* Augmentin ES-600*	Liq/Chew	BID	1,2,3,4,5
(Clavulanate kills resistant bacteria strains)				
Penicillin V-K	Pen VeeK, V-cillinK*	Liquid	BID-QID	5
CEPHALOSPORINS				
Cefdinir	Omnicef*	Liquid	QD/BID	1,2,3,5
Cefixime	Suprax*	Liquid	Qday	1,3,4
Cefprozil		Liquid	BID	1,2,3,4,5
Ceftibuten	Cedax*	Liquid		1,2,5
Ceftriaxone	Rocephin*	injection	QDay	1,2,3,4,5
Cefuroxime	Ceftin*	Liquid	BID	1,2,3,5
Cephalexin	Keflex*	Liquid	TID/QID	3,5
MACROLIDES				
Azithromycin	Zithromax*	Liquid	QD	1,2,3,5
Clarithromycin	Biaxin*	Liquid	BID	1,2,3,5
Erythromycin	E.E.S., Eryped*	Liq/chew	BID/QID	2,3,5
SULFONAMIDES (SULFA)				
Sulfamethoxazole + Trimethoprim	Bactrim, Septra* Sulfatrim, TMP-SMX	Liquid	BID	1,2,4

KEY: Rx? Rx medications are available by prescription only; OTC is over-the-counter.
* A generic is available for this brand-name medicine.

Side Effects:
The most common side effects include:

1.   *Diarrhea.* The antibiotic kills the bacteria causing infection, but also some normal bac-

terial "flora" that helps us digest food in our intestines. Lack of bacterial flora can cause malabsorption (i.e. upset stomach). ANY antibiotic can cause this problem.

2. *Yeast Infections.* Again, the antibiotic kills both bad bacteria and certain bacterial flora that live in our mouths and on our skin. Lack of normal bacteria predisposes a person to yeast infections in the mouth (thrush) and in the genital area (yeast diaper rash).

Allergic Reactions:

A true allergic reaction to these medications includes hives, lip swelling, or difficulty breathing. About 25% of patients who are allergic to the Penicillin family will also be allergic to the Cephalosporin family.

Rare Adverse Reactions:

1. Stevens-Johnson syndrome (severe allergic reaction)
2. C. difficile colitis (bacterial super-infection in intestines)

Antifungals:

GENERIC	BRAND	DOSE	USAGE	AGE LIMIT	RX
Fluconazole	Diflucan*	QD x 2 wks	Thrush	None	RX
Griseofulvin*	Fulvicin	QD x 1month	Scalp Ringworm	None	RX
	Grifulvin				
	Grisactin				

Side effects: nausea, headache, rash, stomach upset

Griseofulvin can cause skin sensitivity to sunlight. Used with caution in patients with Penicillin allergy.

Helpful Hint

Griseofulvin is absorbed better when taken with something rich in fat (milk, ice cream...)

Antihelminthics (For Pinworm Infections):

GENERIC	BRAND	DOSE	AGE LIMIT	RX
Albendazole	Albenza*	2 doses, 2 weeks apart	over 1 mo	RX
Mebendazole	Emverm	1 dose may repeat	over 2 years	RX
Pyrantel	Pin-X/Reese's	2 doses, 2 weeks apart	over 2 years	OTC

Side effects: stomach upset, headache

KEY: Rx? Rx medications are available by prescription only; OTC is over-the-counter.

* A generic is available for this brand-name medicine.

Reality Check

Often the whole family gets treated when one child has pinworms.

Amebicides (For Giardia Infection):

GENERIC	BRAND	AGE LIMIT	Rx
Albendazole	Albenza*	1 mo	RX
Metronidazole	Flagyl*	None	RX
Nitazoxanide	Alinia*	Over 1 yr	RX

Side effects: nausea, diarrhea, hives, metallic taste, dizziness

Antivirals:

GENERIC	BRAND	DOSE	USED FOR	AGE LIMIT	Rx
Acyclovir	Zovirax*	4-5x daily	Varicella Oral herpes, Zoster	None	RX
Oseltamivir	Tamiflu*		Influenza	2 weeks old	RX

Side effects: stomach upset, insomnia, headache, moodiness.
Adverse reactions: kidney failure with acyclovir—patient needs to be well hydrated

KEY: Rx? Rx medications are available by prescription only; OTC is over-the-counter.
* A generic is available for this brand-name medicine.

BOTTOM LINE

Because antiviral medications work by preventing replication of the virus, the medication must be started within 48 hours of when the illness began. Otherwise, it will have no effect on the course of the illness.

8. Nutrition

Vitamin supplements for children aged birth to one are used for specific situations. These include Vitamin D for newborns who drink less than 32 oz a day of formula and exclusively breastfed infants, and iron for children with iron-deficiency anemia. A multivitamin for general well being of infants is not routinely prescribed.

Vitamins

Vitamin D supplements:

BRAND NAME	INGREDIENTS	DOSE	Rx?
Tri-Vi-Sol*	Vitamins A, D, C	1 ml/day	OTC
Vi-Daylin	Vitamins A, D, C	1 ml/day	OTC
D-Vi-Sol	Vitamin D	1 ml/day	OTC
Biogaia Protectis	Vitamin D + Probiotics	5 drops	OTC

MEDICATIONS

? ?

Iron Supplements:

Iron is a necessary ingredient to carry oxygen on red blood cells. Babies are born with a stockpile of iron from their mothers. However, by six months of age, they need to consume iron in their diets to meet their daily needs (11mg/day for ages six to 12 months). Some babies need an iron supplement in addition to their food intake (see Chapter 5, Nutrition & Growth, for details of iron containing foods).

Multivitamins often contain iron (see chart above). The dose of iron in multivitamins made for infants is 9-10 mg of iron per daily dose. This meets the daily nutritional needs of a six to 12 month old. If a child has iron deficiency anemia, they need daily nutritional iron requirements PLUS an additional amount to fill back up their depleted iron stores. The only way to get the higher dose of iron is to use the specific products listed below.

Iron Replacement Therapy

Brand Names: Fer-In-Sol*, Feosol*, Icar, Niferex
Dose: Comes in drops 15mg iron per 1 ml. Dose is based on weight. Your doctor will calculate it for you. There are also syrups for older kids, which can be confusing!
Rx: These drugs are OTC, but are behind your pharmacist's counter so they can help you select the appropriate product.
Side effects: constipation, black looking poop, nausea, stomachache, temporary teeth staining

Helpful Hints

◆ You can avoid staining the teeth by shooting the medicine in the back of the throat. If the teeth do become stained, use baking soda on a toothbrush to remove the stains.

◆ Vitamin C improves the absorption of iron. Calcium interferes with the absorption of iron. So if you are offering a drink with the iron medicine, offer juice—not milk.

◆ If you give the iron AFTER a meal, there is less stomach upset.

9. Respiratory Problems

Asthma

Asthma medications are divided into rescue medications and preventative/long term control medications. The rescue medicines are used as needed (with a certain interval between doses). A child is placed on preventative medicine if they:

1. need rescue medicine more than twice a week
2. have activity affected by asthma flare-ups
3. have problems at night more than twice a month

The idea is to get the asthma under control, then cut back on the amount of medications needed to minimize flare ups.

For information on asthma and home nebulizers, see Chapter 14, Common Diseases.

MEDICATIONS

Rescue medicines

GENERIC	BRAND	DOSE	RX
Albuterol (Nebulizer)		Syrup TID Q4 hrs	Rx
Levalbuterol	Xopenex*	Nebulizer solution TID	Rx

Side effects: Increased heart rate, palpitations, nervousness, insomnia, nausea, headache.

Preventative/Long term control medicines

GENERIC	BRAND	DOSE	RX	AGE LIMIT
Inhaled corticosteroid				
Budesonide	Pulmicort*	Nebulizer BID	Rx	over 6 months
Leukotriene antagonist				
Montelukast	Singulair*	Chew tab QHS	Rx	over 6 months
Granule packets				

KEY: Rx—Rx medications are available by prescription only; OTC is over-the-counter.
* A generic is available for this brand-name medicine.

Side effects:
1. Inhaled corticosteroid: sore throat, nosebleeds, cough, thrush (see below for more information).
2. Leukotriene antagonist: stomach upset, headache, dizziness.

medications

MAKE THE CALL: ASTHMA CONCERNS

If your child needs their rescue medicine more frequently than it has been prescribed, CALL YOUR DOCTOR. Here are some important points to consider:
1. Your child is air hungry and needs to be evaluated by a doctor See Chapter 15, First Aid.
2. Administering asthma medicine more frequently than recommended can be dangerous. A doctor's office or hospital can administer asthma medicine more often than prescribed because a medical provider can be monitoring a patient for side effects of the medicine.
3. If a child is having that much trouble breathing, it is likely that they need to receive oxygen in addition to medication, which is only available in a medical facility.

Helpful Hint

◆ Pulmicort respules (a grainy substance dissolved in liquid) can be administered in a nebulizer machine. Pulmicort is very effective for younger children and has significantly fewer side effects than its oral counterpart.

◆ Always rinse your child's mouth after they have taken an inhaled steroid. It reduces the incidence of thrush.

◆ Steroid medications are always used cautiously. Steroids given by mouth (liquid/pill) are more likely to cause systemic side effects if given for a long time (more than one to two weeks). Inhaled steroids (nebulizer or inhaler) have significantly fewer side effects because only a small amount is absorbed into the bloodstream. As with any medication, the risks of taking these medications are weighed against the potential benefit of therapy for the disease.

Risks of long-term steroid use:
1. Mood change
2. Stomach upset
3. Intestinal bleeding
4. Impaired body's stress responses (HPA axis suppression: hypothalamic-pituitary-adrenal)
5. Bone demineralization (Osteopenia)
6. Weight gain, hair growth (Cushingoid features)
7. Cataracts
8. Growth suppression. Numerous studies show that children who have to take inhaled steroids on a daily basis are about 1cm shorter than their peers. However, children with chronic problems with asthma also have poor growth. Studies have not concluded whether or not these children have "catch up growth" when steroids are discontinued. (*Shared*)

Preventing RSV infection in premature babies
If you have a baby who has graduated from a Neonatal Intensive Care Unit, you may already know that RSV (bronchiolitis) can be a serious lung infection for a premature infant.

A product to prevent RSV infection is called Synagis (generic name is palivizumab). This is a synthetic antibody given by a monthly injection during the peak of RSV season (November to April). The antibody provides immunity for a period of 30 days.

Children who are at risk for more severe cases of RSV are:
1. Babies born prematurely, prior to 29 weeks gestation and under 12 months or age at the start of RSV season.
2. Children with chronic lung disease under age one.
3. Children with congenital heart disease.
4. Children with certain immune deficiencies.

Children who are more likely to get RSV infection include:
1. Babies under age six months when RSV season begins.
2. Babies in daycare.
3. Multiple births.

4. Babies with school age siblings.
5. Babies exposed to smoking.

The American Academy of Pediatrics recommends monthly Synagis injections during RSV season for the following babies:

1. Children under age two years with chronic lung disease (requiring treatment within six months of RSV season)
2. Babies under 12 months of age with chronic lung disease of prematurity.
3. Babies born at less than 29 weeks gestation and less than one year of age at the start of RSV season.
4. Babies at or under 12 months of age with severe types of congenital heart disease.
FYI: Babies with weakened immune systems, airway abnormalities, or neuromuscular disease may also qualify for Synagis during RSV season.

Cough And Cold Medicines

The Food and Drug Administration has banned the sale of all over-the-counter cough and cold remedies for children under four years of age. Yes, there are still "children's" cough and cold products on the market, but they all now warn "do not use in children under four years of age."

Bottom line: please do NOT buy these products and then guess-timate what dose to give to your baby. There is a reason these products are not made for young children anymore. They were never very effective in doing what they claimed to do, and the risk of adverse side effects is greater than for older kids and adults. We will point out the products that are generally safe for infants.

Decongestant

These medications reduce or relieve congestion in the nose. They can be taken by mouth (absorbed into bloodstream) or sprayed into the nose.
Oral decongestants: Pseudoephedrine, phenylephrine, ephedrine.
Side effects: Insomnia, restlessness, dizziness, high blood pressure, heart rhythm disturbances.

Nasal spray: Oxymetazoline (Afrin), Phenylephrine (Little Remedies for Noses)
Side effects: stinging, burning, nosebleed, rebound nasal congestion with prolonged use (more than 4 days)
Note: Little Remedies for Noses is approved for use in children ages two years and up.

Nasal spray: Saline. This is a safe and effective product for all ages, starting at birth.
Side effects: None! Saline is salt water. It is effective in loosening mucus and can be used as often as needed.

Antihistamine

These medications combat the effect of histamine in the body. Histamine is released as an allergy response and causes nasal congestion. Antihistamines are frequently found in cough and cold medicines because they are sedating, improve the cough suppressant effect, and dry up a runny nose.

Common ingredients: brompheniramine, chlorpheniramine, diphenhydramine, (promethazine— Rx only), carbinoxamine

Side effects: sedation, dry mouth, blurred vision, stomach upset, paradoxical excitement in infants. Note: Diphenhydramine (Benadryl), cetirizine (Zyrtec), and loratidine (Claritin) syrup are all generally safe for use in babies ages six months of age and up. They effectively treat allergic reactions. They are not used to treat symptoms of the common cold.

Expectorant

These medications make thick mucous looser. By doing this, the mucous in the bronchial tubes (lungs) can be coughed up more easily. These medications do not suppress the cough.

Common ingredients: guaifenesin

Side effects: sedation, stomach upset, headache

Cough Suppressant

These medications reduce the brain's "cough center" activity. These products are not recommended when someone has pneumonia.

Common ingredients: Dextromethorphan, carbetapentane

Side effects: drug interactions with psychiatric medications.

Helpful Hints

A study published in the journal, Pediatrics, looked at 100 children who took over-the-counter cough medicines and whether they slept better or not. The verdict: nobody slept better (child or parent). Since kids do about the same with or without cough medicine, don't feel like you are missing out because infant cough and cold remedies are off the market.

The decision to take infant cough and cold remedies off the market came after three deaths of infants under six months of age who had about 14 times the recommended dose of pseudoephedrine decongestant in their bloodstream. We'll say it again: over-the-counter cough and cold meds should NOT be given to kids under age four, unless instructed by your doctor.

New Parent 411

If you feel like you must try something to help your baby, Zarbee's natural baby cough syrup is a safe bet. Does it work? Well, studies show it does have a placebo effect for the parent. We are not so sure about its effect on the child. The active ingredient is agave nectar (NOT honey).

Cold Medicines For Breastfeeding Moms

Cold medicines and breastfeeding: Decongestant nose sprays (like Afrin) are usually okay for a day or two as are antihistamines. Some cough medicines are NOT okay. Pseudoephedrine, a popular decongestant, may reduce milk supply by 25%.

10. Skin (Dermatologic) Products

1. Antibiotic creams are used for wound care and minor bacterial infections (impetigo, mild cellulitis).

2. Antifungal creams are used for fungus infections (ringworm, yeast infection, jock itch, athlete's foot) on the skin.
3. Scabicides and pediculocides are used for scabies and head lice.
4. Steroids are used for contact irritations (bug bites, poison ivy, local allergic reactions), seborrhea, cradle cap, and eczema. Steroids are divided into classes by their potency. Doctors always try to use the lowest potency if possible. The higher the potency, the more the risk of side effects (the high potency products can get absorbed into the bloodstream).
5. Anti-inflammatories are FDA approved for kids over age 2 with eczema.
6. Diaper rash creams form a barrier between the irritated skin and recurrent insults caused by pee and poop.

Antibiotic Cream

GENERIC	BRAND	Rx
Bacitracin, Polymyxin B	Polysporin*	OTC
Used for minor cuts, scrapes, irritations		
Mupirocin	Bactroban*, Centany	Rx
Used for impetigo and cellulitis		
Neomycin,Polymixin, Bacitracin	Neosporin*	OTC
Used for minor cuts, scrapes, irritations, and superficial burns		
Retapamulin	Altabax	Rx
Used for impetigo and cellulitis.		
Silver Sulfadiazine	Silvadene*	Rx
Antibiotic salve used for second-degree burns		

Side effects: Burning, stinging, itching.

Antifungal Cream

Uses:
1. Yeast diaper rash (monilial dermatitis)
2. Ringworm of skin (tinea corporis)
3. Athlete's foot (tinea pedis)
4. Jock itch (tinea cruris)

GENERIC	BRAND	USED FOR	AGE LIMIT	Rx
Clotrimazole 1%	Lotrimin AF*	1, 2, 3, 4	None	OTC
Ketoconazole 2%	Nizoral*	1,2,3,4	Over 2 yrs	Rx
Miconazole	Vusion*	1	Over 4 wks old	Rx
	Micatin*	1,2,3,4	None	OTC
	Triple Paste AF	1,2,3,4	None	OTC
Nystatin	Mycostatin*	1	None	Rx
Econazole	Spectazole*	1,2,3,4	None	Rx

KEY: Rx—Rx medications are available by prescription only; OTC is over-the-counter. * A generic is available for this brand-name medicine.

Reality Check
Ringworm of the scalp (called tinea capitis) requires an antifungal medication by mouth for four to eight weeks. The fungus gets imbedded in the hair follicles and will not respond to an antifungal cream.

Scabicides And Pediculocides

GENERIC	BRAND	USED FOR	AGE LIMIT	RX
Acetic acid	Klout	Head lice	None	OTC
Benzyl Alcohol	Ulesfia	Head lice	Over 6 mos	RX
Crotamiton	Eurax	Scabies	None	RX
Ivermectin	Sklice	Head lice	Over 6 mos	RX
Malathion	Ovide*	Head lice	Over 6 yrs	RX
Permethrin 1%	NIX*	Head lice	None	OTC
Permethrin 5%	Elimite*, Acticin	Head lice, scabies	None	RX
Pyrethrum***	A-200*, Pyrinyl* RID, Pronto*	Head Lice	None	OTC
Spinosad	Natroba	Head lice	Over 6 mos	RX

* A generic is available for this brand-name medicine.
**Medication has significant side effects/potential for seizures. Other medications are better alternatives.
***Medication is derived from the chrysanthemum flower. Avoid use with a ragweed allergy.

Side effects: burning, itching, redness, rash

Helpful Hints for Head Lice
1. Use OTC products as directed. I know you are grossed out, but don't overdose the medicine.
   2. Don't use more than one medicine at a time.
3. Use the nit combs every three days.
4. Wash clothing and bed linens in hot water and dry on the hot cycle.
5. Soak combs and hairbrushes in rubbing alcohol for one hour.
6. See Appendix B, Complementary Medications, for other possible remedies.

Reality Check
◆ When head lice enters your home, treat any family member who has an itchy scalp.
◆ When scabies enters your home, treat *all* family members, regardless of whether they have symptoms or not.

Steroids

◆ Low potency: can be used for longer periods (months) of time without side effects, okay to use on the face
◆ Mid potency: okay to use for short periods (weeks) of time without side effects, use with doctor's recommendation on the face
◆ High potency: okay to use for limited period (days) of time without side effects, do not use on the face

Note: None of these steroid creams are FDA approved for use under age two years. But they are used routinely by medical providers who feel that they are safe and efficacious.

GENERIC	BRAND	POTENCY	DOSE	Rx/OTC
Hydrocortisone 0.5%	Cortaid, etc*	Low	BID	OTC
Hydrocortisone 1%	Cortaid, etc*	Low	BID	OTC
Hydrocortisone 2.5%	Hytone*	Low	BID	Rx
Triamcinolone 0.025%	Aristocort, Kenalog*	Low	BID	Rx
Desonide 0.05%	Desowen*	Mid	BID	Rx
Hydrocortisone valerate	Westcort*	Mid	BID	Rx
Hydrocortisone butyrate	Locoid*	Mid	BID	Rx
Mometosone furoate	Elocon*	Mid	QD	Rx
Triamcinolone 0.1%	Aristocort, Kenalog*	Mid	BID	Rx
Betamethasone	Diprolene*	High	BID	Rx
Diflorasone diacetate	Psorcon*	High	BID	Rx
Fluocinonide	Lidex*	High	BID	Rx
Triamcinolone 0.5%	Aristocort, Kenalog*	High	BID	Rx

KEY: Rx? Rx medications are available by prescription only; OTC is over-the-counter. * A generic is available for this brand-name medicine.

Side effects: skin irritation, decreased pigmentation, thinning of skin
Rare adverse reactions:
HPA axis (adrenal gland suppression)—only with high potency steroids

Emollients

GENERIC	BRAND	DOSE	Rx/OTC
Crisaborole	Eucrisa	BID	RX
Pimecrolimus	Elidel	BID	Rx
Tacrolimus -.03%, 0.1 %	Protopic*	BID	Rx

Side effects: burning, redness, itching
Rare adverse reactions: worsens warts, herpes, and chicken pox infections
Note: FDA approved for use in kids over the age of two years.

Another class of eczema medications repairs the skin's top layer and reduces inflammation and

MEDICATIONS

? ?

itching. Brand names include Mimyx, Atopiclair, Epiceram, Promiseb, Prumyx, and Pruclair. They are Rx only (and pretty pricey).

Side effects: burning, redness, itching

Rare adverse reactions: Atopiclair, Promiseb, and Pruclair are derived from the shea nut, so allergic reactions are possible.

Diaper rash creams

The idea behind all of the products listed below is to provide a barrier between the skin and moisture (pee and poop). When applying these creams and ointments, it is key to apply liberally and frequently.

Diaper rash creams

A+D ointment	OTC
Boudreaux's Butt Paste	OTC
Dr. Smith's Diaper Ointment	OTC
Silvadene	Available by Rx only. Used for rash that looks like a burn.
Triple Paste	OTC
Vaseline	OTC
Zinc Oxide (brands: Desitin, Balmex)	OTC

BOTTOM LINE

Many pediatricians have a secret recipe of salves and barrier creams that pharmacies will make especially for them. If none of these over-the-counter products are working, it's time to visit your pediatrician for some help.

Want to know more information about medications and get updated safety alerts? Head to the FDA's website at www.fda.gov/drugs/drug-safety-and-availability/ drug-alerts-and-statements. In an effort for the FDA to provide more transparency, consumers can check on post-marketing drug studies, adverse events reporting, and learn how to report problems with medications.

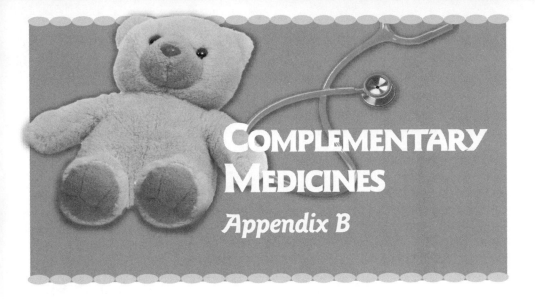

COMPLEMENTARY MEDICINES
Appendix B

While it seems there is a drug for just about every malady, sometimes there's not. That may leave you frustrated as a parent. And some families fear that medications will have harmful side effects. This leads some to search out a "natural" or "alternative" remedy for their children.

Complementary and integrative therapies are big business (over $7 billion annually in the U.S.). Some of these treatment options have real merit and the science to back them up. Those are the therapies we will present to you. While there are many more choices in your local organic grocer's aisle, we are sticking to our comfort zone and our mantra: show us the science.

As a consumer, you also need to know a few things about natural or herbal remedies:

1. **Are they effective?** There are very few scientific studies that prove with statistical significance that herbal remedies work. The National Center for Complementary and Integrative Health, part of the National Institutes of Health, is starting to investigate many of these products.

2. **Are they safe?** There are no required clinical research trials that test herbal products on humans to prove that they are safe before they are sold to the public. Herbal remedies fall into the category of "foods" by the FDA (Food and Drug Administration). This is a convenient loophole for herbal product manufacturers. This means that they do not need to do any of the scientific research that a pharmaceutical company does to market their medications. This is based on federal legislation called the Dietary Supplement Health and Education Act of 1994. Attempts to revise this act have failed in the past due to political pressure (and money) from the dietary supplements lobbying group. (*NPR*)

3. **Are production standards uniform?** Production is not standardized. The potency and purity of the product may vary tremendously. This is especially true for products that contain expensive herbs (e.g. ginseng). In fact, herbs produced in China are often laced with unlabeled products such as steroids and antibiotics to make them more potent. Also know that developing countries may sell products that are contaminated with mercury, arsenic, and lead. (*Kemper*) And, in the United States, researchers found that only 7% of the studied Echinacea supplements complied with FDA labeling standards and some of the supplements contained no measurable amounts of Echinacea! (*Gilroy*)

4. **Can I trust the label?** The claims on the label for marketing purposes do not require scientific evidence that the information is accurate. Bottom line: consumers don't have any protection against misleading information.

Compare herbs to traditional medicine. Many traditional medications are based on naturally occurring products. Penicillin is derived from a mold. Digoxin, a popular heart drug, is based on the digitalis plant. It is true that certain naturally occurring products have medical value. The difference between herbs and medications is *how they are tested and regulated*. Some herbs have absolutely no therapeutic value. And some herbs are so potent, they can be harmful. Just because it's natural, doesn't mean it is safe.

Consider alcohol and tobacco. Both have known effects on the body. Both are legal for use. But long term, chronic use of these products also can cause problems. Alcohol and tobacco are as natural as the herbs you are trying. No one knows what long-term problems *some* herbs can create.

We suggest you look at reliable resources to examine the evidence before you try these complementary meds. A good place to start is the National Center for Complementary and Integrative Health (nccih.nih.gov).

BOTTOM LINE

Just because it's natural doesn't mean it's safe. Get educated about these products before using them.

Q. Is it safe to use VapoRub on my baby when they have a cold?

No. Besides, it's not clear that it even helps.

The most popular brand on the market, Vicks VapoRub, is a combination of camphor, menthol, and eucalyptus oil. It is approved for use in children ages two and up (because camphor has the potential for causing seizures in young children when it is absorbed through the skin).

Once your child is at least two, you are welcome to try it and see if it works. People often report that they can breathe better when they use VapoRub because of the cool sensation in their nostrils. However, the medication does not stop snot production. Parents subjectively noted in one recent study that their snot-nosed-VapoRub-treated children coughed less and slept better than those who got treated with a placebo (a.k.a. Vaseline). And the VapoRub treated group of parents slept better. But note: over 85% of parents in the study correctly guessed if their child was using VapoRub or Vaseline. So, take the study results with a grain of salt. (*Paul*)

Q. I love using essential oils. Are they safe to use with my baby?

Essential oils (aromatherapy) are generally considered safe to use. The therapeutic benefits seem to be most established for stress reduction—which most babies don't really need! While naturopaths tout numerous other health benefits of essential oils, the data is much murkier on these aromas as miracle cures. Using these products is probably okay, with one caveat. I have had a few patients who have started wheezing from being exposed to essential oils in their home. Kids with reactive airways disease/asthma can be very sensitive to scents!

PRObiotics and PREbiotics

Probiotics and prebiotics are touted as having numerous potential health benefits. But what are they?

What are PRObiotics?

These are "good germs" (bacteria or yeast) that help the body digest food. They are found naturally in yogurt, kefir, kombucha, tea, and sauerkraut. They also come in liquid, capsules or powder form. One dose has about 1000 times more "germs" than what is in a serving of yogurt. Note: the good germs are only present when you ingest them. So once a person stops taking them, the benefits go away.

What are PREbiotics?

These are complex starches or polysaccharides in food that help the gut grow the good bacteria mentioned above. This is what sustains the healthy gut environment. Prebiotics are found naturally in whole grains, honey (a no-no under age one), bananas, garlic, onions, leeks, and artichokes. Other food and beverage products are fortified with them. Note: prebiotics basically provide the nesting ground for good germs. So, even if someone doesn't take pre-biotics everyday, the benefits have longer lasting effects.

Does your baby need these products?

There's been quite a bit of hype about the health benefits of both pro- and prebiotics. Formula companies have jumped on the bandwagon: some products contain both prebiotics and probiotics now.

These "good germs" seem to reduce antibiotic-associated diarrhea and diarrhea from stomach viruses in infants as young as one month of age. Probiotics may also be useful for eczema, colic, and intestinal problems in premature babies.

However, it's debatable whether a daily dose is useful or not. More research is definitely needed to know when, what type, how much, and how often these products should be used for proven health benefits.

Which product should I buy?

Probiotic products are mostly bacteria from the Lactobacillus acidophilus, Lactobacillus GG or Bifidobacterium families that are similar to the germs that naturally live in our guts. A few probiotics are actually yeast-based, like Saccaromyces sp. Specific products include: Lactinex (Lactobacillus acidophilus and Lactobacillus bulgaricus), Culturelle (Lactobacillus GG), Lactobacillus reuteri, and Florastor (Saccaromyces).

Do all probiotics have the same effectiveness?

Frankly, we don't really know. Probiotics research is really in its infancy. Lactobacillus reuteri is the probiotic that was specifically used in the study done on reduction of colic in infants (see Chapter 11 for details). Lactobacillus rhamnosus and Lactobacillus GG have proven results in reducing diarrhea from rotavirus infection. Saccaromyces boulardii is also effective for diarrhea.

So, will your local warehouse club version of probiotics prevent your child's diarrhea or colic? We don't have the answers yet—the research is still evolving. Join our online community for the latest updates at Baby411.com.

complementary meds

COMP MEDS

? ?

Do probiotics need to be refrigerated, or need any other special care?

Many need to be refrigerated for the germs to stay alive. Check the packaging on the item you purchase.

Give probiotics and antibiotics at different times. Otherwise, the good germs will be killed off.

If you are adding probiotics to infant formula, do not warm the bottle over 100°F, or you will kill off the good germs.

Are these products safe for my baby to use?

Despite the general belief that these products are safe, there are some serious safety concerns, particularly with young children and those with immune deficiencies. There have been a few cases of bloodstream infections among people with chronic illness. There is also some evidence that newborns and young children who take L rhamnosus have a greater risk of wheezing later in life. (*Kopp*) You also need to know that some probiotics contain cow's milk proteins, which could lead to an allergic reaction for a baby with a milk protein allergy. (*Moneret-Vautrin*) FYI: The only probiotic that is FDA approved for use in formula is B. lactis. Other probiotics are not regulated for children.

How much and how often should I give probiotics to my baby?

Well, we're kinda shooting from the hip here since there are no official recommendations.

Products like Biogaia or Gerber Soothe can be given once a day. Just follow the directions on the package.

Since newborns acquire their baby microbiome over the first few months of life, it makes sense to use probiotics for the first two or three months of life to jumpstart that process. That is also the most common time that babies demonstrate symptoms of colic, which probiotics may help alleviate.

What about PREbiotics?

Prebiotics are certainly safe and they are the building blocks for good germs. So, serve up another helping of bananas or whole grains to your baby who has started solid foods. Is it worth it to buy prebiotic-supplemented formula? It's certainly not a bad idea, but we have to see more data before we recommend it over other products on the market.

Homeopathic Remedies

These are products containing diluted ingredients that are listed in the *Homeopathic Pharmacopeia of the United States* (HPUS). But according to the National Center for Complementary and Integrative Health, "A product's compliance with requirements of the HPUS, ...does not establish that it has been shown by appropriate means to be safe, effective, and not mis-branded for its intended use."

For more information on herbal and homeopathic remedies, check out *The Holistic Pediatrician*, by Kathi J. Kemper, M.D. (see Appendix F). She is a well-respected pediatrician who has done a great deal of research on alternative therapies.

The National Center for Complementary and Integrative Health, a branch of the National

Institutes of Health, also has a useful website at nccih.nih.gov/health/herbsataglance.htm

Home Remedies

Not every ailment requires a trip to the pharmacy. Here is a list of household items and remedies that often provide symptomatic relief for various problems.

Abdominal pain/gas/colic

Give your child a bath. The warm water is soothing. Playing in the bathtub is also a nice distraction technique.

Bruises

Pull out a bag of frozen vegetables and place on the site.

Common Cold (URI)

Make your own saline (salt water) nose drops. Take 1/2 teaspoon of salt and add to 8 oz. of water. Use as much as needed.

Chicken soup. Every culture has their own recipe, and for good reason. The high salt and water content is good for hydrating a child with a fever.

Pull out the humidifier. This moistens the air your child breathes, and loosens the mucous in their nose.

Cradle cap

Massage olive oil into the scalp. Then lift off the plaques.

Croup

Take your child into the bathroom. Close the door. Turn on the shower for ten to 15 minutes. The warm mist will help relax the airway.

If this technique doesn't work, walk outside with your child. The cold night air will often shrink up the swollen airway. It also changes the scenery for your child, which has a therapeutic effect too.

Croup usually occurs in the wintertime. If you live in a warm climate, this might not work for you.

Diaper rash

Good old petroleum jelly (Vaseline) works well. It provides a barrier between the skin and moisture.

Leave your baby open to air (diaper-less) in a safe place inside or outside your house.

Use a blow dryer on the lowest setting to dry baby's bottom.

Some doctors recommend applying liquid antacids (milk of magnesia, kaopectate) to the diaper rash. It might be worth a try.

COMP MEDS

? ?

Vomiting and Diarrhea

Make your own Pedialyte solution. Here is the recipe:

4 cups of water

1/2 tsp of salt

2 Tbsp. of sugar

1/2 tsp of instant Jell-O powder for flavor

Ear infections

Use a heating pad on low setting up to the ear.

To prevent swimmer's ear, you can make your own "Swim-ear" drops. The alcohol will dry up the water left in the ear canal. The vinegar changes the pH of the ear canal so bugs won't want to grow there. Here's the recipe:

2 drops rubbing alcohol

2 drops of vinegar

Eye stye

Place a warm tea bag over the eyelid. It is soothing and reduces the swelling.

Sore throat

Make a milkshake or smoothie (depending on the age of your child). Cold drinks feel good and are a nice way to get the fluid intake in. This idea makes me very popular with my patients.

Warts

Try duct tape. A study showed that smothering the warts suppresses the growth of the virus that causes them. Apply a new piece of duct tape to the wart nightly and leave on for the day. It takes about six weeks.

Reality Check: Clean your humidifier

Clean your humidifier properly every few days or else you will be spewing dust particles and germs into the nursery. Be sure to check the instructions that came with your humidifier for details.

DR B'S OPINION: COMPLEMENTARY MEDICINE

As we discussed in the introduction to this book, our mantra on complementary and alternative medicine for your baby is SHOW US THE SCIENCE. If a complementary therapy is shown to be effective in a reputable scientific study, then we are happy to recommend it. But if it is just snake oil or an online myth, we won't hesitate to say so.

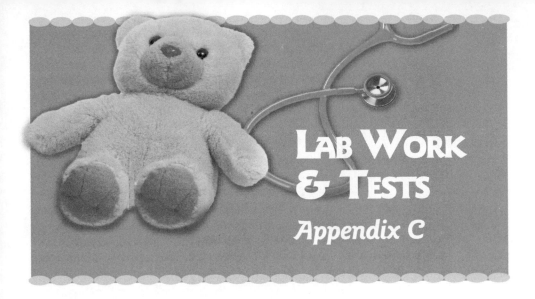

LAB WORK & TESTS
Appendix C

When The Parent Wants Tests Done

Parents frequently ask their doctor to order lab work on their child. Doctors are less interested in getting lab work done if they are comfortable in making a diagnosis. But doctors also know that a parent may bring their child in for the common cold and are actually concerned that the child has leukemia or some other devastating diagnosis. In medical terms, this is called "The Hidden Agenda." It's perfectly fine to have that agenda—you are a parent. But don't keep it a secret. Your doctor won't laugh at you. What we will do is make sure that your child does not have the problem that is keeping you up at night worrying.

What you need to know is that there is no one "test" that will uncover every disease that you have concerns about (like a total body CT scan or a comprehensive blood test panel).

What we might do is order a particular test that would help to diagnose or rule out the concern you have.

When The Doctor Wants Tests Done

Pediatricians can frequently make a correct diagnosis of illness in a child without any tests. I wish I could say it's because we are so much smarter than our other doctor colleagues. The truth is, childhood illnesses are often infections that follow classic patterns. And rashes, which occur more in kids than adults, are helpful in determining the cause of illness.

When do doctors order a test?
1. When there is something about the child's illness history or examination that may indicate a bacterial infection.
2. When there is a concern infection is bacterial and cultures are needed to know what bug it is (so it can be treated appropriately).
3. When a child has a fever with no obvious source.
4. When a baby under three months has a fever.
5. When your doctor thinks your child has a broken bone.
6. When your doctor feels a hip "click" in a newborn. Testing (hip ultrasound) will verify they don't have a congenitally dislocated hip.

7. When a child is vomiting bile or has intractable vomiting.
8. When a child has blood in their poop.
9. When a child has pain when they urinate.
10. When a child's head size is enlarging across percentiles (in other words, the head is growing much faster than expected).
11. When a child's head size is *not* enlarging.
12. When a child is failing to thrive (not gaining weight).
13. When a child wheezes for the first time and it doesn't sound like RSV bronchiolitis.
14. If an abnormality is found during a regular exam (such as distended abdomen, swollen testes).
15. When a child is drinking or urinating excessively.
16. When a child has excessive bruising.
17. When a child has petechiae.
18. When a child has a persistent fever (five days or more).
19. When a newborn is jaundiced to the level below the belly button.
20. When a child is disoriented.
21. When a child has a seizure for the first time.
22. When a child appears dehydrated and the doctor needs to decide how dehydrated they are (that is, do they need to be admitted to the hospital and get IV fluids).
23. When a child bleeds excessively—with cuts or nosebleeds.
24. When a mother has Blood Type O. Your doctor needs to know the baby's blood type so the doctor can be prepared for potential newborn jaundice problems.
25. When your doctor thinks a child has pneumonia and want to confirm it.
26. When a parent is worried.
27. When a child is limping.
28. When a child has recurrent bacterial infections (not just ear infections) such as pneumonia, sinus infections, skin infections.
29. When a child has chronic or severe problems with wheezing.
30. Anytime a child is jaundiced out of the newborn period.
31. When a child has a heart murmur that does not sound like an innocent heart murmur.
32. When a child has an irregular heartbeat.
33. When a child has a bladder or kidney infection.
34. When a child has swallowed a non-food object.

With that said, here are the most common tests we order and what they mean.

Imaging Studies

Ultrasound

The beauty of ultrasonography is that no radiation is used. The technology involves use of sonar waves and computer imaging. Doppler flow studies in addition to ultrasound pictures are helpful in looking at blood flow. Ultrasound pictures can be limited, however. Gas and fat obstructs the view.

? ?

LAB WORK

Abdominal. Looks at the anatomy of the liver, gallbladder, spleen. Not as good at looking at intestines. Detects pyloric stenosis, intussusception, gallstones, masses.

Head. Looks for bleeding inside the skull. Wand is placed on top of the anterior fontanelle (soft spot) to see inside. Not used once fontanelle has closed. Detects intraventricular hemorrhage (IVH), a problem that can occur in babies born prematurely.

Hip. Looks at the hip joint. Detects hip dislocations (Developmental Dysplasia of Hips or DDH) in infants under four months of age.

Heart (echocardiogram with Doppler). Looks at the anatomy of the heart and the great blood vessels coming off of the heart. Detects heart defects.

Kidney (renal). Looks at the anatomy of the kidneys. Detects evidence of enlargement, fluid collection (hydronephrosis), and infection.

Pelvic. Looks at anatomy of the ovaries, uterus, bladder. Detects ovarian cysts, masses. Also detects location of a testes if it has not descended into the scrotum.

Spine. Looks for spina bifida, an abnormal formation of the spine

Testicular, with Doppler flow. Looks at the anatomy of the testes. Detects a twisted testes and can assess blood flow to the testes. Also detects some hernias.

Plain x-rays

X-rays use diffraction of low doses of high-speed electrons (radiation) to project an image. Solid or fluid filled objects appear white and air appears clear. As a general rule, plain x-rays are better at detecting bone problems, and less helpful at assessing problems with "soft tissues."

Abdomen. Looks at the anatomy of the intestines, liver, spleen. Detects intestinal obstructions, malrotations, constipation. Can detect some foreign bodies (swallowed objects that are metal).

Chest. Looks at the anatomy of the heart, lungs, ribs. Detects fluid (blood, pus) in lungs, masses in lungs, enlargement of the heart, rib fractures, foreign inhaled objects.

Extremities. Looks at the bones of the arms and legs. Detects fractures (broken bones), fluid or swelling occasionally. Less helpful in detecting problems with muscles, tendons, and joints.

Neck. Looks at the anatomy of the throat (epiglottis, tonsils, adenoid, trachea). Detects swelling of these areas, location of some swallowed objects.

Skull. Looks at the anatomy of the skull bones. Detects craniosynostosis, fractures.

Sinus. Looks at the anatomy of the sinus cavities of the face. Detects *acute* sinus infections by identifying an air/fluid level. Not helpful in detecting chronic sinus infections.

Spine. Looks at the anatomy of the vertebrae from the neck to the buttocks. Detects fractures, slipped discs, scoliosis.

CT/MRI with or without contrast

Computerized Tomography (CT) uses x-ray technology (radiation) to look at cross sectional slices of the body in a two-dimensional picture. Due to the significant amount of radiation exposure with a CT scan, physicians are very selective about ordering these studies. Magnetic Resonance Imaging (MRI) uses a magnetic field to detect the body's electromagnetic transmissions. MRI's produce narrow slices of the body without radiation. As a general rule, CT and MRI scans are better at detecting abnormalities with soft body tissues and less helpful with bone problems. The decision to perform a CT versus an MRI is based on the particular problem that is being assessed.

Abdomen. Looks at the anatomy of the liver, spleen, pancreas, gallbladder, intestines, kidneys. Detects masses, tumors, abscesses—including appendicitis, fluid collections, trauma.

Chest. Looks at the anatomy of the lungs and heart. Detects masses, tumors, fluid collections, congenital abnormalities, trauma.

Extremity. Looks at the anatomy of the arm or leg. Detects fractures, torn ligaments, masses, tumors, osteomyelitis (infection).

Head. Looks at the anatomy of the brain. Detects masses, tumors, obstruction of spinal fluid flow (hydrocephalus), evidence of stroke (cerebrovascular accident), evidence of trauma, bleeding.

Lymph node. Looks at the anatomy of a concerning (swollen) lymph node. Detects pus (infection), masses, congenital cysts.

Pelvic. Looks at the anatomy of the ovary, uterus, bladder. Detects masses, tumors, fluid collections.

Sinus. Looks at the anatomy of the sinus cavities. More helpful imaging study than plain x-rays. Detects obstruction to flow in the sinuses, chronic sinus infections, masses/polyps.

Special studies

Barium swallow/Upper GI. Looks at the anatomy of the upper gastrointestinal tract (esophagus, stomach, upper small intestine). Detects anatomic abnormalities, hiatal hernias, pyloric stenosis, ulcerations, narrowings. Although gastroesophageal reflux may be seen (barium goes backwards), it doesn't tell you the severity of the reflux. It also does not rule out reflux as a diagnosis.

Bone scan. Nuclear medicine study (uses a radio-isotope to be visualized on x-ray). Looks at the all of the bones of the body in one study. Hot and cold "spots" detect areas of inflammation. Detects: infection, tumors, avascular necrosis, child abuse.

DMSA Scan. Special nuclear medicine study that uses a radio-isotope dye visualized on x-ray. Looks for scarring of the kidneys. Detects: chronic kidney scarring and damage due to kidney infections.

Voiding Cystourethrogram. Looks at the flow of urine from kidney to ureters to bladder to urethra. Detects vesicoureteral reflux in children prone to bladder infections. (*Gunn*)

Laboratory Tests

Blood tests

Amylase. This test looks at the level of an enzyme that the pancreas makes. Detects: pancreatitis

Basic Metabolic Panel. This is a battery of tests that includes *sodium, potassium, chloride, bicarbonate, blood urea nitrogen, creatinine, glucose.* This combination of tests assesses body fluid and salt (electrolyte) balance as well as kidney and adrenal function.
Detects: Dehydration, kidney dysfunction, diabetes, hypoglycemia, adrenal dysfunction

Bilirubin. This test assesses the level of this substance circulating in the bloodstream. Newborns uniquely have higher levels than any other time in life because:

1. Newborn metabolism is not functioning at 100%.
2. Newborns are not eliminating bilirubin in their stool yet.
3. Newborns have bilirubin load due to prematurity, birth trauma, or blood type incompatibility.

A total level is assessed as well as *direct* and *indirect* levels. These indicate the cause of the total elevation. Beyond the newborn period, any evidence of jaundice prompts a lab evaluation.
Detects: Hyperbilirubinemia, Hepatitis, Biliary Atresia, gallstones, hemolytic anemia

Blood culture. see below

Blood sugar (glucose). This test assesses the body's metabolism of sugar. A random level above 110 is concerning for diabetes. In newborns, a level less than 40 is concerning for hypoglycemia. Levels less than 60 in children is concerning for hypoglycemia.
Detects: Hypoglycemia in large birth weights, babies whose mothers have gestational diabetes or diabetes, body temperature irregularities, lethargy
Detects in children: Diabetes, hypoglycemia

Blood type. This test determines what proteins sit on the surface of a patient's red blood cells. There are A and B proteins. The AB blood type means both A and B protein are present. The O blood type means there are no proteins present. Rh typing refers to the presence (+) or absence (-) of another type of protein that sits on the red blood cell surface. These tests are necessary when a blood transfusion is needed. In an emergency situation, however, everyone gets O (-) negative blood. Most hospitals no longer test a newborn's blood type on a routine basis.

C-Reactive Protein (CRP). This is a substance that circulates in the bloodstream when there is an inflammatory process going on. It is one of several "acute phase reactants" whose numbers change by at least 25% when there is active inflammation. It is not specific for any one disease, but it is accurate. It detects inflammation, infection, trauma, or tumors.

Cholesterol level. See lipid panel

Complete Blood Count (CBC). This refers to a test that looks at the number of white blood cells, red blood cells, and platelets that are circulating in the bloodstream.

1. *White blood cell count (WBC).* These cells fight infection, but also rise with inflammation. An elevated count is concerning for a bacterial infection. A depressed count is due to decreased bone marrow production (where white blood cells are made)—usually caused by viral infections (e.g. influenza, mononucleosis).

2. *White blood cell count differential.* Not only is the number of white blood cells counted, but the types of white blood cells are identified in a CBC. The types of cells also give your doctor clues as to the disease process going on.

♦ *Neutrophils (PMN's)-* Cells that fight bacteria. If more than 50% of the WBC's are this type, the likelihood of a bacterial infection is greater.

♦ *Lymphocytes*: Cells that fight viruses. If more than 50% of the WBC's are this type, the likelihood of viral infection is greater.

♦ *Eosinophils*: Cells that fight parasites. Also revved up by allergies. If more than 10-15% of these cells are present, it prompts an investigation.

3. *Hematocrit/Hemoglobin.* These measurements assess the amount of red blood cells in the circulation. Low levels detect anemia.

4. *Platelet count.* These cells help clot the blood. A low level detects a cause for bleeding problems. A low level can also suggest bone marrow suppression (where platelets are made) or an autoimmune disorder. Platelet counts can be elevated with infection or inflammation.

FYI: When all three cell lines (white, red, platelet) are depressed, there is a concern for leukemia.
Uses: infection, inflammation, leukemia, anemia, bleeding disorder

Comprehensive Metabolic Panel. This is a large battery of tests that assesses adrenal, kidney, liver, gallbladder, fluid and electrolyte balance, and a measure of general nutrition. These tests include:

Albumin   Alkaline phosphatase
Alanine Aminotransferase (ALT)   Aspartate Aminotransferase (AST)
Bicarbonate   Bilirubin
Blood Urea Nitrogen (BUN)   Calcium
Chloride   Creatinine
Glucose   Phosphorous
Potassium   Sodium
Total Protein

Detects: Liver dysfunction, hepatitis, gallbladder dysfunction, kidney dysfunction, dehydration, diabetes, adrenal dysfunction, malnutrition.

Chromosome analysis. This test assesses a patient's chromosomes, the part of each cell that contains genes. Blood, tissue, or an amniotic fluid sample can be tested.
Detects: Chromosomal abnormalities related to developmental delays/congenital defects; determines the sex of a baby born with ambiguous genitalia.

Coagulation studies. These tests detect an abnormality in the clotting "cascade" or chain of events that allow blood to clot. These tests include:
Bleeding Time, Factor levels, Prothrombin time (PT), Partial thromboplastin time (PTT)
Detects: Bleeding disorders—such as Hemophilia, von Willebrand's disease

Coombs test. This test looks for antibodies (reaction) to a person's blood type. In newborns whose mothers have O Blood type, many hospitals perform a Coombs test on the baby routinely. There is some mixing of mother's and fetus's blood in the placenta, which can cause a Type O mother's blood to create antibodies to a type A or B baby. These antibodies can potentially kill some of the baby's red blood cells creating an extra bilirubin load in the newborn.
Detects: Blood type incompatibility in newborns

Electrolytes. See Basic Metabolic Panel

Erythrocyte Sedimentation Rate (ESR). This test looks at how fast it takes for red blood cells to settle at the bottom of a test tube. It is a very nonspecific test, but an elevated level suggests further testing. It is a non-specific sign of inflammation.
Detects: inflammation, infection, malignancy, anemia

Liver function tests. This is a battery of tests that evaluates how the liver is working. It looks at products the liver is in charge of metabolizing and producing. Some tests look at the breakdown product of liver cells (but these products are also seen in muscle breakdown) so they are not specific in detecting liver disorders.

Alanine Aminotransferase (ALT)	Albumin
Aspartate Aminotransferase (AST)	Bilirubin
Total protein	

Detects: Hepatitis, liver failure, drug toxicity, heart attack.

Monospot/EBV titers. For monospot, see rapid assays below.
Epstein-Barr Virus (EBV) titers detect a person's immune response (antibodies) to an EBV infection (mononucleosis). Because different types of antibodies are formed through the course of infection, this test differentiates a recent infection and a prior one.
Detects: Acute mononucleosis, prior mononucleosis.

Lipid panel/cholesterol. This battery of tests looks at how the body metabolizes fat. Poor fat metabolism is associated with coronary artery disease (heart disease) in later life. In children, often a random (non-fasting) cholesterol level is an acceptable screening test. If that level is elevated, a full panel is done with the child fasting prior to the test. Tests:

Cholesterol	HDL
LDL	Triglyceride level

Detects: Hypercholesterolemia, hepatitis, metabolic disorders, bile duct obstruction, nephrotic syndrome, pancreatitis, hypothyroidism

LAB WORK

? ?

Reticulocyte count. Reticulocytes are baby red blood cells. They circulate in the bloodstream while they mature. This test looks at the number of these present in the blood. A high level suggests good bone marrow production in response to anemia.
Detects: Body's response to anemia

Thyroid function tests. This is a battery of tests that assesses the function of the thyroid gland. An indirect way of testing thyroid gland function is to look at a Thyroid Stimulating Hormone (TSH) level, a hormone produced by the pituitary gland. If the thyroid gland is not functioning well (hypothyroidism), the TSH level is elevated to stimulate the gland to work harder. This is a test included in all state metabolic screens to detect congenital hypothyroidism.

T3 (triiodothyronine) level	Thyroxine Binding Globulin
T4 (thyroxine) level	Free T3, Free T4 levels
TSH	

Detects: Hypothyroidism, Hyperthyroidism

Viral titers. There are a few viruses for which a patient's antibody response can be detected. These tests are useful to make a diagnosis or confirm immunity to a particular virus.

CMV	Hepatitis A, B, C
HIV	Parvovirus
Rubella	Syphilis
Toxoplasmosis	Varicella

Urine tests

Urinalysis. This is a test that looks at the components of urine and detects any abnormal components. Urine is normally a sterile fluid, thus should not contain any bacteria or white blood cells (which fight infection). Urine does not break down sugar or protein, so it should not contain any of those substances. Urine is produced in the kidneys, so some abnormalities will point to a kidney dysfunction.

In children, obtaining a urine specimen can be a challenge. A urine specimen needs to be clean to be able to make any decisions based on its findings. The preferred method of obtaining this specimen is to insert a small catheter in the urethra of a non-toilet trained child. If the reason for testing urine is not to look for infection, a collection bag may be placed over the urethra. Tests:

Specific gravity	pH
Color, odor	White Blood Cells
Red Blood Cells	Glucose
Protein	Nitrite
Microscopic analysis for bacteria	

Detects: Bladder infection, dehydration, kidney disease, diabetes, adrenal dysfunction, metabolic disorder, kidney stones

Skin tests

PPD. This is the preferred test for exposure to tuberculosis. PPD stands for purified protein derivative, which refers to a synthetic protein "signature" that belongs to the tuberculosis bacteria. If a person has had an exposure to tuberculosis, their antibodies will also respond to this skin test. A positive test requires further evaluation and testing.

Stool tests

Occult blood. This test detects blood in the stool. A small amount of stool (poop) is placed on a special developing card. When a processing fluid is added to the specimen, it turns blue in the presence of blood.
Detects: Gastrointestinal bleeding (e.g. food allergy, infection, ulcer, inflammatory bowel disease, polyp)

Spinal fluid (CSF) tests

Cerebrospinal fluid (CSF) is a liquid that bathes the brain and spinal cord. It transports important chemicals through the central nervous system. A specimen of this fluid helps diagnose viral infection, bacterial infection, tuberculosis meningitis (infection of the tissues protecting the brain), brain infection, and obstruction of the spinal fluid collecting system.

CSF is obtained by performing a lumbar puncture or "spinal tap." This sounds scary, but it is a similar concept to having an epidural placed in childbirth. A small needle is inserted between two vertebrae in the back. A small amount of fluid is collected, and then the needle is removed.

We look at the pressure of the fluid, the appearance of the fluid (should be clear/watery), the sugar/protein levels, and if there are any cells in the fluid (white, red, bacteria).

A culture of the fluid is also done (see below).

Sweat test

A specimen of sweat is obtained by warming the skin on the arm or thigh and obtaining a small amount of sweat.
Detects: Cystic Fibrosis

Cultures

This group of tests takes a particular body fluid and incubates it (creates ideal growing conditions for bugs). If there is a germ in a specimen, there is a chance to identify it. Germs that grow are very accurate for infection growing in the patient (except for contaminated/dirty specimens). But, lack of growth in culture does not necessarily rule out an infection.

Most germs will grow out in a culture within three days. Fungus infections, however, may take up to one month to grow.

Blood. Detects BACTERIAL infections
Urine. Detects bacterial infections
Spinal fluid. Detects primarily BACTERIAL infections, some VIRAL infections
Stool. Detects BACTERIAL, PARASITE, AMOEBA infections
Throat. Detects BACTERIAL infection
Sputum. Detects BACTERIAL infection

Abscess. Detects BACTERIAL infection
Viral. Detects limited number of VIRAL infections (such as Herpes, Varicella, Chlamydia)
Fungal. Detects FUNGUS infections

Rapid Antigen Tests

These tests detect a protein or toxin that is made by a virus or bacteria. It is most accurate when someone has symptoms. A positive test is accurate in confirming infection. A negative test does not rule out infection because it depends on the quality of the specimen. Medical offices offer rapid antigen testing. Home COVID-19 tests are also rapid antigen tests.

Testing has a 15-30 minute turnaround for results.

Rapid antigen tests for: RSV, COVID-19, Flu A and B, rotavirus, infectious mononucleosis, Strep throat

Molecular Assay (NAAT)

This rapid test detects the nucleic acid (DNA or RNA) of the virus. It is most accurate and useful when someone has symptoms. A positive test confirms an active infection. Medical offices offer NAAT testing.

Testing has 15-30 minute turnaround for results.

NAAT tests for: Flu A and B, COVID-19

PCR (Polymerase Chain Reaction)

These tests accurately detect the presence of genetic material (DNA or RNA) of some viruses, bacteria, fungi, and parasites that cause infection. The technology amplifies even the smallest amount of infectious material present so a PCR test can produce a positive test very early in illness. PCR testing is generally done at outside lab facilities, emergency departments, or hospital settings.

Testing has a 1-8 hour turnaround for results.

PCR tests for: Influenza A and B, Rotavirus, COVID-19, RSV

Multiplex PCR (Biofire and others)

This test uses the same PCR technology but can simultaneously screen for multiple viruses (and some other germs) that cause respiratory and gut infections. Few pediatric practices perform these tests because they are expensive and not universally covered by insurance plans.

Testing has a 1hour turnaround for results.

Respiratory PCR panel tests for:

—Viruses: Influenza A and B, several coronavirus strains, COVID-19, Parainfluenza strains, RSV, adenovirus, rhinovirus, enterovirus, human metapneumovirus

—Bacteria: Bordatella pertussis (whooping cough), Bordatella parapertussis, Chlamydia pneumoniae, Mycoplasma pneumoniae

Gastrointestinal PCR panel tests for 22 viruses, bacteria, parasites that cause severe gastroenteritis including norovirus, rotavirus, E.coli, Salmonella, C. difficile, and Giardia.

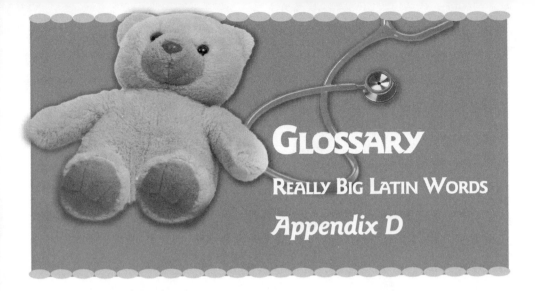

GLOSSARY

REALLY BIG LATIN WORDS

Appendix D

Abdominal tumors. There are some solid tumors that occur more frequently in children than adults. These include Wilm's tumor and neuroblastoma. Patients with these tumors may (not always) have enlarged, firm bellies with a mass that can be felt. Other symptoms include weight loss, lack of appetite, or unexplained fevers.

ABO incompatibility. See Coombs test in Lab section.

Accessory Nipple. See supernumerary nipple.

Acholic stool. Official term for a clay-colored poop. In isolation, it may have no significance. But, it can indicate a problem with the biliary system (liver, gallbladder, pancreas) if it is associated with other symptoms—particularly jaundice (yellowing) of the skin. Diagnoses can include hepatitis infection and biliary atresia. If you see this, check in with your doctor.

Acne (neonatal). Skin inflammation due to hormonal changes in the newborn period. Onset is usually by four weeks of age and lasts until about eight weeks of age.

Acute abdomen. Term that refers to an emergency requiring surgical intervention to alleviate an intestinal problem. Examples of these problems include: appendicitis, intussusception, intestinal obstruction.

Acute life threatening event (ALTE). Term that describes an episode of lack of breathing (apnea) that requires intervention to resume spontaneous breathing. If an event like this happens, a thorough evaluation is done to determine the cause of the event.

Acute otitis media. Infection in the middle ear space. This is primarily caused by bacteria. When the infection comes up quickly, it is called "acute." Symptoms include fever, cranky mood, and vomiting. Occasionally, children may also seem dizzy. Ear infections that smolder for a long period of time are called "chronic" and do not have the same symptoms.

Acrocyanosis. The blue discoloration frequently seen on the hands and feet of newborns. This is due to the body circulation transitioning from fetal to newborn. It does not indicate any problem with the heart or circulatory system. Blue discoloration only on the feet or legs (not hands) can be a sign of a circulation problem (Coarctation of the Aorta) and needs to be evaluated.

Air hungry. The inability of a person to get enough oxygen in with each breath. The person then tries to get more air in with each breath by using chest wall muscles and increasing the number of breaths taken per minute. This is also known as **respiratory distress**.

Ambiguous Genitalia (also known as Disorders of Sex Development). It's hard to tell whether the baby has male parts or female parts. We'll test chromosomes, hormone levels, and get an ultrasound to look for internal genitalia (ovaries/uterus or undescended testes).

Amblyopia. (Known as lazy eye). A reduction of vision in an eye that is not correctable with glasses. This problem can be caused by a weakness of an eye muscle (strabismus). It is important to detect this eye problem early (under age two or three years) so it can be treated.

Anal fissure. A crack in the anus opening usually due to passage of a hard poop. The crack causes discomfort and occasionally blood in the diaper or on a diaper wipe.

Anaphylactic reaction. An allergic response to exposure to a particular item (that is, medication, food). The response is extremely serious and life-threatening. These body responses include: difficulty breathing, heart failure, loss of blood pressure.

Anemia. A reduced amount of hemoglobin that carries oxygen on red blood cells. Because the body is less capable of getting oxygen, symptoms include tiredness, pale appearance, and quick fatigue.

Ankyloglossia (tongue tie). The tongue is attached to the base of the mouth too close to the tip. Not all babies with tongue tie need intervention. If it is so tight that it interferes with feeding or talking, the tissue band can be clipped. This is more likely to be a problem if the tip of the tongue is forked.

Anomaly. Fancy word for abnormality, usually malformed prior to birth (congenital anomaly).

Anterior Fontanelle. See Fontanelle.

Antibiotic induced colitis. Inflammation of the lower part of the intestine which, rarely, can be caused by antibiotics. Symptoms of colitis include blood and mucous in the poop, diarrhea, and cramping. If someone has been on an antibiotic just prior to the onset of these symptoms, a specimen of poop can be checked for this problem.

Apnea. Pause, or temporary absence in breathing. Frequently babies born prematurely have these events when they just plain forget to breathe. This is called **apnea of prematurity**. Preemies eventually outgrow this problem. Until they do, they are placed on an apnea monitor which alarms when breathing stops. Some babies also need caffeine (in medication form) to stimulate them to breathe.

Appendicitis. Inflammation of a small piece of the intestine called the appendix. The appendix is usually located in the lower RIGHT side of the belly, but this varies occasionally. When the appendix gets swollen, symptoms include: vomiting, diarrhea, fever, and abdominal pain that worsens over time. Appendicitis is extremely rare in the birth to age one group.

Asperger's Syndrome. A term that is no longer used to describe a developmental disorder that is part of the Autism Spectrum Disorders. Historically, children with Asperger's have better communication and language skills than those more severely affected.

Asthma. The swelling of the big and little airways in the lungs. The swelling can occur due to allergic response. The episodes happen intermittently. Symptoms include: coughing and labored breathing (respiratory distress).

Atopy. A classic triad of allergic disorders: eczema, asthma, and seasonal allergies (termed "allergic rhinitis"). Not everyone is unlucky enough to have all three problems, but some people are.

Atresia. Means that something is completely absent or is significantly narrowed
    Anal atresia. Anus (opening of the intestines to the outside).
    Biliary atresia. Bile ducts.
    Choanal atresia. Nasal/throat.
    Duodenal atresia. Small intestine.
    Esophageal atresia. Esophagus.
    Ileal atresia. Small intestine.
    Tricuspid atresia. Heart valve.

Autism Spectrum Disorders (ASD). A developmental disorder that is characterized by poor or no language development, lack of normal social skills and repetitive self-soothing behaviors. The disorder has a genetic basis in at least 10-15% of the cases. The diagnosis encompasses the broad range from mild to severely affected individuals.

Autosomal dominant. A genetically inherited trait that requires only one parent to have an abnormal gene to pass it on to a child. If one parent carries an autosomal dominant gene, the chances are 50% that a child inherits the gene.

Autosomal recessive. A genetically inherited trait that requires both parents to have the gene to pass it on to a child. If both parents are carriers of the autosomal recessive gene, the chances are 25% that they will have an affected child. If both parents have the disease, chances are nearly 100% that they will have an affected child.

Bacterial gastroenteritis. (See gastroenteritis)

BAER. Brainstem Audio Evoked Response. An objective hearing test that measures the electrical activity of the inner ear in response to sound. This is a universal screening test done on newborns. It is recommended by the American Academy of Pediatrics and currently mandated in most states.

Balanitis. An inflammation of the tip of the penis, which becomes inflamed an irritated. Balanitis can be caused by an infection.

Bilirubin Induced Neurologic Dysfunction (BIND). A serious consequence of jaundice. Bilirubin collects in the brain, causing permanent damage.

Bladder infection (see UTI)

Blocked tear duct. See nasolacrimal duct obstruction.

Blood in stool. A symptom that may be caused by a variety of reasons. Blood can be found in poop due to skin irritation (diaper rash), a crack or tear in the anus (see anal fissure), inflammation in the intestine (milk protein allergy), intestinal infection (see gastroenteritis), or intestinal obstruction (intus-

glossary

susception). As you can see, the problem may be a minor or serious one. It always should be checked out by your doctor.

Brain tumor. Abnormal mass of cells that grow in the brain tissue. Although not all tumors are malignant (fast growing, aggressive), even benign tumors can be life threatening depending on the location that it arises. Symptoms in infants and young children include morning headaches accompanied by vomiting, increasing head size, behavior changes, imbalance, seizures, and new onset eye abnormalities.

Branchial cleft cyst. An abnormality in fetal development of the throat that results in a cyst that occurs on the neck

Breath-holding spell. An episode where a child holds their breath when upset or angry. Usually occurs after one year of age. The episode ultimately results in a child losing consciousness and regaining normal breathing. Rarely, these episodes are due to anemia—but worth checking out if the episodes occur frequently.

Breech position. Occasionally, a baby will decide to exit the womb with their butt, foot, or feet first—instead of the usual head first (vertex) position. Because this can increase the risk of complications at delivery, it is preferable to deliver these babies by C-section. Babies who are breech in the womb, particularly girls, have a *slightly* increased risk of having **hip dysplasia** (also known as developmental dysplasia of the hips or DDH). There is an association between abnormal formation of the hips as a fetus leading to the unusual butt/foot first position for delivery. See **hip dysplasia.**

Bronchiolitis. Swelling in the tiny airways in the lungs (bronchioles). In children, this is caused primarily by a virus called RSV (Respiratory Syncytial Virus). When the little airways are swollen, it can be difficult to exchange oxygen poor air with oxygen rich air. In severe cases, particularly infants under a year of age or those born prematurely, some children need medication to reduce the swelling (see bronchodilators in medication appendix) and supplemental oxygen.

Bronchitis. Swelling in the larger airways of the lungs (bronchi). In children, this swelling is usually caused by a virus or bacterial infection.

Broncopulmonary dysplasia (BPD). Term used to describe chronic lung disease that occurs primarily in babies who are born prematurely who require prolonged breathing assistance with a mechanical ventilator. The longer the baby is dependent on mechanical ventilation, the poorer the prognosis. Babies with BPD may have poor lung function, wheezing, and higher risk of severe complications with Respiratory Syncytial Virus (RSV) infection. Lung function, however, usually improves over the first several years of life.

Cafe au lait spots. As the name implies, these are light brown (coffee with milk) colored birthmarks. They occur in babies of all races. Most of the time, there is no significance to these marks. When a child has more than five of these birthmarks, there may be an association with a disorder called **neurofibromatosis.**

Carotinemia. A benign yellow discoloration of the skin due to a large dietary intake of carotene containing foods (carrots, sweet potatoes). The whites of the eyes remain white, as opposed to what is seen with jaundice—**see jaundice.**

? ?

GLOSSARY

Cataracts. A clouding of the eye's lens. This can occur at birth (congenital cataracts). If a newborn has cataracts, it can be detected by the lack of a 'red reflex' on an eye examination. A referral to a pediatric ophthalmologist is made.

Celiac disease. A disorder of the intestines which causes poor digestion and absorption of foods. The underlying problem is due to an abnormal response to 'gluten' containing foods (e.g. wheat, oat, rye grains). The classic symptoms of this disorder include foul smelling, chronic diarrhea and failure to thrive (lack of weight gain). Treatment is a lifelong gluten-free diet.

Cephalhematoma. Literally, a head bruise. This often occurs in newborns as a result of birth trauma. Some of these bruises are quite large and take one to two months to completely go away. In the process of healing, these areas can become very hard and firm. Since the bruise is a collection of blood, it sometimes creates an additional bilirubin load and can lead to jaundice in some newborns.

Cerebral palsy. An abnormality of the brain center that controls muscle tone and movement. Cerebral palsy does not cause any abnormalities in IQ. However, there are children who have *both* intellectual disability AND cerebral palsy.

Choanal atresia. Lack of communication between the back of the nasal passages and the throat. This can occur in one or both sides of the nose. If both sides are blocked, a newborn will have severe breathing problems. Newborns only know how to breathe through their noses for the first four months of life.

Clavicle (collar bone) fracture. When Mom is small and baby is big, it can be difficult to get the baby out of the birth canal. The baby's shoulder pulls out and can break the clavicle (collar bone) in the process. It heals nicely without a cast. The area can feel crunchy under the skin, then it feels like a hard lump. The lump is healing bone and goes away after several weeks.

Cleft lip and palate. The roof of the mouth and/or the upper lip does not completely form in a fetus. These defects can occur together or separately in 1 in 1000 births. There is some hereditary predisposition. Rarely, this defect is associated with other congenital defects. Frequently, a team of providers manage babies with these defects (Ear, Nose, and Throat doctors, Plastic Surgeons, Dentist, and Occupational Therapists). See Appendix F for web sites on this issue.

Club foot. An abnormality in the formation of the foot of the fetus. The result is a stiff foot that turns markedly inwards. Pediatric orthopedic surgeons are consulted and a cast is made to correct the position of the foot.

Coarctation of the Aorta. A narrowing or kink in the great artery (aorta) that leaves the heart and supplies the body with oxygen rich blood. This is a defect that occurs during fetal development (prior to birth). If the abnormality is severe, it is diagnosed in newborns who have weakened/no pulse in the legs. If the abnormality is small, it may go undetected until later in life. It is repaired by surgery.

Colostrum. A first "milk" that a mother produces. This product is rich in antibodies and cells. It has fewer calories than mature milk which arrives on about the fourth day after birth.

Conductive hearing loss. Difficulty hearing due to a problem with the transmission of sound waves to the part of the ear that controls hearing. Sound waves can be blocked due to fluid sitting behind the eardrum (see serous obits media) or a significant amount of earwax sitting in the ear canal. The

GLOSSARY

? ?

good news about conductive hearing loss is that the problem can usually be fixed and normal hearing is restored.

Congenital. This refers to an abnormality in the *formation* of a certain organ/body part that occurs in the development of an unborn fetus. These abnormalities may be due to either hereditary problems or environmental exposures during pregnancy. The lay term for these disorders is **birth defect.**

Congenital Adrenal Hyperplasia. An abnormality in the gland that produces steroids in the body (adrenal gland). This can cause severe metabolism problems of body salts. This abnormality is routinely tested in the newborn metabolic screen.

Congenital heart disease. A defect in the structural development of the heart or the great vessels that attach to the heart. Because heart development occurs in the first trimester of pregnancy, many congenital defects can be identified on a prenatal ultrasound. Some abnormalities will resolve on their own. Some require surgical repair. The disease incidence is 1:1000. The most common defects are the least serious ones. Remember, there is a difference between an innocent heart murmur (no defect) and a pathologic murmur (caused by congenital heart disease).

Congenital nevus. (Known as moles, birthmarks) A mark on the skin which is present at birth, or appears within the first year of life. The most concerning moles are ones larger than 10 to 20 cm (really big) that are present at birth. These have more potential risk of skin cancer and removal is usually advised.

Congestive heart failure. When the heart is unable to perform adequately, the blood flow accumulates in the lungs and liver. So, symptoms of heart failure include shortness of breath and enlarged liver size. In children, symptoms include failure to thrive, sweating with feedings, shortness of breath, and excessive fatigue.

Conjunctivitis. An inflammation of the lining of the eyelid. Otherwise known as "pink eye." The inflammation can be caused by a virus, bacteria, allergies, or irritation. All types of conjunctivitis cause redness and some discomfort. Here are the major types of conjunctivitis:
Allergic. An allergic response usually due to a sensitivity to something in the air (e.g. pollens). Usually causes watery, somewhat itchy eyes. Antihistamines treat the symptoms.
Bacterial. A bacterial infection in the eye (often accompanied by ear and sinus infection). Causes thick yellowish eye discharge and may even cause the eyes to be caked over or "matted." Antibiotic eye drops treat the infection.
Viral. A viral infection in the eye (that may be accompanied by a sore throat). Causes watery and very itchy eyes.
Irritation. Eyes become inflamed because of a chemical irritant (e.g. shampoo).

Constipation. The texture of poop is significantly hard, and is passed either in small pieces or in a very large mass of small pieces stuck together. Contrary to popular belief, constipation is NOT defined by the infrequency of poop (although this can contribute to the problem). There is no defined length of interval for which a person needs to poop—it can vary considerably. If the poop is soft when it comes out, your baby is unlikely to be constipated.

Craniosynostosis. A baby's skull bones have gaps that allow for the brain's growth in the first one to two years of life. This abnormality is a premature closure of the gaps (sutures) that occurs in about 1 in 1800 children. The reason why this occurs is unknown, but is not due to any birth trauma or complication. Early closure can cause deformities in the skull and facial shape, inhibition of brain growth, and increased pressure within the skull.

Cystic Fibrosis (CF). This is a genetic disease that causes body glands to produce abnormal secretions. Lung, sinus, pancreas, intestine, and reproductive organ problems occur because of it. One in 20 Caucasians are carriers of this genetic abnormality. The disease incidence is 1:1600 for Caucasian babies (it is much less common in other races). Many women now receive genetic testing during pregnancy for CF.

Developmental Dysplasia of the Hip (DDH). See hip dysplasia.

Diarrhea. Frequent passage of watery or very soft poop. In a breastfed baby, diarrhea is defined more by the dramatic increase in frequency of poop than by the texture.

Duodenal atresia. Congenital abnormality of the first part of the small intestine to form. It's often associated with other abnormalities. Babies are diagnosed with this disorder before birth by an abnormal ultrasound (extra amniotic fluid found) or shortly after birth when they start vomiting bile. This requires surgical repair.

Eczema. A skin disorder that causes redness and scaling. The underlying problem seems to be allergic in nature, and children with eczema have flare-ups with exposure to perfumed products and certain chemicals. Eczema can be associated with other allergic disorders such as asthma, seasonal allergies, and food allergies but it can also occur without any other problems.

Egocentric. The inability to see things from someone else's point of view. This is a child's view of the world from age two to about seven years.

Emesis. The technical term for vomit.

Enamel hypoplasia. A thinning of the enamel of the teeth found in babies who are born prematurely. And there appears to be less "catch up" growth of that enamel in babies born prematurely compared to their full term peers. This may result in increased risk of cavities.

Encephalitis. Brain inflammation usually caused by a virus or a bacterial infection.

Engorgement. The Milkman Cometh. Period of excessive breast milk production around three to five days after childbirth. Women's breasts feel full and often uncomfortable until milk demand and milk supply equilibrate.

Epispadias. Congenital abnormality of the formation of a boy's urethra (tube connecting the bladder to the outside). The hole is located on the top side of the penis, instead of in the center. This requires surgical repair.

Epstein's pearls. Tiny cysts (white bumps) found on the roof of the mouth in newborns. These are common, non-problematic, and go away on their own.

Erb's palsy. An injury to the nerves that supply the arm. This occurs as a result of a difficult delivery requiring the baby's head to be pulled forcefully. On examination, the arm will hang limp. The nerve injury usually heals in a year, but may require surgery or physical therapy.

Eruption Hematoma. This is just a bruise under the gum line that can occur as the tooth is breaking through the gums. It can look pretty darn impressive—swollen and blue or purple. No worries. It means a tooth will be arriving soon.

Erythema toxicum neonatorum. A normal newborn rash that looks like flea bites (white pimple with red around it). These tiny bumps come and go.

Esophagitis. The inflammation of the upper part of the gastrointestinal system (esophagus).

Expressive language delays. A child whose ability to speak words is behind their peers. A child with this delay may have completely normal ability to understand and process language that they hear (see receptive language).

Failure to thrive. When a baby or child falls below the 3rd percentile on the weight curve. When the problem is a chronic one, height and head size also drop on the growth curves. Failure to thrive prompts a thorough medical evaluation.

Fat necrosis. An occasional complication from vaccination injection. As a needle goes through the fat under the skin, it can injure it and create a firm lump. This lump may be present for several weeks after the injection is given. It is painless and not harmful.

Flaring (nostrils). When an infant or young child is having trouble breathing (respiratory distress), they will use any additional methods their body can to get in more air. Nostrils will flare with each breath to try to capture more air. Thus, this is a red flag for respiratory distress.

Flat angiomata. Official term for an "angel kiss" birthmark on the forehead or eyelids. These are flat, reddish colored marks that eventually fade. The color becomes more dramatic with crying or anger.

Fomites. Objects handled by a person with an infection that subsequently allows passage of the germs to someone else.

Fontanelle. A space between the bones of the skull that allows room for the baby's head to pass through the birth canal and room for the baby's brain to grow after birth. The main fontanelle is on top of the head (anterior) and is sometimes called the baby's "soft spot." There is a smaller fontanelle in the back of the head (posterior). The anterior fontanelle closes between nine to 18 months of age.

Food poisoning (see gastroenteritis)

Foreign body/object. Term used to describe an object which has no place being where it is in someone's body. Kids have a way of putting objects like small toys in their noses, ears, etc. as well as swallowing them.

Foremilk. A breastfeeding term used to describe the milk that is released in the first several minutes of nursing. It is less fatty than what comes out later (see **hindmilk**). If your breastfed baby is a snacker, they may not be getting the richer milk. For these babies, it is better to nurse on one breast per feeding.

Frenulum. The tissue that connects the tongue to the base of the mouth. (see **ankyloglossia**).

Frenulectomy. The process of clipping the tissue at the tongue base to correct a 'tongue tie' or ankyloglossia. This procedure can be performed in an office setting if the baby is less than a few weeks old.

Galactosemia. A rare metabolic disorder that makes a baby unable to digest galactose, a milk sugar. Newborns are routinely tested for this disorder in the state metabolic screen. If present, a baby needs a special formula diet. Breastmilk contains galactose, so it is not possible to breastfeed. Babies who have galactosemia and continue a normal diet can have intellectual disabilities.

Gastroenteritis. An inflammation of the stomach and intestines caused by either a virus or bacteria. The inflammation can cause both vomiting and diarrhea. Viral gastroenteritis is commonly known as the "stomach flu" and tends to cause watery diarrhea. Bacterial gastroenteritis is commonly known as "food poisoning" and tends to cause diarrhea mixed with blood or mucous.

Gastroesophageal reflux (GER, acid reflux). The backflow of food and liquids from the stomach into the esophagus (and often all the way to the mouth). This is a common problem for newborns up to age one year. The muscle that separates the esophagus and the stomach (lower esophageal sphincter) is relatively loose in infants, allowing food to travel down to the stomach (good) and back up to the esophagus (not good). Once food contents make it to the stomach, they are mixed with stomach acid. So, when this partially digested food goes backwards, the stomach acid can irritate the esophagus, cause discomfort, and sometimes wheezing or coughing (GERD—Gastroesophageal Reflux Disease). Most babies outgrow this problem by age one.

Gingivostomatitis. Inflammation and irritation of the gums and lining of the mouth caused by the Oral Herpes virus. The amount of inflammation is usually extensive and may lead to refusal to eat or drink anything.

Glaucoma. Increased pressure behind the eye. Babies with hemangiomas near the eye need to be evaluated by an ophthalmologist because they are at risk for glaucoma.

Heart murmur. A noise heard in addition to the normal heart sounds audible with a stethoscope. The murmur can be due to normal heart function (termed innocent, benign, or transitional). Or, it can be due to a structural defect of the heart or great blood vessels coming off of the heart (termed pathologic). The type of noise, location of the noise, and other abnormalities found on physical examination help determine the cause of the murmur. All murmurs do not require an echocardiogram and a cardiologist evaluation to determine the cause.

Hemangioma. See Strawberry Hemangioma.

Hemolytic Uremic Syndrome. (Also known as HUS). A group of medical problems caused by some food poisoning (E coli, Shigella) infections. The problems include severe anemia, low platelet count, and kidney failure. HUS typically occurs in children ages four months to four years of age.

Hemophilia. A genetically inherited blood clotting disorder. People with this disorder lack a chemical clotting "factor" that impairs the body's chain reaction to clot blood when bleeding occurs. In general, this is a disease of males and women are only carriers (i.e. not affected) because the gene for the disorder is on the "X" chromosome.

Henoch-Schonlein Purpura. See Immunoglobulin A Vasculitis.

Hernia. The term used to describe a bulging out of tissue or organ where it is not supposed to be. It occurs due to a weakness of a muscle wall. The most common types include:
Diaphragmatic hernia—abdominal organs protrude into chest
Femoral hernia—intestines protrude into thigh
Inguinal hernia—intestines protrude into groin
Umbilical hernia—intestines protrude into belly button
The risk of all hernias is that the organ that is bulging out will get stuck in that position and cut off the blood supply to it. Umbilical hernias rarely get stuck (incarcerate), thus rarely require any treatment.

Hemorrhagic disease of the newborn. See Vitamin K Deficiency Bleeding.

Hindmilk. Another breastfeeding term. This refers to the fattier milk that comes out after several minutes of nursing. This milk can actually look yellow (like fat). Don't be alarmed—it's good stuff.

Hip dysplasia. Also known as congenital hip dysplasia, or developmental dysplasia of the hip. This is a congenital abnormality where the leg bone is out of its socket at the hip. It is easily treated with a brace if detected in the first few months of life. Babies who are **breech** have a slightly higher risk of having this disorder.

Hirschprung's disease. A congenital abnormality where the nerves of the rectum (intestinal exit) don't form. As a result, newborns cannot poop (stool) without assistance. Infants with severe constipation may have a partial defect and are also tested for this disorder. Treatment is surgical.

Histamine. A chemical compound the body produces in an allergic response. Histamine causes the characteristic "allergy symptoms" that people experience such as hives, itchy eyes, and congestion.

Human Papilloma Virus (HPV). A virus that is transmitted through sexual contact. HPV can live in the undersurface of the foreskin of an uncircumcised man. HPV is also a known factor in the development of cervical cancer in women.

Hydrocele. A fluid collection in a boy's scrotum. Rarely, it is associated with a **hernia**. Most of the time, the fluid is present at birth and goes away on its own by six months of life. It makes the boy's scrotum look unusually large.

Hydrocephalus. An abnormally large collection of cerebrospinal fluid (CSF), the fluid that bathes the brain and spinal cord. This can be caused by excessive production, blockage of the collection pathway, or decreased absorption in the body. Symptoms include: bulging fontanelle (soft spot), headache, vomiting, enlarged head size, loss of developmental milestones, and abnormal neurologic exam.

Hypospadias. A congenital abnormality where the urethra (tube that connects the bladder to the outside) opening is on the underside of the penis instead of in the middle. This requires surgical repair, usually after six months of age. Because the foreskin is used to perform the repair, these babies are not circumcised.

Hypothyroidism. A poorly functioning thyroid gland produces a suboptimal level of thyroid hormone. Thyroid hormone is an essential chemical needed for body metabolism. Babies with congenital hypothyroidism can become intellectually disabled if they are not treated. This is one of the screening tests performed in the state metabolic screen. The incidence of congenital hypothyroidism is one in

4000 newborns.

Idiopathic Thrombocytopenic Purpura (ITP). The destruction of platelets due to an autoimmune response in the body. Can occur after a viral illness. Because platelets are needed to clot blood, a low count causes bruising and **petechiae**. Some children need medication to help the body increase platelet production in the body, others bounce back on their own. The good news is that almost 90% of kids do beautifully and have no further problems after the one episode.

Immunoglobulin A Vasculitis. (Formerly known as Henoch-Schonlein Purpura). Inflammation of the blood vessels (vasculitis) after a viral illness. Symptoms include a dramatic rash of raised bruised areas on the legs. Joint pain, abdominal pain, and blood in the urine also occur. Although the disease sounds and looks serious, 90% of children recover completely without any treatment. Occurs mostly in children aged four to 10 years.

Imperforate Anus. A congenital abnormality where the anus (opening of the intestines to the outside) does not form completely. This abnormality is often associated with a combination of abnormalities called VATER syndrome. It is repaired surgically.

Inflammatory Bowel Disease (IBD). Chronic swelling of the intestinal lining that results in bloody diarrhea. Crohn's Disease and Ulcerative Colitis are types of IBD. It is rare for a child under age two years to be diagnosed with this disorder.

Inguinal hernia. (see **hernia**)

Inhaled steroid. Medication used to control chronic asthma symptoms. The medication is administered via a machine that aerosolizes it (nebulizer) or via a hand-held "inhaler." The inhaled method is preferable because most of the medication goes to the location it is intended to help (i.e. the lungs). Very little of the medicine gets absorbed into the bloodstream—this means there is less of the unwanted side effects and more therapeutic benefit.

Intestinal obstruction. This is a general term to describe the blockage of the intestine. The gastrointestinal tract is like a big pipe, and in these terms, obstruction is a clogged pipe. This can occur due to intussusception, volvulus, malrotation (congenital defect), and hernias. Because the area is blocked, blood flow to the intestines decreases and may cause death of that tissue. This is a surgical emergency or an "acute abdomen." Symptoms include distended belly, vomiting bile.

Intraventricular hemorrhage (IVH). Bleeding within the brain area called the ventricles due to a weak, fragile matrix of blood vessels and blood pressure changes in premature babies. Premature babies born before 32 weeks gestation or less than three pounds are at risk for IVH, which most often occurs in the first five days of life. Some bleeds may be minor and have no significant long term consequences. Severe bleeds can be potentially fatal or have significant neurologic effects.

Intussusception. When a piece of intestine telescopes upon itself creating an intestinal obstruction. The most common time this occurs is between six and 18 months of age. Symptoms include intermittent abdominal pain with pulling up of the legs. Vomiting, and poop that looks like "currant jelly" also occur. This is an emergency. Diagnosis (and treatment) can be done with a special radiological study.

Jaundice. Yellowing of the skin and the whites of the eyes due to a collection of body garbage called bilirubin. The newborn period is a unique time in life that causes a "normal" jaundice. Outside of the newborn period, jaundice is NOT normal. It requires a thorough medical evaluation to look for the cause.

Kawasaki Disease. An illness that causes the body's blood vessels to swell (vasculitis). The cause is unknown. Occurs mostly in children under two years of age. Symptoms include: fever for five or more days straight, rash on the palms and soles, peeling skin on the fingertips, pink eye, bright red lips/tongue, swollen lymph nodes in the neck, general body rash, and irritable mood. The most severe complication is swelling of the arteries that supply the heart (coronary artery aneurysm). This disease is one of the reasons that doctors want to see a child who has had a fever for five consecutive days or more.

Kernicterus. See Bilirubin Induced Neurologic Dysfunction.

Labial adhesion. A condition where the labia minora (smaller lips) of the vaginal opening get stuck together. This happens in little girls because they do not make estrogen hormone yet (pre-puberty). The amount of tissue that is stuck can vary. The problem is that the urethra (opening for the bladder) is located beneath the labia. If the lips are almost completely fused shut, estrogen cream (RX) is applied so that the urine can flow out more easily. Once the labia are unstuck, it is prudent to put Vaseline on the area at diaper changes to prevent them from re-sticking. All girls outgrow this condition once they hit puberty.

Laryngomalacia. A floppy airway. Some babies are born with relaxed throat tissue. When they breathe in, they make a high pitched squeaky noise (**stridor**). Babies outgrow this condition, often by age one. These babies get evaluated by an ear, nose, and throat specialist just to confirm the diagnosis. It does not affect their breathing and no treatment is needed.

Leukemia. Abnormal production of body's blood cells which then leads to failure of the bone marrow to produce normal blood cells necessary for body functioning. Symptoms include: fever, fatigue, paleness of the skin, excessive bruising, **petechiae**, and joint pain.

Macrocephaly. Official term to describe a big head. Most of the time, a child's big head is due to their genes (i.e. someone else in the family has a big head). But, if the head size percentile is enlarging or if there are other concerning symptoms, a doctor may evaluate the head with an imaging study to rule out **hydrocephalus** or a **brain tumor**.

Malabsorption. When the intestine is not performing its job of digesting food. The result is a watery, foul smelling diarrhea. Some causes of chronic malabsorption are **celiac disease** and **cystic fibrosis**. This deserves to be checked out.

Malrotation. A congenital abnormality in the development of the intestines. The abnormal position creates a problem with blood flow to the intestines as well as potential for obstruction of food transit. Newborns with this problem have vomiting, constipation, and abdominal pain. Treatment is surgical.

Masturbation. A normal behavior of exploring one's sexual organs. Both boys and girls do it.

Meconium. The first poop a newborn passes. Black, tarry, sticky. Some babies will pass this first poop before birth during a stressful labor. If the meconium is seen prior to birth, a baby will have their nose, mouth, and throat suctioned at delivery to prevent passage of this stuff into the lungs (called **meconium aspiration syndrome**).

Meconium ileus. A failure of the newborn's poop (**meconium**) to pass because of abnormally thick intestinal secretions. This condition is associated with **cystic fibrosis**.

Meconium plug. A delay in passing of the newborn's first poop (**meconium**). This usually responds to rectal stimulation (e.g. taking a rectal temperature).

Meningitis. Inflammation of the tissues that line the brain and the spinal cord. This can be caused by a virus, bacteria, or by tuberculosis. Symptoms include: headache, vomiting, TRUE IRRITABILITY (i.e. inconsolable), bulging fontanelle (soft spot), fever, neck stiffness, seizures, **petechiae**. This is a medical emergency.

Metabolic disorder. A broad term that describes disorders in breaking down foods (see metabolic storage disease below). These disorders are different than endocrine disorders, which involve abnormal levels of body hormones (e.g. thyroid disease, diabetes, adrenal disease).

Metabolic Storage Disease (Inborn Errors of Metabolism). A group of diseases that all cause an inability to break down certain food products. As a result, byproducts of metabolism accumulate. In some of these disorders this accumulation goes to body parts (liver, heart, brain, kidney, eye) causing permanent damage or even death. The more common storage diseases are tested for on the state metabolic screens (**PKU, galactosemia**).

Microcephaly. The technical term for a small head. Head size is often hereditary. Families with small heads have small headed babies. However, if a child's head size percentile is plateauing or decreasing, an imaging study may be done to look for **craniosynostosis**.

Milk protein allergy. Milk contains protein, sugar, and fat. Some babies (about 2%) have an allergy to the protein component that causes inflammation and irritation of the intestine lining. This leads to diarrhea that can be mixed with blood or mucous. A significant percentage of babies who are allergic to milk protein are also allergic to soy protein. The good news—most kids outgrow this problem.

Milia. A normal newborn rash on the nose that look like pinpoint white dots. These go away on their own.

Miliaria. A normal newborn rash that looks like prickly heat. This goes away on its own.

Mongolian Spots. A bruise like discoloration found on the buttocks of darker pigmented newborns. These spots fade over several years. No treatment is needed.

Murmur. (see heart murmur)

Nasolacrimal Duct Obstruction (blocked tear duct). Babies have narrow tear ducts that lead out to the corner of the eyes. Occasionally, the tube gets clogged. Tears, which are usually watery, get thick from being backed up. The result—goopy fluid that comes out of the eyes. This can happen intermittently for the first year of life. You can help open up the duct by massaging gently just below the corner of the eye near the nose. I usually refer patients to an eye doctor if this is happening beyond a year of age. The difference between blocked tear ducts and pink eye (infection) is that the eye is not red or irritated.

Natal Teeth. Every once in a blue moon, a baby is born with a tooth. These usually fall out spontaneously and the real baby teeth come in at the normal time, between 6-12 months.

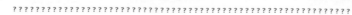
Nevus Flammeus (Stork bite, angel kiss). These are newborn birthmarks located at the nape of the neck, eyelids, and forehead. They are bright pink in color. The marks on the face fade over the first year of life. The marks on the neck can last forever. These marks are not associated with cancer.

Neural tube defects. A congenital abnormality of the brain/spinal cord development. Many of these disorders can be detected prenatally via an abnormal AFP test or an ultrasound. These disorders vary in severity. The most severe form is lack of brain formation (anencephaly). The least severe form is **spina bifida occulta** (see **sacral dimple**), where there is completely normal nerve function.

Neurofibromatosis (NF). A genetic disorder (gene defect) that causes tumors of the tissue covering nerves. Babies are often born without symptoms, although some will have three or more **cafe au lait spots** at birth. As a child grows, they develop numerous (more than five) cafe au lait spots and freckles in the armpit and groin areas. The tumors on the nerves grow later and can be seen as large bumps under the skin. Most of these tumors are benign (not cancerous), but can occur in dangerous places (e.g. eye, ear, brain, kidney). Children with this disorder are seen regularly by a number of doctors. FYI: The diagnosis of NF is not made on the presence of cafe au lait spots alone—this is only one of several symptoms and signs. Most children with a few cafe au lait spots do not have NF.

Newborn acne. (see acne)

Newborn nasal congestion. All newborns have snotty noses. They will sneeze, snort, cough, and snore. This lasts for four to six weeks. If it does not interfere with feedings or sleep, do nothing. If it is causing a problem, use saline nose drops to flush the nose before feedings or bedtime.

Nursing caries. These are cavities—the result of feeding a baby during the night after their teeth come in. If you don't wipe teeth off after a midnight snack of breast milk/formula/milk (which all contain sugar), the sugar will sit on the teeth and make a nice place for plaque and subsequent cavities.

Omphalitis. A belly button infection. The umbilical stump and skin surrounding it looks red and swollen. There is a foul odor coming from it. If this occurs in a newborn, it usually requires admission to a hospital for intravenous (IV) antibiotics.

Orbital cellulitis. A serious infection that involves the tissue surrounding the eye. It is caused by a sinus infection that spreads into the area. Symptoms include: limited eye motion, bulging of the eyeball, eyelid swelling, eye pain, and fever. This is the reason that doctors want to see children who have eyelid swelling and a fever.

Orthotic. A custom-made shoe insert designed by a podiatrist to provide arch support for people who are flat-footed. The AAP does not currently recommend orthotics for babies and young children.

Otitis media. Literally, middle ear inflammation. Acute otitis media refers to an active infection that came up shortly before it is diagnosed in the office. Serous otitis media (or otitis media with effusion) refers to residual fluid that remains after the active infection is over.

Otitis externa. (Otherwise known as swimmer's ear) Literally, external ear inflammation. This is really an infection of the skin that lines the ear canal. It is caused by water that pools in the ear canal and allows germs to grow. Symptoms include pain with touching the ear itself, swelling and redness of the canal, and sometimes a fever. This is uncommon in the under one age group.

? ?

GLOSSARY

Paraphimosis. The foreskin gets stuck behind the head of the penis in an uncircumcised boy. This causes lots of swelling and pain.

Pathologic Heart Murmur. (see Heart Murmur)

Penile adhesions. The head of the penis sticks to the shaft skin. In boys who are circumcised, it is important to visualize the edge of the head at diaper changes and clean the area of any debris (smegma). If the skin starts to get stuck together, try gently pulling down at the base of the penis to separate the area.

Perforated eardrum. Occurs with severe middle ear infection. A small hole in the eardrum lets the pus drain. It is the equivalent of a pimple popping and draining. Pus and blood will be seen draining out of the ear canal.

Periodic breathing. Newborns do not breathe in a regular pattern. They breathe 30 to 60 times a minute, but very erratically. There may be a stretch of several pants in a row, then a long p-a-u-s-e, then a big breath. That is normal, as long as that pause is less than ten seconds.

Phenylketonuria (PKU). A metabolic disorder routinely tested on the state metabolic screen. It is a genetic defect in an enzyme that breaks down phenylalanine. The incidence is one in 10,000. People with this disorder need to have a special diet. See **metabolic storage disease**.

Phimosis. Inability to pull the foreskin of an uncircumcised boy's penis back. In severe cases, circumcision is necessary to fix the problem.

Phototherapy. The term used for treatment of moderate-severe jaundice (hyperbilirubinemia). A jaundiced baby is placed in a blue light source (either via "bili" blanket or bank of lights). The lights help to break-down the bilirubin. For babies who are mildly jaundiced, we do NOT recommend placing an undressed baby near a sunny window in the house. It doesn't help and makes the baby uncomfortable.

Pneumonia. Lung inflammation caused primarily by infection. Both viruses and bacteria can cause pneumonia. The tiny air sacs (alveoli) fill up with pus and prevent air exchange. Symptoms include fever, cough, chest pain, and respiratory distress.

Polydactyly. When there are more than five fingers or toes on a hand or a foot. The extra digit can be removed.

Port wine stain. This is a large, red/purple, flat birthmark that occurs on one side of the face or limb. These do not fade over time and are mostly a cosmetic issue. If the birthmark covers the eyelid, a child is evaluated for glaucoma. Any time it occurs on the forehead or eye, a child is also evaluated for a brain abnormality (**Sturge-Weber syndrome**).

Posterior urethral valves. A congenital defect of the formation of the urethra (tube that connects the bladder to the outside). There are valves that normally push the urine (pee) outwards. In this condition, the valves push the urine backwards into the urinary tract. This is rare, and only occurs in boys.

Post-tussive emesis. The Latin words for "after-cough" vomiting. Babies and young children have over-active gag reflexes. So a forceful cough might bring up lunch. All vomiting in children is not due to an upset stomach.

Preauricular pits and tags. Minor congenital defects of the formation of the external ear. The pits are due to remnants of a cyst that occurred prior to birth. Pits are rarely associated with hearing disorders. The tags are extra pieces of skin. If severe, these can be removed for cosmetic reasons.

Pseudostrabismus. The false appearance that a child looks cross-eyed or has a lazy eye due to the child's facial structure. Babies and young children are often referred to a pediatric ophthalmologist for concerns of a lazy eye (**esotropia, amblyopia**) and are ultimately diagnosed with this benign entity. But, it is better to be on the safe side and check out any concerns.

Pustular melanosis. A normal newborn rash found in darker pigmented babies. The original rash looks like little pimples. As the lesions fade, they leave a temporary brown freckle. Some babies have hundreds of these freckles. They go away on their own.

Pyelonephritis. An infection of the kidneys. In an acute infection, a child has fever, back pain, and pain with urination. Infants under two months of age with a bladder infection routinely get admitted to the hospital because there is a greater risk of the infection extending into the kidneys.

Pyloric stenosis. A narrowing of the outlet from the stomach to the small intestine due to a congenital abnormality in the muscle (pylorus). Babies (more commonly males) will have projectile (REALLY IMPRESSIVE) vomiting at every feeding starting between two and four weeks of life. The vomiting may start out in a small way, but progressively gets worse and more projectile. Delay in seeking medical attention results in dehydration. Treatment is surgical, by making a cut in the muscle.

Refractive errors. This fancy term means that one cannot focus an image perfectly in the eye (retina). It includes near-sightedness, far-sightedness, astigmatism, and amblyopia.

Respiratory Distress. This is the term used to describe a child who is air-hungry. If a child cannot successfully get enough oxygen in with each breath, they will breathe faster, heavier, and use chest wall muscles to get as much air in as possible. This equates to a child who is panting, grunting, flaring his nostrils, and retracting (sucking in of the ribcage).

Respiratory Syncytial Virus (RSV). This is a virus that causes different symptoms depending on the age, and health status of the person. Healthy adults may have an RSV infection and feel like they have a cold. A premature baby may have complete respiratory collapse and need hospitalization. A healthy six-month-old may have a ton of nasal secretions, wheeze, and breathe at twice their normal respiratory rate but not have any distress. RSV shows up every year between November and April in the northern hemisphere.

Retinoblastoma. A malignant tumor of the eye that occurs in babies. Fortunately, this is quite rare. This is one of the important reasons we do an eye exam in the nursery.

Retinopathy of Prematurity (ROP). Incomplete growth of blood vessels in the eyes due to premature birth. Babies born at less than 32 weeks gestation are at the greatest risk of ROP. The growth of the blood vessels need to be monitored regularly by a pediatric ophthalmologist to head off any abnormalities, such as retinal folding/detachment, or permanent vision defects.

Retractions. The term used to describe the sucking in of the ribcage when a child has **respiratory distress**. Retractions occur when the body starts using the chest wall muscles to pull more air in with each breath. With phone encounters, we will ask you to look at how your child is breathing to tell us if they have retractions.

Rickets. Malformation of growing bones in children most commonly due to Vitamin D deficiency. Vitamin D is necessary for calcium to be deposited into the bone (which makes them hard). Bones will form with a bent shape because they are softer than they should be.

Ringworm. (see fungal infections in Chapter 13, "Infections")

Rooting reflex. This is a newborn 'primitive' reflex that causes a baby to turn their head if you stroke their cheek. It is an instinctive mechanism that encourages eating. Babies lose this primitive reflex by three to six months of age.

Sacral dimple. This is a tiny divot, or dimple in the lower portion of the back. These can be associated with a minor abnormality of neural tube development called spina bifida occulta. The L5-S1 vertebrae bone is slightly abnormal but the spinal cord (nerve) is formed normally. Most babies with sacral dimples are unaffected and do not need evaluation or treatment.

Seborrhea. (Also known as dandruff, cradle cap) A skin problem that causes greasy, flaky, and sometimes red skin in areas where 'sebaceous glands' reside—typically the scalp, ears, beside the nose, eyebrows. Many babies are afflicted with this and outgrow it. Teenagers can also get seborrhea and have it for a lifetime. Treatment includes anti-dandruff shampoos, low potency steroid creams/lotions, and vegetable oil to loosen up the flakes in the scalp.

Sensory Processing Disorder. A constellation of behaviors stemming from an inability to process and adapt to stimuli of the five senses. Children with this disorder have trouble with activities of daily living and social encounters (aversion to textured foods, dislike of socks and tags on clothing, avoidance of messy activities, avoidance of being touched...) Diagnosis occurs most frequently in pre-school or school aged children.

Serous otitis media. Fluid in the middle ear space. This fluid can be present several weeks to months after an acute infection (i.e. ACUTE otitis media). This fluid is sterile (free of bugs), but has the potential to get re-infected. Antibiotics are not usually necessary or helpful to clear the fluid.

Shoulder dystocia. This refers to a difficult delivery where the shoulders are forcefully pulled to get the baby out. This happens to a mom with a small pelvis or a big baby. Occasionally, the collar bone (clavicle) breaks during delivery. It heals nicely without any residual problems.

Sickle cell anemia. A hereditary abnormality of the red blood cell structure, causing impaired oxygen carrying capacity and increased destruction of the red blood cells.

Sinusitis. (see Chapter 13, "Infections")

Skin tags. These are tiny pieces of raised skin that can occur anywhere on the body. In the newborn, they are most frequently found in front of the ear (**preauricular tag**) or on the vagina. They are not problematic and require no intervention.

Spina Bifida. A congenital abnormality of the spinal cord development. There is a spectrum of severity of the defect. Most severe defects cause paralysis of the legs and body parts supplied by the affected

? ?

GLOSSARY

nerves (bowel, bladder function). The incidence of spina bifida is decreasing as more women are taking pre-natal vitamins (folic acid) during pregnancy. See **neural tube defects.**

Stevens-Johnson Syndrome. A serious allergic reaction that can be fatal.

Strabismus. An abnormal alignment of the eyes.

Strawberry Hemangioma. A birthmark made of a collection of blood vessels. The vessels grow and enlarge for the first few years of life. So, the birthmark gets bigger. The good news—the vessels shrink up and disappear, usually by age five years. Surgery is usually not done to remove these. However, laser therapy may be helpful for lesions on the eyes, nose, or lips. Cool trend: using topical medication to shrink the blood vessels.

Stridor. A squeaky, high pitched noise with breathing in that can be heard without a stethoscope. In newborns, it is usually caused by **laryngomalacia.** In any other situation, it is a sign of respiratory distress at the level of the throat. Children with severe **croup** infection have a very swollen airway if they have stridor. If your child has stridor, call your doctor immediately.

Stork Bites. see Nevus Flammeus

Sturge Weber syndrome. A serious disorder that includes brain abnormalities in combination with a port wine stain on the face. Brain atrophy, seizures, and paralysis can occur.

Subconjunctival hemorrhage. Broken blood vessel on the surface of the eye. Most often, this occurs in a newborn after delivery. It's not serious (even though it can look worrisome to a new parent). It can take a few weeks to resolve on its own.

Supranumerary nipple (accessory nipple). These are extra, nonfunctional nipples found along the same vertical line as the nipples themselves. They are not problematic. They can be removed for cosmetic reasons.

Supraventricular Tachycardia (SVT). The heart beats at an extraordinarily faster pace (over 200 beats per minute) because a faulty electrical circuitry in the heart. The abnormality may be detected if a baby appears pale, has trouble feeding, or is extremely irritable.

Syndactyly. Two or more fingers or toes are fused either partially or fully together. The severity of the defect determines whether treatment is required.

Thrush. (see Chapter 13, Infections)

Tongue-tied (see ankyloglossia)

TORCH infections. This is an acronym for the standard tests that are done in Mom's prenatal evaluation. They include: Toxoplasmosis, Syphilis, Rubella, Cytomegalovirus (CMV), Hepatitis B, HIV, and Herpes. In certain situations, Varicella (chickenpox) and Parvovirus are also tested. If Mom has been infected, or is a carrier of the Hepatitis B virus, her baby receives not only the Hepatitis B vaccine at birth, but also a shot of medicine to prevent passage of infection.

Torticollis. Literally means, "twisted neck." When it occurs in newborns, (about 1 in 100 babies), it is called congenital torticollis. It occurs more commonly in babies who are born in breech presentation. It usually becomes noticeable by two to four weeks of age, when the baby's head appears tilted to one side. Occasionally, a knot is felt in the neck where the neck muscle is tensed and tightened. Rarely, these babies have other associated issues like hip dysplasia or strabismus. If left untreated, babies can develop asymmetry of the face and skull. Treatment includes muscle stretching exercises and encouraging the baby turn his head in the opposite direction.

Transient Tachypnea of the Newborn (TTN). A common cause of mild respiratory distress in the newborn. Fetuses swallow amniotic fluid while in the womb. When a baby is born vaginally, that fluid gets squeezed out as the baby passes through the birth canal and cries for the first time. Rarely, some of that fluid remains in babies delivered vaginally. More commonly, babies delivered by C-section have this problem. The good news is that the babies all do just fine. They breath faster than normal and may need a little oxygen for the first hour of life.

Transitional heart murmur. The term for a benign, flow murmur heard in the first 24 hours of life. As a baby is born, the fetal heart circulation changes over to the newborn circulation. There are a series of valves that close off the fetal blood pathways and open pathways to the lungs. We often hear the turbulence of blood flow as this is happening. It's nothing to worry about. If a murmur is heard after 24 hours of life, or has a different quality or location that it is heard, your doctor will evaluate it further.

Transmitted upper airway noise. Noise that comes from the nose that is heard and felt in the lungs. When there is a moderate amount of nasal congestion (snot) in the nose, the air going through it makes a loud noise as it passes through. Since babies and young children don't know how to blow their noses, this is often a unique occurrence in this age group.

Tuberculosis. (Known as TB. Previously known as "consumption"). Infectious lung disease that causes nodules in the lungs, but can spread to the lymph nodes and brain. The scary part of the disease is that people can be infected or be "carriers" of the infection without showing symptoms. People with active infection classically have fever, cough, weight loss, night sweats, and blood in the mucous they cough up. Although TB is less common than it used to be, it occurs in urban populations and immigrants from Asia, Africa, and Latin America.

Umbilical hernia. See **hernia.** These are very common in newborns, particularly African American babies. The size of the hernia can be quite large, but the intestine almost never (I've had one patient) gets stuck (incarcerated). These are caused by weak abdominal muscles which will get stronger as the baby starts using them. Most of these hernias resolve on their own. If the hernia is still present by age two, I'll refer a child to a pediatric surgeon for repair. Old Wives Tale: You do not need to bandage the hernia or place a coin on it to make it go away. Your baby will fix the problem when they start doing Ab crunches.

Undescended testes. Failure of the male sex organs to descend into the scrotum in the newborn male. (In fetal development, they grow in the pelvic area, then travel down to the scrotum.) Often, the testes will come down on their own by six months of life. If they don't, a surgical procedure is performed to affix the testes in the scrotum. Testes in the pelvis are at slightly higher risk for testicular cancer, and make it awfully difficult to perform a monthly self-testicular exam in that location.

Uric acid crystals. A waste product found in the urine. When the urine is concentrated (low water volume), the uric acid will pull itself out of the urine solution and can be found in crystal form in the diaper. It looks like brick dust and tends to alarm parents who think it is blood. It is an indication of mild dehydration—so aggressive feeding is the only treatment.

glossary

Urinary tract infections (UTI). An infection in the urinary bladder. It is difficult to diagnose a bladder infection in babies because they do not complain that it burns when they urinate. Sometimes fever and irritability are the only symptoms. It is a good idea to obtain a urine specimen on babies who have a fever with no obvious source of infection.

Vaginal discharge. Newborn girls often have vaginal discharge due to fluctuating hormone levels. Older girls who have vaginal discharge prior to puberty need to be evaluated for infection.

Ventricular Septal Defect (VSD). The most common type of congenital heart defect (abnormal formation of the heart in the fetus). In this defect, a hole is present in either the muscle wall or tissue between the two large chambers (ventricles) of the heart. A murmur is detected due to the blood flow that crosses between the chambers. Most of these holes close on their own with no medical intervention. Children with VSD's are followed by pediatric cardiologists until the hole closes.

Vernix. A cheesy, greasy white coating found on the skin of newborns. It will wash off at your baby's first bath.

Vesicles. Pinpoint, fluid filled blisters seen classically with chickenpox, shingles, and herpes infections. In chickenpox, these lesions appear in crops over a period of a few days.

Vesicoureteral reflux (VUR). An abnormality in the urinary tract system that causes urine to track backward towards the bladder and kidneys. This urine is not sterile, thus these children are predisposed to bladder and kidney infections. VUR is classified by the severity of how extensively the urine tracks in the wrong direction. Grade 1 is mildest and Grade 5 is the most severe. Many children outgrow this disorder, but it can take several years (up to age seven). Children with severe reflux (Grades 4-5) may need surgical repair to prevent scarring and permanent kidney damage. About 70% of children with Grade 3 reflux outgrow it on their own. Virtually all children with milder forms (Grades 1-2) outgrow VUR without any intervention. There is a hereditary predisposition to this disorder.

Vitamin K Deficiency Bleeding (VKDB). A relatively common (one in 200) problem of newborns who have a Vitamin K deficiency. Infants with this disorder can have severe bleeding. Because of this risk, all newborns receive a shot of Vitamin K shortly after they are born.

von Willebrand Disease. A genetically inherited bleeding disorder that affects both the platelets and the blood clotting chain reaction. People with this disorder have frequent, excessive nosebleeds, easy bruising, and heavy periods.

Whooping Cough. (See pertussis in Chapter 12, Vaccines.)

Yeast infection. (See thrush, yeast diaper rash in Chapter 13, Infections.)

References for this section are footnoted in Appendix F, Footnotes.

REFERENCES

RECOMMENDED READING, WEB SITES & MORE

Appendix E

Q. How do I know if an online resource or media platform has reliable medical information?

Yes, there are so many useful resources for people seeking healthcare information. But there are also many grifters and bots running misinformation machines. How do you tease out what is fact vs fiction? Here are a few thoughts:

1. Find out who has created the platform. Is there contact information?
2. What is the purpose of the platform?
3. Who are the experts giving the advice?
4. What references are cited? Citations should be listed from scientific journals. Original sources should be transparent and easy to find.
5. Be suspicious of information that is opinionated or seems biased. Look for several *reliable* sources that confirm and validate the content.
6. Be suspicious of products that are touted as cure-alls or miracles.
7. Make sure the information is current. The content should be reviewed/updated regularly.
Source: ImmunizationInfo.org

Reality Check
80% of people who Google for information online do not bother to check the source of the information they are reading. Know your source. Fact check before believing everything you read!

Reliable web sites

For starters, go to our website at baby411.com for a wealth of useful information, a visual library of rashes and diseases (see Bonus Material), parent chat room, and links to reliable websites (several of which are listed below).

Adoption

University of Minnesota, Adoption Clinic	adoption.umn.edu
Centers for Disease Control	cdc.gov/immigrantrefugeehealth/index.html

Allergies

American Academy of Allergy, Asthma, and Immunology	aaaai.org
Food Allergy Network	foodallergy.org
Allergy and Asthma Network	allergyasthmanetwork.org

Complementary Therapies

National Center for Complementary and Integrative Health	nccih.nih.gov

Breastfeeding

Kelly Mom	Kellymom.com
Dr. Jack Newman	breastfeedingonline.com
Drugs and Lactation Database	ncbi.nlm.nih.gov/books/NBK501922/

Cancer

National Cancer Institute	cancer.gov

Car Seats

National Highway Traffic Safety Administration	NHTSA.gov
American Academy of Pediatrics	HealthyChildren.org
National Safe Kids Campaign	safekids.org

Child Development

Centers for Disease Control	cdc.gov/actearly
Zero to Three	zerotothree.org

Cord blood banking

General info	parentsguidecordblood.com
National Marrow Donor	Bethematch.org

Diabetes

American Diabetes Association	diabetes.org

General medical information

American Academy of Pediatrics	aap.org
American Academy of Pediatrics for parents	healthychildren.org
Food and Drug Administration	fda.gov
Mayo Clinic	mayoclinic.com
Parents Magazine	parents.com
Centers for Disease Control	cdc.gov

Heart defects

Cincinnati Children's Hospital   cincinnatichildrens.org/patients/child/encyclopedia/defects

Lung Problems

American Academy of Allergy, Asthma, and Immunology   aaaai.org

Nutrition

Centers for Disease Control	cdc.gov
American Dietetic Association	eatright.org

Skin Disorders

National Eczema Association   nationaleczema.org

Supplemental Newborn Screening

March of Dimes	Marchofdimes.com
Mayo	mayoclinic.com

Travel Health

Centers for Disease Control   cdc.gov/travel

Vaccinations

American Academy of Pediatrics	HealthyChildren.org
Immunization Action Coalition	immunize.org
Centers for Disease Control	cdc.gov/vaccines/parents/index.html
Children's Hospital of Philadelphia	Chop.edu/centers-programs/vaccine-education-center

references

? ?

REFERENCES

National Organizations

*There is a support group for virtually every medical disease and syndrome. The organizations below should be able to link you to a specific organization to meet your particular needs.

American Academy of Pediatrics, healthychildren.org

Centers for Disease Control and Prevention, cdc.gov

Easter Seals, easter-seals.org

March of Dimes Birth Defects Foundation, modimes.org

National Center on Birth Defects and Developmental Disabilities, cdc.gov/ncbddd

ZERO to THREE: National Center for Infants, Toddlers, and Families. zerotothree.org

Growth Chart: Boys (Birth to 24 months)

Birth to 24 months: Boys
Length-for-age and Weight-for-age percentiles

NAME _____

RECORD # _____

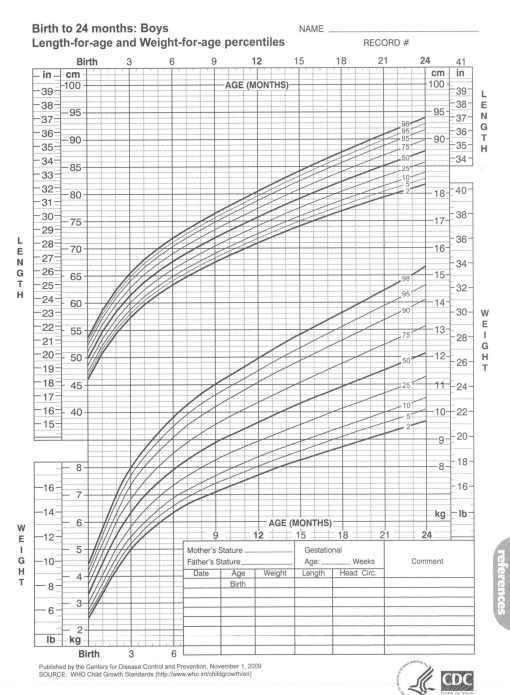

Published by the Centers for Disease Control and Prevention, November 1, 2009
SOURCE: WHO Child Growth Standards (http://www.who.int/childgrowth/en)

Growth Chart: Girls (Birth to 24 months)

Birth to 24 months: Girls
Length-for-age and Weight-for-age percentiles

NAME _____

RECORD # _____

Published by the Centers for Disease Control and Prevention, November 1, 2009
SOURCE: WHO Child Growth Standards (http://www.who.int/childgrowth/en)

Head Circumference: boys

Birth to 24 months: Boys
Head circumference-for-age and
Weight-for-length percentiles

NAME _____

RECORD # _____

Published by the Centers for Disease Control and Prevention, November 1, 2009
SOURCE: WHO Child Growth Standards (http://www.who.int/childgrowth/en)

REFERENCES

Head Circumference: girls

Birth to 24 months: Girls
Head circumference-for-age and
Weight-for-length percentiles

NAME _____

RECORD # _____

Published by the Centers for Disease Control and Prevention, November 1, 2009
SOURCE: WHO Child Growth Standards (http://www.who.int/childgrowth/en)

? ?

REFERENCES

Preemie growth chart

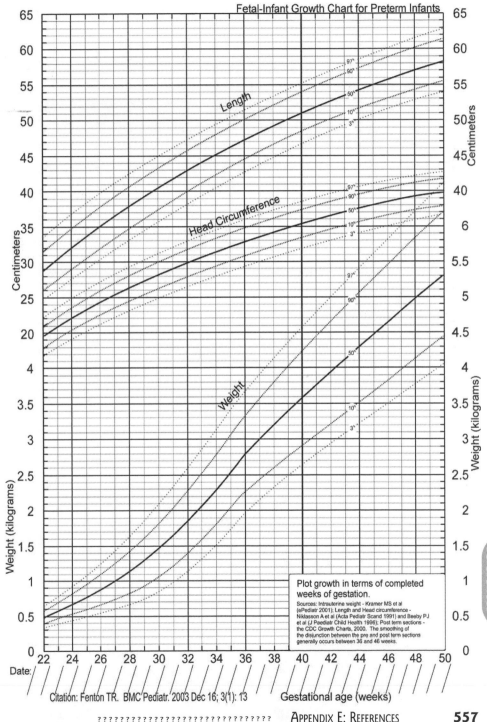

Fetal-Infant Growth Chart for Preterm Infants

Plot growth in terms of completed weeks of gestation.

Sources: Intrauterine weight - Kramer MS et al (ePediatr 2001); Length and Head circumference - Niklasson A et al (Acta Pediatr Scand 1991) and Beeby PJ et al (J Paediatr Child Health 1996); Post term sections - the CDC Growth Charts, 2000. The smoothing of the disjunction between the pre and post term sections generally occurs between 36 and 46 weeks.

Date:

Citation: Fenton TR. BMC Pediatr. 2003 Dec 16; 3(1): 13

Gestational age (weeks)

FOOTNOTES
Appendix F

Chapter 1: Birthday

Abrams SA. Calcium and phosphorus requirements in newborn infants. In Rose BD (Ed), UptoDate, Waltham, MA, 2007.

American Academy of Pediatrics Policy Statement: Initial medical evaluation of an adopted child. *Pediatrics* 1991; 88(3): 642-44.

American Academy of Pediatrics Section on hematology/oncology and section on allergy/immunology. Cord blood banking for potential future transplantation. *Pediatrics* 2007;119:165-170.

American Academy of Pediatrics Clinical Report: Late Preterm Infants: a population at risk. *Pediatrics* 2007;1389-1400.

AAP Task Force on Circumcision: Circumcision Policy Statement. Pediatrics Vol 130 (3) Sept 2012: 585-586.

American Academy of Pediatrics Policy Statement. Newborn and Infant Hearing Loss: Detection and Intervention. *Pediatrics* 1999; 103(2): 527-530.

American Association of Blood Banks. AABB.org. Accessed May 11, 2015.

American Urological Association. Circumcision. auanet.org/about/policy-statements/circumcision.cfm. Accessed May 11, 2015.

Auger N, etal. Neonatal phototherapy and future risk of childhood cancer. Int J Cancer. 2019 Oct 15;145(8):2061-2069.

Centers for Disease Control. CDC.gov. Accessed May 11, 2015.

Collins S, etal. Effects of circumcision on male sexual function: debunking a myth? J Urol 2002 May; 167 (5): 2111-12.

Foundation for the Accreditation of Cellular Therapy. FACTWebsite.org. Accessed May 11, 2015.

Hoffman B, etal. Unsafe from the start: critical misuse of car safety seats for newborns at initial hospital discharge. Abstract presentation, American Academy of Pediatrics, October 13, 2014. San Diego, CA.

Kim D, etal. The effect of male circumcision on sexuality. *BJU* Int 2006 Nov 28, PMID 17155977

Martinez F. The "coming of age" of the hygiene hypothesis. Respiratory Sciences Center, University of Arizona, Respiratory Research, April 2001.

Masood S, etal. Penile sensitivity and sexual satisfaction after circumcision: are we informing men correctly? *Urol Int.* 2005:75 (1): 62-6.

Melinda Gates interview, USA Today, April 2019)

Morris BJ, Krieger JN, Klausner JD. CDC's male circumcision recommendations represent a key public health measure. Glob Health Sci Pract. 2017;5(1):15-27.

Newman TB, etal. Childhood seizures after phototherapy. Pediatrics. Oct 2018 142 (4)

Pasquini, et al: The Likelihood of Hematopoietic Stem Cell Transplantation (HCT) in the United States: Implications for Umbilical Cord Blood Storage. American Academy of Pediatrics. *Pediatrics* 1999 July; 104 (1): 116.

Quinn TC. Circumcision and HIV Transmission. *Current Op In ID* 20(1).33-38 2007

Schulte R, etal. Rise in late onset vitamin K deficiency bleeding in young infants because of omission or refusal of prophylaxis at birth.Pediatr Neurol. 2014 Jun;50(6):564-8. Epub 2014 Feb 28.

Shaheed K. Monitoring growth of preterm NICU graduates. In Basow D (Ed), UptoDate, Waltham, MA, 2011.

Sturgeon PE. Care of the neonatal intensive care graduate. In Basow D (Ed), *UptoDate*, Waltham, MA, 2011.

Tobian AA, etal. Male circumcision for the prevention of HSV-2 and HPV infections and syphilis. *NEJM*.

2009;360(13):1298-309.

Wickremasinghe AC, etal. Neonatal phototherapy and infantile cancer. Pediatrics June 2016, 137 (6)

Wu, YW Risk of autism associated with hyperbilirubinema and phototherapy, pediatrics oct 2016 138 (4)OCT 2016 138 (4)

Chapter 2: You and Your Baby's Doc

American Academy of Pediatrics. AAP.org. Accessed May 11, 2015.

Chapter 3: Parenthood

Celedon, et al: Day care attendance, respiratory tract illnesses, wheezing, asthma, and total serum IgE level in early childhood. *Archives of Pediatric and Adolescent Medicine* 2002; 156: 241-245.

Huston AC, Aronson, SR: Mothers' Time With Infant and Time in Employment as Predictors of Mother-Child Relationships and Children's Early Development. *Child Development* 2005;76 (2):467-482.

Kamper-Jorgensen M, etal. Population-based study of the impact of childcare attendance and hospitalizations for acute respiratory infections. *Pediatrics* 2006;118:1439-1446.

Chapter 4: Hygiene

American Academy of Pediatrics. Guidelines for Perinatal Care. 5th Ed. Elk Grove Village, IL: 2002

American Academy of Pediatrics Policy Statement: Oral Hygiene. *Pediatrics* 2003; 111(5): 1113-1116.

American Academy of Pediatrics. Sun Safety. HealthyChildren.org. Accessed Feb 20, 2022.

Baron ED, etal. Selection of sunscreen and sunprotective measures. In UpToDate, Post TW (Ed), UpToDate, Waltham, MA. (Accessed on Sept 1, 2017)

Chang WU etal. Six children with allergic contact dermatitis to methylisothiazolinone in wet wipes (baby wipes). Pediatrics 2014; 133 (2) e434-438.

Fradin, MS: Comparative efficacy of insect repellant against mosquito bites. *New England Journal of Medicine* 2002; 347: 13-18.

Integrated Management of Pregnancy and Childbirth. Pregnancy, Childbirth, Postpartum and Newborn Care: A guide for essential practice. World Health Organization. 2nd Ed. 2006.

Wall Street Journal May 20, 2003. PD8.

Witorsch RJ, etal. Personal care products and endocrine disruption. A critical review of the literature. Crit Rev Toxicol 2010 Nov 40 suppl.

Zupan J, etal. Topical umbilical cord care at birth. *Cochrane Database Syst Rev* 2004;(3):CD001057.

Chapter 5: Nutrition & Growth

American Dental Association. ADA.org, Fluoride and Infant Formula Frequently Asked Questions, indexed 3/22/07.

American Academy of Pediatrics Clinical Report. Persing J, etal. prevention and management of positional skull deformities in infants. *Pediatrics* 2003;112(1):199-202.

American Academy of Pediatrics Committee on Nutrition: Pediatric Nutrition Handbook, 7th Ed. Elk Grove Village, IL, 2013.

American Academy of Pediatrics Section on Breastfeeding. Breastfeeding and the use of human milk. *Pediatrics.* 2012;129:e827-e841

Baker RD, Greer FR, and AAP Committee on Nutrition. Diagnosis and prevention of iron deficiency and iron-deficiency anemia in infants and young children (0-3 years of age) *Pediatrics* 2010;126:1040-1050.

Behrman, RE. Editor: Nelson Essentials of Pediatrics. Philadelphia: WB Saunders, 1990.

Bernbaum JC. Primary Care of the Preterm Infant. St. Louis: Mosby,1993.

CDC accessed May 1, 2019

Gartner LM, et al: American Academy of Pediatrics. Prevention of rickets and Vitamin D deficiency. New guidelines for Vitamin D intake. *Pediatrics* 2003;111(4):908-910.

Hollis BW, etal. Maternal versus infant vitamin D supplementation during lactation: a randomized controlled trial. Pediatrics 2015. Oct 136 (4) 625-34.

Huh SY, etal. Timing of solid food introduction and risk of obesity in preschool aged children. *Pediatrics* 2011;127:e544-e551.

Institute of Medicine, 2010 iom.edu/Reports/2010/Dietary-Reference-Intakes-for-Calcium-and-Vitamin-D.aspx

Nield LS, etal. Odd skull shapes: head's up on diagnosis and therapy. *Consultation for Pediatricians.*

November 2006:701-709.

Taylor SN, etal. Vitamin D: benefits for bone, and beyond. *Contemporary Pediatrics* 2006;23(11):70-82.

Van Wijk RM, etal. Helmet therapy in infants with positional skull deformation: randomized controlled trial. BMJ 2014;348:g2741.

West D. Lowmilksupply.org. Accessed February 15, 2015.

Chapter 6: Liquids

American Academy of Pediatrics Committee on Nutrition: Soy protein-based formulas: recommendations for use in infant feeding. *Pediatrics* 1998;101:148-153.

American Heart Association, etal. Dietary guidelines for children and adolescents: a guide for practitioners. *Pediatrics* 2006;117(2):544-59.

Bazzano AN, etal. A review of herbal and pharmaceutical galactogogues for breastfeeding. Oschner J. 2016 Winter. 16 (4): 511-524.

Barnes GR, Lethin AN, Jackson EB, et al. Management of breastfeeding. *JAMA*.1953;151:192.

Calello DP, etal. MMWR. Notes from the Field: Vitamin D deficient rickets and severe hypocalcemia in infants fed a homemade alkaline diet formula-Three states. August 2020-Feb 2021. Weekly/August 20, 2021/70(33);1124–1125

Centers for Disease Control. E. sakazakii infections associated with the use of powdered infant formula-Tennessee 2001. *MMWR* 2002;51:297-300.

Centers for Disease Control, Breastfeeding Report Card 2015. CDC.gov accessed May 11. 2015.

Chandran L. Is there a role for long-chain polyunsaturated fatty acids in infant nutrition? *Contemporary Pediatrics* 2003;20(2):107-124.

Danner SC. Breastfeeding the neurologically impaired infant. Waco, TX: *NAACOGS Clin Issu Peri Womens Health Nurs.* 1992;3(4):640-6.

Georgieff M. Taking a rational approach to the choice of formula. *Contemporary Pediatrics* 2001;18(8):112-130.

Hernell, O, etal. Clinical benefits of MFGM for infants and children. J Peds 2016; 173S:S60.5.

Heyman MB, Abrams SA, AAP Committee on Nutrition. Fruit juice in infants, children, and adolescents: current recommendations. Pediatrics June 2017 139 (6)

Huggins K: The Nursing Mother's Companion. Third Revised Ed. Boston: The Harvard Common Press, 1995.

Human Milk Banking Association of North America, February 2011

Jasani B, etal. Long chain polyunsaturated fatty acid supplementation in infants born at term. Cochrane Database of Systematic Reviews March 2017 DOI: 10.1002/14651858.CD000376.pub4

LactMed, Cannabis. Drugs and Lactation Database. November 2021. https://www.ncbi.nlm.nih.gov/books/NBK501587/

Lawrence, RA: Breastfeeding: A Guide for the Medical Profession, 5th ed. St. Louis: Mosby, 1999.

Montgomery-Downs HE, etal. Infant feeding methods and maternal sleep and daytime functioning. *Pediatrics* 2010 DOI: 10.1542/peds 2010-1269.

Mueller NT, etal. The infant microbiome development: mom matters. Trends Mol Med. 2015 Feb 21 (2): 109-117

O'Connor NR, etal. Pacifiers and breastfeeding: a systematic review. *Arch Pediatr Adolesc Med* 2009;163(4):378-382.

Perez SE, etal. Human Sars-CoV-2 Antibodies up to six months after vaccination. Pediatrics (2022) 149 (2): e2021054260.

Riordan J, Auerbach KG. Breastfeeding and Human Lactation. Sudbury: Jones and Bartlett Publishers, 1999.

Sampson, HA. Food Allergy, Part 1. Immunopathogenesis and clinical disorders. *J Allergy Clin Immunol* 1999; 103:717-28.

Sicherer S, etal. Maternal consumption of peanut during pregnancy is associated with peanut sensitization in atopic infants. *JACI* 2010;126(6):1191-1197.

Suitor CW. Nutrition care during pregnancy and lactation: new guidelines from the IOM. *J Am Diet Assoc* 1993;93:478.

Vennemann MM, etal. Does breastfeeding reduce the risk of Sudden Infant Death Syndrome? *Pediatrics* 2009;123(3):e406-e410.

Weizman Z, etal. Effect of a probiotic infant formula on infections in child care centers: comparison of two probiotic agents. *Pediatrics* 2005;115(1):5-9.

West D. Physician's Breastfeeding Triage Tool Kit. International Lactation Consultant Association. Copyright 2006. Adapted with permission.

Chapter 7: Solids

American Academy of Pediatrics Committee on Nutrition: *Pediatric Nutrition Handbook*, 6th Ed. Elk Grove Village, IL, 2009.
Bird JA, etal. Prevention of food allergy: beyond peanut. JACI 2019;143:545-7.
Celiac Disease Foundation, Celiac.org accessed May 4, 2019.
Du Toit G, etal. Early consumption of peanuts in infancy is associated with a low prevalence of peanut allergy. *JACI* 2008;122(5):984-91.
Du Toit G, et al. Randomized trial of peanut consumption in infants at risk for peanut allergy. N Engl J Med. 2015;372:803-813
Eigenmann PA, et al: Prevalence of IgE mediated food allergy among children with atopic dermatitis. *Pediatrics* 1998;101(3):e8.
Fleisher DM, etal. Primary prevention of allergic disease through nutritional interventions. JACI 2013; V1(1):29-36.
Greer FR, etal. Effects on early nutritional interventions on the development of atopic disease in infants and children: the role of maternal dietary restriction, breastfeeding, timing of introduction of complementary foods, and hydrolyzed formulas. *Pediatrics* Jan 2008;121:183-191.
Hill ID. Celiac disease in children. In: UpToDate, Basow DS (Ed). UpToDate.com. Waltham, MA 2013.
Hsiao K, etal. Long term clinical and immunological effects of probiotic and peanut oral immunotherapy after treatment cessation: 4-year follow-up of a randomised, double-blind, placebo-controlled trial. The Lancet: Child and Adolescent Health. Volume 1, No. 2, p97–105, October 2017
Huh SY, etal. Timing of solid food introduction and risk of obesity in preschool-aged children. *Pediatrics* 2011;127:e544-e551.
National Food Allergy Survey 2009-10
NIAID. Guidelines for the diagnosis and management of food allergy in the U.S., December 2010.
Ruffner MA, etal. Food protein induced enterocolitis syndrome: insights from a large referral population. JACI 2013;1(4):343-49.
Sampson HA. Food allergy. *J Allergy Clin Immunol* 2003;111(12):540-547.
Sampson HA. Food-induced anaphylaxis. In *UpToDate*, Basow, DS (Ed), UpToDate, Waltham, MA, 2011
Snell-Bergeon JK, etal. Early childhood infections and the risk of islet autoimmunity: the diabetes autoimmunity study in the young (DAISY). *Diabetes Care.* 2012 Dec;35(12):2553-8.
Wood, RA. The natural history of food allergy. *Pediatrics* 2003;111(6):1631-1637.

Chapter 8: The Other End

American Urological Association. Pediatric VUR Clinical Practice Guidelines Panel. Report on the Management of VUR in Children.1996.
American Urological Association. Management and screening of primary vesicoureteral reflux in children. 2010.
Finnell SME, etal. Diagnosis and management of an initial UTI in febrile infants and young children. Pediatrics 2011;128(3):e749-770.
Friedman AL. Acute UTI. What you want to know. *Contemporary Pediatrics* 2008;25(10):68-75.
McClung HJ, et al: Constipation and dietary fiber intake in children. Pediatrics 1995;96:999-1001.
Nelson SP, etal. One-year followup of gastroesophageal reflux during infancy. *Pediatrics* 1998;102(6):e67.
Nelson SP, etal. Prevalence of symptoms of gastroesophageal reflux during infancy. A pediatric practice-based survey. Pediatric Practice Research Group. *Archives Of Pediatrics And Adolescent Medicine.* 1997;151(6):569
Orenstein SR. Symptoms and reflux in infants: infant gastroesophageal reflux questionnaire revised (I-GERQ-R)—utility of symptom tracking and diagnosis. *Curr Gastro Rep* 2010 Dec;12(6):431-6.
van der Pol RJ, etal. Efficacy of proton-pump inhibitors in children with gastroesophageal reflux disease: a systematic review. *Pediatrics* 2011;127:925–935.

Chapter 9: Sleep

American Academy of Pediatrics, SIDS Task Force, press conference, October 10, 2005.
Coleman-Phox K etal. *Arch Ped Adol Med* 2008;162:963.
Duncan JR, etal. Brainstem serotonergic deficiency in SIDS. *JAMA* 2010;303(5):430-437.
Ferber R. *Solve Your Child's Sleep Problems.* New York: Simon & Schuster, 1985.
Kleitman N. *Sleep and Wakefulness*, 2nd Ed. Chicago: University of Chicago Press,1963.

Mindell JA, etal. Behavioral treatment of bedtime problems and night wakings in infants and young children. *Sleep* 2006;29(10):1263-1276.

Okami P, et al. Outcome correlates of parent-child bed sharing: an eighteen-year longitudinal study. *Dev and Behav Pediatrics* 2002;(23)4:244-253.

Paterson DS, etal. Multiple serotonergic brainstem abnormalities in sudden infant death syndrome. *JAMA* 2006;296(17):2124-2132.

Paul IM, etal. Mother-infant room-sharing and sleep outcomes in the INSIGHTstudy. Pediatrics. 2017;140(1):e20170122

Price AMH, etal. Five-year follow-up of harm and benefits of behavioral infant sleep intervention: randomized trial. *Pediatrics.* 130(4) 2012: p643-651.

Rao MR, etal. Long-term cognitive development in children with prolonged crying. *Arch Dis Child* 2004;89:989-992.

Rechtman LR, etal. Sofas and infant mortality. Pediatrics 2014 pediatrics.org/cgi/doi/ 10.1542/peds.2014-1543

Stifter CA, etal. The effect of excessive crying on the development of emotion regulation. *Infancy* 2002; 3(2): 133-152.

Thach BT, etal. Deaths and injuries attributed to infant crib bumper pads. *Jnl Peds* 2007;(4)28:271-74.

Touchette E. Lecture at annual meeting of the Associated Professional Sleep Societies, 2003.

Willinger M, etal: Trends in infant bed sharing in the United States, 1993-2000: The National Infant Sleep Position study. *Arch Ped Adol Med* 2003;157(1):43-49.

Chapter 10: Developmental Milestones

American Academy of Pediatrics website aap.org/immunization/families/safety.html
American Academy of Pediatrics, Committee on Public Education. Children, Adolescents, and television. *Pediatrics* 2001;107:423-426.

American Academy of Pediatrics. Health supervision for children with Down syndrome. *Pediatrics* 2001;107:442.

AAP, Council on Communications and Media. Media and young minds. Pediatrics Nov 2016, 138 (5)

Anderson DR, Pempek TA. Television and very young children. *American Behavioral Scientist* 2005;48(5):505-522.

Atladottir HO, etal. Autism after infection, febrile episodes, and antibiotics during pregnancy: an exploratory study. *Pediatrics.* 2012; 130(6) e1447-1454.

Brainerd, C. *Piaget's Theory of Intelligence.* Englewood, NJ: Prentice-Hall, 1978.

Brenner RA, etal. Association between swimming lessons and drowning in children: a case-controlled study. *Arch Ped Adol Med* 2009 Mar;163(3):203-10.

CDC.gov, Accessed May 5, 2019

Chahrour M, etal. MECP2, a key contributor to neurological disease, activates and represses transcription. *Science* 2008 May 30;320(5880):1224-9.

Cheslack-Postava etal. Closely spaced pregnancies are associated with increased odds of autism in California sibling births. *Pediatrics* 2011;127(2)

Chyi LJ, etal. *J Peds* 2008;153;25-31

Croen LA, etal. Maternal and paternal age and risk of autism spectrum disorders. *Arch Ped Adol Med* 2007 Apr 161(4):334-40.

Dehaene-Lambertz G, etal. Functional organization of perisylvian activation during presentation of sentences in preverbal infants. Proceedings of the National Academy of Sciences, France, 2006. Pnas.org/cgi/doi/10.1073/pnas. 0606302103

Fatemi SH, etal. Maternal infection leads to abnormal gene regulation and brain atrophy in mouse offspring; implications for genesis of neurodevelopmental disorders. *Schizo Res* 2008;99(1-3):56-70.

Goodwyn SW, etal. Impact of symbolic gesturing on early language development. 2000;24;81-103.

Harder AF. Learningplaceonline.com.

Hyman SL, etal. Identification, evaluation, and management of children with autism spectrum disorder. American Academy of Pediatrics. Pediatrics. 145 (1) January 2020.

Jamain S, etal. Mutations of the X-linked genes encoding neuroligins NLGN3 and NLGN4 are associated with autism. *Nature Genetics* 2003;34:27-29.

Kaiser Family Foundation, 2003.

Krakowiak P, etal. Maternal metabolic conditions and risk for autism and other neurodevelopmental disorders. *Pediatrics.* 2012. 129 (5) e1221-1128.

Limperopoulos C, etal. Positive screening for autism in ex-preterm infants: prevalence and risk factors.

Pediatrics Apr 2008; 121:758-65.

Maestro S. *Psychopathology* 1999; 32(6):292-300.

Mills JL, etal Elevated levels of growth-related hormones in autism and autism spectrum disorder. *Clinical Endocrinology* 2007;67(2):230-7.

Suren P, etal. Association between maternal use of folic acid supplements and risk of autism spectrum disorders in children. *JAMA*. 2013 Feb 13;309(6):570-7.

Vandewater EA, Bickham DS, etal. Time well spent? Relating television use to children's free-time activities. *Pediatrics* 2006:117:181-191.

Volk HE, etal. Traffic-related air pollution, particulate matter, and autism. *JAMA Psychiatry.* 2013; 70(1):71-77.

Zubler JM, etal. Evidence-informed milestones for developmental surveillance tools. Pediatrics 149 (3) March 2022:e2021052138

Chapter 11: Temperament and Soothing

Harriett Lane Handbook, 2002.

High P: Data compiled at Infant Development Center, Brown Univ, 2003.

Jaafar SH, Jahanfar S, Angolkar M, Ho JJ. Pacifier use versus no pacifier use in breastfeeding term infants for increasing duration of breastfeeding. *Cochrane Database of Systematic Reviews* 2011, Issue 3. Art. No.: CD007202. DOI: 10.1002/14651858.CD007202.pub2.

Kurcinka MS. Raising your Spirited Child: A Guide for Parents Whose Child is More Intense, Sensitive, Perceptive, Persistent, Energetic. Harper, 1998.

Perry R, et al. Nutritional supplements and other complementary medicines for infantile colic: a systematic review. Pediatrics, April 2011. 127:720-733. Robertson J, etal. The Harriett Lane Handbook. A Manual for Pediatric House Officers. 17th Ed. Philadelphia: Mosby, 2005.

Savino F, etal. Lactobacillus reuteri vs. simethicone in the treatment of infantile colic: a prospective randomized study. *Pediatrics* 2007;119:e124-130.

Thomas A, Chess S. *Temperament and Development.* New York: Brunner/Mazel 1977.

Viggiano D. *Arch Dis Child* 2004;89:1121-1123.

Chapter 12: Vaccinations

American Academy of Pediatrics Technical Report: Mercury in the environment: implications for pediatricians. *Pediatrics* 2001; 108 (1): 197-205.

Bloomberg.com accessed March 21, 2022 bloomberg.com/graphics/covid-vaccine-tracker-global-distribution/

Centers for Disease Control website at cdc.gov/vaccines/pubs/pinkbook/ pink-appendx.htm#appg Accessed on March 8, 2009.

CDC.gov, MMWR 2021National Immunization Survey; cdc.gov/mmwr/volumes/70/wr/mm7041a1. htm#T1_down

CDC.gov cdc.gov/mumps/vaccination.html accessed March 20, 2022

CDC. Increase in measles cases January 1- April 26, 2019. MMWR 68(17); 402–404-HRSA.gov May 7, 2019

Communicable Disease Surveillance Center, London, 2007.

Dept of Health and Human Services, Agency for Toxic Substances and Disease Registry, Tox FAQ's for Aluminum, Sept 2008.

Dept of Health and Human Services, Agency for Toxic Substances and Disease Registry, Tox FAQ's for Formaldehyde, June 1999.

DeStefano F, etal. Increasing exposure to antibody-stimulating proteins and polysaccharides in vaccines is not associated with risk of autism. *Journal of Pediatrics* 2013. DOI 10.1016/j.jpeds.2013.02.001

Eick AA. Maternal influenza vaccination and effect on influenza virus in young infants. *Arch Ped Adol Med* 2011 Feb;165(2):104-11.

EPA. Mercury study report to Congress: Vol 4: An assessment of exposure to mercury in the US; 1997. www.epa.gov/mercury.

Fenn EA: Biological warfare in eighteenth century North America: beyond Jeffrey Amherst. *Journal of American History* 2000; (86) 4: 1552-1580.

HRSA accessed March 20, 2022 hrsa.gov/vaccine-compensation/data/index.html

Johns Hopkins Hospital, Bloomberg School of Public Health, Institute for Vaccine Safety. Vaccinesafety.edu/cc-exem.htm.

Mills JL, etal Elevated levels of growth-related hormones in autism and autism spectrum disorder. *Clinical Endocrinology* 2007;67(2):230-7.

Mitkus RJ, etal. Updated aluminum pharmacokinetics following infant exposures through diet and vaccination. *Vaccine* 2011;29:9538-9543.

Nelson K. *Pediatrics* 2003;111(3):674-678.

Newsweek at newsweek.com/id/185853

O'Brien MA, etal. Parental refusal of pertussis vaccination is associated with an increased risk of pertussis infection in children. *Pediatrics* 2009;123(6).

Offit P. Addressing parents' concerns: Do multiple vaccines overwhelm or weaken the infants' immune system? *Pediatrics* 2002;109:124.

Offit P. *Pediatrics* 2003;112(6):1394-1401.

Omer SB, etal. Geographic clustering of non-medical exemptions to school immunization requirements and associations with geographic clustering of pertussis. *Am J Epidemiology* 2008;168(12)1389-96.

Omer SB, etal. Vaccine refusal, mandatory immunization, and the risks of vaccine preventable disease. *NEJM* 2009;360(19):1981-8.

Pickering LK, editor. *Red Book: 2006 Report of the Committee of Infectious Diseases.* 27th ed. Elk Grove Village, IL: American Academy of Pediatrics, 2006.

Reis EC, et al: Taking the sting out of shots: control of vaccination-associated pain and adverse reactions. *Pediatric Annals* 1998;27(6):375-386.

Schechter R, etal. Continuing increases in autism reported to California's developmental services system: mercury in retrograde. *Arch Gen Psychiatry* 2008;65(1):19-24.

Schuval S. Avoiding allergic reactions to childhood vaccines (and what to do when they occur). *Contemporary Pediatrics* 2003; 20(4): 29-53.

Smith M, etal. On time vaccine receipt in the first year does not adversely affect neuropsychological outcomes. *Pediatrics* 2010;125:1134-1141.

Thompson WW, etal. Early thimerosal exposure and neuropsychological outcomes at 7 to 10 years. *NEJM* 2007;357:1281-1292.

UCLA website at library.ucla.edu/libraries/biomed/smallpox/

Vaccine Education Center, Children's Hospital of Philadelphia. Parent PACK Newsletter, June 2008.

Wakefield A.J, et al: Ileal-lymphoid-nodular hyperplasia, non-specific colitis, and pervasive developmental disorder in children. *Lancet* 1998;351:637-641.

Chapter 13: Infections

Baker RB. Is ear pulling associated with ear infection? *Pediatrics* 1992;90:1006-7.

CDC.gov accessed March 26, 2022.

Chai G, etal. Trends in outpatient prescription drug utilization in U.S. children 2002-2010. *Pediatrics* 2012;130:23-31.

Donowitz L. Infection control in the office: keeping germs at bay. *Contemporary Pediatrics* 2000;17(9):47.

Dowell SF. Seasonal variations in host susceptibility and cycles of certain infectious diseases. *Emerg Infect Dis* 2001;7(3):369-74.

Hoberman A, etal. Treatment of acute otitis media in children under two years of age. *NEJM* 2011. 364(2):105-115.

Kimberlin DW, editor. Red Book: 2021-2024 Report of the Committee of Infectious Diseases, 32nd ed. Itasca IL: American Academy of Pediatrics, 2021.

Leader S, etal. RSV coded hospitalizations, 1997-1999. Ped Inf Dz J. 2002:21:629.

Mangione-Smith RM, et al. The relationship between perceived parental expectations and pediatrician antimicrobial prescribing behavior. *Pediatrics* 1999;103:711-718.

MMWR March 4, 2011 Vol 60(3)

Peter G. Bacterial resistance in office practice: the need for judicious antimicrobial therapy. Lecture at 25th Annual Pediatric Postgraduate Symposium, Houston, 2003.

Pickering LK, editor. *Red Book: 2006 Report of the Committee of Infectious Diseases,* 27th ed. Elk Grove Village IL: American Academy of Pediatrics, 2006.

Post JC, et al: Is pacifier use a risk factor for otitis media? *Lancet* 2001;357:823-4.

Rosenfeld RM, etal: Clinical efficacy of antimicrobial drugs for acute otitis media: meta-analysis of 5400 children from thirty-three randomized trials. *Journal of Pediatrics* 1994;124:355-67.

Chapter 14: Diseases

Allmers H, etal. Acetaminophen use: a risk for asthma? *Curr All Asthma Rep* 2009;9(2):164-7.

Bakkeheim E, etal. Paracetamol in early infancy: the risk of childhood allergy and asthma. *Acta Paediatrica* 2011;100(1):90-96

Barrow Neurological Institute, St Joseph's Hospital and Medical Center, Phoenix AZ and Cranial Technologies, Phoenix AZ. 2008.

Beasley R, etal. Association between paracetamol use in infancy and childhood, and risk of asthma, rhinoconjunctivitis, and eczema in children aged 6-7 years: analysis from Phase Three of the ISAAC programme. *Lancet* 2008;372(9643):1039-48.

Behrman, RE. Editor: *Nelson Essentials of Pediatrics*. Philadelphia: WB Saunders, 1990.

CDC.gov Accessed March 30, 2022 cdc.gov/ncbddd/sicklecell/documents/fs_splenicinfarcts_lay.pdf

Expert Panel Report II: *Guidelines of the Diagnosis and Management of Asthma*. 1997.

Fleisher G, Ludwig S, editors: *Pediatric Emergency Medicine*, 3rd Ed. Baltimore: Williams and Wilkins, 1993.

National Institutes of Health website at nhlbi.nih.gov/guidelines/asthma/

Ownby, D. et al: Exposure to dogs and cats in the first year of life and risk of allergic sensitization at six or seven years of age. *JAMA* 2002;288(8):963-972.

Persky V, etal. Prenatal exposure to acetaminophen and respiratory symptoms in the first year of life. *Ann Allergy Asthma Immun* 2008;101(3):271-8.

Snell-Bergeon JK, etal. Early childhood infections and the risk of islet autoimmunity: the diabetes autoimmunity study in the young (DAISY). *Diabetes Care*. 2012 Dec;35(12):2553-8.

Stein RT. Early-life viral bronchiolitis in the causal pathway of childhood asthma: is the evidence there yet? *Am J Respir Crit Care Med* 2008;178(11):1097-8.

Stellwagen L, etal. Look for the "stuck baby" to identify congenital torticollis. *Contemporary Pediatrics* May 2004;21:55.

Chapter 15: Safety

Adgent MA etal. "A longitudinal study of estrogen-responsive tissues and hormone concentrations in infants fed soy formula," *Journal of Clinical Endocrinology and Metabolism*, online March 1, 2018.

American Academy of Pediatrics Committee on Environmental Health: *Pediatric Environmental Health, 2nd ed*. Elk Grove Village, IL: American Academy of Pediatrics, 2003.

American Academy of Pediatrics Committee on Nutrition: *Pediatric Nutrition Handbook*, 6th Ed. Elk Grove Village, IL, 2009.

American Cancer Society cancer.org/cancer/cancercauses/othercarcinogens/athome/cellular-phones accessed April 5, 2015.

American Red Cross, Accessed May 12, 2019

Canfield RL, etal. Intellectual impairment in children with blood lead concentrations less than 10 mcg/dl. *NEJM* 2003 Apr 17;348(16):1517-26.

Centers for Disease Control at cdc.gov/nceh/clusters/fallon/organophosfaq.htm.

Centers for Disease Control accessed April 8, 2013. cdc.gov

Center for Science in the Public Interest at cspinet.org/reports/chemcuisine.htm.

Council on Environmental Health. American Academy of Pediatrics. Policy Statement Chemical-Management Policy: Prioritizing Children's Health. *Pediatrics* 2011;127:983-990.

Food and Drug Administration at FDA.gov accessed May 25, 2009.

Forman J, Silverstein J, AAP Committee on Nutrition, AAP Council on Environmental Health. Organic foods: environmental advantages and disadvantages. *Pediatrics* 2012;130:e1406.

Goldman LR. Chemicals and children's environment: what we don't know about risks. *Environ Health Perspect* 1998;106(suppl 3):875-880.

Li D, etal. Microplastic release from the degradation of polypropylene feeding bottles during infant feeding preparation. Nature Food 2020; 1:746-754National Institutes of Health. Niehs.nih.gov/emfrapid/booklet/home.htm.

Sherburn RE, Jenkins RO. Used cot mattresses as potential reservoirs of bacterial infection:*J Appl Microbiol* 2008 Feb;104(2):526-33.

Chapter 16: First Aid

American Academy of Pediatrics: The management of acute gastroenteritis in young children. *Pediatrics* 1996; 97(3):424-35.

Crocetti M. Fever phobia revisited: have parental misconceptions about fever changed in 20 years?

Pediatrics 2001;107(6):1241-6.

Fleisher, G., Ludwig, S, editors. *Pediatric Emergency Medicine*, 3rd Ed. Baltimore: Williams and Wilkins, 1993.

Gunn VL, Nechyba C, editors. *The Harriet Lane Handbook: A Manual for Pediatric House Officers*, 16th ed. Philadelphia: Mosby, 2002.

Pantell RH, et al. Clinical Practice Guideline: Evaluation and Management of Well-Appearing Febrile Infants 8 to 60 Days Old. Pediatrics. 2021;148(2):e2021052228

Paul I, Beiler J, Vallanti J, Duda L, King T. Placebo Effect in the Treatment of Acute Cough in Infants and Toddlers: A Randomized Clinical Trial. JAMA Pediatrics. 2014;168(12):1107-1113

Appendix A: Medications

American Academy of Pediatrics Committee on Nutrition. *Pediatric Nutrition Handbook*, 4th ed. Elk Grove, IL: American Academy of Pediatrics, 1998.

Hale T. Medications and Mother's Milk. *A Manual of Lactational Pharmacology*, 17th ed. Amarillo: Pharmasoft Publishing, 2017.

Murphy JL. editor: *Prescribing Reference for Pediatricians: Spring-Summer 2007*. New York: Prescribing Reference, Inc., 2007.

Shared PJ, etal. The effect of inhaled steroids on the linear growth of children with asthma: A meta-analysis. *Pediatrics* 2000;106(1):E8.

Appendix B: Complementary Medicines

Barrett BP, et al: Treatment of the common cold with unrefined Echinacea. A randomized, double blind, placebo-controlled trial. *Annals of Int Medicine* 2002;137(12):939-46.

Das SK, et al. Deglycyrrhizinated liquorice in aphthous ulcers. *J Assoc Physicians India* 1989;37(10):647.

Eeles R: The effect of menthol on nasal resistance to airflow. *J Laryng Otol* 1983;97:705-9.

Fetrow CW, etal. Professional's Handbook of Complementary and Alternative Medicines, 3rd Ed. Philadelphia: Lippincott, Williams and Wilkins, 2004.

Fox N. Effect of camphor, eucalyptol, and menthol on the vascular state of the mucous membrane. *Arch Oto HNS* 1027(6):112-122.

Gardiner P. Longwood Herbal Task Force website:www.mcp.edu/herbal/

Gilroy CM, etal. Echinacea and truth in labeling. *Archives of Internal Medicine* 2003;163:699-704.

Hederos C, Berg, A. Epogram evening primrose oil treatment in atopic dermatitis and asthma. *Arch Dz in Childhood* 1996;75:494-7.

Horrobin DF. Essential fatty acid metabolism and its modification in atopic eczema. *Am Jnl Clin Nutrition* 2000;71(supp):367s-372.

Kemper, KJ: *The Holistic Pediatrician. A pediatrician's comprehensive guide to safe and effective therapies for the 25 most common ailments of infants, children, and adolescents*, 2nd ed. New York: HarperCollins, 2002.

Kopp MV, etal. Randomized, double-blind, placebo-controlled trial of probiotics for primary prevention: no clinical effects of Lactobacillus GG supplementation. *Pediatrics* 2008;121:e850-6.

Land M. Probiotics, hype or helpful? *Contemporary Pediatrics* 2008;(25)12:34-42.

Moneret-Vautrin DA, etal. Probiotics may be unsafe in infants allergic to cow's milk. *Allergy* 2006;61:507-8.

Mowrey DB. Motion sickness, ginger, and psychophysics. *Lancet* 1982;91:655-7.

National Institutes of Health. National Library of Medicine, Medline Plus. nlm.nih.gov/medlineplus accessed April 26, 2013.

National Public Radio. Politics and lobbying in the US nutritional and dietary supplements industry. National Public Radio, All Things Considered, June 23, 2003.

Paul IM, etal. Vapor rub, petrolatum, and no treatment for children with nocturnal cough and cold symptoms. Pediatrics. 2010;126:1092-99.

Perry R, etal. Nutritional supplements and other complementary medicines for colic: a systematic review. *Pediatrics* 2011;127:720-733.

Rodriguez-Bigas M. A comparative evaluation of aloe vera in the management of burn wounds in guinea pigs. *Plastic Reconst Surg* 1988;81:386-9.

Schmid R, et al. Comparison of seven commonly used agents for prophylaxis of seasickness. *Jnl Travel Med* 1994;1;203-6.

Singh M, etal. Zinc for the common cold. Cochrane Database Review. 2011. Issue 2.

Teelucksingh S. Potentiation of hydrocortisone activity in skin by glycyrrhetinic acid. *Lancet* 1990;335 (8697):1060-3.

Weizman Z, et al. Efficacy of herbal tea preparation in infantile colic. *Journal of Pediatrics* 1993;122:650-2.

Appendix C: Lab Tests

Gunn VL, Nechyba C, editors: *The Harriet Lane Handbook: A Manual for Pediatric House Officers*,16th ed. Philadelphia:Mosby,2002.

Loeb S, editor: *Clinical Laboratory Tests: Values and Implications*. Springhouse, Pennsylvania: Spring House,1991.

Appendix D: Glossary

Behrman RE, Kliegman R. *Nelson Essentials of Pediatrics*. Philadelphia: W.B.Saunders, 1990.

Cloherty JP, Stark AR. *Manual of Neonatal Care*, 3e. Boston: Little Brown, 1992.

Shelov, SP. *Your Baby's First Year*. New York: Bantam, 1998.

Urdang Associates. *The Bantam Medical Dictionary*. New York: Bantam, 1981.

INDEX

A+D ointment, 512
AAFP (American Academy of Family Physicians), 325
AAP. *See* American Academy of Pediatrics (AAP)
Abacavir, 356
abdomen, 8–9, 520–522
abdominal pain, 437–439, 517
ABO incompatibility, 17, 20
abscess culture, 528
accessory nipples, 10
accuracy of information, xvi–xvii
acetaminophen (Tylenol): and asthma, 391; correct dosing of, 466–469, 497; and fevers, 368, 463–469, 497; in first aid kits, 435; and on-call doctors, 434; for teething, 91, 155, 494; using with antibiotics, 489; and vaccinations, 325, 327; and viral infections, 367
acetic acid, 510
acholic stool, 209
acidic foods, 194
acidophilus, 140
acid reflux (GERD). *See* gastroesophageal reflux (GER) and disease (GERD)
ACIP (Advisory Committee on Immunization Practices), 325
acne, 84, 475, 517
ACOG (American Congress of Obstetricians and Gynecologists), 4
acrocyanosis, 8
Acticin, 510
Actifed, 492
acupuncture, 513
acute abdomen, 217, 437–439
acute life threatening event (ALTE), 449
acute otitis media, 379–380
Acyclovir, 356, 368, 370, 503
Adair, Steven, 92
adaptability, and temperament, 299
additives, 409
adenoldltls, 365, 452
adenovirus, 385
ADHD (attention deficit hyperactivity disorder), 410, 415–416

adjusted age, 42, 94, 102, 181, 280
adjuvants, 345
adoption, 45–46, 151, 550
adrenal gland dysfunction, 523, 524, 526
adrenal gland insufficiency, 56
Advanced Practice Providers, 61
adverse reactions, 320, 323, 327–328, 332, 341–342, 344, 493, 502–503
Advil. *See* ibuprofen (Motrin, Advil)
Advisory Committee on Immunization Practices (ACIP), 325
Affordable Care Act, 143
Afrin, 441, 507, 508
agave nectar, 452, 508
agenesis of the corpus callosum, 280
aggression, 298
AIDS: and bacterial infections, 362. *See also* HIV
air hungry, 390, 446–447, 451, 505
air pollution, 277, 409, 423
Albendazole, 502–503
Albenza, 502–503
albumin, 345
albuterol, 366, 392, 488, 505
alcohol, 149, 352–353, 369, 409, 495, 514, 518
Alinia, 503
All Clear Free, 85
allergic reactions: to antibiotics, 324, 326, 501; and asthma, 194, 200, 390, 404; calling the doctor for, 439–440; and exposure to environmental hazards, 409; and histamines, 194–195, 440, 508; hives, 193–195, 200, 213, 439, 471, 474–475; and introduction of solid foods, 190, 193–194, 439–440; to medications, 501–502, 512; prevention of, 201–202; and rashes, 439–440; steroids for, 509
allergies/allergens: and antihistamines, 508; and blood in poop, 209, 213; and casein, 158; to cow's milk, 133, 146–147, 161, 166, 170, 186, 193–197, 213, 305; dairy, 110, 146–147, 196–197; and diarrhea, 193, 453; drug allergies, 474; and dust mites, 377; and ear piercing, 89; and eczema, 161,

183, 186, 195, 199, 201, 213, 393, 398–399, 404, 439, 471, 474; and fluid in ears, 378; and formulas, 160, 161, 213; genetic predispositions to, 391; and introduction of solid foods, 180, 183, 186, 190, 193–194, 195–202, 207, 439–440; medications for, 439–440, 493; metal, 89; and milk protein, 167, 194, 194–197, 516; and on-call doctors, 434; outgrowing, 194, 196, 202; to peanuts, 148, 194–197, 196–198; and probiotics, 516; and rashes, 471, 473; and red eyes, 460; seasonal, 393, 400, 404–405, 460; testing for, 201–202, 524; and vaccinations, 324, 327–328; websites on, 147, 196, 405, 550

Allergy Asthma Technology Ltd., 405

All Free and Clear, 84

Altabax, 509

ALTE (acute life threatening event), 449

alternative dairy products, 176

alternative therapies. See complementary therapies

aluminum, in vaccines, 345–347

aluminum hydroxide, 498

aluminum salts, 345–347

Alzheimer's disease, 346

Amazon.com, 75, 81, 153, 225

ambiguous genitalia, 10, 524

amblyopia, 42, 284, 389

Ameda Comfort Gel Pads, 138

American Academy of Family Physicians (AAFP), 325

American Academy of Pediatric Dentistry, 92

American Academy of Pediatrics (AAP): and ASD, 278; and avoiding juice, 174–175; and belly button cleaning, 80; and bladder infections, 219–220; breastfeeding guidelines from, 114–115, 120, 154; and car seats, 29, 428; and circumcision, 27; contact information for, 552; and cord blood banking, 25; and crib bumpers, 237–238; and developmental milestones, 268; DHA recommendations for nursing mothers, 107; and Down syndrome, 279; and ear infections, 380, 382; and family beds, 115, 241, 243; and feeding schedules, 102; and fluoride, 108, 494; formula recommendations of, 157–158, 165–166; and hearing screenings, 16, 56; and introduction of solid foods, 181, 186, 197, 199; iron guidelines from, 105, 156, 183; and jaundice, 20; and media use, 291–293, 295; milk recommendations, 175; and

orthotics, 400–401; and pacifiers, 302–303; policy statements of, 57, 292–293; and preemies discharge from hospital, 41; and RSV immunization, 507; and SIDS, 236–237, 237–238, 241, 243; and sleep positioners, 238; and sunscreen, 85; and swim classes, 294–295; and teeth cleaning, 92; thermometer recommendations from, 466; vaccine recommendations from, 325, 336, 337, 349; and vision screening, 390; and vitamin D, 104; and walkers, 287; and well child visits, 55–56. See also pediatricians

American Academy of Pediatrics Breastfeeding Committee, 181

American Academy of Pediatrics Nutrition Committee, 168, 181

American Academy of Pediatrics SIDS Task Force, 234

American Cancer Society, 414

American Congress of Obstetricians and Gynecologists (ACOG), 4

American Dental Association (ADA), 107–108, 170, 493–494

American Red Cross, 153

American Sensors, 423

American Urological Association, 27, 220

amino acids, 158–159, 162

amniocentesis, 3

amniotic fluid, 82–83

amoxicillin, 363–364, 382, 501

Amoxil, 501

amylase, 522

anal atresia, 9

anaphylactic reaction, 193–194, 200, 327, 439–440

anemia: and aluminum poisoning, 346; and celiac disease, 198; and cutting the umbilical cord, 4; and failure to thrive, 103; and food poisoning, 373; and iron deficiency, 103, 105, 182, 313, 395–397, 503–504; and sickle cell disease, 396; tests for, 46, 56–57, 105, 526

anesthesia, 391

anesthetic creams, 325

angel kisses, 11

animal bites, 476

ankyloglossia, 7, 137

antacids, 212, 498–499, 517

anterior fontanelle, 6, 95–96, 217, 454, 480–481, 521

antibacterial soaps, 352–353

antibiotic creams/ointments, 121, 139, 372,

445, 477, 508–509, 512
antibiotic ear/eye drops, 12, 373, 459–460, 495–497
antibiotics: allergies to, 324, 326, 501; and bacterial infections, 362, 371–375, 463, 501–502; and blood in poop, 443; and diarrhea, 386, 501–502, 515; ear/eye-drops containing, 12, 373, 459–460, 495–497; and ear infections, 380–384, 386–388, 391, 495–496; in food, 409, 411–412; and food poisoning, 373; and fungal infections, 376; generic, 487; and Group A Strep, 488; and mastitis, 131, 140; and organic certification, 189; over-prescription of, 364; resistance to, 323, 337, 363–364, 375, 376, 379, 382–383, 387, 412–413, 434, 460, 501; and Strep B infection, 18, 374–375; and Strep pneumoniae, 337; using leftover, 488–489; using with fever medications, 489; in vaccines, 345; and viruses, 323, 358, 362, 363; and VUR, 219–220. See also medications
antibodies: in breast milk, 113–114, 141, 150; in colostrum, 34, 124; and EBV, 525; and exposure to viruses, 353; in formulas, 160; and measles, 329; and RSV, 366; and vaccinations, 322, 326
anti-circumcision groups, 25, 27
antifungals, 81, 131, 140, 376, 502, 509–510
antihelminthics, 502
antihistamines, 201, 358, 387, 391, 399, 440, 493, 507–508. See also histamines
anti-inflammatories, 398, 509
antimicrobials, 168
antiseptics, 80
anti-vaccine movement, 319, 319–320, 320, 323, 331, 342
antivirals, 503
anus: abnormal formation of, 9; and blood in poop, 209, 442; and constipation, 206; and HPV, 26; pinworm eggs on, 378; rashes on, 367; and viruses, 354; wiping, 89, 218–219
anxiety: and breastfeeding, 120; and infant weight loss, 15, 120; at mealtime, 192; and mother/baby separation, 132–133, 290, 298, 312–313; stranger, 288, 298, 312–313
aorta, 8
APGAR test, 5
apnea, 8, 39, 42–43, 239, 448–449, 452
apnea of prematurity (AOP), 39, 42–43
appendicitis, 437
ARA (arachidonic acid), 159, 160

Arachidonic Acid (ARA), 159, 160
arbetapentane, 508
areolas, 118, 121, 123, 137–138, 145
Aristocort, 511
arms, examination of, 10, 521–522
aromatherapy, 514, 517
arsenic, 185, 409, 413, 513
artificial ingredients, in formulas, 168–169
artificial sweeteners, 186, 415
asbestos, 429
ascorbic acid, 416
ASD. See autism spectrum disorders (ASD)
AskLenore.info, 151
Asperger's syndrome, 273–274
aspirin, avoiding, 465, 497
Association for Children with Down syndrome, 279
Association of Women's Health Obstetric and Neonatal Nurses, 82
asthma: and advantages of breast milk, 114; and allergic reactions, 194, 200, 390, 404; and aromatherapy, 514, 517; calling the doctor about, 505; and coughing, 452, 505; diagnosis of, 390–391; and eczema, 393, 400; environmental triggers for, 409; and GERD, 216; long-term consequences of, 393; medications for, 366, 390, 392, 488, 504–506; and nebulizers, 60; outgrowing, 393; and respiratory distress, 448; and RSV, 365–366; and smoking, 391, 423; treatment of, 392–393; and vaccinations, 339
athlete's foot, 376, 509
Atopiclair, 512
atopy, 393, 400
atresia, 7
attachment parenting, 65, 254–255, 255–256
attention deficit disorder (ADD), 300
Attention Deficit Disorder (ADD), and ASD, 274
attention deficit hyperactivity disorder (ADHD), 410, 415–416
attention span, 409
auditory processing disorder, 267
Augmentin, 501
AuPairAmerica.com, 72
au pairs, 68–69
Auro-Dri, 495–496
authoritarian parenting, 65
autism spectrum disorders (ASD): and aluminum, 346; causes of, 276–278; developmental milestones and, 275; diagnosis

of, 273–278, 343–344; environmental triggers for, 275, 277, 410; genetics and, 276–
277; and jaundice, 21; and phototherapy,
21; and preemies, 42, 277; red flags with,
275; screening for, 56, 273, 275; therapy
for, 278; and vaccinations, 274, 277, 320,
343–344; websites on, 275, 278
autoimmune disease, 104, 403
autonomy, 282
autosomal dominant/recessive, 395
Aveeno, 85, 399
Avent bottle nipples, 172
Axid, 213, 498
azithromycin, 501
AZT, 356

Baby411.com, xviii
Baby Anbesol, 494
babybargains. com, 30
baby blues, 37
The Baby Book (Sears), 251, 256
Baby Brezza Formula Pro, 172
baby carriers, 229–231, 284
baby foods: and baby-led weaning, 182;
commercial, 183; compared to food, 179;
cost of, 183, 189; home made, 183, 188,
412, 414; non-GMO, 414; and nutrition,
93; organic, 189–190, 320, 412; rice cereal, 185; in squeezable packages, 188–189.
See also foods
BabyFormulaExpert.com, 157, 164
Babyganics, 80
baby-led weaning, 182
Baby Merlin Sleep Suit, 240
baby monitors, 239, 246, 249, 259
Baby Numz-it, 494
Baby Oragel, 494
baby proofing, checklist for, 422
babysleep.com, 253
baby wipes, 36
Bacitracin, 509
back injuries, 481
Back to Sleep campaign, 234–235, 286
backup plans, and childcare, 75
bacteremia, 18
bacteria: and bladder infections, 218–220,
385; in bottled water, 174; described,
360; and diarrhea, 453, 501–502; drug-
resistant, 323, 337, 363–364, 372, 375,
379, 382–383, 385, 387, 412–413, 434,
460, 501–502; and ear infections, 378–
379, 382–388, 387; and eye ointment for
newborns, 12; and fungal infections, 375–

376; HIB, 333; and intestinal infections,
453, 502; in mattresses, 427; plaque as,
92; in poop, 89, 203; and prebiotics, 168,
516; and thrush, 90, 140, 376, 502; in ure-
thras, 89, 218–219, 361, 374; in urine, 526;
and vaccinations/vaccines, 322–323, 330,
333, 336–337, 345; in water filters, 417
bacterial conjunctivitis, 373, 388
bacterial enteritis, 217
bacterial gastroenteritis, 453, 457
bacterial infections: and antibiotics, 362,
371–375, 463, 501–502; compared to viral
infections, 361–362, 364–365; contagiousness of, 362; diagnosis of, 354, 364; and
ear infections, 365, 371–373, 375, 378–
379, 382–388, 385–388, 464; of the eye,
459–460; and fevers, 361–362, 364–365,
369, 374, 463, 464; and green snot, 358,
363; identifying, 362, 364–365; and
influenza, 338–339; of intestines, 453, 502;
and laboratory tests, 519–520, 522–528;
medications and medication resistance,
323, 337, 360, 362–365, 372, 375, 379,
382–383, 385, 387, 412–413, 434, 460,
501–502; methods of introduction into the
body, 361; of nipples, 131, 133, 139; and
pacifiers, 303–304; and rashes, 471, 472–
473; respiratory, 446; seasonal patterns of,
372–373, 375, 386; secondary, 338–339,
361–362, 364–365, 371–372, 464; and
vaccinations, 322–323, 330, 333, 336–337,
345
bacterial meningitis, 337–338, 385
Bactrim, 501
Bactroban, 509
BAER (brainstem audio evoked response), 7
balanitis, 26
Balmex, 81, 512
barium swallow imaging study, 214, 522
barking cough, 367, 447–448, 452
barley, 403
Barracuda feeding behavior, 124
bassinets, 229, 241, 244, 263, 426
Batelle Sleep School, 256
baths: baby's first, 82–83; and ear infections,
381; and eczema, 85, 399; and fevers,
465, 469; as home remedy, 517; and passing gas, 222; and soothing, 302; and
stitches, 478; ten step method for, 83
BBQ, 416, 429
beans, 110–112, 182–183, 191, 196, 209, 455
bedding, 234–237, 241, 377, 405
bedtime: and last feeding, 175; and sleep

routines, 242–247, 249, 253, 254–255, 260–263; and teething pain, 91; and wired baby, 251

behavior: abnormal or confused, 479–480, 484; and artificial food coloring, 415–416; and ASD, 274, 276; and cartoon watching, 293; and childcare, 66–67; and discipline, 297, 308–312; feeding, 124, 134; learned, 108; nervous, 505; and parenting style, 66; rewarding good, 311; and sleep, 255, 259; and social development, 288; and temperament, 297

Bell, Edward, 488

belladonna, 91, 494–495

belly button, 9, 35, 79–81

Benadryl. See diphenhydramine (Benadryl)

Benefiber, 499

benzene, 409

benzyl alcohol, 510

beta agonists, 505

Betamethasone, 511

BeTheMatch.org, 23

Biaxin, 501

bifidobacterium, 106, 114, 306, 515

bile, 216, 456–457, 520

bili blanket/bed, 21

bilirubin, 15, 19–22, 35, 126, 188, 335

Bilirubin-Induced Neurologic Dysfunction (BIND), 20

bilirubin test, 15, 20–22, 523

BIND (Bilirubin-Induced Neurologic Dysfunction), 20

binky. See pacifiers

biochemical abnormalities, and SIDS, 236

Biogaia, 516

BioGaia ProTectis, 104, 106, 307, 500, 503

biopsies, 214

birth canal, 19

birth complications, 18–19

birth control, breastfeeding and, 114

birthing centers, 5–6, 82

birthmarks, 11

birth trauma, 13

birth weight: and breastfeeding, 15, 19, 125–126; and feeding/elimination tracking, 40; and growth charts, 94; and powdered formulas, 170; and preemies, 42, 43; and sleeping through the night, 120

bismuth subsalicylate, 456

bisphenol-A (BPA), 409, 430

biting, 298, 313–314

black tar poop, 14, 204, 209. See also meconium

bladder, 10, 521

bladder infections: as bacterial, 218–220, 385; and circumcision, 26; description, diagnosis, and treatment of, 374; and diaper changes, 89, 218–219; and laboratory tests, 520, 526; medications for, 501; and stomach ache, 437; and vomiting, 457; and VUR, 219–220, 522

blankets, 21, 41, 235, 237–238, 249

blebs, 130

bleeding: and bruising, 440–441; and circumcision, 29; in esophagus, 217; and eye injuries, 481–482; and face or scalp wounds, 479; and head injuries, 479–482, 484; and laboratory tests, 520, 525; and mouth injuries, 482; newborn girls' vaginas, 9; nipples, 118, 123, 131, 136, 138; nosebleeds, 441, 451, 482, 484, 505, 507; postpartum, 126; and stitches, 477–479; vitamin K deficiency bleeding, 11

blessed thistle, 134, 492

blindness, 333, 334

blisters, 445, 472, 475–476

blood: and anemia, 395; biomarkers for ASD in, 275; cord blood banking, 4, 17, 22–25, 64, 550; in diapers, 15, 146, 218; infections of, 40, 337, 375; lead in, 275; in pee, 218; in poop, 166, 194, 196–197, 204–205, 209, 213, 338, 373, 442–443, 453, 520, 527; in spit up, 216–217; and spread of viral infections, 371; vomiting, 442, 458

blood blisters, 484

blood cell abnormalities, and rashes, 471

blood clotting, 11–12, 440

blood count: and Down syndrome, 279; and infection, 361; and international adoption, 46; laboratory tests for, 523–524; white blood count, 356, 361, 365, 372, 523

blood culture, 6, 527

blood in stool, 166, 194, 196–197, 204–205, 209, 213, 338, 373, 442–444, 453, 520, 527

blood pressure: and advantages of breastfeeding, 114; as breastfeeding complication, 126; and decongestants, 507; screening test for, 56; and taking vital signs, 435

blood sugar: as diabetes cause, 403; low, 125; and malunggay, 134; in preemies, 40; testing, 18, 523

blood tests, 15–20, 198, 396, 522–526

blood type, 17, 520, 523, 525

Blue Baby Syndrome, 8, 215, 414, 476
blue cohosh, 492
board books, 253, 296
Bobbie formula, 169
body mass index (BMI): and ASD, 277–278; and diabetes, 403; and growth charts, 94; and overweight, 109–110; screening test for, 56
bone injuries, 483–484, 519, 521–524
bone marrow, 22–23, 395, 440–441, 524
bone problems, 402, 506, 521
bone scans, 522
books: for ages birth to one year, 295–296; board, 253, 296; on child development, 295–296; on colic, 307; and language development, 287, 289, 291; on preemies, 42; Reach Out and Read program, 286; on sleep, 253–256; on vaccinations, 352
booster shots, 326, 331, 333, 334, 337, 352
Boston Children's Hospital, 254, 394
BOTOX injections, 402
bottled water, 107–108, 170–171, 174, 494
bottle propping, and ear infections, 379
bottles: and BPA, 424–425, 430; breast milk in, 44, 116, 119, 125–126, 132–133, 139, 141–144, 153, 155, 191–192; and food poisoning, 373; introducing, 143–144; paced bottle feeding, 111, 119, 126, 144; recommended, 172; refusing, 144; sterilizing, 171; water in, 173–175. See also formulas; weaning
botulism, 186
Boudreaux's Butt Paste, 81, 512
bovine growth hormone, 176, 412–414
bowel obstruction, 205, 209, 338, 344
bowlegged, 284, 400
boy parts, 87–89. See also genitals
BPA (bisphenol-A), 409, 424–425, 430
braces, 304, 400
brain damage: and bilirubin levels, 20, 126; and body temperature, 461, 462, 469; and ear infections, 382; and low blood sugar, 125; and neurotoxins, 409; from shaking, 307; and Zika virus, 371
brain development: and ASD, 275–278; and DHA, 106, 148, 164; and dietary fats, 175; and head size, 95; and lead exposure, 410; and methylmercury exposure, 416–417; and MFGM, 168; Piaget's stages of, 281–282; and preemies, 39; and skulls, 6, 95; and sleep, 250; and vaccinations, 352
brain disorders: and measles, 333; vaccines and, 333. See also meningitis

brain hemorrhages, 11–12
brainstem audio evoked response (BAER), 7
brain tumors: and anterior fontanelle, 95, 217; and eye problems, 390; and radiation, 424; and vomiting, 457
branchial cleft cyst, 8
BRAT diet, 456
breads, 112, 113, 207–208
breast enlargement, in newborns, 10
breastfeeding: AAP guidelines for, 114–115, 120, 154; and adoption, 46, 151; advantages of, 114; advice from lactation consultants, 15, 36, 41, 116–118; and allergy prevention, 200–201; and appearance of baby poop, 204; and availability of formulas, 159; and baby's dietary needs, 100; and baby vomiting blood, 442; and blood in poop, 443; and blood sugar testing, 18; and breast reduction surgery, 145; and cancer rates, 114, 154; and cleaning teeth, 92, 252; and colic, 306; common questions and concerns, 128–141; and cost of formula, 114, 158–159, 160, 161, 167–168; and cough/cold medications, 508; and COVID-19, 149–150; and cow's milk, 132, 146, 155, 157–162, 194; and drinking water, 146–147; and ear infections, 155, 384; and eating fish, 417; and elimination, 34; encouraging, 115, 117, 159, 160; and family bed, 242, 256; first, 82; and fluoride in water, 107, 494; formal evaluation of, 115; frequency of, 32–33, 41, 117–120, 120–122, 155–157, 172–173; and gastroesophageal reflux, 116, 132, 153–154; and growth charts, 94; and growth spurts, 100–101; help with, 37, 61; Linda Hill's tips on, 118, 123, 132–133, 135, 139–141, 144, 155, 304; and infant weight loss, 15, 19, 60, 120, 124, 126, 128, 156, 227; insufficient milk supply, 116; and introducing solid foods, 103, 106, 181, 185, 191–192; and iron supplements, 105–106, 156, 180, 182–183, 396; and jaundice, 20–22, 120, 126; and late preterm infants, 125, 133–134, 152–153; medications to avoid, 149; and mother/baby separation, 132–133, 144; and mother's diet, 145–149, 212; and newborns' tiredness, 13–14, 32, 34, 36, 39–41, 44, 117, 122, 172–173; and obesity, 109; overview of first year, 155–157; and pacifiers, 115, 128–129, 259, 303–304; painful, 14, 115, 121, 123–124, 128, 130–

131; and pain medications, 122; and pee in diapers, 218; pillows for, 123, 145; positions for, 121, 122–123, 126, 131, 136, 153; and preemies, 39, 44, 105, 116, 120, 133–134, 151–152; preference for one breast, 119, 129; problems with, 130–131; reasons for stopping, 115–117; red flags with, 122; and rehydration solutions, 500; and returning to work, 116, 150, 166; and rooming in with newborns, 13; safety of medications taken when, 491–492; scheduling classes for, 64; science of, 117; and SIDS, 114, 236; and sleep, 115–116, 121, 127, 129, 156, 227–228, 229, 241, 243, 244, 246; and supplementation with formula, 21–22, 42, 44–45, 113, 115, 118, 124–129, 129, 150, 152–153, 166, 168; and thrush, 90, 376; timeline for first month, 117–120; and tongue tie, 7; and vitamin supplements, 103, 105, 132; and vomiting, 457; weaning, 140, 154–155, 157, 173, 182; websites on, 124, 134, 151, 550

breast implants, breastfeeding and, 145
breast milk: and acid reflux, 211; advantages of, 114; and allergy prevention, 200–201; aluminum in, 347; applied to painful nipples, 139; and baby poop appearance, 34, 126, 204; in bottles, 44, 116, 119, 125–126, 132–133, 139, 141–144, 153, 155, 191–192; BPA in, 424; breast milk/formula decision, 113; calories in, 99, 160, 181; compared to formulas, 132–133, 157–160; DHA in, 106–107, 148, 160, 164; and diarrhea, 455; fat content of, 150, 160, 181; frozen, 132–133, 141–143, 153; insufficient supply of, 116; iron in, 105–106, 156, 180, 182–183, 396; lack of fiber in, 207; lactoferrin in, 168; and mastitis, 131, 140; medications to stimulate production of, 46, 116, 151; milk fortifier, 44–45; milk transfer, 134–135, 153; mixed in cereal, 185; mother's pain medications in, 122; and nutrition, 93, 100–101, 104; overproduction of, 130, 133, 135; pesticides in, 411; prebiotics/probiotics in, 167–168, 306; production of, 34, 44–45, 119–120, 125–129, 141, 145, 147, 151, 153, 155, 227, 252, 492, 508; pumping, 44, 100, 103, 116, 125–143, 143–149, 150, 152–153, 154–155; pumps for, 127, 132, 143, 150, 152; quantity consumed per feeding in first year, 155–157; and rice cereal, 102; sale of, 151; secreted by newborns, 10; and solid food, 103, 106, 156–157, 179, 187; sour-smelling, 142, 149–150; storage of, 127, 132, 141–143, 150, 153; sugar in, 160, 161, 162, 164; time frames for using stored, 143; unacceptable substitutes for, 155; underproduction of, 130, 133–135; and vitamin D, 104, 157, 181, 500, 503; and vomiting, 217; water in, 173–174; and weaning, 155; zinc in, 111
breast pumps, 127, 132, 143, 150, 152
breast reduction surgery, 145
breasts: alternating feedings on, 129, 135, 151; and arrival of mature milk, 118; cancer of, 114, 154; enlarged in mothers, 115, 135–136; preference for one over the other, 119, 129; small, 145
breast shells, 119, 137
breath-holding spells, 313, 395
breathing: and air hungry diagnosis, 446–447, 451, 505; and allergic reactions, 439–440; calling the doctor for problems with, 446–449, 447–448; environmental hazards to, 408–409; and meconium in the lungs, 19; and nasal congestion, 450–451; and nose injuries, 482; periodic, 8, 31, 448; and polio, 332; and preemies, 39, 42–43; rapid, 395; red flags with, 31, 448; respiration rate, 5–6, 435–436; stopped, 448; and Strep B infection, 18; trouble with, 5–6
breath odors, 406, 470
breech position births, 10, 402
brick dust. See uric acid crystals
bris ceremonies, 22, 25, 28
broken bones, 482–484
brompheniramine, 507
bronchiolitis (RSV), 43, 354, 365–366, 385, 390–391, 446, 448–449, 506–507
bronchitis, 446
bronchodilators, 392
bronchopulmonary dysplasia (BPD), 43
Brown, Mark, 386
bruising: and bone injuries, 484; calling the doctor about, 440–441; and delivery trauma, 6, 35; and head injuries, 480–482, 484; home remedies for, 517; and laboratory tests, 520; Mongolian spots, 11; and petechiae, 471; and teething, 91
Budesonide, 392, 505
bulb syringes, 31–32, 442, 451
burns, 445, 470, 509
burping, 118, 151, 153, 204, 220–221

index

burrito wraps, 237–238, 402. *See also* swaddling
Burt's Bees, 169
Butler, Ginny, 353
ByHeart, 169
ByHeart formula, 169–170

cabbage leaves, for engorgement, 136
café au lait spots, 11
caffeine, 43, 91, 146
Cal-Ben's Seafoam, 85
calcium: in alternative dairy products, 176; consuming, 101, 110; in formulas, 164–165, 168; and iron supplements, 106, 397, 504; and preemies, 44, 165
calcium carbonate, 498
calories: in alternative dairy products, 176; average calorie intake, 111; in breast milk, 99, 160, 181; in colostrum, 124; in formulas, 10, 44, 99, 160, 181, 202; high calorie diets, 44, 99, 103, 125, 165, 181; needed by infants, 98–100; needed by nursing mothers, 147; in rice cereals, 187
camphor, 359, 517
campylobacter infection, 453
cancer: and advantages of breastfeeding, 114, 154; and artificial sweeteners, 415; and BPA, 424; breast, 114, 154; and circumcision, 26; and cord blood banking, 22; endometrial, 114; environmental triggers for, 409, 413, 421; and fluoride, 108; liver, 335; ovarian, 114; and smoking, 409; and sunblock, 85–86; and vitamin D supplements, 104; websites on, 550
cannabis use, 148
capillary refill, 454
CAP-RAST test, 201
carbamide peroxide, 496
carbcarbinoxamine, 507
car beds, 45
carbohydrates, 157, 160, 176
carbon dioxide, 234
carbon monoxide, 409, 423
carcinogens, 409, 416, 421–422
Care.com, 68
carotinemia, 188
carpeting, hazards with, 420–421, 423
carrageenan additive, 165
car rides, soothing with, 229, 231, 301–302
car seats, 29–30, 41, 45, 96, 116, 358, 428, 550
Cartoon Network, 293
Carvalho Fisheries, 417, 430

casein, 158–160, 162, 163, 200
casts, for broken bones, 483–484
cataracts, 6, 506
catch-up growth, 44, 61–62, 94, 99, 506
cavities, 45, 92, 493–494
C. difficile infection, 453, 498, 499, 502
Cedax, 501
Cefdinir, 501
Cefixime, 501
Cefprozil, 501
Ceftibuten, 501
Ceftin, 501
Ceftriaxone, 501
Cefuroxime, 501
celiac disease, 198, 279, 453
cell phones, 423–424
cellulitis, 372, 508
Centany, 509
center care, 69–70
Centers for Disease Control and Prevention (CDC): and ASD, 278; and child development, 273; and circumcision, 26; contact information for, 552; and developmental milestones, 268; growth charts from, 93–94; National Immunization Program, 349; and pesticides, 421; and spacing of pregnancies, 278; and vaccinations, 320, 325, 327, 333, 334, 336, 339, 347
Cephalexin, 501
cephalhematoma, 6, 20, 96
Cephalosporins, 501–502
CeraVe, 83, 399
cereals: arsenic in, 413; fiber in, 185, 207–208; and GERD, 213; rice, 99, 102, 180, 185, 207–208, 228, 413; and sleep, 228; whole grain, 111–112; zinc and iron in, 111, 183, 185
cerebral palsy, 10
cerebrospinal fluid (CSF), 527
Cetaphil, 399
Cetaphil soap, 83
cetirizine (Zyrtec), 474, 493, 508
chamomile (anthemis nobilis), 306
chemicals, 407–415
chemotherapy, 338, 362
Cherry Mylanta Supreme, 213
chest, examining, 8, 521–522
chest thrusts, 449
chicken, and salmonella, 444
chickenpox (varicella): and aspirin, 497; description, diagnosis, and treatment of, 336–337, 369–370, 472–473; and emollients, 511; medications for, 356, 503; post-

infection return to daycare, 388; and Strep infections, 319, 337; as viral infection, 385

chickenpox (varicella) vaccine, 56, 322, 324, 326, 330, 336–337, 357, 370, 475

chiggers, 377

Child (magazine), 255

childcare: alternatives for, 71–72; and back-up plans, 75; and child development, 66–67; and commuting, 71; cost of, 66–69; and fevers, 462; finding, 68–73; and frequency of illness, 67–68; and infections, 70–71, 387; and lice, 377; and nasal congestion, 451; options for, 67–70; out-of-the-home, 73; and parenting style, 63–64, 66–74; and waiting lists, 67; websites on, 68; and work/life balance, 66–67, 71–76

Child Development, 70

child development, websites on, 550

Children's Health Insurance Program (CHIP), 60

Children's Hospital, Philadelphia, 352

Children's Memorial Hospital, Chicago, 254

Chinese herbs, 513

chlorpheniramine, 507

choanal atresia, 7

choking, 182, 186, 191, 199, 207, 239, 449

cholesterol, 56, 106, 176, 525

chorioamnionitis, 18

Christtakis, Dimitri, 294

chromosomal abnormalities, 276, 278–279

chromosomal microarray (CMA), 275

chromosome analysis, 275, 524

chronic medical problems: coughing, 452–453; and doctor's appointments, 51–52, 58; and nursing mother's medications, 135; and probiotics, 516; and secondary infections, 365. *See also specific diseases*

chronological age, 94, 280

Chronulac, 499

chrysanthemum flower, 510

churches, and childcare, 72, 74

circadian rhythm, 226–227

circumcision: arguments for and against, 25–27, 29; as controversial subject, 25, 66; expert opinions about, 27, 29; and hypospadius/epispadias, 9; and obstetricians, 22, 27; pain medication for, 28–29; and penile adhesions, 27, 29, 88–89, 405; scheduling, 64; wound care for, 28–29, 87–88

citronella, 87

Clarithromycin, 501

clavicle fracture, 8

Clavulanate, 501

clay colored poop, 209

cleaning products: and allergic reactions, 440; as poisons, 420; safety with, 419–420, 430; websites on, 420

cleft lip/palate, 7, 379

Clinical Immunization Safety Assessment Network, 327

clitoris, 10

clostridium botulinum, 186

clothing, 30, 80, 377, 440

clotrimazole, 141, 509

club foot, 11

cluster feedings, 13, 34, 102, 120, 122, 155–156, 227

CMV (Cytomegalovirus), 277, 357

coagulation studies, 525

coarctation of aorta, 8

coconut, 163, 197

codeine, 491

coffee grounds, vomit appearing like, 216–217, 442, 458

cognitive development: from four to six months, 286; and media use, 293; milestones for, 267, 270; Piaget's theories of, 280–282; and reading, 284; from six to nine months, 288

Colace, 496

cold sores, 367–368

cold viruses: and air travel, 314; and antibiotics, 362–363; and asthma, 391; and bacterial infections, 361–362, 372; and breastfeeding, 114, 150; compared to sinus infections, 358, 360, 364–365; and coughing, 358, 452; diagnosis and treatment of, 358; and ear infections, 378–379, 387, 450; and goopy eyes, 459, 460; home remedies for, 517; medications for, 358–359, 507–509; and nasal congestion, 449; questions about, 357–359; and respiratory distress, 446; return to daycare after, 388; seasonal patterns of, 354, 386; and teething, 91; and vaccinations, 325; as viral infections, 385; and vomiting, 457

colic: and crying, 301–302, 306–307; dealing with, 305–307; and gas, 222, 305–306; and GERD, 212–213, 300, 305–306; home remedies for, 500, 517; medications for, 305–306, 500; and probiotics, 30, 106, 167, 306–307, 500, 515–516; and soy formula, 166; and temperament, 298

colostrum, 34, 119–120, 122, 124, 145, 168

comfort objects, 252, 274
comfrey, 492
common cold. *See* cold viruses
community programs for babies, 295
complementary foods, 100, 115, 154, 156, 173
complementary therapies: for colic, 306; herbal remedies, 134, 306, 489, 492, 513–514, 516; and pediatricians, 52, 513, 517, 518; safety and effectiveness of, 513–514, 517; websites on, 514, 516, 550
complete blood count (CBC), 369
comprehensive metabolic panel, 524
compression, 119, 122
compression stripes, 136
computerized tomography (CT) scans, 424, 481, 521–522
concrete operational development, 282
concussions, 480
conductive hearing loss, 383
cone head, 95–96
conflict, 37, 311
congenital hearing loss, 16
congenital heart disease, 8, 40, 394, 506–507
congenital nevus, 11
congestion, calling the doctor about, 450–451
congestive heart failure, 8
conjunctivitis, 373, 388, 459–460, 496
consciousness, loss of, 479–480, 484
consistency, 243–247, 245, 255, 260–261, 309
constipation: and blood in poop, 443; and crying, 301; and fiber, 111, 206, 222; and firmness of poop, 205–206; and formulas, 161; and grunting baby syndrome, 205; and introduction of solid foods, 207; and iron supplements, 504; medications for, 206, 499; and palm olein/oil, 164; and stomach ache, 438
Consumer Product Safety Commission (CPSC), 238, 426, 428
contact naps, 230
convulsions, 469
cooking, 75, 188, 189
Coombs test (ABO incompatibility), 20, 525
co-pays, 60
cord blood banking, 4, 17, 22–25, 64, 550
corneal abrasion, 460, 481, 496
corn syrup, 161–162, 169, 415
Corona Ointment, 81
Cortaid, 511

cortisol, 259
co-sleeping, 242–243, 253, 255, 256, 377
Costco, 162
coughing: and asthma, 452, 505; calling the doctor about, 451–452, 464; and choking, 449; chronic, 452–453; and cold viruses, 358, 452; and measles, 333; medications for, 358, 452, 507–509, 514; and mucous, 331, 446, 447; and petechiae, 441; and transmission of infections, 331–332, 353; typical doctor's questions about, 452; and VapoRub, 517; and vomiting, 452, 457. *See also* whooping cough (pertussis)
coupons, 60
COVID-19: and croup, 447; description, diagnosis, and treatment of, 366; exposure of babies to, 30, 33; and social media, xviii; tests for, 528
COVID-19 vaccinations, 33, 149, 317–319, 340–342, 366
cow milk protein enteropathy, 194
cowpox viruses, 319
cow's milk: allergies to, 133, 146–147, 161, 166, 170, 186, 193–197, 213, 305; alternative dairy products compared to, 176; and breastfeeding, 132, 146, 155, 157–162, 194; compared to toddler formulas, 168; in formulas, 157–162, 165–170, 305; introducing, 175; in probiotics, 516; proteins in, 146–147, 160–167, 170, 186, 194, 196–197, 305, 516; as unacceptable substitute for breast milk, 155
coxsackievirus, 354, 367, 371, 472–473
CPR, 45, 191, 419, 429, 435, 449–450, 476
CPSC (Consumer Product Safety Commission), 238
cradle cap, 79, 84–85, 509, 517
cradle hold, 122, 151
craniosynostosis, 6, 95, 96–97, 521
C-Reactive Protein (CRP), test for, 523
Crescent Womb Hammock, 240
cribs, 229, 235, 237–242, 248, 252–253, 257, 263, 426–427. *See also* mattresses
Crisaborole, 511
Cromolyn, 392, 505
Cronobacter sakazakii, 170
cross cradle hold, 123
Crotamiton, 510
croup, 354, 385, 388, 447–448, 517
crying: and choking, 449; and colic, 301–302, 306–307; and postpartum depression, 37; PURPLE, 305–306; and separa-

tion anxiety, 312; and serious medical problems, 301; and sleep problems, 226, 246–247, 249, 254–260, 264, 300; and temperament, 298, 300; and vaccinations, 328

crying it out, 247, 256–259, 264

cry management approach, 301

cryptosporidium, 453

C-sections, 12–13, 19, 36, 96

CT (computerized tomography) scans, 424, 481, 521–522

Culturelle, 456, 499, 515

cultures, 527–528

cups, drinking from, 175

currant jelly stool, 209

Cushingoid features, 506

Cutter Advanced, 86

cystic fibrosis (CF), 9, 393, 527

Cytomegalovirus (CMV), 277, 357

dactylitis, 396

dairy products: allergies to, 110, 146–147, 196–197; and calcium, 110, 176; and chronic diarrhea, 453, 456; environmental hazards in, 411–412; and food poisoning, 444; guidelines for, 112; and introduction of, 101, 183, 184; and iron supplements, 106

daycare: biting at, 314; cost of, 69; and ear infections, 379; finding, 69–70; in-home, 69, 72; licensed day care facilities, 69–70; naps at, 262; and rashes, 336; and RSV, 506; and Strep pneumoniae, 337; waiting lists for, 64

Day-Night Reversal, 227, 231

DDH (developmental dysplasia of the hip), 402, 521

deafness, 333, 334

Debrox, 496

decision making: breastmilk/formula, 113; and childcare, 72; and parenting style, 63; timeline for, 64

decongestants, 314, 358, 387, 391, 435, 441, 507–509

DEET, 86–87, 371

dehydration: and acetaminophen, 465, 497; and anterior fontanelle, 95; and diarrhea, 217, 454–455, 457–458; and fever, 19; and food poisoning, 373; and formula supplementation, 126; home remedies for, 517; IV fluids for, 221; and laboratory tests, 520, 523, 526; and nutrition, 93; and preemies, 40–41; signs of, 217; and stom-

ach viruses, 367–368, 500; and vomiting, 457–458

demineralization, 506

dental care: and injuries to teeth, 482–483; and juices, 174–175; medications for, 92, 107–108, 171, 174, 417, 492–494; and night feedings, 252; and pacifiers, 303–304, 379, 386; for preemies, 45; and sippy cups, 174; teeth cleaning, 92, 96, 108, 175, 252, 504; and tooth eruption, 90, 96

depression, help for, 61

Dermabond, 476, 478–479

dermatitis, contact, 439

Desitin, 81, 512

Desloratadine (Clarinex), 493

Desonide, 511

Desowen, 511

development: and BPA, 424; and comparisons of children, 265–266; definitions of, 266–267; and discipline, 308–312; and environmental hazards, 408–410; motor, 181, 266, 268–273, 283, 285–291, 296; normal, 267; of preemies, 39–45, 45, 264, 268–273; screening test for, 56–57; toys and, 291; websites on, 291, 550. See also specific types of development

developmental checklists, 267–273, 280, 287

developmental delays: and Down syndrome, 278–279; and ECI, 279–280; identifying, 268–269; and laboratory tests, 524; and preemies, 39, 41–42; screening tests for, 267; and sleep training, 259; and texture aversion, 192

developmental dysplasia of the hip (DDH), 402, 521

developmental milestones: and adoption, 46; and ASD, 275; from birth to two months, 283; cognitive, 267, 270; definition of, 267; failure to meet, 273; from four to six months, 285–287; and introduction of solid foods, 180; for language development, 266, 269–272, 274–276; for motor development, 181, 266, 268–272, 283, 285–291, 296; from nine to twelve months, 289–291; and preemies, 41–42, 45, 268–273; regression from, 275–276; from six to nine months, 287–289; and sleep, 248; for social-emotional development, 266–267, 270–272; toilet training, 210; from two to four months, 284–285

developmental stimulation: from birth to two months, 283–284; for four to six months,

index

287; from six to nine months, 288–289, 291–292; from two to four months, 284–285

dextromethorphan, 508

DHA. *See* docosahexaenoic acid (DHA)

diabetes: and advantages of breastmilk, 114; and celiac disease, 198; description of, 403; gestational, 18; and HFCS, 415; and introduction of solid foods, 180, 403; and malunggay, 134; testing for, 18, 57, 403, 523, 526; and vaccinations, 339; and vitamin supplements, 104; websites on, 403, 550

diaper bags, 74

diaper changes: and bladder infections, 89, 218–219; and cleaning circumcision site, 88; and dehydration, 217; detecting urine in, 455; diaper wipes, 80; in first year, 101; and GERD, 211; identifying contents of, 14–15; and new fathers, 36; and torticollis exercises, 401; tracking, 14, 34, 37–39, 218; and tummy time, 97

DiaperFreeBaby.org, 210

diaper rash: and blood in poop, 443–444; calling the doctor about, 475–476, 512; home remedies for, 517; medications for, 509–510, 512; Rash-o-Rama, xviii; treating, 81, 475–476; types of, 81; yeast, 61, 81, 90, 140–141, 376, 385, 472–473, 502, 509–510

diapers, and Elimination Communication, 210

diaper wipes, 80

diarrhea: and abdominal pain, 437–438; and antibiotic use, 386, 501–502, 515; blood in, 443, 453; calling the doctor about, 453–456, 499; and C. difficile infection, 498; and celiac disease, 198, 453; and dehydration, 217, 454–455, 457–458; and fevers, 454–455, 464; and food allergies, 193, 453; and food poisoning, 373, 453; formulas for, 167, 455; home remedies for, 518; and introduction of solid foods, 455–456; and lactose intolerance, 195, 456; and measles, 333; medications for, 456, 499; and norovirus, 369; and parasites, 378, 453; and pee in diapers, 218; as pooping red flag, 205; and probiotics, 456, 515; and Reglan, 498; and rehydration solutions, 500; and rotavirus, 338, 368–369; as side effect of medications, 503; and stomach ache, 437–438; and sugar in juice, 175, 453; and teething, 91; typical doctor's questions about, 453–454;

and viral gastroenteritis, 453; and vomiting, 454–455, 457–458

diets: and allergies, 197; calculating dietary needs, 99–100; and diabetes, 403, 415; and eczema, 85; elimination, 201; and fat, 175–176; high calorie, 44, 99, 103, 125, 165, 181; for nursing mothers, 145–149, 212; and obesity, 108–110; and sour-smelling breast milk, 142

difficult child temperament, 298–299

Diflucan, 502

Digoxin, 514

Dimenhydrinate, 500

diphenhydramine (Benadryl): for allergic reactions, 440, 493; as antihistamine, 201, 507–508; for colic, 500; and coxsackievirus, 367; in first aid kits, 435; and hives, 474; sedating effect of, 314, 399, 493; and weaning, 154

diphtheria, 330

diphtheria vaccine, 322, 331–332

Diprolene, 511

discipline: and behavior, 297, 308–312; and child development, 308–312; and masturbation, 313; as parental responsibility, 63; and physical force, 310; and temper tantrums, 310, 312

discipline management plans, 310

diseases: and exposure to environmental hazards, 409–410; and germs, 351; and vaccines, 320–324, 326. *See also specific diseases*

dislocations, 483–484

Disneyland, measles outbreak at, 333

disorientation, 520

distracted parenting, 293

DMSA scans, 522

DockATot, 240

docosahexaenoic acid (DHA), 159; in breast milk, 106–107, 148, 158–159, 160, 164; in formulas, 106–107, 148, 158–159, 160, 164; and heart disease, 106–107

doctor's office: described, 47; staff at, 58–59, 61. *See also* pediatricians

Doppler studies, 521

doubt, autonomy versus, 282

doulas, 64

Dove soap, 83, 353

Down syndrome, 198, 278–279

Dramamine, 500

dream feeds, 247–248, 255

drooling, 90, 470

drowning, 294–295, 418–419

Dr. Smith's Diaper Ointment, 81, 512
drug interactions, 489
drug resistance, 323, 337, 363–364, 372, 375, 379, 382–383, 385, 387, 412–413, 434, 459, 501–502
dry heaves, 456
dry lips and mouth, 453
dry skin, 85, 398–399
DSM-5, 274
DTaP vaccine, 56, 326–327, 330–331, 353
ducts, 119, 131, 133, 139–140, 145, 154
duodenal atresia, 9
Duphalac, 499
dust mites, 377, 405, 421
D-Vi-Sol, 503
dyes, avoiding, 398–399
dyslexia, environmental triggers for, 410

eardrums, 379–381, 383–384, 386, 387, 391, 482, 496
ears: bruising behind, 480; examining, 7; hair on, 105; piercing, 89; structure of, 379
ear/eye drops, antibiotic, 12, 373, 459–460, 495–497
ear infections: and bacterial infections, 365, 371–373, 375, 378–379, 382–388, 385–388, 464; and breastfeeding, 155, 384; and conjunctivitis, 459–460; doctor's appointments for, 60; and ENT specialists, 384, 386, 386–387; and fluid in ears, 378–379, 382–384, 386–388; frequency of, 386–387; home remedies for, 518; and influenza, 338, 382, 385, 385–386, 451; medications for, 380–384, 391, 495–496, 501; and pacifiers, 303–304, 379, 386–387; and PE tubes, 60, 383–384, 386–388, 491, 495–496; prevention of, 379, 386–387, 518; and Strep pneumoniae, 337, 363, 382, 385; and teething, 91; and travel, 314, 384; and vomiting, 457; wind/ceiling fans and, 362
ear injuries, 482, 484
early childhood intervention (ECI), 279–280
ears, pulling on, 383
ear thermometers, 35, 464
Earth's Best, 161–164, 169
ear wax, 496
Easter Seals, 279–280, 552
easy child temperament, 298
eating, 313, 450. See also breastfeeding; feedings; foods
EBV (Epstein-Barr Virus), 525

Echinacea, 513
echocardiogram, 394
echovirus, 371
ECI (early childhood intervention), 279–280
eco hazards, 407–417; reducing, 429–430
E. coli, 218, 361, 373–374, 385, 444–445
Econazole, 509
eczema: and allergies, 161, 183, 186, 195, 199, 201, 213, 393, 398–399, 404, 439, 471, 474; and asthma, 393, 400; and baths, 85, 399; home remedies for, 518; and introduction of solid foods, 85, 183, 186, 195, 199, 201, 398; medications for, 398–399, 511–512; outgrowing, 400; soaps for, 83, 353; and steroids, 398–399, 509
educational programming, 292–294
E.E.S., 501
eggs: allergies to, 183, 186, 195, 199, 324; and food poisoning, 444; in vaccines, 345
egocentricity, of babies, 281, 309, 312
Elastogel, 121
Elecare, 161, 162–163
electrocardiogram (EKG), 394
electrolyte balance, 458, 499, 523
electrolyte drinks, 455
electromagnetic fields (EMFs), 409, 423–424
Elidel, 399, 511
elimination, 20–21, 34. See also pee; poop
Elimination Communication (EC), 210
elimination diets, 201
elimination table, first week, 38–39
Elimite-5% Permethrin, 377, 510
Elocon, 511
embryonic stem cells, 22
emergency calls: for allergic reactions, 439–440; for anaphylactic reaction, 439–440; and apnea, 448; and choking, 449; and fevers, 463; for neck and back injuries, 481, 484; and pediatricians, 53, 433–434; phone numbers for, 435; for poisoning, 470; and seizures, 476; and swollen or bulging eyes, 460
emergency rooms, 60, 62, 438, 470
Emetrol, 500
emollients, 195, 399, 511–512
emotional development, 266–267, 282
emotional health, 61, 298, 310
Emverm, 502
Emverm (mebendazole), 378
enamel hypoplasia, 45
encephalitis, 327, 333, 336, 367, 371
endocrine disruptors, 409, 425

endocrine problems, 403, 409
endoscopy, 214
energy, and temperament, 299
Enfalyte, 500
Enfamil formulas, 104, 161–164, 166, 166–168
engorgement, 115–116, 118–119, 130, 133, 136, 141
Enspire, 161
enterocolitis/enteropathy, 166
enteroviruses, 355, 371
ENT specialists, 384, 386, 386–387, 496
environmental exposures: to aluminum, 346; and ASD, 277, 410; to chemicals, 407–415; to pesticides, 411–412, 421, 429–430; to pollutants, 275, 277, 397, 407–415; to vaccine ingredients, 346, 352; websites on, 397, 407. *See also specific chemicals and pollutants*
Environmental Protection Agency (EPA): and lead exposure, 397–398; list of hazardous chemicals from, 407; and radon, 421–422
Environmental Working Group, 277, 411
eosinophils, 524
ephedrine, 507
Epiceram, 512
epidemics, 331–332
epiglottitis, 333, 521
Epi-Pens, 200
epispadias, 9
Epsom salts, 139
Epstein-Barr Virus (EBV), 525
Epstein's pearls, 7
Equal, 415
Erb's palsy, 10
erections, 313
ERGO baby carriers, 230
Erikson, Erik, 282
errands, "two stop" rule for, 75
eruption hematoma, 91
Eryped, 501
erythema infectosum (Parvovirus), 370, 385, 472–473
erythema multiforme, 439, 474
erythema toxicum, 11
erythorbic acid, 416
Erythrocyte Sedimentation Rate (ESR), 525
Erythromycin, 501
esophageal pH probes, 214
esophagitis, 442
esophagus, 204, 210–211, 214, 216–217, 442
essential oils, 514, 517
estrogen, 406, 410, 425

eucalyptus oil, 377, 517
Eucerin, 83, 399
Eucrisa, 511
Eurax, 510
European Commission, 413
European formula brands, 162–163, 169
Eustachian tubes, 361, 378–380, 391
Evivo, 307
Excited Ineffective feeding behavior, 124
exercises, for torticollis, 401–402
exercising, 149–150
Exersaucer toys, 287
exhaustion: and breastfeeding, 116, 127, 129, 140, 150; and family beds, 241–242; of newborns, 117–118, 127, 152; and sleep problems, 225, 231, 258; and sleep training, 256
expectorants, 508
expiration dates, of medications, 488
expressive language delays, 266, 273–274, 384, 386
expressive language skills, 266, 270–273
extremities, examining, 10, 521–522
eye contact, avoiding, 273, 274
eye/ear drops, antibiotic, 12, 373, 459–460, 495–497
eye exams, and preemies, 42, 45
eyes: crossed, 284; examining, 6–7, 42, 45; goopy, 451, 459–460; and jaundice, 19
eye infections, 354, 385, 459–460
eye injuries: calling the doctor about, 481, 484; and stitches, 477, 479; and surgical glue, 479
eye problems: calling the doctor about, 459–460; detection of, 389–390; lazy eye, 57, 389–390; from Zika virus, 371
eye stye, home remedies for, 518

failure to thrive, 103–104, 198, 396, 520
family beds, 115, 241–243, 256
family caretaker, 68
family life, and work, 64, 66, 71–76, 258
Family Medical Leave Act (FMLA), 75
Famotidine, 213
Famotidine (Pepcid), 498
fatigue, and anemia, 395
fat necrosis, 327
fats: in alternative dairy products, 176; and brain development, 175; in breast milk, 150, 160, 181; and diarrhea, 455–456, 499; in formulas, 157–160, 164, 175–176; in goat's milk, 176–177; guidelines for, 112
fear: and breastfeeding, 128; of strangers,

288, 298, 312–313
febrile seizures, 465, 469–470, 476
feeder bottles, 172
feedings: ad lib/on demand, 13–14, 34, 102; and air travel, 314; behaviors, 124, 134; and burping, 204; cluster, 13, 34, 102, 120, 122, 155–156, 227; and dehydration, 126; dream feeds, 247–248, 255; and ear infections, 386; and elimination, 34; first feedings, 12–14; formula feeding in first year, 172–173; and GERD, 153–154, 173, 210–211, 212, 213, 216, 305–306; for late preterm infants, 152–153; and low blood sugar, 125; and mastitis, 140; and newborn tiredness, 13–14, 32, 34, 36, 39–41, 44, 117, 122, 172–173; night, 109, 134, 212, 242–243, 247, 249, 250, 252, 255–256, 264, 298; overfeeding, 108; paced bottle, 111, 119, 126, 144; patterns for, 102; poor routines for, 103; and preemies, 39–41, 44–45, 102, 151–152; red flags with, 34; and sleep, 129, 172–173, 175, 227–228, 241, 243, 243–250, 252, 254–255; and sleep routines, 251; and teeth cleaning, 92; tracking, 14, 34, 37–39; and twins, 234; and vomiting, 217, 457. See also breastfeeding
feeding schedules: and late preterm infants, 152–153; and newborns, 101–102; and night nursing, 134, 212; for preemies, 44, 101–102; and sleep, 34, 92, 134, 172–173, 175; and twins, 151
feeding table, first week, 38–39
Feingold Hypothesis, 415
fennel (foeniculum vulgare), 222, 306, 500
Fenugreek, 492
Feosol, 504
Ferber, James, 249, 253–254, 253–255, 257, 259
Ferberizing, 257. See also progressive waiting
Fer-In-Sol, 504
fermented products, 146
Feverall. See acetaminophen (Tylenol)
fevers: and abdominal pain, 437–438; and bacterial infections, 361–362, 364–365, 369, 374, 463, 464; and bladder infections, 219–220; and blood in poop, 443; and breastfeeding, 150; and bruising, 441; and burns, 445; calling the doctor about, 54, 301, 327, 329, 461–470; and circumcision, 29; and cold viruses, 357–359; and contagion, 359, 362; correct dosing of

medications for, 465, 467–468; and coughing, 452–453; and crying, 301; definition of, 461; and dehydration, 19; and diarrhea, 454–455, 464; and influenza, 338; and laboratory tests, 519–520; and mastitis, 131, 139; medications for, 35, 461–469, 497; and nasal congestion, 451; parental misconceptions about, 462; and plugged ducts, 139; and pulse rate, 436–437; and rashes, 471–475; recurring, 463–464; and red eyes, 460; red flags with, 35, 470; and respiratory distress, 447, 449; and roseola, 464; and seizures, 469–470, 476; and stitches, 477, 479; and swollen eyes, 460; and teething, 91, 469; and temperature-taking techniques, 56, 435, 461–462, 464, 466–467, 469; treatment protocol for, 462–464; typical doctor's questions about, 469; and vaccinations, 35, 58, 326–329, 331, 334, 463, 465; and varicella, 336; and viral infections, 357, 361–362, 365–375; and vomiting, 216–217, 458, 464
Fexofenadine (Allegra), 493
fiber: in cereals, 185, 207–208; and constipation, 111, 206, 222; and diarrhea, 455–456, 499; foods containing, 207–209; in formulas, 167, 455; and gas, 222; in peels, 412, 430; requirements for, 110–111, 207
Fifth disease (Parvovirus), 370, 385, 388, 472–473
fine motor development, 266, 271–272, 285–290, 291, 295–296
finger foods, 191
fingers, 301, 484
first aid, 435, 448–449
fish: allergies to, 195; DHA in, 106–107; and food poisoning, 444; iron in, 111; mercury in, 146, 191, 416–417, 430; websites on, 417
Fisher Price Newborn Rock 'n Play, 229
fish oil, 106–107
Flagyl, 503
flame retardants, 409, 418
flaring nostrils, 8, 31, 448, 452
flat angiomata, 11
flat feet, 400–401
flat heads, 95–97, 238–240, 240
flat nipples, 119, 137
flora: normal, 360–361, 502. See also bacteria
Florastor, 515
flu. See influenza

index

Fluconazole, 502
fluid, in ears, 378–379, 382–384, 386–388
fluid intake, 408, 457. *See also* dehydration
Fluocinonide, 511
fluoride, 92, 107–108, 171, 174, 417, 492–494
fluoride supplements, 107–108, 174, 493–494
fluorosis, 107, 494
Flushield, 324
Fluvirin, 324
Fluzone, 324, 339
folate, 176, 395, 396
folic acid deficiency, 278
fomites, 352, 368–369
Food Allergy Network, 196, 201
FoodAllergy.org, 147
Food and Drug Administration (FDA): and anti-inflammatories, 509; arsenic recommendations by, 413; and complementary therapies, 513; and cough and cold medications, 358, 507; drug safety website of, 512; and formula requirements, 158, 164; and GERD medications, 212; and GMOs, 414; and goat's milk formulas, 161, 166, 170; and immunoregulators, 399; mercury recommendations of, 191; and off-label use, 489; and Phenergan, 500; prescription labeling guidelines from, 491; and probiotics, 516; and reflux medications, 498; and regulation of herbs, 134; and steroid use, 501; and teething medications, 91, 494–495; and vaccinations, 322–323, 327, 338, 339–340, 344
food challenge, 98, 202
food coloring, 415–416, 459
food diversity, 180
food fights, 313
food intolerance, 195, 453. *See also* allergies/allergens
food poisoning, 217, 373–374, 385, 388, 444–445, 453, 457. *See also* gastroenteritis
foods: allergenic, 195–196; antibiotics in, 409, 411–412; calcium content of, 110; complementary, 100, 115, 154, 156, 173; DHA in, 148; and dietary restrictions for nursing, 145–149; encouraging introduction of, 180, 182, 186; enjoying mealtime, 181, 185, 191–192, 212; environmental hazards in, 408–417; expectations for one-year olds, 192–193; gassy, 147; guidelines for, 111–112; HFCS in, 415; hidden allergens in, 146, 196, 200; liquid, 113, 191–

192; malabsorption of, 103; overview of first year, 192–193; prebiotics in, 515–516; restaurant, 109, 111; solid, 93, 100–103, 105–106, 109, 115, 156–157, 175, 180–202, 207, 439–440; stuck in airway, 390; textured, 182, 192; and toddler formulas, 168; vitamin D in, 103–104; and weaning, 182. *See also* baby foods; *specific foods*
football hold, 34, 122–123, 151
foreign body/objects, 452–453, 460, 520
foremilk, 119, 150, 205
foreskin, 25–27, 88–89
formaldehyde, 345–346
formal operational development, 282
formulas: after first year, 177; aluminum in, 347; and baby poop appearance, 34, 204–205; and baby's first feedings, 13; and blood sugar testing, 18; BPA in, 424; and breastfeeding difficulties, 116; breast milk/formula decision, 113; calcium in, 164–165, 168; calories in, 10, 44, 99, 160, 181, 202; changing, 165–166; compared to breast milk, 132–133, 157–160; comparison of various brands, 162–163; cost of, 114, 157–160, 161–164, 167–170, 177; cow's milk based, 157–162, 165–170, 305; DHA in, 106–107, 148, 158–159, 160, 164; and diarrhea, 167, 455; DIY, 62; fats in, 157–160, 164, 175–176; feeding for first year, 172–173; and fluoride in water, 107–108, 171, 174; and frequency of pooping, 205; freshness of, 169; generic, 169; and GERD, 167, 173, 211, 213; goat's milk, 17, 155, 158–159, 161, 162, 166, 170; gourmet, 167–168; history of, 158–159; incorrect preparation of, 103; iron in, 105, 160, 180, 182–183, 396; lactoferrin in, 168; liquid concentrate, 107; with MFGM, 168; mixed in cereal, 185; mixing with water, 158, 167, 170–171, 493–494; and nutrition, 17, 93, 100–101, 157–158, 177; and obesity, 109; organic, 158, 161–162, 164–165, 169, 411–412; palmitic acid in, 163, 164; powder, 107, 165, 170–171; prebiotics in, 168, 515, 516; and preemies, 41, 44–45; probiotics in, 158, 167, 306–307, 515; ready-to-feed, 171; and rehydration solutions, 500; and rice cereal, 102; and solid food, 103, 105, 179, 185; soy, 158–166, 162–163, 165–166, 410; supplementing breastfeeding, 21–22, 41, 44–45, 113, 115, 118, 124–129, 129, 150, 152–153, 166, 168; toddler, 164, 168, 170; vitamin D in,

181, 500; and vitamin supplements, 104–105, 158, 164; and vomiting, 217; and water temperature, 167; and weaning, 155, 173; websites on, 157; zinc in, 111

Formvirisen, 357

four C's, avoiding, 111

FPIES (Food Protein-Induced Enterocolitis Syndrome), 194

Fragile X Syndrome, 276–277

free range parenting, 65

frenulectomy, 137

frenulum, tight, 7

fruits: fiber in, 111, 208; and food poisoning, 373, 444–445; guidelines for, 112; and introduction of solid foods, 184, 187; pesticides in, 411–412

fully hydrolyzed protein formulas, 158–163

Fulvicin, 502

fungal infections: description, diagnosis, and treatment of, 375–376; laboratory tests for, 528; medications for, 81, 131, 140, 364, 376, 502, 509–510; and rashes, 471, 472–473; as source of illness, 385; and thumb sucking, 304

fungi, 174, 345, 364

fussiness: and bladder infections, 374; and changing formulas, 165; and cold viruses, 360; and colic, 305; and fevers, 463; and formula selection, 161; and GERD, 211–212; and milk allergies, 146, 212; and mother's exercise, 149–150; and nasal congestion, 451; and nursing mother's diet, 147–148, 212; and red eyes, 460; and supraventricular tachycardia, 395; and vaccinations, 326

Gagnon, Tricia, 74

gag reflex, 182, 239, 449, 457

galactogogues, 134

galactosemia, 56, 166, 410

Galbreath, Laurie, 74

garden hoses, 419

gas: and breastfeeding, 147; and changing formulas, 165; and colic, 222, 305–306; and crying, 301; definition of, 203–204; and GERD, 212; helping baby pass, 222; home remedies for, 517; medications for, 500; and milk allergies, 146; and probiotics, 106, 222; and stomach ache, 438; and sucking, 221

gastritis, 442

gastroenteritis, 205, 217, 368–369, 438, 453, 457

gastroesophageal reflux (GER) and disease (GERD): and apnea, 449; and breastfeeding, 116, 132, 153–154; and colic, 212–213, 300, 305–306; and crying, 301; diagnosing, 211–216; and formula feeding, 167, 173, 211, 213; and hiccups, 221; and laboratory tests, 522; medications for, 213–214, 498–499; and nasal congestion, 450; outgrowing, 216, 264; and pediatricians, 167, 211–214, 264; and preemies, 43; and probiotics, 106, 213; questionnaire for, 215–216; red flags with, 210–211; and sleep, 102, 132, 173, 213–214, 237, 239, 257, 264; and teething, 91; tests for, 213–214, 220; treating, 213–214, 216; and vomiting, 211, 213, 457; and weight loss, 103; and wheezing, 216, 391

gastrointestinal problems: laboratory tests for, 522; medications for, 498–500; and preemies, 40, 43. See also colic

gastrointestinal viruses, 368–369, 385

Gatorade, 217, 458, 500

Gaviscon, 498

gelatin, 324, 345

gel balls, in diapers, 15

gel pads, 139

gender differences: and ASD, 276–277; and bladder infections, 218–219, 374; and BMI, 109; and DDH, 402; and growth charts, 94, 553–557; and soy formulas, 410; and toilet training, 210

generic formulas, 169

generic medications, 60, 487–488, 490. See also specific medications

genetically modified organisms (GMOs), 158, 169, 414

genetic disorders: and ASD, 276–277; and cord blood banking, 22, 24; cystic fibrosis, 393; diabetes, 403; and global developmental delays, 273; and sickle cell trait, 395–396

genetic mutations, 277, 409

genetic predispositions, 391, 404, 423

genital herpes (HSV-2), 26, 367

genitals: ambiguous, 10, 524; burns on, 445; caring for, 79, 89, 218–219, 374; examining, 9–10; playing with, 313; problems with, 405–406; and yeast infections, 502. See also circumcision; penises

gentle parenting style, 65

gentle sleep training, 255–256

Gerber formulas, 106, 161–164, 166, 168

Gerber Pediatric Electrolyte, 500

index

Gerber Soothe, 307, 516
German measles, 277, 334, 472–473
germs: in digestive tract, 306, 456, 515; and fomites, 352; and laboratory tests, 527–528; limiting newborns' exposure to, 33, 462; and pacifiers, 303–304; and painful nipples, 139, 140; in poop, 203; and pre-chewing, 189; as source of disease, 351; and Strep pneumoniae, 337; and vaccinations/vaccines, 320, 322–323, 330, 345–346. See also antibiotics; bacteria; infections; probiotics; viruses
gestational diabetes, 18
Giardia, 378, 385, 388, 453, 503
ginger (Zingiber officinale), 222, 306, 500
gingivostomatitis, 367
girl parts: caring for, 89, 218–219, 374, 405–406. See also genitals
global developmental delays, 273
glossary, 533–552
Glow Baby, xix, 14, 34, 120
glue, closing wounds with, 476, 478–479
gluten, 180, 198
glycerin bullet, 206, 499
glycine, 345
GMOs. See genetically modified organisms (GMOs)
goat's milk: and allergies, 197; compared to cow's milk, 176–177; in formulas, 17, 155, 158–159, 161, 162, 166, 170
goat's rue, 134
goiters, 188
Golacta.com, 134
goodie bags, 314
goose egg bumps, 481
Gourmet feeding behavior, 124
gourmet formulas, 167–168
gradual sleep training, 253–255, 257
grains, 111, 184, 198, 207, 208, 403
grandparents, 68, 116, 235, 292
grape jelly-appearing poop, 438, 443, 454
Grifulvin, 502
grilling, 416
gripe water, 222, 500
Grisactin, 502
Griseofulvin, 502
gross motor development, 266, 270–273, 285–291, 291, 295. See also large muscle development
Group A Strep (Strep throat), 362, 383, 385, 488–489, 501
Group B Strep, 17–18, 361, 362, 374–375, 385, 463

growth: and allergies, 197; catch-up, 44, 61–62, 94, 99, 506; charting, 44, 93–94, 99, 103, 553–557; daily, 98; and Down syndrome, 279; in first year, 98; height prediction, 94–95; and nutrition, 93; rate of, 98; spurts, 100–101; and steroid use, 506
growth charts, 44, 93–94, 99, 103, 553–557
growth plates, 483
Grunting Baby Syndrome, 205
grunting sounds, 8, 31, 35, 205, 448, 452
guaifenesin, 508
guar gum, 499
guilt, 74, 255, 258, 282
gums, 7
Gunter, Jennifer, 42
gut absorption, and environmental hazards, 408
gut bacteria, 361
gut building, 114
Guthrie, Robert, 36
Gymboree, 294

haemophilus influenza, 373
haemophilus influenza B (HIB), 319, 333
haemophilus influenza B (HIB) vaccine, 56, 322, 324, 330, 333, 353
haemophilus influenza non-typable, 382, 385, 396, 459
hair, 240, 506
Hale, Thomas, 135, 491
Halo Bassinet Swivel Sleeper, 230
Halo SleepSack, 237
hand-foot-and-mouth, 354, 371, 385, 388, 472–473
hand-me-downs, 426
hands, burns on, 445
hand sanitizers, 80, 352–353, 369, 372
Happiest Baby on the Block (Karp), 307
Happy Baby, 169
hay fever, 404
HCAs (heterocyclic amines), 416
headaches: and asthma medications, 505; and cold viruses, 360; and head injuries, 480; and Parvovirus, 370; as reaction to medications, 502–503, 508; and Reglan, 498; and vomiting, 457
heads: baby carriers' support for, 284; examining, 521–522; flat, 95–97, 237–238; shape of, 6, 96
Head and Shoulders, 85
head banging, 274–275
head circumference, 555–556
head control: developmental milestones for,

266; and holding newborns, 34, 41; and preemies, 41, 45; and torticollis, 401–402

head injuries: and bleeding, 479–482, 484; calling the doctor about, 54, 479–481; and CT scans, 424, 481; and vomiting, 457–458

head lice, 377–378, 388, 509–510

head size: and ASD, 277; charting, 93–95; and laboratory tests, 520

head trauma, 476, 479–481

health care, decision-making for, 64, 66

health issues: and Down syndrome, 279; and environmental exposures to chemicals, 407–417, 419–420; and GMOs, 414; and hospitalization of newborns, 5

Healthy Sleep Habits, Happy Child (Weissbluth), 254–255

hearing, 7, 283, 380, 382–384

hearing tests, 15, 16, 42, 56, 279

heartburn: and colic, 300, 305–306; and crying, 301; diagnosis and treatment of, 211–214; formulas for, 167; and sleep, 102, 239. *See also* gastroesophageal reflux (GER) and disease (GERD)

heart defects: diagnosing, 8, 394, 521; and Down syndrome, 279; ultrasound imaging of, 8, 521; websites on, 394, 551; and Zika virus, 371

heart disease: and advantages of breast-feeding, 114; and DHA, 106–107; and fiber, 110; and RSV, 366; and vaccinations, 339

heart murmurs, 8, 394, 520

heart rate: and asthma medications, 505; and decongestants, 507; and laboratory tests, 520; of newborns, 5, 395; and taking vital signs, 435–437

height, 93–95

Heimlich maneuver, 429, 449

helmets, 95–97, 239

hematocrit, 56, 524

hematomas, 6, 20, 91, 96

hematopoietic stem cells, 23

hemoglobin, 395–396, 524

hemolytic anemia, 523

hemolytic uremic syndrome (HUS), 373, 444–445

hemophilia, 440, 525

hepatitis A, 46, 335

hepatitis A vaccine, 56, 322, 330, 335, 353, 357

hepatitis B, 46, 151, 335

hepatitis B vaccine: aluminum in, 347; and celiac disease, 198; as inactivated vaccine, 322; and preemies, 43; and prevention of viral infections, 323, 357; scheduling, 330, 335–336; as standard care, 16, 18

hepatitis C, 46

herbal remedies, 134, 306, 489, 492, 513–514, 516

herbal supplements, 134

herd immunity, 320–321

hernias, 521

herpes, 352, 356, 475, 511

herpes stomatitis, 385, 388

Herpetic Whitlow, 472–473

heterocyclic amines (HCAs), 416

hiatal hernias, 216, 522

HIB. *See* haemophilus influenza B (HIB)

hiccups, 33–34, 204, 221

high chairs, 185

high fructose corn syrup (HFCS), 161, 164, 415

high-maintenance children, 299, 301

Hill, Linda, breastfeeding tips from, 118, 123, 132–133, 135, 139–141, 144, 155, 304

hindmilk, 119, 150, 153, 205

HIPAA, 62

HIPP formulas, 162–163

hips, 10, 34, 238, 402, 521

Hirschprung's disease, 9

histamine receptor antagonists, 213

histamines, 194–195, 213, 440, 474, 508. *See also* antihistamines

hitting, 298

HIV: and adoption, 46; and bacterial infections, 375; and circumcision, 25–26, 28; medications for, 356; and purchased breast milk, 151

hives: and allergic reactions, 193–195, 200, 213, 439, 471, 474–475; calling the doctor about, 439, 474–475; description and treatment, 474–475; as side effect of medications, 474–475, 502–503

HMO (Human Milk Oligosaccharide), 168

Hoag Hospital, 82

holiday/Christmas lights, safety with, 418

The Holistic Pediatrician (Kemper), 516

Holle formulas, 162–163

home: baby-proofing checklist for, 422; environmental hazards in, 409

Homeopathic Pharmacopeia of the United States (HPUS), 516

homeopathic remedies, 516, 516–517

homeopathic teething tablets, 91, 494–495

homeopathy, 513

home remedies, 500, 517–518

Honest Company, 80

honey, 180, 186, 452, 515

hormones: and acne, 84; and ASD, 277; and blood in diapers, 15, 218; and body temperature, 461; bovine growth hormone, 176, 412–414; and breast enlargement in newborns, 10; and breastfeeding, 115, 145; and cradle cap, 84; and endocrine disruptors, 409; in food, 409, 411–414; and growth plates, 483; and insufficient milk supply, 116; and organic certification, 189; and oxybenzone, 86; postpartum, 36, 37; and rashes in newborns, 11, 35, 471, 475; thyroid, 188; Thyroid Stimulating Hormone, 526. *See also specific hormones*

hot tubs, 419

housekeepers, 72

house rules, 309

HPA axis suppression, 506, 511

HPUS (Homeopathic Pharamacopeia of the United States), 516

Huggins, Kathleen, 141

Human Milk Banking Association of North America, 151

Human Milk Oligosaccharide (HMO), 168

human papillomavirus (HPV), and circumcision, 26

human papillomavirus (HPV) vaccine, 26, 357

Hume, Mary C., 319

humidifiers, 85, 358, 359, 367, 517, 518

hunger drive, 112

hunger strikes, 112, 155

hydrocele, 9

hydrocephalus, 217

hydrocortisone cream, 85, 399, 435, 511

hydrolyzed formulas, 158–163, 166

hydronephrosis, 220, 521

hydroureter, 220

Hydroxyzine(Atarax), 493

hygiene: and bladder infections, 218–219; and circumcision, 26; and head lice, 510; and humidifiers, 517; and infection prevention, 43, 369, 371, 372–373, 387, 477; and yeast infections, 140

hygiene products, *See also* cleaning products

Hyland's Teething Tablets, 494–495

hyperthermia, 461, 465

hyperthyroidism, 526

hyphema, 481

hypoallergenic, breastfeeding as, 114

hypoallergenic formulas, 157, 159–160, 161, 213

hypoallergenic shampoos, 84

hypoglycemia, 125, 523

hypospadias, 9, 410

hypothyroidism, 56, 103, 526

Hytone, 511

ibuprofen (Motrin, Advil): and breastfeeding, 136; correct dosing of, 466–469, 497; and fevers, 369, 464–469, 497; in first aid kits, 435; for teething, 91, 494; and viral infections, 367

Icar, 504

identity, role confusion versus, 282

idiopathic thrombocytopenic purpura (ITP), 441, 471

IgA antitissue transglutamate, 198

IgA endomysial antibody, 198

I-GERQ-R score, 214

ILCA (International Lactation Consultant Association), 303

ileus, 205

ILikeMyTeeth.org, 108

imaging studies, 424, 481, 520–522

imitation, 290

immobilization, of broken bones, 483–484

immune compromise: and bacterial infections, 360, 362, 375; and chickenpox, 336; and COVID-19, 366; and fungal infections, 375; and powdered formulas, 170; and probiotics, 106, 516; and RSV, 506–507; and vaccinations, 322, 324, 339–340

immuneglobulin A vasculitis, 441

immune response: and asthma, 390; and diabetes, 403; and fever, 462; and infections, 354, 378, 474; and introduction of solid foods, 198, 403; and rashes, 474; and vaccines, 43, 322, 324, 326, 329, 331, 334–345, 352

immune systems: and allergies, 195; and bacterial infections, 362; and celiac disease, 198; and COVID-19, 340–341; and fevers, 461–462; and rashes, 474; and vaccinations, 319, 322–325, 324, 325; and viral infections, 354, 360, 366

immunity: and chickenpox vaccine, 336, 370; and COVID-19 vaccinations, 341; and exposure to viruses, 30, 353; herd, 320–321; and influenza vaccine, 339; and pertussis, 331; and rhinoviruses, 358; and vac-

cination requirements, 325–326
immunization: and adoption, 46; and RSV, 507; schedule, 56–57; and stitches, 477, 479; and vaccinations, 325–326, 331–332; and well child checks, 58
Immunization Action Coalition, 349, 352
immunoregulators, 399
impetigo, 372–373, 388, 472–473, 508
inactivated vaccines, 322, 326, 339
inappropriate programming, 292
incarcerated hernia, 437
inclined sleep products, 229
independent play, 293–294
industry: inferiority versus, 282; waste from, 417
infant CPR classes, 45, 191, 435
Infant Formula Act (1986), 165
InfantProctocolitis.org, 147
Infant Swimming Resource (ISR), 295, 296
infections: and animal bites, 477; and apnea, 449; and appearance of poop, 209; of the belly button, 80–81; and blood in poop, 209, 338; of blood of, 40, 337, 375; and burns, 445; and childcare, 70–71, 387; and circumcision, 25–26, 28; cronobacter sakazakii, 170; and ear piercing, 89; exposure to, 30, 353; and fever, 219–220, 329, 357, 361–362, 365–375, 461–462, 463, 464; and fluid in ears, 378–379; HIB, 333; and immune response, 354, 378, 474; intestinal, 167; kidney, 219–220, 374, 457, 463, 520–524, 522, 526; and laboratory tests, 361, 364, 519–520, 524, 526–528; lung, 333, 358–359, 372, 385, 393, 446–449; and lymph nodes, 359–360; mastitis, 139–140, 150; mumps, 334; of nipples, 131, 133, 139; and petechiae, 441; and preemies, 40, 43; and purchased breast milk, 151; and rashes, 471, 474; and red eyes, 460; reducing by breastfeeding, 114; of respiratory system, 150, 446–449; rubella, 334; and runny noses, 450–451, 464; screening test for, 57; and sickle cell disease, 396; as source of disease, 351; of umbilical stump, 35, 81–82, 330; and unusual body odors, 406; UTI, 10, 26, 89, 218–220, 374, 463; and vaccinations, 322–324, 325–326, 329–342, 354; of the womb, 17–18, 150; of wounds, 477–479; yeast, 61, 81, 84–85, 90, 131, 133, 140–141. See also bacterial infections; bladder infections; ear infections; fungal infections; viral infections;

specific diseases
inferiority, 282
infertility, 342
inflammatory bowel disease (IBD), 114, 453
influenza: and abnormal genetic development, 277; and aspirin, 497; and asthma, 391; description, diagnosis, and treatment of, 338–340, 365; and ear infections, 338, 382, 385–386, 451; laboratory tests for, 528; medications for, 503; and nasal congestion, 450; and respiratory distress, 446; seasonal patterns of, 43, 353–354, 387; and sinus infections, 372; as viral infection, 385; and white blood cell count, 356
influenza vaccines: allergic reaction to, 324; CDC recommendations for, 339; as inactivated vaccines, 322, 339; and polyethylene glycol, 346–347; and preemies, 43, 45; for prevention of flu, 365; schedule for, 330; and stomach flu, 453
ingestions, 470, 476
inguinal hernia, 9
inhaled steroids, 392, 505–506
in-home daycare, 69, 72
initiative, guilt versus, 282
injuries, 440, 448
inoculation. See vaccinations/vaccines
insect bites, 460, 509
insect repellents, 86–87, 371, 421
insomnia, 503, 505, 507
Inspired Start, 199
instincts, going with, 55, 63–64, 68
Institute of Medicine (IOM), 146, 344
insulin, 227, 403
insurance: and breast pumps, 143; and circumcision, 28; and Down syndrome, 279; and hearing tests, 16; and pediatricians, 50, 52–53, 55, 58; and vision screenings, 57, 390
intellectual development: and anemia, 105; checklist for, 269–270; and Down syndrome, 278–279; and exposure to environmental hazards, 408, 413; and HIB, 333; and mumps, 334
intensity, and temperament, 299
International Committee on Taxonomy of Viruses, 352
International Lactation Consultant Association (ILCA), 303
International Pediatric Sleep Education Task Force, 248
interventions, sleep issues and, 254, 258, 260–261

intestinal obstruction, 437, 457
intestines: and anti-diarrheal medications, 456; and asthma medications, 506; bacterial infections of, 453, 502; blockage of, 216–217; and blood in poop, 209; and C. difficile colitis, 502; and celiac disease, 198; and cystic fibrosis, 393; and gas, 203–204; infections of, 167; kinks in, 209; malrotation of, 9; and measles, 333; pinworms in, 378; x-rays of, 521
intoeing, 400
intravenous fluids, as jaundice treatment, 21
intraventricular hemorrhage (IVH), 42, 521
intussusception, 205, 209, 338, 344, 437, 521
inverted nipples, 119, 137
iodine, 188
IOM (Institute of Medicine), 146, 344
IPV vaccine, 56, 324, 330, 332
iron: in breast milk, 105–106, 156, 180, 182–183, 396; in cereals, 111, 183, 185; in cow's/goat's milk, 176–177, 396; in formulas, 105, 160, 180, 182–183, 396; and introduction of solid foods, 180, 182, 202, 396; and lactoferrin, 168; need for, 105, 111, 180, 182–183; and preemies, 44–45, 105–106; and vitamins, 111, 504
iron deficiency anemia, 103, 105, 182, 313, 395–397, 503–504
iron replacement therapy, 504
iron supplements, 105–106, 156, 396–397, 503–504
irritants, 409, 421
irritation, 460, 509
iScreen, 389
isoflavones, 410
Isomil DF formula, 455
Ivermectin, 510

jaundice: abnormal, 19–21; and bilirubin test, 15; and blood type incompatibility, 17; and breastfeeding, 20–22, 120, 126; compared to carotinemia, 188; and dehydration, 21, 126; and laboratory tests, 520, 523; normal, 19, 35; and preemies, 40; and skin, 11, 19–20, 35; treating, 21–22; and umbilical cord cutting, 4
Jenner, Edward, 319
jock itch, 376, 509
Johnson's baby shampoo, 83
juices: avoiding, 111, 174–175; and chronic diarrhea, 453; and food poisoning, 444; and iron absorption, 111; iron supplements in, 397, 504; and nutrition, 93, 174–

175

Kabrita formulas, 162–163, 170
Kao-electrolyte, 500
Kaopectate, 456, 517
Karp, Harvey, 241, 307
Kawasaki disease (KD), 472–473
Keflex, 501
Kemper, Kathi J., 516
Kenalog, 511
kerion, 376
kernicterus, 20
Ketoconazole, 509
Kiddie, 423
kidney disease, 103, 375
kidney infections: and bladder infections, 374; and fevers, 463; and laboratory tests, 520–524, 522, 526; and vomiting, 457; and VUR, 219–220
kidneys: and adverse reactions to medications, 503; and diabetes, 403; examination of, 10, 522; failure of, 373; and failure to thrive, 103; malformation of, 9, 219; screening test for, 57; ultrasound imaging of, 521
kidney stones, 526
King of the Sea tuna, 417, 430
Kirkland formulas, 162, 164
Klout, 510
knock-kneed, 400
Kondremul, 499
Kosher salt, 188
Kroger, 413
Kunik, Randy, 303

labels, 200, 514
labia, 9, 89, 406
labial adhesion, 405–406
laboratory tests, and bacterial/viral infections, 361, 364, 519–520
lactase, 167, 453
lactase deficiency, 166
lactation consultants (LCs): advice from, 15, 36, 41, 116–118; bottle nipple recommendations, 172; and breast reduction surgery, 145; and herbal supplements, 134; and late preterm infants, 153; and nipple issues, 121, 137; and preemies, 44, 116; scheduling, 64; and tongue tie, 138; and yeast infections, 141
lactation services, 143
lactic acid, 149–150
Lactinex, 499, 515

Lactobacillus, 361, 456, 499
Lactobacillus acidophilus, 515
Lactobacillus bulgaricus, 515
Lactobacillus GG, 500, 515
Lactobacillus reuteri, 106, 167, 222, 306, 500, 515
Lactobacillus rhamnosus, 515
lactoferrin, 168
lactoglobulin, 200
lactose free diet, and diarrhea, 195, 456
lactose free formulas, 167
lactose intolerance, 161, 167, 195, 301, 453, 456
lactose sugar, 160, 161, 164, 167, 176–177, 345, 453
lactulose, 499
La Leche League, 141
Lancet, 415
language development: and ASD, 274–276, 343; from birth to two months, 270, 283; checklist for, 269–270; description of, 266; and ear infections, 383–384, 386; and ECI, 279; from four to six months, 285–287; and media use, 292, 294; and methylmercury exposure, 416; from nine to twelve months, 272, 291; from six to nine months, 271–272, 288–289; and temper tantrums, 312; from two to four months, 270–271, 284–285
lanolin, 81, 119, 121, 137, 139
Lansoprazole, 213, 498
large babies, 99, 103, 401, 523
large muscle development, 42, 266, 270–273, 279, 295. See also gross motor development
laryngomalacia, 7
larynx, 446–447
latch: assistance establishing, 36, 115, 121; difficulties of, 115–116; and engorgement, 130, 135–136, 141; and nipple pain, 136–138; and nipple shields, 41; and nursing position, 123; tips for a comfortable, 123; and tongue tie, 137
late preterm infants (LPI): and breastfeeding, 125, 133–134, 152–153; and clothing, 80; concerns with, 39–41; and developmental delays, 280; and jaundice, 19
laundry detergents, 85, 440
lawns, pesticides on, 421
Lawrence, Ruth, 150
lazy eye, 57, 389–390
LCs. See lactation consultants (LCs)
lead: in herbal remedies, 513; in holiday

lights, 418; as neurotoxin, 57, 409–410; screening test for, 56–57, 397–398; in water, 409, 417
lead poisoning, 275, 395, 397–398
LEAP Study, 197, 199
learning disabilities: and developmental delays, 280; and expressive language delays, 273; and preemies, 39
Lebenswert formulas, 162–163
Legendairymilk.com, 134
legs, 10, 402, 521–522
legumes, 184, 196, 209
let down, 119, 136, 149, 154
lethargy, 122, 217, 328, 441, 454, 470, 480
leukemia, 23–24, 421, 441, 471, 524
leukotriene antagonists, 505
Levalbuterol, 505
lice, 377–378, 385, 509–510
licensed vocational nurse (LVN), 61
licorice, 306
Lidex, 511
Lieberman, Allen, 183
lifetime burden, of environmental hazards, 408
life/work balance, 64, 66, 71–76, 258
light sensitivity, 274, 502
limping, 402, 470, 483, 520
Lindane, 510
Linden, Dana, 42
lipase, 142
lipid panel/cholesterol, 525
lipids, 159
lips, stitches in, 477
lip sucking, 303
lip swelling, 439, 474, 502
Little Gym, 294
Little Remedies for Noses, 441, 507
Little Tummys, 500
live attenuated vaccines, 321–322, 326, 332, 336
liver, 126, 335, 456, 497
liver function tests, 525
location, and environmental hazards, 408
lockjaw, 331
Locoid, 511
Lomotrin AF, 81, 509
Looking Out for Number Two (Vartabedian), 106
loperamide (Immodium), 456
Loratadine (Claritin, Alavert), 474, 493, 508
lotions, 83–84
lower respiratory infections, description of, 446

index

low-maintenance children, 299
lungs: and asthma, 390, 392; and coughing, 446, 452–453; and meconium, 19; and preemies, 39, 42–43
lung infections: bacterial, 372, 385; and cold viruses, 358–359; and cystic fibrosis, 393; measles, 333; and respiratory distress, 446–449. *See also* haemophilius influenza; haemophilus influenza B (HIB); haemophilus influenza non-typable; pneumonia; RSV (respiratory syncytial virus)
lung problems, websites on, 551
lutein, 164
Lyme Disease, 86, 472–473
lymph nodes, 359–360, 522
lymphocytes, 356, 524
lymphoma, 23, 421

Maalox, 367
McCarthy, Jenny, 276
macroencephaly, 95
macrolides, 501
magnetic resonance imaging (MRI), 424, 521–522
malabsorption, 198, 209
Malathion, 377, 510
malnutrition, 517
malrotation, of intestines, 9
maltodextrin, 161–162, 164
malt soup, 499
Maltsupex, 499
malunggay, 134
manicures, baby, 79
March of Dimes Birth Defects Foundation, 552
massage, 140, 222, 302, 306, 308
mastitis, 131, 133, 139–140, 150
mastoiditis, 382
masturbation, 313
maternal age, and insufficient milk supply, 116
maternity leave, 72, 144, 150
mattresses, 237–238, 242, 263, 358, 427
mature milk, 119–120, 122, 124, 206
Mayo Clinic, contact information for, 17
MCV 4 vaccine, 338
measles, 319, 321, 326, 329, 333–334, 472–473
measles (MMR) vaccine, 274, 326, 329, 334, 343, 357
meats: antibiotics in, 413; and food poisoning, 373, 444; grilling, 416; guidelines for, 112; and introduction of solid foods, 183–

185; iron in, 105, 111, 182–183; nitrates/nitrites in, 416; zinc in, 111, 183
Mebendazole, 502
meconium, 4, 9, 14, 18, 34, 36, 204–205, 209
meconium plug, 9, 205
MECP2 gene, 277
Medela breast pumps, 127
media use, 292–294, 549
medical abbreviations on prescriptions, 490
medical histories, 46, 236, 328, 402
medical information, websites on, 551
medical passports, 328
medical provider, 61
medications: age restrictions for taking, 463, 489, 493, 497, 501, 507–508, 511; allergic reactions to, 501–502, 512; for allergies, 439–440, 493; for anaphylactic reaction, 439; antibiotic ear/eye drops, 12, 373, 459–460, 495–497; for asthma, 366, 390, 392, 488, 504–506; avoiding while nursing, 149; and baby's sleeping through air travel, 314; for bacterial infections, 362–365; and breastfeeding, 135, 140–141; for burns, 445; for cold viruses, 358–359, 507–509; for colic, 305–306, 500; compared to complementary therapies, 513; for constipation, 206, 499; correct dosing of, 465–469, 488–489, 493, 497, 498–499, 504; cost of, 60; for coughing, 358, 452, 507–509, 514; for dental care for, 92, 107–108, 171, 174, 417, 492–494; for diarrhea, 456, 499; and drug resistance, 323, 337, 363–364, 372, 375, 379, 382–383, 385, 387, 412–413, 434, 459, 501–502; for ear infections, 380–384, 391, 495–496, 501; for eczema, 398–399, 511–512; for eye problems, 496–497; for fever, 35, 369, 461–469, 463–469, 497; for fungal infections, 81, 131, 140, 376, 502, 509–510; generic, 60, 487–488, 490; for GERD, 213–214, 498–499; for Giardia, 503; herbal remedies, 134, 306, 489, 492, 513–514, 516; and hives, 474–475, 502–503; in home first aid kit, 435; for labial adhesions, 406; for mastitis, 131, 140–141; and medical passport, 328; for nasal congestion, 493; and on-call doctors, 434–435; over-prescription of, 364; over-the-counter, 388, 490; for pain, 28–29, 122, 497; for pinworm, 378, 502; and preemies, 43; and rashes, 474–475, 509–510, 512; safety with, 491–492; for scabies, 377; for skin

problems, 501, 508–512; to stimulate breast milk production, 46, 116, 151; for teething, 91, 155, 492, 494–495; tips for administering, 488; for torticollis, 402; for viral infections, 322–324, 356–357, 365–371, 503; for vomiting, 500; and weaning, 155. *See also* vaccinations/vaccines

Medications and Mother's Milk (Hale), 135, 491

melanin, 86

melatonin, 226

meningitis: as bacterial infection, 337–338, 385; and bladder infections, 374; and bruising, 441; description, diagnosis, and treatment of, 217, 333, 374–375, 472–473; and ear infections, 382; as enterovirus, 371; and fevers, 219, 463; Meningococcal, 349; and mumps, 334; and petechiae, 471; and Strep B infection, 18, 374–375; and Strep pneumoniae, 337, 337–338, 375; and vaccinations, 326, 337–338, 354; and vomiting, 217, 457

Meningitis Angels, 354

Meningococcal meningitis, 349, 354

menopause, 114

menstruation, 150, 395, 406, 413–414

menthols, 517

mercury: in fish, 146, 191, 416–417, 430; in herbal remedies, 513; in vaccines, 344–346, 352

mesenchymal stem cells, 23

metabolic disorders: and apnea, 449; and developmental delays, 273; diabetes, 403; and failure to thrive, 103, 396; screening tests for, 16–17, 46, 56, 393, 395, 523, 526; and soy formulas, 410; and unusual body odors, 406; and vomiting, 457

metabolic storage disease, 8

metabolism, and ASD, 278

metals, 275

methamphetamines, 507

methemoglobinemia, 414, 494

Methicillin Resistant Staph Aureus (MRSA), 372, 385

methylchloroisothiazolinone (MCI), 80

methylmercury, 409, 416–417, 430

metocloparamide, 498

metric system conversions, 98–99

Metronidazole, 503

MFGM (Milk Fat Globule Membrane), 168

Micatin, 509

Miconazole, 509

microcephaly, 95, 371

microchips, implanting, 343

microplastics, 425

middle ear infections, 379–384, 383, 386

milia, 11

miliaria, 11

milk: and calcium, 110; cow's, 133, 146–147, 155, 157–162, 160–170, 175, 186, 193–197, 213, 305, 516; environmental hazards in, 411–412; guidelines for, 112; and iron supplements, 397; organic, 176, 408, 411–414; raw, 176, 374; whole, 101, 112, 155, 157, 168, 173, 175, 193, 414

Milk Fat Globule Membrane (MFGM), 168

milk transfer, 134–135, 153

Milley, Frankie, 349, 354

Milley, Ryan, 354

Mimyx, 512

Mindell, J., 259

mineral oil, 499

minerals, 158, 161

mint tea, 306

Miracle Blanket, 238

Miralax, 499

MIS-C (multisystem inflammatory syndrome), 342

mites, 364, 376–377, 385, 421

mixed temperament, 298

MMR vaccine: allergies to, 324; and ASD, 274, 343; and disease prevention, 357; as live attenuated vaccine, 322, 326, 334; and rashes, 475; scheduling, 329, 334

mohel, 22, 28

moisturizers, 85, 398–399

molds, 421

Molecular Assay (NAAT), 528

moles, 11

Molluscum contagiosum, 472–473

Mometosone furoate, 511

Mom's Day Out programs, 74

Mongolian spots, 11

monilial dermatitis. *See* yeast diaper rash

mononucleosis, 525, 528

monospot, 525

Montagu, Mary Wortly, 319

Montelukast, 505

moods, 299, 503, 506

moraxella, 382

Moringa oleifera, 134

Moro, Debby, 75

moro reflex, 10

Moser, C., 352

mosquitoes, 86–87, 371

Mother's Milk Banks, 151

index

mothers/mothers-in-law, help from, 36–37
motion detectors, 239
motor development, 181, 266, 270–273, 285–291, 295–296, 312
Motrin. *See* ibuprofen (Motrin, Advil)
mouth: abnormalities of, 134–135; babies putting things in, 296, 353; bacteria in, 361, 502; burns to, 470; caring for, 90–92; examining, 7; injuries to, 482; and pacifiers, 303; viral infections of, 367–368, 385
movement, soothing with, 229–230
MRI (magnetic resonance imaging), 424, 521–522
mRNA vaccines, 340–343
MSG, 345
mucous: and asthma, 390; and coughing, 331, 446, 447; in diarrhea, 453–454, 499; and expectorants, 508; and humidifiers, 359; and respiratory distress, 446; saline nose drops for, 30–31, 60, 358, 435, 450–451, 507, 517; as symptom of viral infection, 354, 358, 361, 446, 451
multiple births. *See* twins
multiple language speakers, 290
multiplex PCR testing, 355–356, 528
multisystem inflammatory syndrome (MIS-C), 342, 366
multivitamins, 45, 106, 503–504
mumps, 334, 357
Mupirocin, 509
Murine, 496
muscle problems, 400–402
muscles: development of, 42, 266, 270–273, 279, 295–296; sphincter, 210–211, 216; tightening of, 401
mutagens, 409
Mycostatin, 509
Mylanta, 498
Mylicon drops, 211, 221–222, 500

NAEYC (National Association for the Education of Young Children), 70
nails, 79, 367, 484
nanny/au pair, 68–69, 72
naps: frequency and duration of, 260–263; missing, 249; for new parents, 36; and school schedules, 262; at six to twelve months, 233–234, 261–262; and sleep rituals, 254, 261; and two to four months, 230, 232–233, 234, 244–246, 261–262; and two to six months, 261–262; and Weissbluth sleep training, 254–255
nap schedules, 243–247, 245, 261

nasal congestion: and asthma medications, 505; and breastfeeding, 155; calling the doctor about, 450–451; and decongestants, 507; medications for, 493; in newborns, 7; saline nose drops for, 31, 60, 358, 435, 450–451, 517
nasal sprays, 507
nasolacrimal duct obstruction, 7, 459
natal teeth, 7
National Allergy Supply Inc., 405
National Association for the Education of Young Children (NAEYC), 70
National Asthma Education and Prevention Program, 392
National Center for Complementary and Integrative Health, 513–514, 516
National Center on Birth Defects and Developmental Disabilities, 552
National Highway Transportation Safety Administration, and car seats, 30
National Institute of Allergy and Infectious Diseases, 181, 197
National Institutes of Health (NIH), 104, 416, 513, 516, 517
National Lead Information Center (NLIC), 397
National Marrow Donor website, 23
National Newborn Screening & Genetics Resource Center, 16
National Sleep Foundation, 264
National Transportation Safety Board, 314
National Vaccine Program Office, 352
Native Americans, 379, 403
Natroba (spinosad), 377, 510
naturopaths, 517
nebulizers, 60, 366, 392, 504–506
neck injuries, 481, 484
necks: examining, 8; and torticollis, 96–97, 401–402; and tummy time, 97, 402; x-rays of, 521
neck stability, and Down syndrome, 279
neck stretching exercises, 97, 401–402
neglectful parenting, 65
Neisseria meningitides, 338
Neocate, 161–162, 162–163
Neomycin, 324, 345, 509
neonatal acne, 11
neonatal intensive care unit (NICU), 5, 39, 43–45, 99, 506
Neosporin, 445, 509
nervous behavior, 505
nervous system, 10, 229–230, 238, 277, 300
Nestle, formulas from, 158

nettle leaf, 134
neural tube defects, 10, 371
neurological development: and aluminum
poisoning, 346; and lead, 57, 409–410;
and preemies, 39, 42, 45, 264; and
Reglan, 498; and sleep, 252–253, 257,
259, 264
Neuropro, 161
neurotoxic effects, of DEET, 87
neurotoxins, 409
neutrophils (PMNs), 361, 524
nevus flammeus, 11
newborn holds, 34, 122–123
New England Journal of Medicine (NEJM),
xviii, 148, 382
nicotine, 148
Niferex, 540
night feedings: and family beds, 242–243,
256; and GERD, 212; and overweight,
109; and sleep, 241, 243, 298; trained
night feeders, 134, 249, 250, 252; and
twins, 264
night wakenings, 226, 231, 244, 251–252,
298
NIH (National Institutes of Health), 104, 416
nipples: biting, 313–314; bleeding, 118, 123,
131, 136, 138; for bottles, 172; cracked,
118–119, 121, 123, 131, 137–140, 304, 442;
enlargement of newborn's, 10; flat, 119,
137; healing, 128; infections of, 131, 133,
139; inverted, 119, 137; and lanolin, 81,
121; and latch, 41, 123, 136–138; painful,
115, 123–124, 128, 130–131, 136–139, 304;
relief for, 130; supranumerary, 10; and
thrush, 90, 376
nipple shells, 137
nipple shields, 41, 119, 121, 128, 135, 137–
138, 152
Nirmatrelvir, 357
Nitazoxanide, 503
nitrates, 414
nitrites, 414, 416
nitrosamines, 416
nits, 377
NIX, 510
Nix shampoo, 377
Nizatidine, 213, 498
Nizoral AD shampoo, 85
Nizoral antifungal cream, 509
non-REM sleep, 226
non-verbal communication, 269–270, 288,
290
norovirus, 369, 385

nose, 361, 372, 446, 450–451. See also nasal
congestion
nosebleeds, 441, 451, 482, 484, 505, 507
nostrils, flaring, 446, 448
Nuk pacifiers, 303–304
numbing products, 28, 91, 325, 494
Numzit, 91
nursemaid's elbow, 484
nurse practitioners (NPs), 61
nurses, 54, 61–62, 433–434
nursing. See breastfeeding
nursing caries, 92
The Nursing Mother's Companion
(Huggins), 141
Nutramigen, 161
Nutrasweet, 415
nutrition: and adoption, 46; in alternative
dairy products, 176; and anemia, 395;
and ASD, 278; for baby's first six months,
179; for baby's first year, 99–101; in breast
milk, 93, 100–101, 104; and breast
milk/formula decision, 113–114; and failure
to thrive, 103; first year, 99–101; and formulas, 17, 93, 100–101, 157–158, 177; and
growth, 93; infant, 98–101; and introduction of solid foods, 180–181, 181, 195; and
juices, 93, 174–175; and limiting baby's
sleep, 227; and liquids, 101, 193; and milk
supply, 133; overview of first year, 192–
193; sources of nutrients, 110–112; and
spacing of pregnancies, 278; and stored
breast milk, 143; supplementing with vitamins and minerals, 503–504; and toddler
formulas, 168; vitamins supplementing, 93,
103–106, 148; websites on, 551. See also
specific nutrients
Nystatin, 509

obesity: and AAP milk recommendations,
175; and advantages of breastmilk, 114;
and ASD, 278; avoiding, 111; and diabetes, 403; environmental triggers for,
410; and four C's, 111; and HFCS, 415;
and introduction of solid foods, 180; and
media use, 292; and nutrition, 93; preventing, 109–110
object permanence, 286, 307
obstetricians (OB): and circumcision, 22, 27;
and cord blood banking, 22, 24; and
mastitis, 140; and meconium in amniotic
fluid, 19; and metabolic screening tests,
17; and painful nipples, 140; and umbilical
cord cutting, 4

occult blood, 527
odors: of belly button, 35, 81; of pee, 219, 406; and poisoning, 406, 470; of poop, 209, 406; of sour milk, 142, 149–150; unusual body, 406
Odwalla apple juice, 445
Offit, Paul, 341, 352
off-label use, 489
Off Skintastic, 86
Oil of Lemon Eucalyptus, 86
ointments, 12, 81, 139
OIT (oral immunotherapy), 200
oleic, 163, 164
oligosaccharides IgA, 114
olive oil, 139, 377, 517
Omega fatty acids, 106–107, 158, 164, 417
Omeprazole, 213, 498
Omnicef, 501
omphalitis, 35, 81
on-call etiquette, 433–434
Ondansetron (Zofran), 500
on demand eating, 13–14, 34, 102
online shopping, 75
ophthalmologists, 390
Oppenheimer Toy Portfolio, 296
oral exploration, and environmental hazards, 408
oral herpes stomatitis (HSV-1), 367–368, 503
oral immunotherapy (OIT), 200
oral motor development, 181, 266, 286, 288, 290
oral polio vaccine, 322
Orange (teething gel), 91
orbital cellulitis, 460
Oregon Health and Science University, 30
organic certification, 189, 414
organic foods: baby foods, 189–190, 320, 412; cost of, 169, 176, 189, 411–412
organic formulas, 158, 161–162, 164–165, 169, 411–412
organic mattresses, 427
organic milk, 176, 408, 411–414
organophosphates, 409, 421
orthodontic problems, 303–304
orthotics, 400–401
Oseltamivir, 356, 503
osteomalacia, 352
osteopenia, 506
osteoporosis, 115
OTC (over the counter) medications, 490
otitis externa, 380, 495
otoscopes, 381
ovaries, 521

overeating, 108
overproduction of breast milk, 130, 133, 135
over the counter (OTC) medications, 388, 490
overweight, and BMI, 109–110
Ovide, 510
oxidation, 142
oxybenzone, 86
oxygen, 5, 105, 396, 505
oxymetazoline, 507

PABA, 86
paced bottle feeding, 111, 119, 126, 144
pacifiers: and breastfeeding, 115, 128–129, 259, 303–304; and ear infections, 303–304, 379, 386; and SIDS, 128, 236, 241, 302–303; and sleep, 128, 244–245, 249, 251, 303–304; and sleep routines, 249, 251; and soothing, 301–303; and tooth decay, 92; and yeast infections, 131
pain: abdominal, 437–439, 517; and breast-feeding, 14, 115, 121, 123–124, 128, 130–131; and ear infections, 384, 386; and food poisoning, 373; and GERD, 212–213; medications for, 28–29, 122, 497; nipple, 115, 123–124, 128, 130–131, 136–139, 304; and rotavirus, 338; and swimmer's ear, 381; and teething, 91, 155; with urination, 520; and vaccinations, 325, 326; and yeast infections, 131
pale complexion, and anemia, 395
palivizumab, 506
palmar grasp, 10
palmitic acid, breast milk and, 163, 164
palm oil, 163, 164
palpitations, 505
pancreas, 393, 403, 522
pandemic, 317, 320–321, 323, 328
parainfluenza, 354
paraphimosis, 26, 89
parasites, 46, 322, 364, 378, 385, 453, 524
parental age, and ASD, 277–278
parent at home, 63, 67
parent-child relationships, 64–66, 259
parenting: attachment, 65, 251–252, 255–256; and childcare, 63–64, 66–74; and children's temperament, 298–299; and developmental delays, 280; help from in-laws, 68; and laboratory tests, 519; and media use, 291–294; and over-prescription of antibiotics, 364; questions about, 63–64; and sleep problems, 246, 250, 254, 258; stay-at-home, 67; styles of, 64–

66; and testing of newborns, 12; tips for new fathers, 36; and vaccinations, 64, 319–322, 325–326, 328–329, 347–349; and vitamin K shots, 11–12

ParentsGuideCordBlood.com, 24

partial wakening, 226, 249

Parvovirus, 370, 385, 472–473

pasteurization, 151, 158, 176, 374, 413, 445

pathologic murmurs, 394

patient portals, 52–53, 55, 62

Paxlovid, 357

PBS (Public Broadcasting System), 293

PCBs (polychlorinated biphenyls), 409, 417

PCR (Polymerase Chain Reaction) testing, 528

PCV 13, 56, 337–338, 375

peanuts, allergies to, 148, 194–197, 199

Pedialyte, 60, 217, 455, 457–459, 500, 517–518

pediatricians: and abdominal pain, 437–439; and adoption, 46; and anterior fontanelle, 95, 480; and apnea, 449, 452; and ASD, 278; and Autism Toolkit from, 275; and bad odors, 406; and Benadryl for babies, 314; and bladder infections, 219–220; and bleeding, 197, 440; and blood in poop, 443; and bone injuries, 483–484; and breastfeeding difficulties, 117; and breath-holding spells, 313; and bruising, 440–441; and burns, 445; calling, 433–436; choosing, 47–48, 55; and circumcision, 27; and colic, 305, 307; communication with, 53–54, 61–62, 433–435, 436–439; and complementary therapies, 52, 513, 517, 518; and depression, 61; and developmental concerns, 267, 279; and diaper rash creams, 475–476, 512; and diarrhea, 453–456, 499; and DYI formulas, 169; and ear infections, 380–383, 384, 391; and ear injuries, 482; and ECI, 279; and eczema, 398–399; and emergency calls, 53, 433–434; and eye problems, 284, 389–390, 459–460; and fevers, 54, 301, 327, 328, 461–470; and finger/toe injuries, 484; first meeting with, 6; and GERD, 167, 211–214, 264; and heart problems, 394; and hives, 439, 474–475; and insurance, 50, 52–53, 55, 58; and introduction of solid foods, 182, 186; and iron deficiency anemia, 396–397; and laboratory tests, 519–520; medical review by, 47–48; and metabolic screening tests, 17; and muscle/bone problems, 402; and nasal con-gestion, 450–451; and night feedings, 250; and nose injuries, 482; and off-label use of medications, 489; on-call, 54, 433–435; and over-prescription of antibiotics, 364; and painful nipples, 140; and pain relievers, 325, 327; and phone diagnoses, 436; and poisoning, 470; and pooping problems, 205–206; and preemies, 41–43; and prioritizing phone calls, 436–437; questions for, 48–57; and respiratory distress, 446–449; running late, 50–51; scheduling visits with, 58–59; and seizures, 476; selecting, 55, 64; as source of information, xvi; and swaddling, 238; and temperament/discipline issues, 297; and trauma, 479–481; and uric acid crystals in pee, 218; and use of toddler formulas for infants, 165; and vaccinations, 319, 324, 326, 328, 334, 343–345, 348; and viruses, 351, 354–356; and vomiting, 216–217; and vomiting blood, 442; and walkers, 287; and well child appointments, 50–51, 55–56, 59; and wounds needing stitches, 476–477, 479. *See also* American Academy of Pediatrics (AAP)

Pediatrics (journal), 508

Pediavision, 389

pediculocides, 509–510

pee: abnormal stream of, 89, 220; blood in, 218; and circumcision, 28; definition of, 203; and dehydration, 217; and diabetes, 403; and diaper rash creams, 509, 512; and laboratory tests, 522; odors of, 219, 406; phthalates in, 426; and spread of Zika virus, 371; white blood cells in, 361. *See also* pee; urination

peeling, 412, 430

pelvis, examining, 521–522

penicillin, 337, 375, 382, 501–502, 514

penile adhesions, 27, 29, 88–89, 405

penises: and ambiguous genitalia, 10; and bladder infections, 219; and circumcision, 25–29, 88–89, 405; environmental triggers for problems with, 410; erections, 313; hidden, 27, 88; penile adhesions, 27, 29, 88–89, 405; uncircumcised, 88–89

Pentacel, 324

Pen VeeK, 501

Pepcid, 213

Pepto-Bismol, 210, 456

perforated eardrum, 381–382, 384, 496

perfumes, avoiding, 83, 85, 398–399

periodic breathing, 8, 31, 448

Perkin Elmer, contact information for, 17
Permethrin, 510
permissive parenting, 65
persistence, and temperament, 299
personality development, 269–270, 287, 289–290, 299–300
pertussis. *See* whooping cough (pertussis)
pervasive developmental disorder, not otherwise specified (PDD-MOS), 273
pervasive developmental disorders (PDD), 192, 273
pesticides, 164, 176, 189, 377, 409, 411, 421, 429–430
petechiae, 373, 440–441, 463, 470, 471, 472–473, 475, 520
petroleum jelly, 81, 83, 87, 194, 406, 435, 467, 517–518
pets, and food poisoning, 373, 444
PE tubes (pressure equalization tubes), 60, 383–384, 386–388, 491, 495–496
Pfizer-BioNTech mRNA, 340
Phazyme, 500
Phenergan, 500
phenol, 345
phenylephrine, 507
phenylketonuria (PKU), 16, 46, 56
Philips Avent Soothie, 128, 304
phimosis, 89
phosphorated-carbohydrate, 500
phosphorous, 44, 165
phototherapy, 21
phthalates, 409, 425–426
physical activity, 111
physical therapy, and torticollis, 97, 402
physician assistants (PAs), 61
phytoestrogens, 409
Piaget, Jean, 281
picaridin, 86–87, 371
Pimecrolimus, 511
pincer grasp, 191
pink eye, 333, 373, 382, 459–460, 496
pinworms, 378, 385, 388, 502
Pin-X, 378, 502
Pityriasis rosea, 472–473
placenta, 4, 11, 23–24
plaque, 92
plastics, harmful chemicals in, 424–426
platelet count, 440–441, 524
playgroups, 61, 329, 359
playmats, 421
plugged ducts, 119, 131, 133, 139–140, 154
Pneumococcus vaccine, 375, 396
pneumonia: and chickenpox, 336; and fevers, 463; and influenza, 338–339; and laboratory tests, 520; as lower respiratory infection, 446; medications for, 501; misconceptions about, 31; and secondary bacterial infections, 365, 372, 464; and Strep B infection, 18; and weather, 362
pneumonia vaccine, 396
Poison Control, 429, 435, 470
poisoning: emergency calls for, 470; and seizures, 476; and unusual body odors, 406, 470; and vomiting blood, 442
poison ivy, 460, 509
poisons: cleaning products as, 420; vaccines for, 322
polio, 332, 371
polio vaccine, 332, 357
pollens, 405
pollutants, environmental exposures to, 275, 277, 397, 407–415
polycarbonate, 430
polychlorinated biphenyls (PCBs), 409, 417
polycyclic aromatic hydrocarbons (PAHs), 416
polydactyly, 10
polyethylene glycol, 346–347, 499
Polymixin, 509
Polymox, 501
Polymyxin B, 324, 509
polypropylene, 425
Polysporin, 509
polyvinyl chloride, 419
Poly-Vi-Sol with Iron, 105
pools, 419
poop: appearance of, 34, 126, 146, 194, 196–197, 203–206, 209, 397, 438, 442–443, 454, 504; and bacterial infections, 361; black-looking, 504; and bladder infections, 218–219; blood in, 166, 194, 196–197, 204–205, 209, 213, 338, 373, 442–443, 453, 520, 527; and constipation, 111, 161, 164, 205–207; and diaper rash creams, 509, 512; and food poisoning, 373; frequency of pooping, 205–206; and introduction of solid foods, 209; and iron supplements, 397; and jaundice, 19–21, 126; and mature milk, 120; meconium, 4, 9, 14, 18, 34, 36, 204–205, 209; odors of, 209, 406; and palm oil, 164; and preemies discharge from hospital, 41; red flags with, 205; and rotavirus, 368; snotty-looking, 146, 194, 196–197, 209; and tracking diaper changes, 14, 34, 37–39, 218; transit time for, 203–206; and UTIs,

89; watery, 167, 453–454; worrisome poops for older babies, 209. *See also* diarrhea; stool

port wine stains, 11

positional plagiocephaly, 95–96, 240, 284

positive parenting, 65

positivity, and discipline, 311

posterior fontanelle, 96

posterior urethral valves, 10

postpartum bleeding, 126

postpartum depression, 37, 61

post-tussive emesis, 457

potty seats, 210

powders, avoiding, 81, 512

PPIs (proton pump inhibitors), 213, 498

preauricular pits and tags, 7

prebiotics, 168, 515–516

pre-chewing, 189

The Preemie Primer (Gunter), 42

Preemies: The Essential Guide for Parents of Premature Babies (Linden), 42

preemies: and apnea, 449; and ASD, 42, 277; and bacterial infections, 362; books for parents of, 42; and breastfeeding, 39–41, 44–45, 105, 116, 120, 133–134, 151–152; and caffeine, 146; and car seats, 30, 41, 45; and catch-up growth, 44, 94, 99; concerns with, 39–45; developmental checklist for, 268–273, 280; feeding, 40–41, 44–45, 101–102, 151–152; formulas for, 165; and GERD, 43; growth chart for, 44, 557; high calorie diets for, 99, 125, 165, 181; and introduction of solid foods, 181; and iron, 44–45, 105–106; and laboratory tests, 523; and large muscle development, 42; and parents' fear of germs, 33; and powdered formulas, 170; and probiotics, 106, 515; and purchased breast milk, 151; and respiratory distress, 448; and RSV, 365, 506–507; sleeping through the night, 264; and soy formulas, 166; and supplementation with formulas, 125, 165; and zinc in food, 111

pregnancies: and Group B Strep, 374–375; spacing of, 277–278; and vaccinations, 339–340; and viral infections, 370; and Zika virus, 371

prenatal consultation, 48–49

pre-operational development, 281

prescriptions: and off-label use, 489; and on-call doctors, 434–435; reading, 490

preservatives, 339, 344–345, 352, 415–416

pressure, and petechiae, 441, 471

pressure equalization (PE) tubes, and ear infections, 60, 383–384, 386–388, 495–496

Prevacid, 213, 498

Prevident, 494

Prevnar: aluminum in, 347; and antibiotic resistance, 323, 363; as inactivated vaccine, 322; and limiting infections, 387; and sickle cell disease, 396; and Strep pneumoniae, 337, 337–338, 375, 382; and vaccination schedules, 56

Prilosec, 213, 498

primary care provider, 61

private parts: caring for, 79, 89, 218–219, 374. *See also* genitals

probiotics: and allergies, 516; and colic, 30, 106, 167, 306–307, 500, 515–516; and diarrhea, 456, 515; in formulas, 158, 167, 306–307, 515; and gas, 106, 222; and GERD, 106, 213; and mastitis, 140; in vitamins, 104, 503; and yeast infections, 131, 141

Procrastinator, feeding behavior, 124

product recalls, 229

progressive waiting, 254, 259

projectile vomiting, 211, 438, 458

prolactin, 133

Promethazine, 500

Promiseb, 512

proteins: and allergies, 167, 194, 196–197, 199, 201, 516; in alternative dairy products, 176; and ASD, 277; in breast milk, 160; comfort, 166; in cow's milk, 146–147, 160–167, 170, 186, 194, 196–197, 305, 516; in formulas, 157–161; gentle, 166, 170; gluten, 198; guidelines for, 112; lactoferrin, 168; and sickle cell disease, 395–396; and vaccines, 322

proton pump inhibitors (PPIs), 213, 498

Protopic, 399, 511

Pruclair, 512

Prumyx, 512

prune juice cocktail, 206

pseudoephedrine, 154, 492, 508

pseudostrabismus, 390

Psorcon, 511

psychiatric medications, 508

puberty: and bovine growth hormone, 413–414; early, 413–414; and growth, 94; and growth plates, 483; precocious, 176

Public Broadcasting System (PBS), 293

public health, concept of, 318

Pulmicort, 392, 505–506

pulse, 8, 435–437. *See also* heart rate
pulse oximeter, 436–437
PurAmino, 161
Purell, 353
PURPLE crying, 305–306
pus: and burns, 445; and circumcision, 29; and ear infections, 380–381, 383–384; and infected wounds, 477–478, 479; and nipple infections, 139; and ringworm, 376; and stitches, 477; from umbilical stump, 35
pustular melanosis, 11
PVC, 330
pyelonephritis, 10
pyloric stenosis, 211, 216, 437, 457, 521–522
Pyrantel, 378, 503
Pyrethrum, 510
Pyrinyl, 510

Q-tips, 496
quality time, 66–67, 70
quilts, 235, 237

RabAvert, 324
rabies vaccine, 324
racemic epinephrine, 367
radiation, 409, 424
radio frequency emissions, 409
radon, 408, 409, 421–422
ragweed, 510
rapeseed, 163
rapid antigen tests, 528
rapid extinction, 254–255, 259
rapid eye movement (REM) sleep, 226
rapid sleep training, 255–256, 257
rashes: and allergic reactions, 439–440; and antifungals, 502; and bruising, 440–441; calling the doctor about, 61, 471–476; causes of, 471; and fevers, 469–470; and food allergies, 194; and measles, 329; in newborns, 11, 36, 471, 475; poison ivy, 460, 509; prevalence in children, 519; return to daycare after viral, 388; roseola, 369, 385, 464, 472–473; severe, 81; typical doctor's questions about, 471; and vaccinations, 326, 334, 336, 475; and viral infections, 364, 367, 369–371, 471; websites on, xviii, 60, 367, 375, 471. *See also* diaper rash; eczema
Rash-o-Rama, xviii, 60, 472–473
RAST testing, 201
raw honey, 180
raw milk, 176, 374
Reach Out and Read program, 286

reactive airway disease, 391, 517
reading, 284, 286
receptive language skills, 266, 270–272, 274
recliners for infants, 426
rectal thermometers, 206
red blood cells, 105, 395–396, 414
Red Cross, swimming lessons and, 295
red eyes, 284, 460
red face, 205, 331, 448, 452
reflexes, 10, 283
reflexology, 306
Reflo drinking cups, 174
refractive errors, 42, 57
Reglan, 498
regularity, and temperament, 299
regurgitation. *See* vomiting
rehydration, 217, 500
REM (rapid eye movement) sleep, 226
Remsdesivir, 357
repellents, 86–87
repetitive behaviors, 273, 274
reproductive system, environmental triggers for problems with, 409–410
resale shops, 428
rescue medications, 504–506
respiration rate: and air hungry diagnosis, 446–447, 451; and coughing, 452; of newborns, 5, 448; and poisoning, 470; and taking vital signs, 435–436
respiratory distress: and allergic reactions, 502; and coughing, 452; examination for, 8; and lung infections, 446–449; and pneumonia, 371; and poisoning, 470; and RSV, 365; when to call the doctor, 446–449
respiratory droplets, and transmission of infections, 30, 351–358, 353, 365–370, 370, 375, 390
respiratory issues: and GERD, 216; medications for, 504–509; and preemies, 39, 42–43
respiratory syncytial virus. *See* RSV (respiratory syncytial virus)
respiratory system: infections of, 150, 446–449; and influenza, 338
respiratory viruses. *See* cold viruses; *specific respiratory viruses*
Rester feeding behavior, 124
Retapamulin, 509
reticulocyte count, 526
retinoblastoma, 6
retinopathy of prematurity (ROP), 42
retractions, respiratory, 8, 31, 452

Rett Syndrome, 277
reverse osmosis filters, 417, 494
Reye's syndrome, 456, 497
rheumatoid arthritis, 114
rhinoviruses, 354, 357–358, 385, 391
rice cereal, 99, 102, 180, 185, 207–208, 228, 413
Ricelyte, 458
rice milk, 155, 197
rice starch, 167, 213
ricin, 470
rickets, 103–104
RID, 510
ringworm, 376, 385, 388, 472–473, 509–510
Rocephin, 501
rocking, 229–230, 244–247, 248, 252, 254, 255, 258, 301
Rocky Mountain Spotted Fever, 471, 472–473
role confusion, identity versus, 282
rolling over, 266, 286
room sharing, 115, 236, 241
rooting reflex, 10
roseola (herpes virus 6), 369, 385, 464, 472–473
Rotarix, 338
Rotateq, 338
rotavirus: description, diagnosis, and treatment of, 56, 368–369; and laboratory tests, 528; and probiotics, 515; seasonal patterns of, 354; vaccine for, 322, 338, 344, 357, 369; as viral infection, 385
RSV (respiratory syncytial virus): and apnea, 449; description, diagnosis, and treatment of, 365–366; and ear infections, 451; and laboratory tests, 528; as lower respiratory infection, 446–447; and nasal congestion, 451; prevention of, 506–507; seasonal patterns of, 43, 354, 506–507; Synagis injections for, 43, 507; as viral infection, 385; and wheezing, 365, 390–391, 446–447
rubella, 277, 334, 357
runny noses: and allergies, 404–405; and decongestants, 508; and head injuries, 479–482; and infections, 450–451, 464; and red eyes, 460; and teething, 91. See also mucous
Rx symbol, 490

Saccaromyces sp., 515
Saccharin, 415
sacral dimple, 10

safety: of antihistamines, 508; baby-proofing checklist for, 422; and cleaning products, 419–420, 430; of complementary therapies, 513–514, 517; FDA's drug safety website, 512; of fish/seafood, 416–417; and fluoride, 494; of GMOs, 414; and holiday/Christmas lights, 418; house rules for, 309; of medications, 491–492; of probiotics, 516; and toys, 428; of vaccines, 322–323, 344–348, 352; and walkers, 287, 481; water, 294–295, 418–419
safety gates, 263
Safeway, 413
safflower oil, 163, 164
sage, 492
saline, nose drops, 30–31, 60, 358, 435, 450–451, 507, 517
salmonella, 373, 385, 444, 453
salt, 180, 188, 190, 416, 458
sample medications, 60
sandboxes, 428–429
SARS-CoV-2. See COVID-19
scabicides, 509–510
scabies, 376–377, 385, 388, 472–473, 509
scales, weighing, 153
scarlet fever, 472–473
scarring, and ear piercing, 89
scents, 83, 85, 517
SCID (Severe Combined Immune Deficiency), 338
screening tests: and adoption, 46; for ASD, 56, 273, 275; decision-making about, 64; for developmental delays, 267; and Down syndrome, 279; for GERD, 213–214, 220; for Group B Strep, 375; for iron deficiency, 105; for lead exposure, 56–57, 397–398; for metabolic disorders, 16–17, 46, 56, 393, 395, 523, 526; for newborns, 15–18, 42, 279; nurses performing, 61; for sickle cell disease, 395; VCUG test, 220, 522; for vision, 46, 56–57, 389–390; websites on, 551; and well child visits, 56–57, 64
screen time, limiting, 292–293
scrotum, 438
seafood. See fish
Sears, Bob, 251
Sears, William, 256
sea salt, 188
seasonal allergies, 393, 400, 404–405, 460
seasonal patterns of illnesses, 43, 353–354, 365–370, 372–373, 375, 386, 398–399, 506–507, 540

seasonings, 180, 188, 190, 198
seborrhea, 84–85, 509
Sebulex, 84
secondary bacterial infections, 338–339, 361–362, 364–365, 371–372, 464
sedating effect, from medications, 305, 314, 358, 399, 498, 508
seizures: and camphor, 359, 517; definition of, 476; febrile, 465, 469–470, 476; and fever, 469–470, 476; and head injuries, 480–481; and laboratory tests, 520; and Lindane, 510; and low blood sugar, 125; and phototherapy, 21; and poisoning, 470; vaccinations and, 327, 328
self, concept of, 281, 290
Selsun Blue, 84
senna, 499
Senokot, 499
sensitivity, and temperament, 299
sensorimotor development, 281, 284, 296
sensory processing disorder, 192
separation anxiety, 132–133, 290, 298, 312, 312–313
sepsis, 40, 337, 463
septal hematoma, 482
Septra, 501
serotonin, 236
serous fluid, 383
serous otitis media, 383
serving sizes, 109–112, 202, 207–209
Seventh Generation Free and Clear, 84
Severe Combined Immune Deficiency (SCID), 338
sexually transmitted infections, 25–26, 28, 335, 361, 371
sexual pleasure, 27, 28
shampoos, 83–84, 84–85
Shannon, Michael, 430
shea nut, 512
shellfish. See fish
shigella, 373, 453
shingles, 336, 356, 370, 472–473
shoes, 291, 400
shoulder dystocia, 8
shoulders, examining, 8
show us the science, xviii
sick child appointments, scheduling, 51–52, 57–59
sick leave policy, 75
sickle cell disease, 46, 56, 375, 395–396
side effects, 213
side-lying hold, 123
SIDS. See sudden infant death syndrome

(SIDS)
sign language, 289
Silber, Seth, 91
Silvadene, 445, 509, 512
Silverstone, Alicia, 189
silver sulfadiazine, 509
simethicone, 222, 500
Similac formulas, 161–162, 164, 166, 167
singing, 229, 252, 258, 301
Singulair, 392, 505
sinuses, examining, 521
sinus infections: compared to cold viruses, 358, 360, 364–365; and conjunctivitis, 459–460; and laboratory tests, 520, 521; medications for, 501; orbital cellulitis, 460; and secondary bacterial infections, 338–339, 365, 371–372, 464; and Strep pneumoniae, 337, 385
sinusitis, 360, 452
sippy cups, 174
skim milk, 175, 414
skin: abnormalities in newborns, 10, 11; bacteria on, 361; and burns, 445; dry, 85, 398–399; and fungal infections, 375–376; and jaundice, 11, 19–20, 35; sensitive, 84, 398, 474–475; and surgical glue, 478–479; yellow, 188, 335
skin creams, 83–84
skin disorders, websites on, 551
skin infections: bacterial, 372–373, 385; and laboratory tests, 520; medications for, 501, 508–512; seasonal patterns of, 354; swimmer's ear, 380. See also eczema
skin tags, 7
skin tests, 201
skin to skin contact, and sleep, 230, 255
skin turgor, 454
Sklice (ivermectin), 377, 510
skull fractures, 481–482
skulls: and brain development, 6, 95; molding of, 96; pressure in, 217; x-rays of, 521
slapped cheek (Parvovirus), 370, 385, 472–473
sleep: adult and newborn compared, 226–227; books about, 253–256; and breastfeeding, 115–116, 121, 127, 129, 156, 227–228, 229, 241, 243, 244, 246; and cough/cold medications, 508; and coughing, 452; and crying, 226, 246–247, 249, 254–260, 264, 300; Day-Night Reversal, 227, 231; and developmental milestones, 248; devices for, 238–241; and diphenhydramine, 314, 399, 493; and Down syn-

drome, 279; and ear infections, 386; establishing good sleep habits, 244–245, 254; and feedings, 129, 172–173, 175, 227–228, 241, 243–250, 252, 254–255; and feeding schedules, 34, 92, 134, 172–173, 175; Ferber sleep training, 253–255, 257, 259; and formula supplementation, 129; and GERD, 102, 132, 173, 213–214, 237, 257, 264; and head injuries, 480; and heartburn, 102, 237; and mastitis, 140; and milk production, 134; Mindell sleep training, 255–256, 259; naps effecting nighttime, 263; and nasal congestion, 450–451; and newborns, 13–14, 32, 34, 36–37, 227–230; and nicotine, 148; and night feedings, 241, 243, 298; and pacifiers, 128, 244–245, 249, 251, 303–304; patterns of, 102; and postpartum depression, 37; and preemies, 45; products for, 229–230; and rapid extinction, 254–255, 255; red flags with, 34; requirements for birth to two years, 230–234; and room sharing, 241; science of, 225–227, 254; Sears sleep training, 251, 255; and SIDS, 95, 236; SLEEP plan, 260; sleep training failure, 257–258; and soothing, 15, 246–247, 249–251, 257–258, 300; ten commandments for, 244–245; and torticollis, 401–402; tracking, 40; transitions in, 246–248, 256; types of, 226; websites on, 253; Weissbluth on, 254–255, 259

sleep aids, 236–239

sleep cycles, 226, 246, 248, 250, 260

sleep deprivation, 37, 116, 129, 225, 254, 452

sleeping through the night: average age for, 228; and birth weight, 120; and GERD, 102, 264; and introduction of solid foods, 180; and pumping, 156

sleep patterns, 226–228, 230–234

sleep position: devices for, 238; and head shape, 95–97; and SIDS, 95, 231, 234–236, 238, 239, 241, 243, 286; and skin to skin contact, 230, 255

sleep routines: bad, 248–252; and bedtime, 242–247, 249, 253, 254–255, 260–263; and early risers, 253; family bed versus solitary sleep, 242–243; for naps, 254, 261; and night wakenings, 226, 231, 246, 251–252, 298; and pacifiers, 249, 251; and parenting styles, 254; and progressive waiting, 254; setting up, 229, 242–247, 254–256, 260; and skin to skin contact,

230, 255; and sleep regression, 250; and twins, 234, 258, 263–264

SleepSack, 237

sleep schedules, disrupted, 91, 243, 245, 249, 252

sleep training, 248–260, 254–259

slings, 426

slow to warm up temperament, 298, 312

small muscle development, 42, 266, 271–272, 279

smallpox vaccine, 318–319, 321–322, 357

smartphones. See media use

smegma, 27, 88

smoking: and asthma, 391, 423; breastfeeding and, 148; and ear infections, 379, 387, 518; and indoor air pollution, 409, 423, 430; and RSV risk, 507; and SIDS, 236, 242

smothering, 241, 252

snacks, 74, 111, 133, 185, 199

Snoo, 229–230, 239, 241

snot: and cold viruses, 358–360, 359, 446; green, 358, 363; saline nose drops for, 30–31, 60, 358, 435, 450–451, 507, 517; and VapoRub, 517; and wheezing, 446–447

soap, 83, 85, 353, 440

social development: and ASD, 274–275; from birth to two months, 283; Erik Erikson's theory of, 282; from two to four months, 285; from four to six months, 286–287; from six to nine months, 288–289; from nine to twelve months, 290–291, 291; milestones for, 266–267, 271–272

social media, and COVID-19, xviii

sodium, 176

sodium benzoate, 415

sodium bicarbonate, 498

sodium caseinate, 200

sofas, sleeping on, 234

soft spot, 6, 95–96, 217, 454, 480–481

solitary sleep, 243

Solka, Shelley, 303

Solve Your Child's Sleep Problems (Ferber), 253–255

Soothies by Lansinoh, 138

soothing: from dads, 246; and help from grandparents, 116; and hiccups, 204; and neurologic issues, 39; self-soothing, 229–230, 247, 249–251, 257–259, 300–301, 313; and sleep, 15, 246–247, 249–251, 257–258, 300; and spoiling, 300–301;

and sucking, 118, 128–129, 155–156, 229, 301–302; ten tricks for, 301–302; and twins, 302
sorbitol, 206
sore throat, 358, 368, 385, 505, 518
soy, allergies to, 197
soy formulas, 158–166, 162–163, 165–166, 410
soy milk, 155, 353
Spectazole, 509
speech impediments, 303
speech therapy, 279
sperm, 277, 410
sphincter muscles, 210–211, 216
spices, 180, 188, 190
spike protein, 341–342
spina bifida, 10, 278, 521
spinal fluid tests, 527
spine: and Down syndrome, 279; examination of, 10; injuries to, 481, 484; spinal manipulations, 513; ultrasound imaging of, 521; white blood cells in fluid of, 361; x-rays of, 521; and Zika virus, 371
Spinosad, 510
spit-up, 34, 167, 210–211, 216–217
spleen, 375, 396
Splenda, 415
splints, making, 482
Spoonful One, 199
Spot (vision screening device), 389
sputum, 527
squealing cough. See stridor
squeezable baby food packages, 188–189
staph, 361, 372, 385
staples, 479
Starbuck's, 413
startle reflex, 236
Steenhagen, Deb, 72
stem cells, 23–24
sterilization, 90, 131, 141, 170–171
sternocleidomastoid muscles, 401
steroid creams, 398–399
steroids: for allergic reactions, 509; and asthma, 392, 505–506; in ear drops, 495; and eczema, 398–399, 509; FDA recommendations for, 501; medications containing, 511
Stevens-Johnson syndrome, 439, 502
Stewart, Jon, 320
stitches, 96–97, 476–479, 482
stomach: bleeding in, 217; sleeping on, 239; stomachaches, 437–439, 458, 502, 504, 505–506, 508; swollen, 437–438

stomach viruses: and acholic stool, 209; as cause of infection, 385; and dehydration, 367–368, 500; description, diagnosis, and treatment of, 368–369; and diarrhea, 453, 456; formulas for, 167; and probiotics, 515; and return to daycare, 388; seasonal patterns of, 354, 369; and vomiting, 217, 457
stool: acholic, 209; definition of, 203; watery, 167, 453–454. See also poop
stool cultures, 46, 527
stool tests, 527
stork bites, 11
Stough, Wendy, 74
strabismus, 42, 389
stranger anxiety, 288, 298, 312–313
strawberry hemangioma, 11
Strep: and chickenpox, 319, 337; contagiousness of, 362; Group A Strep (Strep throat), 362, 382, 385, 488–489, 501; Group B Strep, 17–18, 361, 362, 374–375, 385, 463; as skin bacteria, 361
Strep pneumoniae, 337, 337–338, 354, 363, 375, 382, 385, 396
Streptomycin, 324
stress, 140, 149
stridor, 367, 447–448, 452
strollers, 301–302
Sturge-Weber syndrome, 11
subconjunctival hemorrhage, 6–7, 482
subungual hematoma, 484
succinic acid, 92
sucking: and burping, 204; and ear infections, 384; and gas, 221; reflex in newborns, 10; and SIDS, 234; and soothing, 118, 128–129, 155–156, 229, 301–302; and stimulation of milk production, 145, 153; and teething, 155
sucrose, 345
Sudafed, 154, 489, 492
sudden infant death syndrome (SIDS): and advantages of breast milk, 114, 236; and apnea, 449; and cannabis use, 148; and comfort objects, 252; and crib mattresses, 427; and family beds, 241, 243; and infant loungers, 426; and pacifiers, 128, 236, 241, 302–303; prevention of, 241, 243; risk factors for, 235–241, 243; and sleep position, 95, 231, 234–236, 238, 239, 241, 243, 286
sudden unexplained infant death (SUID), risk factors for, 241, 243
suffocation, 234, 236, 238, 241, 252

sugar: in breast milk, 160, 161, 162, 164; and diabetes, 403; in formulas, 158, 161, 164; in goat's milk, 176–177; and HFCS, 415; in juices, 174–175; in six month old's diet, 190; in solution for colic, 306; and vaccines, 322; and yeast infections, 141
Sulfamethoxazole, 501
Sulfatrim, 501
sulfonamides (sulfa), 501
sunblock, 79, 104
sunflower oil, 163, 164
sunlight, 103–104, 139, 226
sunscreen, 85–86
super-ego, 309
supplementation: and breastfeeding, 21–22, 41, 44–45, 113, 115, 118, 124–129, 129, 150, 152–153, 166, 168; and jaundice, 21–22; and preemies, 41, 44–45
support, and depression, 61
suppositories, 206, 468
supranumerary nipples, 10
supraventricular tachycardia (SVT), 395
Suprax, 501
SurgiSeal, 478–479
sushi, 148
sutures, 96–97, 476–479
swaddling: and hip movement, 34, 237, 402; and sleep, 229–230, 242; and Snoo Smart Sleeper, 238; and soothing, 301; technique for, 236–240
sweating, and sleep, 230
sweat test, 393, 527
sweeteners, 186
swim classes, 294–295
Swim Ear, 495, 518
swimmer's ear, 380–381, 495, 518
swimming, and stitches, 478
swimming lessons, 418–419
Synagis RSV antibody injections, 43, 45, 366, 506–507
synapses, 277
syndactyly, 10
syphilis, 46

Tachypnea of newborn, 8
Tacrolimus, 511
Taking Cara Babies video, 255
talk time, 285, 292–293
Tamiflu, 356, 503
Target, formulas at, 161, 162
tax deductions, breastfeeding, 143
tear ducts, 7, 459
tearing, constant, 460

tea tree oil (Melaleuca alternifolia), 377
teeth: arrival of, 7, 90–91, 95–96; cleaning, 92, 96, 108, 175, 252, 504; and fluoride, 107–108, 493–494; injuries to, 482–483; iron staining of, 397, 504; and juices, 174–175; and night feedings, 252; and solid food introduction, 191
teething: and biting, 313–314; coping with, 90–91, 495; and disrupted sleep, 91, 252; and fevers, 91, 469; medications for, 91, 155, 492, 494–495; and sucking, 155; teething necklaces, 92
television. See media use
temperament, 297–301, 311
temperature: daily fluctuation patterns of, 462, 465; and layered clothing, 100; of newborns, 5–6, 19; and preemies, 39, 41; and SIDS, 233, 242; and taking vital signs, 435–437; techniques for taking, 56, 435, 461–462, 464, 466–467, 469
temper tantrums, 310, 312
Tempra. See acetaminophen (Tylenol)
teratogens, 409
Terrible Twos, 310
testes, 9, 520–521
tests: for allergies, 201–202, 524; for diabetes, 18, 57, 403, 523, 526; for GERD, 213–214, 220; imaging studies, 520–522; laboratory, 519–520, 522–528; for lead exposure, 56–57, 397–398; scheduling, 64; for VUR, 219–220. See also screening tests
tetanus vaccine, 322, 330–331, 477–478
texture aversion, 192
THC, and SIDS, 148
therapists, 22, 274, 278–279
thermometers, 56, 206, 435, 464, 466–467
thimerosal, 339, 344–346, 352
thirst, 112, 147, 403
throat culture, 527
throat infections, 331, 385
throats: examining, 7; and HIB, 333; sore, 358, 368, 385, 505, 518
thrush, 90, 140, 376, 385, 502, 505–506
thumb sucking, 303–304, 313
thyroid, 46, 279, 371, 409
thyroid function tests, 526
tick-borne illnesses, 86, 472–473
tiger parenting, 65
tinea corporis. See ringworm
tinea pedis. See athlete's foot
TIRED study (Trial of Infant Response to Diphenhydramine), 493

index

titanium oxide, 86
TMP-SMX, 501
tobacco, 409, 423, 514
toddler formulas, 164, 168, 170
toes, 10–11, 484
toilet training, early, 210
tongue, 7, 477–478
tongue thrusting, 137, 303–304
tongue-tied, 7, 134–135, 137–138
tonsils, 521
toothbrushes, 397
tooth decay, 92, 107, 174–175, 189, 248, 303
tooth intrusion, 482–483
toothpaste, 92, 108
Topfer formulas, 162–163
torticollis, 8, 96–97, 401–402
touchscreens, educational apps on, 294
Toxic Substance Control Act of 1976, 407
toxins: and bacterial infections, 361; in cord
    blood, 277; environmental exposures to
    chemicals, 407–415; and food poisoning,
    373
toxoids, 322
toyportfolio.com, 296
toys: favorite, 307–308; finding age appro-
    priate, 296; and media use, 294;
    Oppenheimer Toy Portfolio, 296; pesti-
    cides on, 430; from resale shops, 428;
    swapping, 291; and torticollis exercises,
    402; and travel, 314
trachea, 446, 521
trampolines, 429
transient tachypnea of the newborn (TTN),
    19
transitional murmur, 8
transitional objects, 307–308
transmitted upper airway noise, 358–359
transplant rejection, 22
trauma: and apnea, 449; and bruising, 6, 35,
    440; head injuries, 476, 479–481; and red
    eyes, 460; red flags with, 484; and
    seizures, 476
travel: and ear infections, 314, 384; and food
    poisoning, 373; pillows for, 263; and sleep
    disruptions, 245, 252, 261; tips for, 314;
    websites on, 551
tree nuts, 195–196, 202
triage, 437
Trial of Infant Response to Diphenhydramine
    (TIRED), 493
Triamcinolone, 511
Trimethoprim, 501
Trimox, 501
Triple Paste, 512

Triple Paste AF, 81, 509
Tri-Vi-Sol, 503
trust/mistrust, 282
tuberculosis (TB), 46, 453
tuberculosis vaccine, 322
tummy time, 95–97, 235, 240, 284–285, 402
tumors, 9, 95, 217, 390, 424, 457
twins: and breastfeeding, 151; burping, 221;
    and cord blood banking, 23; feeding and
    elimination tracking with, 40; and RSV risk,
    506; and sleep, 234, 258, 263–264; and
    solid food introduction, 192; soothing,
    302; and study of ASD, 276; and torticol-
    lis, 401; toys for, 291; and well child
    appointments, 58
2-phenoxyethanol, 345
two-percent milk, 101, 112, 157, 168, 173,
    175, 193
Tylenol. See acetaminophen (Tylenol)
typhoid fever, 444

ulcers, 367, 439, 442, 473, 517
Ulesfia, 510
Ulesfia (benzyl alcohol), 377
ultrasounds: compared to CT scans, 424;
    and DDH, 402, 521; described, 520; and
    intraventricular hemorrhage, 42, 521; and
    VCUG screening test, 220, 522
umbilical cord: and baby's first bath, 82; and
    cord blood banking, 4, 17, 22–25; cutting,
    4; examining, 9; infection of, 35, 81–82,
    330; toxins in cord blood, 277
umbilical hernia, 9
unconsciousness, 449
underproduction of breast milk, 130, 133–
    135
undescended testes, 9
unilateral laterothoracic exanthem, 472–473
uninvolved parenting, 65
USDA (U.S. Department of Agriculture), 189
U.S. Department of Agriculture (USDA), 189
U.S. Department of Health and Human
    Services, 143, 327
U.S. National Toxicology Program, 415
upper GI bleeding, 442
upper respiratory infections (URI): antibiotics
    and, 364; and asthma, 390; and cough-
    ing, 452; description of, 446; and ear
    infections, 378; home remedies for, 517;
    and runny noses, 405, 450; as viral infec-
    tion, 385. See also cold viruses
urethra: abnormal formation of, 9; bacteria
    in, 89, 218–219, 361, 374; and labial adhe-
    sions, 406; and laboratory tests, 522; and

urine, 203
uric acid crystals, 14, 218
urinalysis, 57, 369, 374, 526
urinary tract defects, 463
urinary tract infections (UTI): and circumcision, 26; description, diagnosis, and treatment of, 374; and diaper changes, 89, 218–219; examination for, 10; and fevers, 463; and VUR, 219–220
urination: and abdominal pain, 437–439; and diabetes, 403; and diarrhea, 454; and laboratory tests, 520; and newborns, 10; and tracking diaper changes, 14, 34, 37–39; and vomiting, 458
urine. *See* pee
urine culture, 527
urologists, and circumcision, 27
utensils, 192
uterus, 521

Vaccination Revealed (Butler), 349, 353
vaccination schedules, 56, 64, 322, 324, 329–340, 347–349, 353
vaccinations/vaccines: additives in, 345; adverse reactions to, 320, 323, 327–328, 332, 341–342, 344, 493, 503; and ASD, 274, 277, 320, 343–344; and bacteria, 322–323, 330, 333, 336–337, 345; combination vaccines, 324, 330–332; controversies about, 317–323, 323, 331, 342–345; for COVID-19, 317–319, 340–342; and FDA, 322–323, 327, 338, 339–340, 344; and fever, 35, 58, 326–329, 331, 334, 463, 465; and hepatitis B, 18; and herd immunity, 320–321; and immune response, 43, 322, 324, 326, 329, 331, 334–345, 352; and infections, 322–324, 325–326, 329–342, 354; keeping record of, 328; medical reasons for delaying or discontinuing, 324–325; mercury in, 344–346, 352; misconceptions about, 320; and parenting, 64, 319–322, 325–326, 328–329, 347–349; for polio, 332; and preemies, 43; preservatives in, 339, 344–346, 352; questions about, 52, 55, 321–329; and rashes, 326, 334, 336, 475; removed from the market, 344; requirements for, 328, 339; for rotavirus, 322, 338, 344, 357, 369; safety of, 322–323; smallpox, 318–319, 321–322, 357; testing of, 322–323; typical side effects of, 326–327, 336; vaccination rates, 321; and viruses, 321–323, 334–342, 344, 357; websites on, 3, 322, 327, 328, 330, 345, 349, 551; for whooping cough,

322, 326, 329–332
Vaccine Adverse Event Reporting System (VAERS), 327, 344
Vaccine Education Center, Children's Hospital of Philadelphia, 349
Vaccine Education Center, 352
vaccine exemptions, religious/philosophical, 325–326
Vaccine Injury Compensation Program (VICP), 327–328
vaccines, safety of, 344–346, 352
Vaccines and Your Child: Separating Fact from Fiction (Offit and Moser), 352
Vaccines For Children program (VFC), 60
VAERS (Vaccine Adverse Event Reporting System), 327, 344
vagina, 9–10, 89, 378, 405–406
vaginal bacteria, 361
vaginal discharge, 9, 218
valerian root, 492
vapocoolant sprays, 325
vaporizers, 359, 392
vapo-rubs, 359, 514
varicella. *See* chickenpox (varicella)
varicella vaccine. *See* chickenpox (varicella) vaccine
Vartabedian, Bryan, 106, 197
Vaseline, 512, 517, 517–518
V-cillinK, 501
VCIP (Vaccine Injury Compensation Program), 327–328
VCUG (voiding cystourethrogram) test, 220, 522
vegan diet, 185, 444
vegetable oil, 84
vegetables: calcium in, 110; fiber in, 110–111, 209; and food poisoning, 373, 444; guidelines for, 112; homemade baby food from, 414; and introduction of solid foods, 184, 187; pesticides in, 411–412, 415, 429–430
vegetarian diet, 159, 165–166, 185, 444
ventricular septal defect (VSD), 394
vernix, 4, 82
vervain, 306
vesicles, 370
vesicoureteral reflux (VUR), 10, 219–220, 374, 522
vibrating chairs/swings, 302
Vicks VapoRub, 517
Vi-Daylin, 503
violence, 292
viral bone marrow suppression, 356
viral exanthems, 369–370, 385, 472–473

viral infections: and acetaminophen, 367; and ASD, 277; and bruising, 440–441; compared to bacterial infections, 361–362, 364–365; croup, 354, 385, 388, 447–448, 517; diagnosis of, 354–356; duration of, 357; and ear infections, 381–382, 387; enteroviruses, 355, 371; of the eye, 459–460; and fever, 357, 361–362, 365–375; gastrointestinal viruses, 368–369, 385; and immune systems, 354, 360, 366; laboratory tests for, 523–524, 526–528; medications for, 322–324, 356–357, 365–371, 503; mosquito-borne, 371; mouth and tonsil viruses, 367–368, 385; and multiplex PCR testing, 355–356; prevention of, 323–324, 357, 379, 386–387, 506–507, 518; and rashes, 364, 367, 369–371, 471; respiratory viruses, 365–367, 385, 446–449; seasonal patterns of, 353–354, 365–370, 372, 372–373, 386; viral exanthems, 369–370, 385, 472–473. See also specific viruses

viral titers, test for, 526

viruses: and antibiotics, 322, 358, 362, 363–364; COVID-19, 30, 33, 149–150, 317–319, 340–342, 354–357, 357; exposure to, 30, 353; and hand sanitizers, 352–353; Hepatitis A, 46, 335; measles, 333–334; polio, 332; questions about, 352–362; as source of disease, 351; transmission of, 30, 331–332, 351–358, 353, 365–371, 375, 386–387; and vaccinations, 321–323, 334–342, 344, 357. See also infections; specific viruses

vision: and antihistamines, 508; and DHA, 148, 164; of newborns, 283; from two to four months, 285

vision screens, 46, 56–57, 279, 389–390

vital signs: checking, 6, 435–437; and preemies discharge from hospital, 41

Vitamin A: in alternative dairy products, 176; breastfeeding and, 146; guidelines for, 112; and introduction of solid foods, 188; supplemental, 503

vitamin B12, 176–177, 395

Vitamin C: in alternative dairy products, 176; guidelines for, 111; iron and, 111, 504; and juices, 174; supplemental, 503

Vitamin D: in alternative dairy products, 176; in breast milk, 104, 157, 181, 500, 503; in formulas, 181, 500; and rickets, 103–104; supplemental, 503

Vitamin K, shots of, 5, 11–12

vitamin K deficiency bleeding (VKDB), 11

vitamins: in formulas, 104–105, 158, 161; for nursing mothers, 132; for preemies, 45; probiotics in, 104, 503; supplementing nutrition, 93, 103–106, 148; supplements for vegetarians, 185

VOCs (volatile organic compounds), 409, 420–421

voiding cystourethrogram (VCUG) test, 220, 522

volatile organic compounds (VOCs), 409, 420–421

vomiting: and abdominal pain, 437–438; blood, 442, 458; and blood in poop, 443; calling the doctor about, 457–458; and celiac disease, 198; and choking, 237; compared to spit-up, 34, 456; and coughing, 452, 457; and diarrhea, 454–455, 457–458; and fevers, 216–217, 458, 464; and food allergies, 194; and food poisoning, 373; and GERD, 211, 213, 457; and head injuries, 480–481, 484; home remedies for, 518; and intestinal malformation, 9; and introduction of solid foods, 182; and laboratory tests, 520; medications for, 500; and norovirus, 369; and pee in diapers, 218; and pneumonia, 372; and poisoning, 470; red flags with, 216–217; and rehydration solutions, 500; and respiratory distress, 447; and stomach ache, 437–438; typical doctor's questions about, 457–458

von Willebrand's disease, 440, 525

VUR (vesicoureteral reflux), 10, 219–220, 374, 522

Vusion, 509

waiting rooms, 49–50, 58

wake windows, 261–262

Walgreens, 434

walkers, 287, 481

walking, 268, 287–288, 400

Walmart, 153, 162, 164, 413

warts, 511, 518

water: for babies with diarrhea, 458; in baby's bottle, 173–175; baby's need for, 173–174; commercially bottled, 107–108, 170–171, 174, 494; drinking when nursing, 146–147; environmental hazards in, 409, 417, 430; filtration systems for, 417; fluoride in, 107–108, 174, 493–494; mixing formulas with, 158, 167, 170–171, 493–494; and night feedings, 252; nitrates in, 414; and PE tubes, 491; purification of, 318; and stitches, 478; and swimmer's ear, 380–381

waterproof mattress covers, 427
water safety, 294–295
weaning, 140, 154–155, 157, 173, 182, 193
weather, and pneumonia, 31
weight: and anemia, 105; and ASD, 277; and celiac disease, 198; charting, 93–94, 99; and correct dosing of medications, 468–469, 498–499, 504; and cystic fibrosis, 393; and developmental delays, 280; in first year, 98, 156; and GERD, 103; and juices, 175; and late preterm infants, 153; and night feedings, 252; and preemies, 40, 43, 45, 94, 152; and steroid use, 506. *See also* obesity; overweight
weight loss: and advantages of breastfeeding, 114; in breastfed infants, 15, 19, 60, 120, 124, 126, 128, 156, 227; concerns about, 120; and dehydration, 217, 454; and diabetes, 403
weight percentiles, 109, 553–557
Weissbluth, M., 254, 259
well child appointments: avoiding unnecessary, 60–61; and developmental concerns, 267, 270; free books at, 286; and iron deficiency screening, 105; scheduling, 50–51, 55–59; screening tests at, 56–57, 64; and sick-child appointments, 52, 59; and twins, 58; and vaccinations, 328
Westcort, 511
West Nile Virus (WNV), 86, 371
wet nurses, 158
wheat, and diabetes, 403
wheezing: and allergies, 200; and aromatherapy, 517; and asthma, 390–393, 505; and GERD, 216, 391; and laboratory tests, 520; and respiratory distress, 447–448; and RSV, 365, 390–391, 446–447; and smoking, 423
whey, 158–163, 163, 200
Which Toys for Which Child: A Consumer's Guide for Selecting Suitable Toys (CPSC), 296
white blood cells, 354, 360, 396, 526
white blood count (WBC), 356, 361, 365, 372, 523
whole milk, 101, 112, 155, 157, 168, 173, 175, 193, 414
whooping cough (pertussis): and apnea, 449; and chronic cough, 453; and respiratory distress, 447–448; vaccine for, 322, 326, 329–332
wills, 64
Witch's Milk, 10
The Womanly Art of Breastfeeding (La Leche League), 141
work: and family life, 64, 66, 71–76, 257; returning to, 100, 116, 150, 166
World Health Organization (WHO): and aluminum in vaccines, 345; and baby formulas, 158; and baby's first bath, 82; carrageenan additive and, 165; and growth charts, 93–94; and influenza vaccines, 339; and polypropylene bottles, 425; and smallpox, 319
worms, 376, 385
wounds: and bacterial infections, 361; circumcisions as, 28–29, 87–88; closing with glue, 476, 478–479; diagnosing infections in, 477–479; herbal remedies for, 514; stitches for, 476–479
Wright, Karen L., 394
wrists, broken, 483
Wymox, 501

Xopenex, 505
X-rays, 364, 367, 372, 402, 481, 483, 521

yawning, 314
yeast: and antibiotic use, 386, 502; and antifungals, 509; and breastfeeding problems, 133, 140–141; and cradle cap, 84–85; and diaper rash, 61, 81, 90, 140–141, 376, 385, 472–473, 502, 509–510; and thrush, 90, 140, 376, 385, 502; in vaccines, 345
yeast diaper rash, 61, 81, 90, 140–141, 376, 385, 472–473, 502, 509–510
yeast infections, 61, 81, 84–85, 90, 131, 133, 140–141
yelling, and discipline, 311
yellow fever vaccine, 324
YF-VAX, 324
yogurt, 140, 146–147, 197, 413, 456, 515
Young, Bridget, 157, 164, 165

Zarbee's baby cough syrup, 452, 508
Zegerid, 498
ZERO to THREE: National Center for Infants, Toddlers, and Families, 552
Zika virus, 86, 371
Zilactin Baby, 494
zinc, 110–111, 185, 517
zinc oxide, 512
Zithromax, 501
Zofran, 500
Zoster, 503
Zovirax, 356, 503
Zyrtec, 201

COME VISIT US AT BABY411.COM!

Rash-O-Rama: Contagious Diseases

Impetigo

WHAT'S ONLINE?

- Rash-o-rama! Check out pictures of common rashes, birth marks and more. Click on BONUS.

- MESSAGE BOARDS with in-depth discussions of hot-button parenting topics.

- Follow us on Twitter @baby411

- Follow us on Facebook.com/Expecting411

How to reach the authors:

- Email: authors@baby411.com

More books by the Fields:

- Baby Bargains: Your Baby Registry Cheat Sheet!

  See it at BabyBargains.com

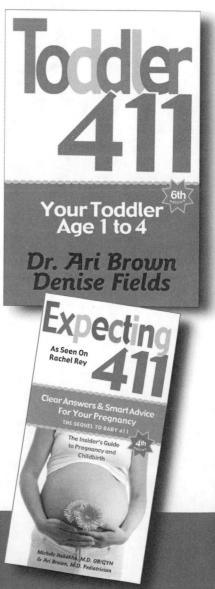